Babesia and Human Babesiosis

Babesia and Human Babesiosis

Editors

Estrella Montero
Jeremy Gray
Cheryl Ann Lobo
Luis Miguel González

MDPI • Basel • Beijing • Wuhan • Barcelona • Belgrade • Manchester • Tokyo • Cluj • Tianjin

MDPI

Editors
Estrella Montero
Laboratorio de Referencia en Investigación y Parasitología
Centro Nacional de Microbiología
Instituto de Salud Carlos III
Majadahonda
Spain

Jeremy Gray
UCD School of Biology and Environmental Science
University College Dublin
Dublin
Ireland

Cheryl Ann Lobo
Blood Borne Parasites
F. Kimball Research Institute (LFKRI) at New York Blood Center
New York
United States

Luis Miguel González
Laboratorio de Referencia en Investigación y Parasitología
Centro Nacional de Microbiología
Majadahonda
Spain

Editorial Office
MDPI
St. Alban-Anlage 66
4052 Basel, Switzerland

This is a reprint of articles from the Special Issue published online in the open access journal *Pathogens* (ISSN 2076-0817) (available at: www.mdpi.com/journal/pathogens/special_issues/Babesia_and_Human_Babesiosis).

For citation purposes, cite each article independently as indicated on the article page online and as indicated below:

LastName, A.A.; LastName, B.B.; LastName, C.C. Article Title. *Journal Name* **Year**, *Volume Number*, Page Range.

ISBN 978-3-0365-4472-4 (Hbk)
ISBN 978-3-0365-4471-7 (PDF)

Cover image courtesy of Javier Conesa

Contents

About the Editors vii

Preface to "*Babesia* and Human Babesiosis" ix

Abhinav Kumar, Jane O'Bryan and Peter J. Krause
The Global Emergence of Human Babesiosis
Reprinted from: *Pathogens* **2021**, *10*, 1447, doi:10.3390/pathogens10111447 1

Jeremy S. Gray and Nicholas H. Ogden
Ticks, Human Babesiosis and Climate Change
Reprinted from: *Pathogens* **2021**, *10*, 1430, doi:10.3390/pathogens10111430 25

Anke Hildebrandt, Annetta Zintl, Estrella Montero, Klaus-Peter Hunfeld and Jeremy Gray
Human Babesiosis in Europe
Reprinted from: *Pathogens* **2021**, *10*, 1165, doi:10.3390/pathogens10091165 39

Nélida Fernández, Belen Revuelta, Irene Aguilar, Jorge Francisco Soares, Annetta Zintl and Jeremy Gray et al.
Babesia and *Theileria* Identification in Adult Ixodid Ticks from Tapada Nature Reserve, Portugal
Reprinted from: *Pathogens* **2022**, *11*, 222, doi:10.3390/pathogens11020222 69

Sam R. Telford, Heidi K. Goethert and Timothy J. Lepore
Semicentennial of Human Babesiosis, Nantucket Island
Reprinted from: *Pathogens* **2021**, *10*, 1159, doi:10.3390/pathogens10091159 81

Heidi K. Goethert
What *Babesia microti* Is Now
Reprinted from: *Pathogens* **2021**, *10*, 1168, doi:10.3390/pathogens10091168 95

Claire Bonsergent, Marie-Charlotte de Carné, Nathalie de la Cotte, François Moussel, Véronique Perronne and Laurence Malandrin
The New Human *Babesia* sp. FR1 Is a European Member of the *Babesia* sp. MO1 Clade
Reprinted from: *Pathogens* **2021**, *10*, 1433, doi:10.3390/pathogens10111433 103

Sarah I. Bonnet and Clémence Nadal
Experimental Infection of Ticks: An Essential Tool for the Analysis of *Babesia* Species Biology and Transmission
Reprinted from: *Pathogens* **2021**, *10*, 1403, doi:10.3390/pathogens10111403 121

Evan M. Bloch, Peter J. Krause and Laura Tonnetti
Preventing Transfusion-Transmitted Babesiosis
Reprinted from: *Pathogens* **2021**, *10*, 1176, doi:10.3390/pathogens10091176 135

Divya Beri, Manpreet Singh, Marilis Rodriguez, Karina Yazdanbakhsh and Cheryl Ann Lobo
Sickle Cell Anemia and *Babesia* Infection
Reprinted from: *Pathogens* **2021**, *10*, 1435, doi:10.3390/pathogens10111435 151

Scott Meredith, Miranda Oakley and Sanjai Kumar
Technologies for Detection of *Babesia microti*: Advances and Challenges
Reprinted from: *Pathogens* **2021**, *10*, 1563, doi:10.3390/pathogens10121563 161

Stephane Delbecq
Major Surface Antigens in Zoonotic *Babesia*
Reprinted from: *Pathogens* **2022**, *11*, 99, doi:10.3390/pathogens11010099 177

Reginaldo G. Bastos, Jose Thekkiniath, Choukri Ben Mamoun, Lee Fuller, Robert E. Molestina and Monica Florin-Christensen et al.
Babesia microti Immunoreactive Rhoptry-Associated Protein-1 Paralogs Are Ancestral Members of the Piroplasmid-Confined RAP-1 Family
Reprinted from: *Pathogens* **2021**, *10*, 1384, doi:10.3390/pathogens10111384 . . . . **191**

Isaline Renard and Choukri Ben Mamoun
Treatment of Human Babesiosis: Then and Now
Reprinted from: *Pathogens* **2021**, *10*, 1120, doi:10.3390/pathogens10091120 . . . . **207**

Pallavi Singh, Anasuya C. Pal and Choukri Ben Mamoun
An Alternative Culture Medium for Continuous In Vitro Propagation of the Human Pathogen *Babesia duncani* in Human Erythrocytes
Reprinted from: *Pathogens* **2022**, *11*, 599, doi:10.3390/pathogens11050599 . . . . **225**

Monica Florin-Christensen, Sarah N. Wieser, Carlos E. Suarez and Leonhard Schnittger
In Silico Survey and Characterization of *Babesia microti* Functional and Non-Functional Proteases
Reprinted from: *Pathogens* **2021**, *10*, 1457, doi:10.3390/pathogens10111457 . . . . **235**

Pavla Šnebergerová, Pavla Bartošová-Sojková, Marie Jalovecká and Daniel Sojka
Plasmepsin-like Aspartyl Proteases in *Babesia*
Reprinted from: *Pathogens* **2021**, *10*, 1241, doi:10.3390/pathogens10101241 . . . . **261**

About the Editors

Estrella Montero

Estrella Montero is currently Head of Laboratory at the Parasitology Reference and Research Department of the National Centre for Microbiology, Spain. She received her PhD in Biological Sciences from the Complutense University, Madrid, Spain, in 2003. During this period, she worked on the molecular biology of helminthiasis under the direction of Drs. Teresa Gárate and Luis Miguel González. Subsequently, she did her postdoc at Lindsley F. Kimball Research Institute (LFKRI) at New York Blood Center where she commenced the study of the erythrocyte invasion process of *Babesia divergens* under the direction of Dr. Cheryl Ann Lobo.

The laboratory of Estrella Montero studies basic aspects of the asexual life cycle of *B. divergens* by the means of modern microscopic tools, integrative omics approaches and molecular biology. She also works on developing diagnostic tools to detect *Babesia* and other piroplasms in humans, domestic and wild animals and ticks. She is currently collaborating on *Babesia* and human babesiosis transmission with Drs. Luis Miguel González and Cheryl Ann Lobo and Professor Jeremy Gray.

Jeremy Gray

Jeremy Gray obtained his PhD in Animal Parasitology from the University of London in 1972 and shortly afterwards took up a lecturing post in University College Dublin, remaining there to teach animal parasitology for more than 30 years, focusing initially on infections of farm animals, and latterly on zoonoses. His research on the tick *Ixodes ricinus* and the pathogens that it transmits (especially *Babesia divergens* and *Borrelia burgdorferi*) commenced soon after his arrival in Ireland. He left the university in 2008, but as an Emeritus Professor and Associate Editor for the journal *Ticks and Tick-borne Diseases* has been able to maintain fruitful working relationships with colleagues at UCD and in many other parts of the world.

Cheryl Ann Lobo

Dr. Cheryl Ann Lobo is a full Member of Lindsley F. Kimball Research Institute (LFKRI) at New York Blood Center and Head of Laboratory of Blood Borne Parasites. She has a long history in molecular parasitology for over 30 years, focusing on parasites that can be transmitted by transfusion - malaria and babesiosis - emerging infectious diseases that are transfusion threats. Her laboratory studies the biology underlying the mechanisms of invasion, intracellular development, multiplication and egress in these intra-erythrocytic parasites, using in vitro culture systems and rodent models of disease, with the eventual goal of developing viable interventions to detect and halt transfusion-transmission of these pathogens.

Luis Miguel González

Luis Miguel González is currently Head of laboratory at the at the Parasitology Reference and Research Department of the National Center for Microbiology, Spain. He received his PhD in Biological Sciences from the University of La Laguna, Tenerife, Spain, in 1993. He has a long experience in developing molecular and serologic tools for the detection of helminthiases and tick borne diseases that affect humans, domestic and wild animals. His laboratory also studies basic aspects of the asexual life cycle of *Babesia divergens* by the means of modern microscopic tools, integrative omics approaches and molecular biology in collaboration with Dr. Estrella Montero.

Preface to "*Babesia* and Human Babesiosis"

Babesia is a genus of intraerythrocytic protozoan parasites belonging to the exclusively parasitic phylum Apicomplexa. There are more than a hundred known species of this genus, occurring mainly in mammals, but also in birds, and all transmitted by ticks, which are blood-sucking arthropods related to spiders. Ixodid (hard-bodied) ticks are vectors of the vast majority of *Babesia* spp., but a small number of babesias are transmitted by argasid (soft-bodied) ticks. For many years, *Babesia* spp. were only known as important parasites of domestic animals and were the first pathogens shown to be transmitted by an arthropod vector when, in 1893, Smith and Kilborne reported the vector role of cattle ticks in redwater fever (babesiosis) in the USA [1]. Human babesiosis was first described in 1957 when it occurred as a fulminant and ultimately fatal infection in a Croatian farmer [2]. More human cases followed over the next 50 years, and at least four taxonomically classified *Babesia* species (*B. divergens, B. duncani, B. microti,* and *B. venatorum*) have now been confirmed as zoonotic pathogens, with some others that have not yet been identified to species.

The main pathological event of infection with these parasites is the destruction of erythrocytes, resulting in haemolytic anaemia with added complications due to the release of toxins and waste products into the bloodstream. Further damage to the host can be caused by cytokine storms as the host's immune system responds to infection. In many respects, the pathology of babesiosis is similar to that of the much better-known disease, malaria, caused by *Plasmodium* spp.

This Special Issue consists of 11 reviews that between them address the global babesiosis situation, the disease in Europe, the history and current status of *B. microti* in the USA, babesiosis in relation to sickle cell anaemia, experimental infections of ticks, transfusion transmission, the significance of major surface antigens, advances in the diagnosis of babesiosis, historical and current approaches to treatment and management, and babesiosis in relation to climate change. Additionally, six research articles are presented addressing the discovery of a new zoonotic genotype of *B. divergens*, the characterisation and function of certain proteins involved in parasite–erythrocyte interaction, the identification of proteases as possible drug targets, the identity of piroplasms in ticks removed from deer in Portugal, and the identification of an alternate growth medium that can support the *in vitro* growth of *B. duncani* in human erythrocytes.

In their review on the worldwide occurrence of human babesiosis, Kumar et al. [Ch. 1] draw attention to the fact that this is an emerging zoonosis, with increasing reports of infections caused by the known zoonotic species in new areas, for example, in China, in addition to cases involving *Babesia* parasites of undetermined species. They conclude that the true number of affected patients is considerably underestimated, particularly in regions where clinical and diagnostic overlap with malaria occurs, and call for improved surveillance and continued research on treatment and prevention. The authors mention climate change as a possible factor in the gradual spread of *B. microti* in the USA, and the role of climate in the epidemiology of zoonotic babesiosis in general is discussed more fully by Gray and Ogden [Ch. 2], with particular reference to climate effects on the vector ticks. While extensive data suggest that global warming is affecting the distribution of the *Ixodes* vectors, no changes in the current occurrence of zoonotic babesiosis can, as yet, be convincingly attributed directly to climate change, though models suggest that this is only a matter of time.

Hildebrandt et al. [Ch. 3] discuss European babesiosis in more detail. Compared with the USA, the disease is relatively rare in Europe, but the authors point out that most cases present as medical emergencies, mainly in immunocompromised patients, and particularly in those that are asplenic. Unusually, an attempt has been made to present data on every recorded case that has occurred in the last two decades, with the hope of shedding new light on both the epidemiology of the disease as well as on diagnosis and management. Most human babesiosis cases in Europe are due to infection with *B. divergens* and *B. microti*, although the true prevalence of the latter is unknown because of the apparent low pathogenicity of European strains of this parasite. There is also uncertainty about the epidemiology of the genuinely pathogenic *B. divergens*, particularly the possible role of red deer as reservoir hosts. This topic is again addressed in a research paper by Fernandez et al. [Ch. 4], who describe a study in which ixodid ticks removed from deer in a Portuguese nature reserve were analysed for piroplasm infections. *B. divergens* sequences were detected that were apparently identical to those associated with human and bovine babesiosis, and it is concluded that the most likely source of these parasites was the deer. Other interesting findings include the association of *Theileria* spp. with *Ixodes ricinus* and the abundant occurrence of an exophilic form of the brown dog tick, *Rhipicephalus sanguineus*.

Babesia microti, the causal agent in the vast majority of cases, particularly in the USA, is the subject of two reviews. Telford et al. [Ch. 5] describe in detail the emergence of this pathogen 50 years ago. This is probably the first time that all the salient facts behind the appearance of this pathogen and the subsequent spread of *B. microti* babesiosis in the USA are presented in detail, which will make interesting and enlightening reading for all babesiologists. A range of interventions are described, and although the extent of their implementation has proved disappointing, the authors remain optimistic that by the centennial of the discovery of "Nantucket fever", technological advances will have resolved many of the control and prevention problems. In the second review on *B. microti*, Goethert [Ch. 6] describes its worldwide diversity, knowledge of which has evidently increased markedly over the decades since the parasite's emergence as a human pathogen. The author argues that because many of the studies on *B. microti* were conducted before the availability of molecular analysis, an understanding of its ecology has been hampered by confusion about parasite identity. *B. microti* has now been taxonomically allocated to five distinct clades within the species complex, but problems with identity evidently persist in some recent studies.

Parasite diversity has also drawn the attention of researchers in the study of *B. divergens*-like pathogens since the occurrence of four human cases in the USA [3, 4, 5, 6] and two in Europe [7, 8]. In some of these reports, the infectious agent was initially identified as *B. divergens*, but subsequent analysis has established that they are all clearly distinct from this species and are currently described as *B. divergens*-like or have been given an abbreviation to indicate the location of the case. Thus, the causal agent of the first of these [3] occurred in Missouri and is described as *Babesia* sp. MO1. In this Special Issue, Bonsergent et al. [Ch. 7] describe an isolate obtained from a case in France, which caused a relatively mild infection, compared with classic *B. divergens* babesiosis. The subsequent molecular analysis determined that the parasite involved, which they name *Babesia* sp. FR1, belongs to the MO1 clade. Their study demonstrates that variations in the severity of suspected *B. divergens* babesiosis [9] may be due to infections with *B. divergens*–like parasites rather than with the classic *B. divergens* of cattle. The reservoir host of *Babesia* sp. MO1 is believed to be the cotton-tail rabbit (*Sylvilagus floridanus*), and while the reservoir host of *Babesia* sp. FR1 is unknown, the European rabbit (*Oryctolagus cuniculus*) is implicated by its high abundance in the habitat where the infection is thought to have been contracted.

The list of zoonotic *Babesia* spp. is gradually lengthening, but it is difficult to determine the tick vector involved in the transmission of parasites known only as isolates from patients. The detection of parasite DNA in ticks is only indicative of vector status and absolute proof requires experimental demonstration of transmission under controlled conditions [10]. A review of the approaches and technologies to achieve such proof is presented by Bonnet and Nadal [Ch. 8], who discuss the application of ticks to both naturally infected and experimental animals, and also the increasing use of artificial tick-feeding systems. They conclude that systems for the experimental infection of ticks are vital tools for the determination of vector competence, enhancing our knowledge of pathogen ecology and of *Babesia* spp. life cycles, and that consideration should be given to the standardisation of artificial-feeding protocols.

Although tick transmission is the primary means by which *Babesia* spp. infect humans, blood transfusions are an increasingly important source of infection, particularly of *B. microti* in the USA. Bloch et al. [Ch. 9] review the history of transfusion-transmitted babesiosis, mainly in the USA, evaluate the evolution of surveillance, assay development, and screening policy in the USA, and suggest that the current American model for the prevention of transfusion babesiosis could form the basis for similar measures in other countries where the perception of transfusion transmission risk is currently low. One of the groups of patients that is particularly prone to haemolysis and requires frequent blood transfusions are those suffering from haemoglobinopathies such as sickle cell anaemia and thalassaemia. Little is known about the course of babesiosis in such patients, but it has been accepted for many years that haemoglobinopathies afford some protection against malaria, and studies on *Babesia* spp. in this context, reviewed here by Beri et al. [Ch. 10], suggest that such conditions also hinder intraerythrocytic growth of parasites. Possible mechanisms for the resistance of sickle cells to *Babesia* spp. are explored and suggestions are made for further studies to identify the possible "Achilles heel" of both *Babesia* and *Plasmodium* spp. that could result in effective interventions.

The detection of *Babesia* parasites in stored blood by molecular methods is an essential component of screening procedures for blood transfusion and is also the most reliable approach for detection of parasites in clinical cases when parasitaemias are low, whereas microscopy in the hands of experienced laboratory staff is useful at higher parasitaemias. Meredith et al. [Ch. 11] address the history, current status, and future prospects for laboratory diagnosis of *B. microti*, with particular emphasis on the application of modern technologies such as exploitation of the CRISPR–Cas system, which markedly increases the sensitivity of nucleic acid test systems. Serological testing for babesiosis has mainly relied on immunofluorescence techniques to detect surface antigens, and increased knowledge of the nature of these surface antigens is important. Delbecq [Ch. 12] reviews the major surface antigens of *B. microti* and *B. divergens*, highlighting their role in both erythrocyte invasion and the immune response. He concludes that the increased knowledge of the major antigens will contribute to the development of vaccines, and of more sensitive serological assays and antigen capture assays that could be used to identify biomarkers for exposure, active infection, and protection. Other antigens, members of the rhoptry-associated protein-1 (pRAP-1) family, are the subject of a work by Bastos et al. [Ch. 13]. These proteins are secretory products of the apical complex in piroplasms, which plays an essential role in cell invasion by the parasite. Rhoptry proteins have not received the attention they should and the study described here suggests the involvement of pRAP-1 in parasite adhesion, attachment, and possibly evasion of the immune response. Antibodies in *B. microti*-infected humans recognise recombinant forms of the two proteins studied, suggesting that they could be candidates for both diagnostic assays and vaccines.

Efficacious drug treatment of patients is central to the management of babesiosis and a review of antimicrobial use in the past and present by Renard and Ben Mamoun [Ch. 14] draws attention to the fact that the currently available drugs are limited and have been repurposed rather than developed specifically as antibabesials. Since they are associated with either significant side effects or the rapid emergence of drug resistance, it is clear that new therapeutic strategies are required. *In vivo* models for antibabesial evaluation using mice, hamsters, and gerbils have been available for some years but continuous culture *in vitro* has been restricted to *B. divergens* up to the present. However, Singh et at., have demonstrated that the DMEM-F12 medium supports the continuous *in vitro* culture of *B. duncani* in human erythrocytes [Ch. 15]. This finding in combination with the development of the 'in culture-in mouse' (ICIM) model of *B. duncani* infection, also conducted by Ben Mamoun's laboratory [11], are major advances and are likely to result in *B. duncani* becoming the species of choice for the discovery of antimicrobials against all the zoonotic *Babesia* spp.

Babesia microti is the predominant zoonotic species and is also arguably the least susceptible to existing antimicrobials [12]. The identification of chemotherapeutic targets in these parasites thus becomes an important research priority. Florin-Christensen et al. [Ch. 16] focus on species-specific proteases and have used bioinformatics to identify genes in the *B. microti* genome that code for these enzymes. They classify 89 proteases into five groups and report that comparisons between *B. microti* and *B. bovis* reveal differences between sensu lato and sensu stricto parasites, reflecting their distinct evolutionary histories, which is probably relevant to their susceptibilities to antibabesials [12]. In another work on proteases [Ch. 17] Šnebergerová et al. investigate aspartyl proteases in *B. microti*, particularly in relation to homologues of known function in other parasites, such as plasmepsins in *Plasmodium* spp. They suggest that analogies with plasmodial plasmepsins indicate piroplasmid aspartyl proteases as potentially important therapeutic targets.

We hope this Special Issue will motivate research scientists to further develop strategies for the prevention and control of babesiosis in the future. Improvements are required in diagnosis, the rigorous typing and identification of *Babesia* parasites, prevention of transfusion transmission, and the discovery of novel antibabesial drugs. The development of safe and effective vaccines for use in humans remains an unrealised goal and is an important research priority.

The researchers who have participated in this Special Issue remind us that zoonotic babesiosis is a complex emerging disease, in which ticks and domestic and wild animals have crucial roles so that environmental factors, particularly in a climate change context, must be taken into account. In the coming years, multidisciplinary collaboration between research groups, the use of digital tools for analysing and sharing essential data about current and new species, the involvement of health authorities in the implementation of surveillance systems, and the development of specific funding strategies for emerging infections such as babesiosis, will be decisive in achieving the necessary goals. Finally, it is imperative to inform and collaborate with veterinary scientists, community health care workers, and the general population in order to determine and reduce the risk of zoonotic babesiosis.

Our sincere thanks to all the authors for their excellent contributions to this book and to the Special Issue assistant Editor, Anne Wang, for her assistance throughout.

References

1. Smith, T.; Kilborne, F.L. Investigations into the nature, causation and prevention of Southern cattle fever.*In Ninth Annual Report of the Bureau of Animal Industry for the Year 1892*; Government Printing Office: Washington, DC, USA, 1893; pp. 177–304.

2. Skrabalo, Z.; Deanovic, Z. Piroplasmosis in man; report of a case. *Doc. Med. Geogr. Trop*. 1957, 9, 11–16.

3. Herwaldt, B.; Persing, D.H.; Précigout, E.A.; Goff, W.L.; Mathiesen, D.A.; Taylor, P.W.; Eberhard, M.L.; Gorenflot, A.F. A fatal case of babesiosis in Missouri: Identification of another piroplasm that infects humans. *Ann. Intern. Med*. 1996, 124, 643–650.

4. Beattie, J.F.; Michelson, M.L.; Holman, P.J. Acute babesiosis caused by *Babesia divergens* in a resident of Kentucky. *N. Engl. J. Med.* 2002, 347, 697–698.

5. Herwaldt, B.L.; de Bruyn, G.; Pieniazek, N.J.; Homer, M.; Lofy, K.H.; Slemenda, S.B.; Fritsche, T.R.; Persing, D.H.; Limaye, A.P. *Babesia divergens*-like infection, Washington State. *Emerg. Infect. Dis.* 2004, 10, 622–629.

6. Burgess, M.J.; Rosenbaum, E.R.; Pritt, B.S.; Haselow, D.T.; Ferren, K.M.; Alzghoul, B.N.; Rico, J.C.; Sloan, L.M.; Ramanan, P.; Purushothaman, R.; et al. Possible transfusion-transmitted *Babesia divergens*-like/MO-1 infection in an Arkansas patient. *Clin. Infect. Dis.* 2017, 64, 1622–1625.

7. Olmeda, A.S.; Armstrong, P.M.; Rosenthal, B.M.; Valladares, B.; del Castillo, A.; de Armas, F.; Miguelez, M.; Gonzalez, A.; Rodriguez Rodriguez, J.A.; Spielman, A.; et al. A subtropical case of human babesiosis. *Acta Trop.* 1997, 67, 229–234.

8. Centeno-Lima, S.; do Rosário, V.; Parreira, R.; Maia, A.J.; Freudenthal, A.M.; Nijhof, A.M.; Jongejan, F. A fatal case of human babesiosis in Portugal: Molecular and phylogenetic analysis. *Trop. Med. Int. Health TMIH* 2003, 8, 760–764.

9. Martinot, M.; Zadeh, M.M.; Hansmann, Y.; Grawey, I.; Christmann, D.; Aguillon, S.; Jouglin, M.; Chauvin, A.; De Briel, D. Babesiosis in immunocompetent patients, Europe. *Emerg. Infect. Dis.* 2011, 17, 114–116.

10. Gray, J.S.; Estrada-Pena, A.; Zintl, A. Vectors of babesiosis. *Annu. Rev. Entomol.* 2019, 64, 149–165.

11. Pal, A.C.; Renard, I.; Singh, P.; Vydyam, P.; Chiu, J.E.; Pou, S.; Winter, R.W.; Dodean, R.; Frueh, L.; Nilsen, A.C.; et al. *Babesia Duncani* as a model organism to study the development, virulence and drug susceptibility of intraerythrocytic parasites *in vitro* and *in vivo*. J. Infect. Dis. 2022, doi:10.1093/infdis/jiac181.

12. Gray, J.; Zintl, A.; Hildebrandt, A.; Hunfeld, K.P.; Weiss, L. Zoonotic babesiosis: Overview of the disease and novel aspects of pathogen identity. *Ticks Tick-Borne Dis.* 2010, 1, 3–10.

About the cover: This image represents *Babesia divergens* parasites and is based on 3D tomograms obtained by cryo-soft X-ray tomography (cryo-SXT) at the Alba Synchrotron, Barcelona, Spain. Cryo-SXT assays were conducted by Drs. Javier Conesa, Daniel Luque, Javier Chichón, Eva Pereiro, Luis M. Gonzalez and Estrella Montero.

Estrella Montero, Jeremy Gray, Cheryl Ann Lobo, and Luis Miguel González
Editors

pathogens

Review

The Global Emergence of Human Babesiosis

Abhinav Kumar [1], Jane O'Bryan [2,3] and Peter J. Krause [1,*]

1 Department of Epidemiology of Microbial Diseases, Yale School of Public Health and Yale School of Medicine, New Haven, CT 06510, USA; abhinav.kumar@yale.edu
2 Department of Obstetrics, Gynecology & Reproductive Sciences, Yale School of Medicine, New Haven, CT 06510, USA; jane.obryan@yale.edu
3 Frank H. Netter MD School of Medicine, Quinnipiac University, North Haven, CT 06473, USA
* Correspondence: peter.krause@yale.edu

Abstract: Babesiosis is an emerging tick-borne disease caused by intraerythrocytic protozoa that are primarily transmitted by hard-bodied (ixodid) ticks and rarely through blood transfusion, perinatally, and organ transplantation. More than 100 *Babesia* species infect a wide spectrum of wild and domestic animals worldwide and six have been identified as human pathogens. *Babesia microti* is the predominant species that infects humans, is found throughout the world, and causes endemic disease in the United States and China. *Babesia venatorum* and *Babesia crassa*-like agent also cause endemic disease in China. *Babesia divergens* is the predominant species in Europe where fulminant cases have been reported sporadically. The number of *B. microti* infections has been increasing globally in recent decades. In the United States, more than 2000 cases are reported each year, although the actual number is thought to be much higher. In this review of the epidemiology of human babesiosis, we discuss epidemiologic tools used to monitor disease location and frequency; demographics and modes of transmission; the location of human babesiosis; the causative *Babesia* species in the Americas, Europe, Asia, Africa, and Australia; the primary clinical characteristics associated with each of these infections; and the increasing global health burden of this disease.

Keywords: babesiosis; *Babesia microti*; epidemiology; immunoepidemiology; case surveillance; babesiosis

Citation: Kumar, A.; O'Bryan, J.; Krause, P.J. The Global Emergence of Human Babesiosis. *Pathogens* **2021**, *10*, 1447. https://doi.org/10.3390/pathogens10111447

Academic Editors: Estrella Montero, Jeremy Gray, Cheryl Ann Lobo and Luis Miguel González

Received: 24 September 2021
Accepted: 30 October 2021
Published: 6 November 2021
Corrected: 23 May 2022

Publisher's Note: MDPI stays neutral with regard to jurisdictional claims in published maps and institutional affiliations.

1. Introduction

Human babesiosis is caused by intraerythrocytic protozoal parasites in the phylum Apicomplexa and is transmitted by hard bodied ticks. It is rarely transmitted through red blood cell transfusion, transplacentally from mother to fetus, and through organ transplantation. Babesiosis is an emerging infection with increasing numbers of cases being reported throughout the world (Figure 1) [1–8].

More than 100 species of *Babesia* have been described that infect a wide array of wild and domestic animals [9,10]. Babesiosis is a significant problem for cattle and has had a major economic impact in several cattle producing countries. Six primary species have thus far been confirmed as human pathogens: *Babesia crassa*-like *agent*, *Babesia divergens*, *Babesia duncani*, *Babesia microti*, *Babesia motasi*, and *Babesia venatorum*. Several other genetically related pathogen substrains have been reported to infect humans, including *Babesia divergens*-like and *Babesia microti*-like pathogens (Table 1).

Human babesiosis is found primarily in the temperate zone. The predominant species is *B. microti*, which is endemic in the northeastern and northern midwestern United States and southwestern China [1,3,4,6]. *B. crassa*-like pathogen and *B. venatorum* are endemic in northeastern China [11,12]. *B. divergens* is found most commonly in Europe [2,5]. Cases of babesiosis have been sporadically reported in Australia [13], Bolivia [14], Brazil [15], Canada [16,17], the Canary Islands [18], Colombia [19], Ecuador [20], Egypt [21], India [22,23], Japan [24], Korea [25,26], Mexico [27], Mongolia [28], Mozambique [8], South Africa [29], Taiwan [30], and Turkey [31] (Table 2).

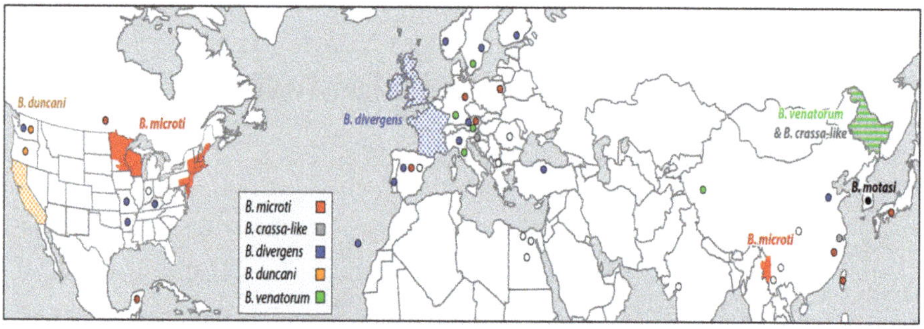

Figure 1. Geographic distribution of major areas of human babesiosis transmission. The map depicts the major areas where human babesiosis has been reported. Additional areas where human babesiosis has been reported but are not shown in the figure are mentioned in the text. Solid colors indicate areas where human babesiosis is endemic. Stippled areas indicate areas where babesiosis is sporadic with ≥10 cases reported. Circles depict areas where 1–10 cases have been reported. Colors distinguish the etiologic agents: *Babesia crassa*-like agent (gray), *Babesia duncani* (orange), *Babesia divergens* (blue), *Babesia microti* (red), *Babesia motasi* (black), and *Babesia venatorum* (green). White circles depict cases caused by *Babesia* spp. that were not characterized. Asymptomatic infections are omitted (adapted from The New England Journal of Medicine, Edouard Vannier, and Peter J. Krause, Human Babesiosis, 2012, 366, 2397. Copyright (2021) Massachusetts Medical Society. Reprinted with permission [1]).

Table 1. First reports of *Babesia* species causing human babesiosis.

***Babesia* Species**	**Year Case Reported**	**Major Region of Transmission**	**Primary Vector**
Babesia microti	1968 [32]	United States (Northeast, northern Midwest)	*I. scapularis*
Babesia divergens	1957 [33]	Western Europe	*I. ricinus*
Babesia duncani	1991 [34]	United States (Farwest)	*D. albipictus*
Babesia venatorum (EU1)	2003 [35]	Europe (Austria, Italy) China	*I. ricinus* *I. persulcatus*
Babesia motasi (KO-1)	2007 [26]	South Korea	unknown
Babesia crassa-like agent	2018 [11]	Northeast China	*I. persulcatus*
Genetic variants			
Babesia divergens-like	1996 [36]	United States	Unknown
Babesia microti-like (TW1)	1997 [30]	Taiwan, Japan	Unknown

adapted from Puri et al. Frontiers in Microbiology, 2021 [37].

Babesia parasites were first described by Victor Babes in Romanian cattle in 1888 [38]. The first human case of babesiosis was described in 1957 by Skrabalo and Deanovic in Yugoslavia and the second in 1968 in California [32,33,39]. The causative *Babesia* species was not determined in either instance. A year later, a third babesiosis patient was reported and the causative species was identified as *B. microti*. The patient was a resident of Nantucket Island in Massachusetts where babesiosis was soon recognized as endemic [40]. Additional cases were reported in the southeastern New England mainland and from there the disease spread eastward, northward, and southward [41–46]. A primary cause of this emergence is thought to be a marked increase in the white-tailed deer population that greatly amplifies the number of vector *Ixodes scapularis* ticks. Other causes include an increase in the human population, home construction in wooded areas, increased recognition of the disease by physicians and the lay public, and improved diagnostic testing [1,39,41]. The emergence of babesiosis has lagged behind that of Lyme disease, even though it is transmitted by the same tick and is sometimes transmitted simultaneously [45,47]. Babesiosis due to *B. microti* is now endemic from Maryland to Maine and in the northern Midwestern states of Minnesota and Wisconsin. A modest number of cases of *B. duncani* have been reported on the West coast [48]. Babesiosis due to a *Babesia divergens*-like pathogen has been identified in patients in five states: Arkansas, Kentucky, Michigan, Missouri, and Washington [36,49–52].

Babesiosis should be suspected in patients who live in or travel through an endemic area or have received a blood transfusion within the previous six months and present with typical symptoms that include fever, chills, sweats, headache, and fatigue [2,53]. The disease is confirmed by identifying *Babesia*-infected red blood cells on thin blood smear or amplification of *Babesia* DNA using polymerase chain reaction (PCR) [1,2,54–56]. Atovaquone and azithromycin (the drug combination of choice) or clindamycin and quinine treatment are usually very effective, although prolonged illness may occur in immunocompromised hosts with a mortality rate as high as 20% [1,2,11,54,57,58].

In this review we focus on the epidemiology of human babesiosis. We will discuss epidemiologic tools used to monitor disease location and frequency, modes of transmission and demographics, the location of human babesiosis, the causative *Babesia* species in the Americas, Europe, Asia, Africa, and Australia, and the primary clinical characteristics associated with each of these infections.

Table 2. World-wide case distribution of human babesiosis *.

Continent/Country	Causative Agent (Number of Cases)
Africa	*Babesia* spp.
Egypt	*Babesia* sp. (4) [21]
Mozambique	*Babesia* sp. (2) [8]
South Africa	*Babesia* sp. (2) [29]
Asia	*B. crassa*-like agent, *B. divergens B. microti*, *B. motasi*, *B. venatorum*
China	*B. crassa*-like agent, *B. divergens B. microti*, *B. venatorum*
India	*Babesia* sp. (1) [22,23]
Japan	*B. microti* (1) [24]
Korea	*B. motasi* (2) [25,26]
Mongolia	*B. microti* (3) [28]
Australia	*B. microti*
New South Wales	*B. microti* (1) [13]
Europe	*B. crassa*-like agent, *B. divergens*, *B. microti*, *B. venatorum*
Canary Islands (Spain)	*B. divergens*-like agent (1) [18]
North America	*B. divergens*-like, *B. duncani*, *B. microti*
United States	*B. divergens*-like, *B. duncani*, *B. microti*
Canada	*B. microti* (1), *B. odocoilei* (2) [16,17]
Mexico	*B. microti* (4), *Babesia* spp. (3) [27,59]
South America	*B. microti*
Bolivia	*B. microti* (9) [14]
Brazil	*Babesia* sp. (1) [15]
Colombia	*Babesia* sp. (1), *B. bovis* (4), *B. bigemina* (2) [19]
Ecuador	*B. microti* (1) [20]

* The well-established *Babesia* spp. that cause human babesiosis in China, Europe, and the United States are listed. The *Babesia* spp. that have been identified in countries where only a few cases of human babesiosis have been identified in case reports or small case series (<10 cases) are also identified. Some causative agents have not been confirmed in larger case series so are not yet accepted as established causes of human babesiosis. *Babesia* sp. designate where a specific species was not identified.

2. Epidemiologic Tools

A number of methods are used to determine the frequency, location, and future emergence of infections, as part of local, state, national, and international disease tracking efforts. Case surveillance is of central importance and other methods, including case reports and case series, provide validation of surveillance data.

2.1. *Case Surveillance*

Public health officials at the local, state, and national levels collect reports of disease cases from physicians, hospitals, and laboratories. Babesiosis is one of about 120 diseases that are nationally notifiable in the United States and it was so designated in 2011. Case surveillance is of primary importance in helping the United States Centers for Disease Control and Prevention (CDC) determine the location of diseases, the number of cases of diseases at various locations, and the appropriate responses to prevent outbreaks (https://www.cdc.gov/nndss/about/index.html, accessed on 27 July 2021) [60–62]. Traditionally, case surveillance has been carried out through physician reporting of notifiable diseases. Recent variations on this standard approach include citizen science participation where members of the public collaborate with scientists to collect samples and data [63].

2.2. *Case Reports and Case Series*

A case report is a description of a single patient that usually includes symptoms and signs, diagnosis, and treatment. It often describes a new disease but can also describe a novel aspect of a well-known disease. Case reports include descriptions of a previously unreported disease or the presence of an emerging disease in a new location, insights into disease pathogenesis, and generation of new hypotheses or new ideas. Limitations include a lack of generalizability, inability to show cause and effect, potential for overinterpretation of the cause or outcome of disease, and a narrow focus on rare aspects of a disease [64].

A case series involves a report of a group of cases (usually more than three) that can provide information about infection transmission, risk factors for disease, diagnosis, treatment, and outcome of disease. Case series are descriptive in nature rather than hypothesis driven and are prone to selection bias and findings are often not generalizable to other populations. Despite these limitations, the publication of case reports and case series is important to raise awareness of emerging infectious diseases. Indeed, the discovery of the first human case of babesiosis was published as a case report [33]. The first reports of endemic human babesiosis were case series, describing infections due to *B. microti* [65], *B. venatorum* [12], and *B. crassa*-like agent [11].

2.3. *Serosurveys*

A serosurvey is a sera screening analysis of a group of people designed to determine the prevalence of infection. Seroprevalence provides a measurement of disease exposure and risk that is based on the antibody response of those tested [60,66–68]. Antibody generally can be detected about two weeks after the onset of infection and may last as little as a year or as long as a lifetime, depending on the infectious pathogen and the immune characteristics of the host. Serosurveys are one of several immunoepidemiologic tools used to improve our understanding of the epidemiology of a disease [69]. They complement case surveillance and have the advantage of capturing both asymptomatic and symptomatic infection [60]. They also inform public health officials of notifiable diseases. Thus, serosurveys are less likely to underestimate the true prevalence of infection than case finding [60,70]. One challenge of serosurveys and case surveillance methods is that antibody assays and case definitions often change over time, altering interpretation of disease trends and incidence of cases [68]. Seroprevalence surveillance may overestimate prevalence of infection if patients are repeatedly surveyed on an annual basis because antibody often persists for more than a year. Unlike case surveillance, seroprevalence does not distinguish between symptomatic and asymptomatic infection and it is symptomatic infection that better estimates the health burden of a disease.

2.4. Ecological Studies

Tick Vector and Mammalian Host Surveillance

Surveillance of tick vectors and/or reservoir hosts can provide a strong measure of risk of pathogen acquisition [3,70–78]. Detection methods include PCR, culture, and antibody testing. Tick vector or reservoir host surveillance only indirectly estimate the prevalence and location of human tick-borne infection but may provide a useful estimate of infection risk that complements results of human studies. In a comparative study of human and tick surveillance, incidence of Lyme disease and babesiosis were determined by reports of physicians to the Connecticut and Massachusetts Departments of Health and by reports of selected research study physicians in private practice in northeastern Connecticut and Nantucket, Massachusetts. The results of the study suggest that tick-borne surveillance can provide an early warning system for the emergence of tick-borne emerging infections [70].

2.5. Genomics

Genomics is an interdisciplinary branch of molecular biology that consists of the study of the structure, function, evolution, mapping, and editing of genomes. It focuses on the characterization and quantification of all the genes and their interactions that affect the function of the organism. The study of genomics has provided important new insights into the genetic basis of pathogen populations, their structure, diversity, evolution, and emergence; as well as pathogenesis, biomarkers of detection, drug resistance markers, targets for novel therapeutics, and vaccines [37,44,79–82].

2.6. Mathematical Modeling

Mathematical modeling is an epidemiologic tool used to study population dynamics and infectious disease transmission [83,84]. Modeling has increasingly been recognized as an important technique used to inform disease prevention and control efforts. Models may range from simple to highly complex, containing any number of parameters and variables depending on the outcome under investigation and data availability. Garner and Hamilton describe the different categories of epidemiologic models, which are classified on the basis of "treatment of variability, chance and uncertainty (deterministic or stochastic), time (continuous or discrete intervals), space (non-spatial or spatial), and the structure of the population (homogeneous or heterogeneous)" [84]. For example, in one study, laboratory and field data were integrated into a mathematical model to determine whether host coinfection with *Borrelia burgdorferi* (the agent of Lyme disease) and *B. microti* significantly increases the likelihood of *B. microti* establishment in a new previously uninfected region [45]. In another study, it was found that a model predicted that tick-borne diseases spread in a diffusion-like manner in the northeastern United States with occasional long-distance dispersal and that babesiosis spread exhibits strong dependence on Lyme disease [41].

3. Modes of Transmission and Demographics of Human Babesiosis

Babesia spp. perpetuate in nature through a tick-vector and mammalian-host cycle [39]. Vectors and hosts differ for each species of *Babesia* and vary geographically but the basic tick–host transmission cycle is similar for all [1]. The life cycle for *B. microti* is shown in Figure 2 with *I. scapularis* as the tick vector but other tick species serve as vectors for other *Babesia* spp. (Table 1). *Peromyscus leucopus* is the primary reservoir for *B. microti* but other small mammals, such as shrews and chipmunks, can also serve as reservoir hosts for *B. microti* and other *Babesia* spp. [39,85]. Similarly, deer and other large mammals are favored hosts for adult ixodid ticks. In some *Babesia* spp., such as *B. divergens*, this transstadial transmission is supplemented by transovarial transmission from mother to egg [7,86]. Deer markedly amplify tick numbers and are largely responsible for the emergence of *Babesia* and other tick-borne infections over the last three decades in the Northeast and northern Midwest regions of the United States [39,70].

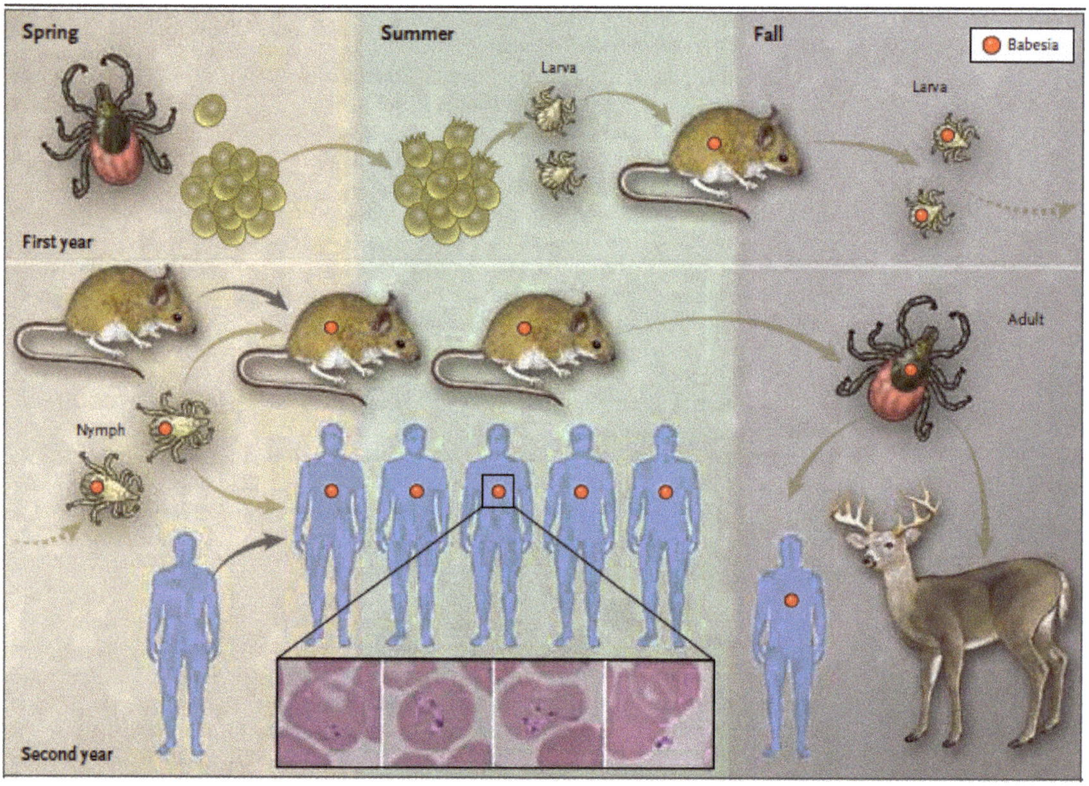

Figure 2. Transmission of *Babesia microti* and stages in the *Ixodes scapularis* tick vector life cycle. Female *I. scapularis* lay 2000–3000 eggs in the spring that hatch in early summer and produce larvae. Larval *I. scapularis* ticks become infected with *B. microti* when they take a blood meal from infected white-footed mice (*Peromyscus leucopus*) or other small rodent hosts in late summer. Fed larvae molt into nymphs and overwinter. During the following late spring, summer, and early autumn, infected nymphs transmit *B. microti* to uninfected mice or humans when they take a blood meal. In the autumn, nymphs molt into adults. Adult males and females preferentially feed and procreate on white-tailed deer (*Odocoileus virginianus*) but rarely on humans. The blood meal provides sufficient protein for female ticks to lay eggs. The tick life cycle is repeated when a new generation of larvae hatch from the eggs in the early spring to complete the tick life cycle. Deer do not become infected with *B. microti*. The inset panels from left to right show a *B. microti* ring form with a non-staining vacuole surrounded by cytoplasm (blue) and two small nuclei (purple), an amoeboid form, a tetrad form (also referred to as a Maltese cross), and an extracellular form (adapted from The New England Journal of Medicine, Edouard Vannier, and Peter J. Krause, Human Babesiosis, 2012, 366, 2397. Copyright (2021) Massachusetts Medical Society. Reprinted with permission [1]).

B. microti are primarily transmitted by *I. scapularis* ticks and rarely through blood transfusion, organ donation, and transplacentally [1,39,87–89]. Babesiosis has been one of the leading causes of transfusion transmitted infection in the United States [87,90]. More than 250 cases have been reported and approximately one-fifth of these cases have been fatal [87]. Blood donor screening for *B. microti* is an effective preventative measure [91,92]. In 2020, the United States Food and Drug Administration recommended donor screening in 14 *B. microti* endemic states and Washington D.C. using approved PCR technologies. Initial data indicate that the numbers of transfusion-transmitted cases has markedly decreased.

Ten cases of congenital babesiosis due to *B. microti* have been described [88,93]. Strong supportive evidence indicates that these cases were not due to transfusion or tick transmission and definitive evidence was available for several cases. Congenital babesia infection is not always severe in neonates and there have been no fatalities. *B. microti* infection also has been reported in two kidney transplant recipients who received kidneys from a single infected kidney donor [89].

The peak age of reported human *B. microti* cases in the United States is between 60 and 70 years of age (Figure 3). Very few cases are reported in children. In contrast, serosurveys show that children are infected as frequently as adults. Children have much milder disease and the diagnosis is more often missed in children. Indeed, about 40% of children are asymptomatically infected compared with about 20% of adults [60,94]. Babesiosis is reported more frequently in males than females, presumably because they are more often exposed to tick-infested areas. Lawn maintenance workers and those with occupational exposure to ticks are at greater risk of tick-borne diseases than the general population.

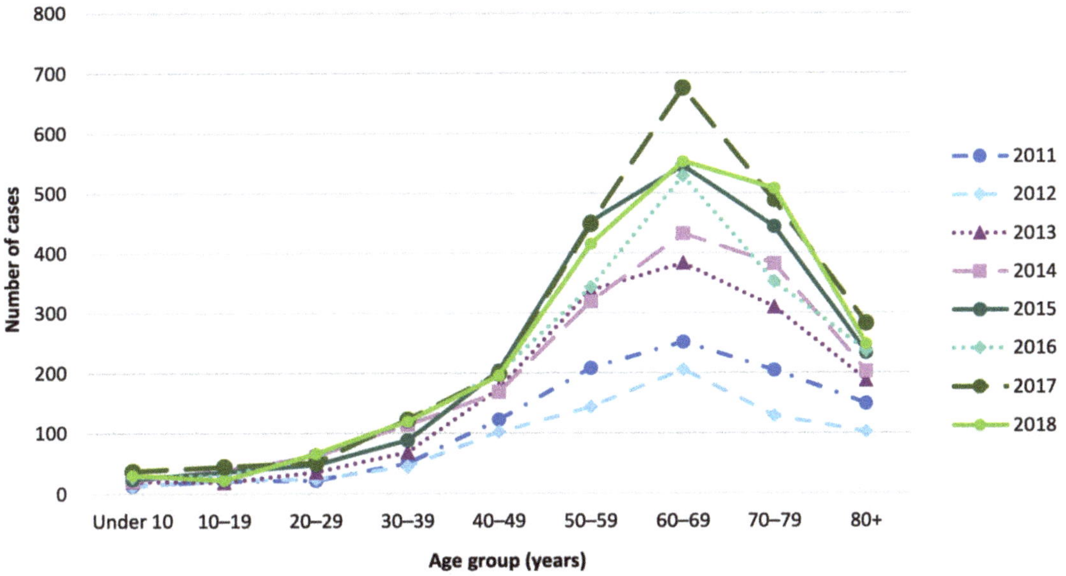

Figure 3. Babesiosis cases by age in the United States. Babesiosis cases reported by age to the Centers for Disease Control and Prevention, United States between 2011 and 2018 are shown. The low numbers of cases in children is due to the mild clinical symptoms resulting from *B. microti* infection rather than exposure to the infection. Almost half of children are asymptomatically infected compared to about a fifth of adults. Thus, *B. microti*-infected children are not diagnosed as frequently as adults (adapted from the Centers for Disease Control and Prevention. Notifiable Diseases and Mortality Tables. MMWR Morb Mortal Wkly Rep 2016, 65(3) [95]).

4. Human Babesiosis in the Americas

4.1. Overview

The first case of babesiosis in the United States was described in 1968 in a California resident, although the species was not identified [32]. Two years later, a case of *B. microti* was described in Nantucket, Massachusetts [40]. Subsequent reports on Nantucket established this island as the first babesiosis endemic site. The disease became known as Nantucket fever [65]. Subsequently, cases were reported on Cape Cod, Massachusetts, and the New England mainland. The reports of babesiosis subsequently broadened from southern New England to include endemic areas from Delaware to Maine [41,42,44,81,82,96,97]. Recent genomic studies have established that the initial source of *B. microti* was not from Nantucket but rather from the mainland in southeastern New England [44,81,82]. A similar emergence of babesiosis in Wisconsin and Minnesota is ongoing [81,98].

The emergence of babesiosis in the Northeast is thought to be due to several factors, including increased recognition of babesiosis by health care workers and the general public, an increase in the human population, construction of homes near wooded areas where ticks abound, and a marked increase in the deer population [41,71,96,97,99–101]. In the late 19th century, the number of deer in the United States had decreased to an estimated 300,000 due to hunting and the loss of forest habitat for farmland. Deer sightings in New England at that time were mentioned in local newspapers [39]. As farming moved to the Midwest and hunting declined, the deer population steadily increased to about 30 million in 2017. An increase in the white-tailed deer population has been accompanied by a marked increase in the *I. scapularis* population and a concomitant increase in the number of cases of Lyme disease, while removal of deer from specific locations has greatly diminished the number of ticks and cases of Lyme disease [39,102–104]. Interestingly, Lyme disease has spread more widely than babesiosis, in part because *B. microti* is less efficiently transmitted than *B. burgdorferi* [41,45]. There are large areas of the Northeast and northern Midwest where Lyme disease is endemic but babesiosis is not. There are no areas where babesiosis is reported in the absence of Lyme disease (Figure 4). Laboratory studies suggest that Lyme disease/babesiosis coinfection enhances the transmission of babesiosis and it has been hypothesized that the establishment of Lyme disease in an area is a prerequisite for the establishment of babesiosis [43,45]. Furthermore, birds can serve as hosts for *B. burgdorferi* but not *B. microti*. Larval ticks may attach and feed on *B. burgdorferi*-infected birds and be deposited hundreds of miles away where they can then establish a new site of infection. Both *B. burgdorferi* and *B. microti* can spread from one infected colony of mice to an adjacent colony but spread in this case is much slower than with birds [39,41].

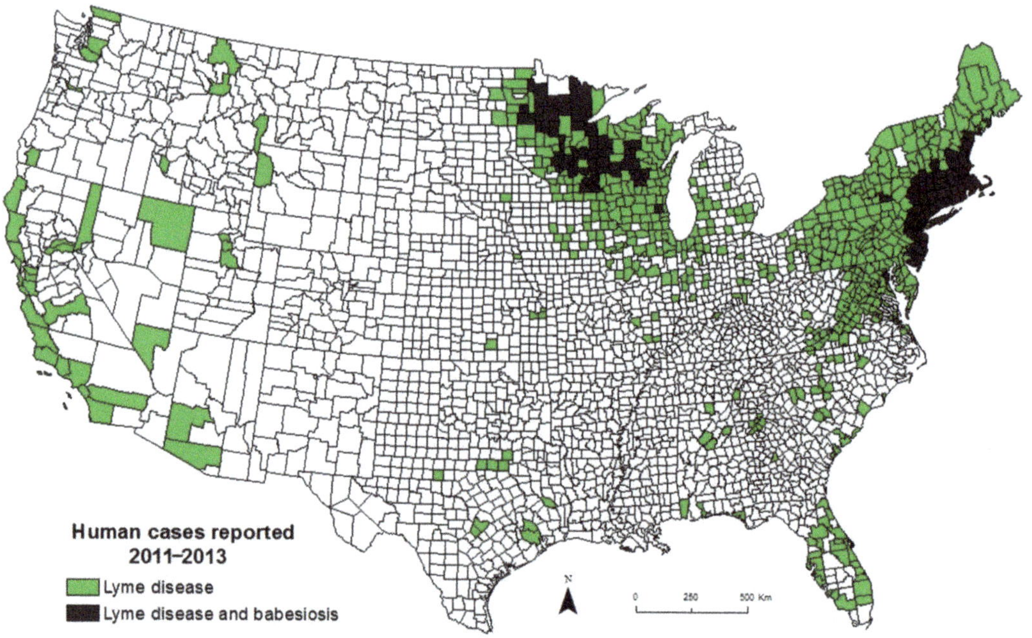

Figure 4. Human babesiosis occurs within Lyme disease endemic areas in the United States. Lyme disease and human babesiosis have been nationally notifiable conditions since 1991 and 2011, respectively. The names of counties that reported cases of Lyme disease and/or babesiosis from 2011 to 2013 were obtained from the Centers for Disease Control and Prevention. Counties with three or more cases of Lyme disease but fewer than three cases of babesiosis are depicted in green. Counties with three or more cases of Lyme disease and three or more cases of babesiosis are depicted in gray. No county reported three or more cases of babesiosis but fewer than three cases of Lyme disease (adapted from Diuk-Wasser M, Vannier E, Krause PJ. Coinfection by *Ixodes* tick-borne pathogens: Ecological, epidemiological, and clinical consequences. Trends Parasitol 2016, 32, 30–42 [43]).

4.2. United States

4.2.1. *Babesia microti* Infection

Currently, 14 states account for the vast majority of babesiosis cases in the United States and most are due to *B. microti*. These states include Connecticut, Delaware, Maine, Maryland, Massachusetts, Minnesota, New Hampshire, New Jersey, New York, Pennsylvania, Rhode Island, Virginia, Vermont, and Wisconsin [46,95]. Geographic modeling suggests that babesiosis will continue to emerge in the United States. The areas presently endemic for babesiosis and Lyme disease are expanding toward each other from the Northeast and Midwest. It has been postulated that a continuous endemic band of these two diseases may someday extend from Minnesota to the East coast. Lyme disease also is expanding into southeastern Canada and this is thought to be due, at least in part, to climate change [105,106].

Clinical manifestations of *B. microti* illness vary from subclinical illness to fulminating disease resulting in death [1,39,60,100,107]. Fever typically develops after a gradual onset of malaise, anorexia, and fatigue and may reach 40 °C (104 °F) [1,96,100,108]. Other common symptoms include chills, sweats, myalgia, arthralgia, nausea, and vomiting. Physical examination of *B. microti*-infected patients reveals fever and occasionally mild splenomegaly, hepatomegaly, or both. Abnormal laboratory findings include hemolytic anemia, elevated renal function and liver enzyme levels, and thrombocytopenia [58,96,100]. The illness usually lasts for a week or two but occasionally several months, with prolonged recovery taking up to 18 months [58,109]. Persistent parasitemia and clinical and microbiological relapse have been described for as long as 27 months after the initial episode, due in part to the development of antibiotic resistance [58,81,110–112]. Severe *B. microti* illness requiring hospital admission is common in patients with splenectomy, malignancy, HIV infection, hemoglobinopathy, chronic heart, lung, or liver disease, organ transplantation, acquisition of babesiosis through blood transfusion, and in newborn infants and the elderly [1,2,4]. Complications include severe hemolytic anemia, congestive heart failure, acute respiratory distress syndrome, disseminated intravascular coagulopathy (DIC), renal failure, coma, and shock [54,100,107].

4.2.2. *Babesia duncani* Infection

In 1991, a 41-year-old resident of Washington State presented with viral-like symptoms and was diagnosed with babesiosis. The causative pathogen was propagated in hamsters and was found to be morphologically similar but genetically and antigenically distinct from *B. microti* [34]. The organism was named WA-1. Eight additional cases of babesiosis with recovery of the same causative *Babesia* pathogen were subsequently reported in California and Washington states. The *Babesia* were found to be morphologically, ultrastructurally, and genetically indistinguishable from one another and were subsequently named *Babesia duncani* [48]. Two additional cases have been described in California and Oregon, respectively. The primary vector is *Dermacentor albipictus* [113]. Limited data suggests that the clinical manifestations of these cases are similar to those of *B. microti*. There is a marked difference in disease severity in hamster and C3H/Hen mouse models, however, as *B. duncani* causes fatal illness while *B. microti* causes mild or asymptomatic infection [114,115].

4.2.3. *Babesia divergens*-Like Infection

In 1996, Herwaldt and colleagues described a fatal case of babesiosis in a 73-year-old asplenic resident of Missouri who was infected with a *Babesia* that shared morphologic, antigenic, and genetic characteristics with *B. divergens*. The patient had previous exposure to cattle. The pathogen was named MO1 [36]. Four similar cases of *B. divergens*-like organisms have subsequently been described, none with exposure to cattle: (i) a 56 year old asplenic male resident of Kentucky who survived [49]; (ii) an 82-year-old asplenic male resident of Washington State with hypertension and secondary renal insufficiency who survived [50]; (iii) an 81-year-old asplenic Arkansas resident with diabetes, coronary artery disease, chronic obstructive pulmonary disease, a history of mitral valve replacement, hypertension, and GI bleeding, who died [51], and (iv) a 60-year old asplenic female resident of Michigan who developed multiple organ failure but survived [52]. These cases were similar to those of *B. divergens* cases from Europe, where almost all have occurred in asplenic individuals and many have died (see below).

4.2.4. Coinfection

Several different human pathogens cycle between *I. scapularis* ticks and mammalian reservoir hosts in the United States, including *Anaplasma phagocytophilum*, *Babesia microti*, *Borrelia burgdorferi*, *Borrelia mayonii*, *Borrelia miyamotoi*, deer tick virus (Powassan virus), and *Ehrlichia muris*-like organism [116]. These pathogens differ in their geographic range within the Northeast and northern Midwest. In areas where two or more pathogens are enzootic, simultaneous infection (coinfection) may occur. In the first case series of coinfection, the frequency and clinical outcome of Lyme disease and babesiosis alone were compared with those of Lyme disease and babesiosis coinfection [47]. Eleven percent of Lyme disease patients experienced coinfection while 72% of babesiosis patients had coinfection. This was expected because of the much larger number of Lyme disease patients compared with babesiosis patients. Lyme disease patients had a greater number of symptoms for longer duration if they were coinfected with *B. microti* [43,47]. The percentage of patients experiencing coinfection varies geographically and depends on the relative incidence of Lyme disease and babesiosis.

In addition to exacerbating human disease severity, *B. microti*-*B. burgdorferi* coinfection appears to increase *Babesia* parasitemia in the natural mouse reservoir, leading to greater transmission of *B. microti* from mouse reservoir to tick vector [45]. This enhancement of otherwise less transmissible *B. microti* may help explain why babesiosis has emerged more slowly than *B. burgdorferi* and is only found in areas of the United States where Lyme disease is endemic. Additional data suggests that coinfection provides a survival advantage for both *B. microti* and *B. burgdorferi* [43].

4.3. *Canada*

The first case of babesiosis in a Canadian resident was reported in 1999 [117]. The patient had traveled to Nantucket, Massachusetts six weeks prior to disease onset, indicating that the *Babesia* sp. identified on blood smear may not have been acquired indigenously. A second case of babesiosis was reported in 2001 in a 53-year-old Canadian resident who most likely acquired infection through blood transfusion from an asymptomatic *B. microti* positive donor [16]. The donor was thought to have acquired his infection in Cape Cod, Massachusetts. The first definitive case of locally acquired babesiosis in Canada was reported in a seven-year-old asplenic resident of Manitoba [17]. The child had not traveled outside Manitoba and never had a blood transfusion. *Babesia* were demonstrated on blood smear and *B. microti* was identified as the causative *Babesia* sp. by PCR. *I. scapularis* ticks infected with *B. microti* have been found in six different localities in Manitoba. Recently, two cases of *Babesia odocoilei* have been described with typical symptoms of babesiosis and positive PCR testing [118].

4.4. *Mexico*

A *Babesia* serosurvey was performed in Las Margaritas, Mexico in 1976. The sera of one third of 101 study subjects reacted against a dog *Babesia* antigen (*Babesia canis*) [59]. Three seropositive residents were found to be infected with *Babesia* when their blood was injected into splenectomized hamsters and *Babesia* were isolated from the hamsters. The *Babesia* species could not be identified. Four decades later, babesiosis due to *B. microti* was described in Yucatan State, Mexico [27]. The four patients ranged in age from 8 to 14 and lived in close proximity to each other in a rural area of eastern Yucatan. All subjects had tick bites or lived in tick-infested areas. All experienced mild to moderate illness with fever and three also experienced fatigue, arthralgia, and myalgia. The diagnosis was confirmed and the infecting species identified by amplification of *B. microti* DNA using PCR. All were given chloroquine and had a full recovery despite the fact that chloroquine is not effective for the treatment of human babesiosis.

4.5. South America

Two cases suggestive of babesiosis were reported in 2003 in South America. One was a 37-year-old resident of Puerto Berrio, Colombia who had fever, chills, sweats, weakness, and bone aches. *Babesia* parasites were identified on thin blood smear. A PCR was not performed but the patient had an antibody titer of 1:64 against *Babesia bovis* antigen [19]. The second case was an asymptomatic 2-year-old from Brazil with hepatoblastoma who had a positive blood smear for *Babesia* [15]. No *Babesia* PCR or antibody testing were performed.

In a survey of 300 residents of two rural towns (Turbo and Necocli) in Colombia where cattle ranching is an important industry, four subjects tested positive for *B. bovis* by PCR, including two who were blood smear positive [119]. Another two residents tested positive for *B. bigemina* by PCR, including one whose blood smear was positive. Three of these subjects were symptomatic with fever and/or headache and three were asymptomatic. Human babesiosis due to *B. bovis* and *B. bigemina* had not previously been described.

Nine cases of asymptomatic *B. microti* infection were discovered among 271 healthy residents of two rural towns in southeastern Bolivia [14]. All nine cases had *Babesia* identified on thin blood smear and further characterized as *B. microti* by PCR and molecular sequencing. All cases were seropositive when tested with a standard *B. microti* immunofluorescence antibody (IFA) assay.

A 72-year-old patient from Ecuador with chronic abdominal pain moved to Chicago and two months later developed fever, chills, headaches, myalgia, dry cough, nausea, vomiting, and diarrhea. He was admitted to the hospital and diagnosed with malaria based on his country of origin, symptoms, a positive blood smear showing intraerythrocytic ring forms (parasitemia 0.5%), and positive *P. falciparum* IgG antibody. A blood sample sent to the CDC was positive for *B. microti* by PCR. His infection resolved on atovaquone and proguanil [20].

In summary, there is evidence of human *B. microti* and other *Babesia* spp. infection in South America. Additional studies are necessary to better define the scope of the problem there, including confirmation of other *Babesia* species causing human infection.

5. Human Babesiosis in Europe

5.1. Overview

The first documented case of human babesiosis anywhere in the world was reported in the former Yugoslavia in 1957 [33]. The affected patient was a splenectomized farmer who succumbed to severe hemolytic anemia. The parasite species was never determined but *B. bovis* was found in the cattle he tended [120]. Since then, more than 50 cases of babesiosis have been reported on the European continent [1,5,121–123]. The predominant pathogen in Europe is *B. divergens*, however, *B. microti* and *B. venatorum* have been identified in a small number of cases [35,124,125]. A case of *B. divergens*-like infection has been reported in the Canary Islands (Spain) [8]. A comprehensive review of human babesiosis in Europe by Hildebrandt et al. (2021) documented a total of 51 autochthonous cases, with 35 attributed to *B. divergens*, 11 to *B. microti*, and 5 to *B. venatorum* [2]. Epidemiologic surveys have indicated widespread distribution of *B. divergens* and its associated tick vector, *Ixodes ricinus*, throughout Europe [126]. Recent seroprevalence reports suggest a much higher clinical incidence than has been described in the extant literature to date [127]. Quantitation of true babesiosis incidence across Europe remains a challenge because symptoms often manifest non-specifically, immunocompetent individuals are frequently asymptomatic, and babesiosis is not a notifiable disease in many countries [128].

5.2. *Babesia divergens*

B. divergens is the primary causative agent of human babesiosis in Europe and is endemic in the European cattle population. Gray (2006) described the ecological landscapes of countries with the highest incidence of bovine babesiosis as having significant tick populations in "rough open hill-land or damp low-lying meadows" and "where woodland frequently abuts cattle pasture" [129]. Over half of the cases of European babesiosis have been reported in France and the British Isles, with at least 10 other countries represented in single case reports [31,122,130–133]. Prevalence of babesiosis is reportedly increasing, and the European Center for Disease Prevention and Control have identified several factors driving this trend: landscape modifications affecting tick populations, deer population growth, human activity in infested areas, and dissemination of pathogens through cattle movement (https://www.ecdc.europa.eu/en/all-topics-z/babesiosis/facts-about-babesiosis, accessed on 27 July 2021). Disease emergence at increasingly northern latitudes in Europe has been recently observed. Mysterud and colleagues analyzed longitudinal tickborne disease incidence data from Norway and found that this emergence is linked to tick vector distribution [134]. *I. ricinus* is the primary vector of *B. divergens* and is widely distributed across Europe [135]. Primary host species include domesticated cattle, [126], roe deer, and other cervids (e.g., moose, red deer, reindeer, sika deer) [136].

B. divergens infections are characterized by fulminant disease and all but a few cases have been reported in asplenic patients [5,123,128]. Factors that predispose patients to severe disease include the extremes of age and other causes of immunocompromised clinical status [122,137]. After an incubation period of 1–3 weeks, *B. divergens* symptoms generally have a rapid progression with high fever, chills, sweats, headache, myalgia, hemolytic anemia, and hemoglobinuria [5]. Mortality associated with *B. divergens* infection, often due to multiorgan failure, was previously estimated to be as high as 42% but is improving. Better outcomes are thought to result primarily from more aggressive therapy, including intravenous antibiotics and the early use of exchange transfusion [5]. Two recent publications have challenged this "classic description of babesiosis in Europe." Martinot et al. described two exceptional cases of severe babesiosis in healthy, young, immunocompetent patients in France, and Gonzalez described a similar case in Spain [123,138].

5.3. *Babesia venatorum*

B. venatorum is an emerging public health concern in Europe due to its widespread zoonotic presence [136]. *B. venatorum*, formerly referred to as *Babesia* sp. EU1, is closely related to *B. divergens* and *B. odocoilei* [35,139]. Wild hosts include roe deer and moose [136]. The parasite has also been detected in captive reindeer and domesticated sheep [75,140–142]. The *I. ricinus* tick acts as both vector and reservoir. Cases in humans have thus far been reported in Austria, Germany, and Italy [35,124]. Case reports have described disease manifestations ranging from mild to moderately severe, which resolve with antimicrobial therapy, even in the setting of asplenia and lymphoma. The clinical presentation of *B. venatorum* infection is generally less severe compared to that of *B. divergens* [5].

5.4. *Babesia microti*

Cases of *B. microti* infection have been reported from Austria, Germany, Italy, Poland, Spain, and Switzerland [35,125,143–146]. The first evidence of human *B. microti* infection in Europe was a report of seropositive residents in Switzerland in 2002 [147]. A number of serosurveys have shown a wide range of *B. microti* seropositivity depending on the location and study population (e.g., general public, forest workers, Lyme disease coinfected subjects). *B. microti* seropositivity has ranged from 0.5% to 32% in study populations in Belgium, France, Germany, Italy, Poland, Sweden, and Switzerland [139,147–153] Furthermore, Hunfeld et al. (2002) reported that IgG seroprevalence rates were higher for *B. microti* (9.3%) than for *B. divergens* (4.9%) among patients exposed to ticks in Germany. [139] These seroprevalence data indicate that there is more human *B. microti* infection in Europe than currently identified.

5.5. Babesia crassa-Like Agent

Babesia crassa is a relatively uncommon *Babesia* species with documented infection in sheep in Iran and Turkey [154]. A single case of *B. crassa*-like infection has been reported in Europe in Slovenia [155]. The patient in question was asplenic and recovered after standard antibiotic treatment. Cases subsequently have been described in China.

6. Babesiosis in Asia

6.1. Overview

Several countries in Asia have reported human cases of babesiosis, including China, India, Japan, Korea, and Mongolia. In addition to previously documented human *Babesia* pathogens, several new *Babesia* species have been found to infect humans. As with any single case report of a novel *Babesia* species or report of a known *Babesia* sp. in a new region, identification of additional cases and pathogen isolation from local tick vectors and mammalian hosts will help confirm original findings [22,156]. The increasing interest and reports of human babesiosis in Asia are likely to reveal additional species and new areas of endemicity.

6.2. China

6.2.1. Human Infection

Outside the United States, the greatest number of human babesiosis cases are reported in China. China is the only country, other than the United States, where babesiosis has been shown to be endemic. Babesiosis in China is considered an emerging public health threat [3,6,157,158]. Among the human *Babesia* spp. identified to date, four (*B. microti*, *B. divergens*, *B. venatorum*, and *B. crassa*-like agent) have been confirmed to cause human infections in China [11,35,159–165]. Studies in western China more than a decade before the first official report of human babesiosis in Yugoslavia described *Babesia*-like intraerythrocytic organisms associated with febrile illness that may have been *Babesia* [6].

6.2.2. *Babesia venatorum*

B. venatorum was found to cause infection over a two year study period in Heilongjiang province in northeastern China, indicating endemic transmission. The majority of tick-borne cases in China are found in this province. Jiang et al. screened 2912 individuals for microscopic, PCR, or animal inoculation evidence of *Babesia* spp. infection in patients who reported a recent tick-bite and who sought hospital care between 2011 and 2014. Results showed that 48 (0.16%) of these patients had *B. venatorum* infection [12]. The *B. venatorum* 18S RNA gene sequences from all 48 patients were identical and differed from European *B. venatorum* parasite isolates by only two nucleotides. These data suggested a common origin of *B. venatorum* spp. in parasites circulating in northeastern China and Europe. Only five cases of *B. venatorum* had previously been identified, four of which were in Europe and one in a child in China [6,35,124,164,166,167].

6.2.3. *Babesia crassa*-Like Agent

A similar study led to the discovery of *B. crassa*-like pathogen as another causative agent of endemic human babesiosis in China. Between May 2015 and July 2016, Jia et al. screened 1125 residents of Heilongjiang Province for evidence of *Babesia* spp. infection who experienced fever and recent tick-bites. Of these participants, 5.0% (58/1125) demonstrated the presence of a novel *B. crassa*-like species in their blood, based on species-specific PCR testing and nucleotide sequencing [11]. *B. crassa*-like parasites were visualized on thin blood smears and showed ring, ameboid (<3 μm in size), and tetrad forms. The authors characterized the severity of disease manifestations as mild to moderate. Interestingly, 7.5% of healthy, asymptomatic residents of the area tested positive for *B. crassa*-like infection, suggesting that many human babesiosis cases due to *B. crassa*-like pathogen go undetected in China [11].

DNA samples also were collected from 1732 adult ticks from May to July 2014 from the same study area. Nine *I. persulcatus* and *Haemaphysalis concinna* ticks showed the presence of *B. crassa*-like species. Blood samples collected from 5 of 1125 sheep contained *B. crassa*-like DNA [11]. The *B. crassa*-like species is phylogenetically related to *B. crassa*, a large *Babesia* parasite of sheep in Turkey and Iran [154,168]. The near full length *B. crassa*-like 18S rRNA gene sequences showed 96.7% and 97.7% sequence similarities with the *B. crassa* sequences, respectively, from sheep in those countries [11].

6.2.4. *Babesia microti*

B. microti is another important *Babesia* sp. that causes human babesiosis in China [158]. Phylogenetic analyses based on the sequences from the 18S rRNA gene have revealed that *B. microti* from China are phylogenetically similar to those from Japan and Switzerland [6]. Clinical cases attributed to *B. microti* have been reported sporadically from Zhejiang, Yunnan, and Guangxi provinces [158,160]. Accurate diagnosis of clinical babesiosis is a challenge where *B. microti* babesiosis and malaria coexist in the same area in southwestern China, specifically Yunnan Province along the China–Myanmar border. The first reported cases of co-infections of *B. microti* and *Plasmodium* spp. were discovered there in 2012–2013 [165]. *B. microti*, *P. falciparum*, *P. vivax*, and *P. malariae* infections were identified among 449 febrile patients. Eight patients (1.8%) had infection with *B. microti* alone while 10 (2.2%) were co-infected with *B. microti* and either *P. falciparum* or *P. vivax* [165]. These results clearly illustrate a possible hidden clinical burden of *B. microti* in malaria endemic areas where babesiosis is not known to exist. Furthermore, patients experiencing febrile illness with intraerythrocytic parasites on blood smear may be misdiagnosed as having malaria when they actually have babesiosis.

B. microti has been shown to be transmitted by blood transfusion in the United States and Japan. Very limited data is available on the transmission risk of *B. microti* in Chinese blood donors. A single case of transfusion-associated babesiosis in China has been reported. *B. microti* was identified as the causative agent [169]. Large scale molecular and serological surveys to assess *Babesia* spp. risk among random blood donors in China are not yet available. A 2016 pilot serosurvey of blood donors in Heilongjiang Province revealed that 13 of 1000 (1.3%) donors had antibodies against *B. microti* parasites by the immunofluorescence antibody assay [161]. This *B. microti* antibody positivity rate is comparable to rates observed in blood donors in endemic areas in the northeastern United States [170]. These results provide further evidence that the prevalence of *B. microti* transmission in China may be significantly higher than currently realized and might be comparable to prevalence in the United States.

6.2.5. *Babesia divergens*

In recent years, laboratory screenings of probable cases of babesiosis in patients presenting to Chinese hospitals with recent tick bites have yielded surprising findings that are suggestive of the presence of novel *Babesia* spp. The first case of *B. divergens* (cattle *Babesia* sp.) infection in China was identified in a patient in 2011. The 18S rRNA gene sequence from this individual had 98.4% similarity with the gene of *B. divergens* in Switzerland [162]. A subsequent study in Gansu Province of 754 patients who visited a hospital for a tick bite between April and March 2016 showed that 10 patients (1.3%) had *B. divergens* infections, based on positive PCR tests [163]. *B. divergens* sequences from this study site were 99.9% identical to sequences of *B. divergens* from Europe. Interestingly, *B. divergens* infection has never been identified in cattle in China, possibly indicating a different reservoir host for this *Babesia* sp. Another salient feature of this study was that all 10 *B. divergens* infected patients were immunocompetent and only two had clinical symptoms at the time of sample collection.

6.2.6. Tick-Vectors and Animal Hosts of *Babesia* spp. in China

Several entomological and molecular studies have allowed quantitation of tick-vector and reservoir host infection rates, as well as geographic distribution of *Babesia* spp. in China. Fang et al. (2015) published a comprehensive overview of tick-borne infections in tick vectors, animal hosts, and humans [3]. The authors reported a total of 33 emerging tick-borne agents that have been identified in mainland China, including 11 species of *Babesia*. Their analyses showed that transmission of *Babesia* spp. is associated with 13 tick species. Although more prevalent in the northeastern regions, *Babesia* spp. were distributed throughout China.

Among *Babesia* spp. that infect humans, *B. venatorum* has been reported in *I. persulcatus* ticks from northeastern China [3]. *B. crassa*-like agent has been detected in *I. persulcatus* and *H. concinna* ticks from sheep in the same area in Heilngjiang Province [11]. *B. microti* has been identified over a broad expanse of China, including, (i) *I. persulcatus* and *H. concinna* ticks and striped field mice and reed voles in Heilongjiang Province, (ii) *H. longicornis* ticks on dogs from Henan Province, and (iii) rodents from Fujian, Zhejiang, Henan, and Heliongjiang provinces. *B. divergens* has been detected in *I. persculcatus, H. concinna,* and *Haemaphysalis japonica* ticks and in striped field mice in Heilongjiang Province. *Babesia* spp. that have not been shown to cause human infection in China include *B. ovis, B. major, B. ovata, B. orientalis, B. motasi, B. caballi, Babesia* sp. Kashi, and *Babesia* sp. Xinjiang [3]. More recently, Xia et al. have performed genotyping of *Babesia* spp. in a total of 2380 *I. persulcatus* and *H. concinna* ticks in a narrow forested area at 30 sampling points in northeastern China based on the 18S rRNA gene sequences [76]. Results showed that 23 (0.97%) of *I. persulcatus* ticks tested positive for five *Babesia* spp.—*B. bigemina, B. divergens, B. microti, B. venatorum* and one novel strain HLJ-80. Thirteen *H. concinna* ticks were positive for the following *Babesia* spp.—*B. bigemina, B. divergens,* three genetic variant forms of HLJ-874, and eight other *Babesia* variants represented by HLJ 242, which were similar to *B. crassa* [76]. The authors concluded that each site contained 5–6 different *Babesia* spp., several of which are capable of infecting humans. Additionally, Kobi-type and Otsu-type *B. microti* have been detected in wild rodents in Yunnan Province [171]. Overall, the presence of a number of *Babesia* spp. and their genetic variants infecting tick vectors and animal hosts indicate a high *Babesia* transmission risk to humans living in different parts of China.

6.3. *India*

A single case of human babesiosis was described in a resident of north central India in 2005. The diagnosis was confirmed by identification of *Babesia* on thin blood smear but the species was not identified. Antigen tests for *Plasmodia* were negative [22,23].

6.4. *Japan*

In 1980, Shiota et al. documented the presence of *B. microti* parasites in blood films collected from Japanese field mice [172]. The only autochthonous case of human babesiosis that has been reported from Japan was in a patient who acquired infection through blood transfusion during admission to Kobi University Hospital, Hyogo Prefecture in 1999 [24]. *B. microti* parasites were confirmed by blood smear microscopy and PCR analysis. The parasite isolated from the index patient's blood sample and from a blood sample inoculated and propagated in SCID mice were identified as a *B. microti*-like parasite, which had a 99.2% sequence homology with the *B. microti* reference strain from the US [24]. Although a blood sample from the implicated asymptomatic donor collected eight months after the index donation was negative for *B. microti* parasites by blood smear microscopy and PCR analysis, inoculation into SCID mice allowed detection of *B. microti* parasites that had sequence identity with the parasite isolate from the blood recipient [173]. *B. microti*-parasites exhibiting a similar genotype as the index patient and the asymptomatic blood donor were also isolated from a field mouse near the donor's residence, indicating enzootic and zoonotic transmission of *B. microti* in the area [173].

Molecular surveillance studies in the presumed *I. persulcatus* tick vector and field mouse reservoir host have demonstrated the presence of *Babesia* spp. throughout Japan with a potential for human transmission [173]. A field survey in Hokkaido Prefecture revealed the presence of *B. divergens* (Asia lineage) parasites in *I. persulcatus.* The presence of *B. microti* (United States lineage) and *B. venatorum* (strain Et65) were also noted in the same tick species [174]. Sika deer (*Cervus nippon*) were shown to carry *B. divergens* parasites in different Japanese prefectures [175]. In a more recent study, hard ticks belonging to the genera Ixodes and Haemaphysalis collected from sika deer in Hokkaido were found to harbor DNA for *B. microti, B. microti* Hobetsu, and *B. divergens*-like (Bab-SD) parasites [176]. Together, these studies suggest a wide-spread presence of *Babesia* spp. in tick vectors, mouse reservoir hosts, and humans in Japan.

6.5. *Korea*

Two cases of human babesiosis have been documented in Korea. In the first case, a blood sample from a patient contained paired pyriform and ring forms of *Babesia* parasites. The parasite isolate was named *Babesia* sp. KO1 and was found to be genetically related to sheep *Babesia* in China [26]. In the second case, a parasite isolate from a symptomatic patient was found to be closely related to *B. motasi*, a sheep parasite. Tick samples collected nearby the patient's residence demonstrated the presence of *B. microti* and *B. motasi* DNA (98% homology) [25]. Limited data is available for the tick-vectors and reservoir hosts of *Babesia* spp. in Korea. In one study, *B. microti* parasites (United States type) were detected by PCR in blood samples from wild animals in Gangwon-do Province [177]. In another study, *B. microti* (United States type) DNA was detected in blood samples from *Apodemus agrarius* (striped field mouse) but was absent from the other small mammals that were screened [28].

6.6. *Mongolia*

A survey of 100 asymptomatic farmers in Selenge province, Mongolia revealed that 7% had *B. microti* antibody and 3% had amplifiable *B. microti* DNA in their blood [28]. In a more recent study, a third of 63 questing *I. persulcatus* ticks were found to be infected with *B. microti* (United States type) in Selenge province in Mongolia [178].

7. Babesiosis in Africa

There have been very few cases of human babesiosis reported on the African continent to date. Human babesiosis caused by unknown species have been described in Egypt and Mozambique [8,21,121]. Two cases of babesiosis due to unknown species were reported in South Africa [29]. A 2018 case study described by Arsuaga et al. illustrates the difficulties of diagnosing babesiosis in the malaria-endemic areas of Cameroon and subsequently, Equatorial Guinea [179]. The complicated travel history of the patient in question coupled with the lack of available surveillance data on ticks and vertebrate reservoirs of *Babesia* species rendered it impossible for the authors to determine the definitive source of infection. Bloch and colleagues attribute the dearth of reported cases in Africa to a lack of surveillance data and to clinical and diagnostic overlap of *Babesia* with *Plasmodium* spp. in endemic areas [161]. In a pilot seroprevalence study, these authors examined seroreactivity among children in the Kilosa district of Tanzania. They concluded that *Babesia* may be present in the area, but that the potential for serological cross-reactivity and false positivity between *Babesia* and *Plasmodium* spp. impedes definitive conclusions about seroprevalence [161].

8. Babesiosis in Australia

A single autochthonous case of human babesiosis has been documented in Australia. Blood smear microscopy and molecular analysis revealed *B. microti* (United States type) as the infecting parasite [13]. A single imported case of babesiosis caused by *B. microti* infection also has been reported [180]. No evidence of *B. microti*-specific antibodies in 7000 blood donors and 29 clinically suspected babesiosis patients was detected in a serosurvey at multiple study sites in eastern Australia, leading the authors to conclude that transmission of *B. microti* is uncommon in this large region [181]. Babesiosis is a prevalent disease in cattle in Australia and is caused by *B. bigemina* and *B. bovis* [182]. Babesiosis is also prevalent in dogs where infecting species are *B. canis*, *B. vogeli*, and *B. gibsoni* [183]. Molecular studies demonstrating a tick-vector and reservoir-host for human *Babesia* spp. are lacking.

9. Conclusions

Human babesiosis is a worldwide emerging health problem that imposes a major disease burden, especially on the expanding older population and immunocompromised patients. Numerous studies indicate that the true number of *Babesia*-infected patients is markedly underestimated. As the infection continues to emerge, the number of affected individuals is likely to increase. Improved surveillance, as well as development of new antibiotics, supportive therapies, and a vaccine will all be important in limiting the impact of this disease.

Funding: We thank the Llura A. Gund Laboratory for Vector-borne Diseases and the Gordon and Llura Gund Foundation for financial support. The funders had no role in the design of the study; in the collection, analyses, or interpretation of data; in the writing of the manuscript, or in the decision to publish the results.

Institutional Review Board Statement: Not applicable.

Informed Consent Statement: Not applicable.

Data Availability Statement: Not applicable.

Acknowledgments: We thank Molly Missonis for her assistance in writing this manuscript.

Conflicts of Interest: The authors declare no conflict of interest.

References

1. Vannier, E.; Krause, P.J. Human babesiosis. *N. Engl. J. Med.* **2012**, *366*, 2397–2407. [CrossRef] [PubMed]
2. Hildebrandt, A.; Zintl, A.; Montero, E.; Hunfeld, K.P.; Gray, J. Human babesiosis in Europe. *Pathogens* **2021**, *10*, 1165. [CrossRef] [PubMed]
3. Fang, L.Q.; Liu, K.; Li, X.L.; Liang, S.; Yang, Y.; Yao, H.W.; Sun, R.X.; Sun, Y.; Chen, W.J.; Zuo, S.Q.; et al. Emerging tick-borne infections in mainland China: An increasing public health threat. *Lancet Infect. Dis.* **2015**, *15*, 1467–1479. [CrossRef]
4. Krause, P.J. Human babesiosis. *Int. J. Parasitol.* **2019**, *49*, 165–174. [CrossRef] [PubMed]
5. Hunfeld, K.P.; Hildebrandt, A.; Gray, J.S. Babesiosis: Recent insights into an ancient disease. *Int. J. Parasitol.* **2008**, *38*, 1219–1237. [CrossRef] [PubMed]
6. Zhou, X.; Xia, S.; Huang, J.L.; Tambo, E.; Zhuge, H.X.; Zhou, X.N. Human babesiosis, an emerging tick-borne disease in the People's Republic of China. *Parasit. Vectors* **2014**, *7*, 509. [CrossRef] [PubMed]
7. Homer, M.J.; Aguilar-Delfin, I.; Telford, S.R., III; Krause, P.J.; Persing, D.H. Babesiosis. *Clin. Microbiol. Rev.* **2000**, *13*, 451–469. [CrossRef] [PubMed]
8. Kjemtrup, A.M.; Conrad, P.A. Human babesiosis: An emerging tick-borne disease. *Int. J. Parasitol.* **2000**, *30*, 1323–1337. [CrossRef]
9. Schnittger, L.; Rodriguez, A.E.; Florin-Christensen, M.; Morrison, D.A. *Babesia*: A world emerging. *Infect. Genet. Evol.* **2012**, *12*, 1788–1809. [CrossRef]
10. Levine, N.D. Taxonomy of the Piroplasms. *Trans. Am. Microsc. Soc.* **1971**, *90*, 2–33. [CrossRef]
11. Jia, N.; Zheng, Y.C.; Jiang, J.F.; Jiang, R.R.; Jiang, B.G.; Wei, R.; Liu, H.B.; Huo, Q.B.; Sun, Y.; Chu, Y.L.; et al. Human Babesiosis Caused by a *Babesia crassa*-Like Pathogen: A Case Series. *Clin. Infect. Dis.* **2018**, *67*, 1110–1119. [CrossRef] [PubMed]
12. Jiang, J.F.; Zheng, Y.C.; Jiang, R.R.; Li, H.; Huo, Q.B.; Jiang, B.G.; Sun, Y.; Jia, N.; Wang, Y.W.; Ma, L.; et al. Epidemiological, clinical, and laboratory characteristics of 48 cases of "*Babesia venatorum*" infection in China: A descriptive study. *Lancet Infect. Dis.* **2015**, *15*, 196–203. [CrossRef]
13. Senanayake, S.N.; Paparini, A.; Latimer, M.; Andriolo, K.; Dasilva, A.J.; Wilson, H.; Xayavong, M.V.; Collignon, P.J.; Jeans, P.; Irwin, P.J. First report of human babesiosis in Australia. *Med. J. Aust.* **2012**, *196*, 350–352. [CrossRef] [PubMed]
14. Gabrielli, S.; Totino, V.; Macchioni, F.; Zuñiga, F.; Rojas, P.; Lara, Y.; Roselli, M.; Bartoloni, A.; Cancrini, G. Human Babesiosis, Bolivia, 2013. *Emerg. Infect. Dis.* **2016**, *22*, 1445–1447. [CrossRef] [PubMed]
15. Rech, A.; Bittar, C.M.; de Castro, C.G.; Azevedo, K.R.; dos Santos, R.P.; Machado, A.R.; Schwartsmann, G.; Goldani, L.; Brunetto, A.L. Asymptomatic babesiosis in a child with hepatoblastoma. *J. Pediatr. Hematol. Oncol.* **2004**, *26*, 213. [CrossRef]
16. Kain, K.C.; Jassoum, S.B.; Fong, I.W.; Hannach, B. Transfusion-transmitted babesiosis in Ontario: First reported case in Canada. *CMAJ* **2001**, *164*, 1721–1723. [PubMed]

17. Bullard, J.M.; Ahsanuddin, A.N.; Perry, A.M.; Lindsay, L.R.; Iranpour, M.; Dibernardo, A.; Van Caeseele, P.G. The first case of locally acquired tick-borne *Babesia microti* infection in Canada. *Can. J. Infect. Dis. Med. Microbiol.* **2014**, *25*, e87–e89. [CrossRef]
18. Olmeda, A.S.; Armstrong, P.M.; Rosenthal, B.M.; Valladares, B.; del Castillo, A.; de Armas, F.; Miguelez, M.; González, A.; Rodríguez Rodríguez, J.A.; Spielman, A.; et al. A subtropical case of human babesiosis. *Acta Trop.* **1997**, *67*, 229–234. [CrossRef]
19. Ríos, L.; Alvarez, G.; Blair, S. Serological and parasitological study and report of the first case of human babesiosis in Colombia. *Rev. Soc. Bras. Med. Trop.* **2003**, *36*, 493–498. [CrossRef]
20. Al Zoubi, M.; Kwak, T.; Patel, J.; Kulkarni, M.; Kallal, C.A. Atypical challenging and first case report of babesiosis in Ecuador. *IDCases* **2016**, *4*, 15–17. [CrossRef]
21. El-Bahnasawy, M.M.; Khalil, H.H.; Morsy, T.A. Babesiosis in an Egyptian boy aquired from pet dog, and a general review. *J. Egypt. Soc. Parasitol.* **2011**, *41*, 99–108. [PubMed]
22. Marathe, A.; Tripathi, J.; Handa, V.; Date, V. Human babesiosis—A case report. *Indian J. Med. Microbiol.* **2005**, *23*, 267–269. [CrossRef]
23. Negi, T.; Kandari, L.S.; Arunachalam, K. Update on prevalence and distribution pattern of tick-borne diseases among humans in India: A review. *Parasitol. Res.* **2021**, *120*, 1523–1539. [CrossRef] [PubMed]
24. Saito-Ito, A.; Tsuji, M.; Wei, Q.; He, S.; Matsui, T.; Kohsaki, M.; Arai, S.; Kamiyama, T.; Hioki, K.; Ishihara, C. Transfusion-acquired, autochthonous human babesiosis in Japan: Isolation of *Babesia microti*-like parasites with hu-RBC-SCID mice. *J. Clin. Microbiol.* **2000**, *38*, 4511–4516. [CrossRef]
25. Hong, S.H.; Kim, S.Y.; Song, B.G.; Rho, J.R.; Cho, C.R.; Kim, C.N.; Um, T.H.; Kwak, Y.G.; Cho, S.H.; Lee, S.E. Detection and characterization of an emerging type of *Babesia* sp. similar to *Babesia motasi* for the first case of human babesiosis and ticks in Korea. *Emerg. Microbes Infect.* **2019**, *8*, 869–878. [CrossRef] [PubMed]
26. Kim, J.Y.; Cho, S.H.; Joo, H.N.; Tsuji, M.; Cho, S.R.; Park, I.J.; Chung, G.T.; Ju, J.W.; Cheun, H.I.; Lee, H.W.; et al. First case of human babesiosis in Korea: Detection and characterization of a novel type of *Babesia* sp. (KO1) similar to ovine babesia. *J. Clin. Microbiol.* **2007**, *45*, 2084–2087. [CrossRef] [PubMed]
27. Peniche-Lara, G.; Balmaceda, L.; Perez-Osorio, C.; Munoz-Zanzi, C. Human babesiosis, Yucatán State, Mexico, 2015. *Emerg. Infect. Dis.* **2018**, *24*, 2061–2062. [CrossRef]
28. Hong, S.H.; Anu, D.; Jeong, Y.I.; Abmed, D.; Cho, S.H.; Lee, W.J.; Lee, S.E. Molecular detection and seroprevalence of *Babesia microti* among stock farmers in Khutul City, Selenge Province, Mongolia. *Korean J. Parasitol.* **2014**, *52*, 443–447. [CrossRef] [PubMed]
29. Bush, J.; Isaäcson, M.; Mohamed, A.; Potgieter, F.; De Waal, D. Human babesiosis-a preliminary report of 2 suspected cases in southern Africa. *S. Afr. Med. J.* **1990**, *78*, 699. [PubMed]
30. Shih, C.M.; Liu, L.P.; Chung, W.C.; Ong, S.J.; Wang, C.C. Human babesiosis in Taiwan: Asymptomatic infection with a *Babesia microti*-like organism in a Taiwanese woman. *J. Clin. Microbiol.* **1997**, *35*, 450–454. [CrossRef]
31. Tanyel, E.; Guler, N.; Hokelek, M.; Ulger, F.; Sunbul, M. A case of severe babesiosis treated successfully with exchange transfusion. *Int. J. Infect. Dis.* **2015**, *38*, 83–85. [CrossRef]
32. Scholtens, R.G.; Braff, E.H.; Healey, G.A.; Gleason, N. A case of babesiosis in man in the United States. *Am. J. Trop. Med. Hyg.* **1968**, *17*, 810–813. [CrossRef]
33. Skrabalo, Z.; Deanovic, Z. Piroplasmosis in man; report of a case. *Doc. Med. Geogr. Trop.* **1957**, *9*, 11–16. [PubMed]
34. Quick, R.E.; Herwaldt, B.L.; Thomford, J.W.; Garnett, M.E.; Eberhard, M.L.; Wilson, M.; Spach, D.H.; Dickerson, J.W.; Telford, S.R., III; Steingart, K.R.; et al. Babesiosis in Washington State: A new species of *Babesia*? *Ann. Intern. Med.* **1993**, *119*, 284–290. [CrossRef] [PubMed]
35. Herwaldt, B.L.; Cacciò, S.; Gherlinzoni, F.; Aspöck, H.; Slemenda, S.B.; Piccaluga, P.; Martinelli, G.; Edelhofer, R.; Hollenstein, U.; Poletti, G.; et al. Molecular characterization of a non-*Babesia divergens* organism causing zoonotic babesiosis in Europe. *Emerg. Infect. Dis.* **2003**, *9*, 942–948. [CrossRef] [PubMed]
36. Herwaldt, B.; Persing, D.H.; Précigout, E.A.; Goff, W.L.; Mathiesen, D.A.; Taylor, P.W.; Eberhard, M.L.; Gorenflot, A.F. A fatal case of babesiosis in Missouri: Identification of another piroplasm that infects humans. *Ann. Intern. Med.* **1996**, *124*, 643–650. [CrossRef]
37. Puri, A.; Bajpai, S.; Meredith, S.; Aravind, L.; Krause, P.J.; Kumar, S. *Babesia microti*: Pathogen genomics, genetic variability, immunodominant antigens, and pathogenesis. *Front. Microbiol.* **2021**, *12*, 2416. [CrossRef]
38. Babes, V. On bacterial haemoglobinuria in cattle. *Comptes Rendus l'Acad. Sci.* **1888**, *107*, 692–694.
39. Spielman, A.; Wilson, M.L.; Levine, J.F.; Piesman, J. Ecology of *Ixodes dammini*-borne human babesiosis and Lyme disease. *Annu. Rev. Entomol.* **1985**, *30*, 439–460. [CrossRef] [PubMed]
40. Western, K.A.; Benson, G.D.; Gleason, N.N.; Healy, G.R.; Schultz, M.G. Babesiosis in a Massachusetts resident. *N. Engl. J. Med.* **1970**, *283*, 854–856. [CrossRef]
41. Walter, K.S.; Pepin, K.M.; Webb, C.T.; Gaff, H.D.; Krause, P.J.; Pitzer, V.E.; Diuk-Wasser, M.A. Invasion of two tick-borne diseases across New England: Harnessing human surveillance data to capture underlying ecological invasion processes. *Proc. Biol. Sci.* **2016**, *283*, 20160834. [CrossRef] [PubMed]
42. Joseph, J.T.; John, M.; Visintainer, P.; Wormser, G.P. Increasing incidence and changing epidemiology of babesiosis in the Hudson Valley region of New York State: 2009–2016. *Diagn. Microbiol. Infect. Dis.* **2020**, *96*, 114958. [CrossRef] [PubMed]

43. Diuk-Wasser, M.A.; Vannier, E.; Krause, P.J. Coinfection by *Ixodes* tick-borne pathogens: Ecological, epidemiological, and clinical consequences. *Trends Parasitol.* **2016**, *32*, 30–42. [CrossRef] [PubMed]
44. Carpi, G.; Walter, K.S.; Mamoun, C.B.; Krause, P.J.; Kitchen, A.; Lepore, T.J.; Dwivedi, A.; Cornillot, E.; Caccone, A.; Diuk-Wasser, M.A. *Babesia microti* from humans and ticks hold a genomic signature of strong population structure in the United States. *BMC Genom.* **2016**, *17*, 888. [CrossRef] [PubMed]
45. Dunn, J.M.; Krause, P.J.; Davis, S.; Vannier, E.G.; Fitzpatrick, M.C.; Rollend, L.; Belperron, A.A.; States, S.L.; Stacey, A.; Bockenstedt, L.K.; et al. *Borrelia burgdorferi* promotes the establishment of *Babesia microti* in the northeastern United States. *PLoS ONE* **2014**, *9*, e115494. [CrossRef]
46. Menis, M.; Whitaker, B.I.; Wernecke, M.; Jiao, Y.; Eder, A.; Kumar, S.; Xu, W.; Liao, J.; Wei, Y.; MaCurdy, T.E.; et al. Babesiosis Occurrence Among United States Medicare Beneficiaries, Ages 65 and Older, During 2006–2017: Overall and by State and County of Residence. *Open Forum Infect. Dis.* **2021**, *8*, ofaa608. [CrossRef] [PubMed]
47. Krause, P.J.; Telford, S.R., III; Spielman, A.; Sikand, V.; Ryan, R.; Christianson, D.; Burke, G.; Brassard, P.; Pollack, R.; Peck, J.; et al. Concurrent Lyme disease and babesiosis. Evidence for increased severity and duration of illness. *JAMA* **1996**, *275*, 1657–1660. [CrossRef] [PubMed]
48. Conrad, P.A.; Kjemtrup, A.M.; Carreno, R.A.; Thomford, J.; Wainwright, K.; Eberhard, M.; Quick, R.; Telford, S.R., III; Herwaldt, B.L. Description of *Babesia duncani* n.sp. (Apicomplexa: Babesiidae) from humans and its differentiation from other piroplasms. *Int. J. Parasitol.* **2006**, *36*, 779–789. [CrossRef] [PubMed]
49. Beattie, J.F.; Michelson, M.L.; Holman, P.J. Acute babesiosis caused by *Babesia divergens* in a resident of Kentucky. *N. Engl. J. Med.* **2002**, *347*, 697–698. [CrossRef] [PubMed]
50. Herwaldt, B.L.; de Bruyn, G.; Pieniazek, N.J.; Homer, M.; Lofy, K.H.; Slemenda, S.B.; Fritsche, T.R.; Persing, D.H.; Limaye, A.P. *Babesia divergens*-like infection, Washington State. *Emerg. Infect. Dis.* **2004**, *10*, 622–629. [CrossRef] [PubMed]
51. Burgess, M.J.; Rosenbaum, E.R.; Pritt, B.S.; Haselow, D.T.; Ferren, K.M.; Alzghoul, B.N.; Rico, J.C.; Sloan, L.M.; Ramanan, P.; Purushothaman, R.; et al. Possible Transfusion-Transmitted *Babesia divergens*-like/MO-1 Infection in an Arkansas Patient. *Clin. Infect. Dis.* **2017**, *64*, 1622–1625. [CrossRef] [PubMed]
52. Herc, E.; Pritt, B.; Huizenga, T.; Douce, R.; Hysell, M.; Newton, D.; Sidge, J.; Losman, E.; Sherbeck, J.; Kaul, D.R. Probable Locally Acquired *Babesia divergens*-Like Infection in Woman, Michigan, USA. *Emerg. Infect. Dis.* **2018**, *24*, 1558–1560. [CrossRef] [PubMed]
53. Ruebush, T.K., 2nd; Juranek, D.D.; Chisholm, E.S.; Snow, P.C.; Healy, G.R.; Sulzer, A.J. Human babesiosis on Nantucket Island. Evidence for self-limited and subclinical infections. *N. Engl. J. Med.* **1977**, *297*, 825–827. [CrossRef]
54. Krause, P.J.; Auwaerter, P.G.; Bannuru, R.R.; Branda, J.A.; Falck-Ytter, Y.T.; Lantos, P.M.; Lavergne, V.; Meissner, H.C.; Osani, M.C.; Rips, J.G.; et al. Clinical Practice Guidelines by the Infectious Diseases Society of America (IDSA): 2020 Guideline on Diagnosis and Management of Babesiosis. *Clin. Infect. Dis.* **2021**, *72*, 185–189. [CrossRef] [PubMed]
55. Grabias, B.; Clement, J.; Krause, P.J.; Lepore, T.; Kumar, S. Superior real-time polymerase chain reaction detection of *Babesia microti* parasites in whole blood utilizing high-copy BMN antigens as amplification targets. *Transfusion* **2018**, *58*, 1924–1932. [CrossRef]
56. Krause, P.J.; Telford, S., 3rd; Spielman, A.; Ryan, R.; Magera, J.; Rajan, T.V.; Christianson, D.; Alberghini, T.V.; Bow, L.; Persing, D. Comparison of PCR with blood smear and inoculation of small animals for diagnosis of *Babesia microti* parasitemia. *J. Clin. Microbiol.* **1996**, *34*, 2791–2794. [CrossRef]
57. Smith, R.P.; Hunfeld, K.P.; Krause, P.J. Management strategies for human babesiosis. *Expert Rev. Anti-Infect. Ther.* **2020**, *18*, 625–636. [CrossRef]
58. Krause, P.J.; Gewurz, B.E.; Hill, D.; Marty, F.M.; Vannier, E.; Foppa, I.M.; Furman, R.R.; Neuhaus, E.; Skowron, G.; Gupta, S.; et al. Persistent and relapsing babesiosis in immunocompromised patients. *Clin. Infect. Dis.* **2008**, *46*, 370–376. [CrossRef] [PubMed]
59. Osorno, B.M.; Vega, C.; Ristic, M.; Robles, C.; Ibarra, S. Isolation of *Babesia* spp. from asymptomatic human beings. *Vet. Parasitol.* **1976**, *2*, 111–120. [CrossRef]
60. Krause, P.J.; McKay, K.; Gadbaw, J.; Christianson, D.; Closter, L.; Lepore, T.; Telford, S.R., III; Sikand, V.; Ryan, R.; Persing, D.; et al. Increasing health burden of human babesiosis in endemic sites. *Am. J. Trop. Med. Hyg.* **2003**, *68*, 431–436. [CrossRef] [PubMed]
61. Hai, V.V.; Almeras, L.; Socolovschi, C.; Raoult, D.; Parola, P.; Pagès, F. Monitoring human tick-borne disease risk and tick bite exposure in Europe: Available tools and promising future methods. *Ticks Tick-Borne Dis.* **2014**, *5*, 607–619. [CrossRef] [PubMed]
62. Lesko, C.R.; Keil, A.P.; Edwards, J.K. The Epidemiologic Toolbox: Identifying, Honing, and Using the Right Tools for the Job. *Am. J. Epidemiol.* **2020**, *189*, 511–517. [CrossRef] [PubMed]
63. Nieto, N.C.; Porter, W.T.; Wachara, J.C.; Lowrey, T.J.; Martin, L.; Motyka, P.J.; Salkeld, D.J. Using citizen science to describe the prevalence and distribution of tick bite and exposure to tick-borne diseases in the United States. *PLoS ONE* **2018**, *13*, e0199644. [CrossRef] [PubMed]
64. Vandenbroucke, J.P. In defense of case reports and case series. *Ann. Intern. Med.* **2001**, *134*, 330–334. [CrossRef]
65. Ruebush, T.K., 2nd; Juranek, D.D.; Spielman, A.; Piesman, J.; Healy, G.R. Epidemiology of human babesiosis on Nantucket Island. *Am. J. Trop. Med. Hyg.* **1981**, *30*, 937–941. [CrossRef] [PubMed]
66. Krause, P.J.; Kavathas, P.B.; Ruddle, N.H. *Immunoepidemiology*; Springer International Publishing: Cham, Switzerland, 2020.
67. Lantos, P.M.; Rumbaugh, J.; Bockenstedt, L.K.; Falck-Ytter, Y.T.; Aguero-Rosenfeld, M.E.; Auwaerter, P.G.; Baldwin, K.; Bannuru, R.R.; Belani, K.K.; Bowie, W.R.; et al. Clinical Practice Guidelines by the Infectious Diseases Society of America, American Academy of Neurology, and American College of Rheumatology: 2020 Guidelines for the Prevention, Diagnosis, and Treatment of Lyme Disease. *Neurology* **2021**, *96*, 262–273. [CrossRef] [PubMed]

68. Levin, A.E.; Williamson, P.C.; Bloch, E.M.; Clifford, J.; Cyrus, S.; Shaz, B.H.; Kessler, D.; Gorlin, J.; Erwin, J.L.; Krueger, N.X.; et al. Serologic screening of United States blood donors for *Babesia microti* using an investigational enzyme immunoassay. *Transfusion* **2016**, *56*, 1866–1874. [CrossRef]
69. Niccolai, L.M.; Ruddle, N.H.; Krause, P.J. Introduction to immunology, epidemiology, and immunoepidemiology. In *Immunoepidemiology*; Krause, P.J., Kavathas, P.B., Ruddle, N.H., Eds.; Springer International Publishing: Cham, Switzerland, 2019; pp. 3–17.
70. Diuk-Wasser, M.A.; Liu, Y.; Steeves, T.K.; Folsom-O'Keefe, C.; Dardick, K.R.; Lepore, T.; Bent, S.J.; Usmani-Brown, S.; Telford, S.R., III; Fish, D.; et al. Monitoring human babesiosis emergence through vector surveillance New England, USA. *Emerg. Infect. Dis.* **2014**, *20*, 225–231. [CrossRef] [PubMed]
71. Smith, R.P., Jr.; Elias, S.P.; Borelli, T.J.; Missaghi, B.; York, B.J.; Kessler, R.A.; Lubelczyk, C.B.; Lacombe, E.H.; Hayes, C.M.; Coulter, M.S.; et al. Human babesiosis, Maine, USA, 1995–2011. *Emerg. Infect. Dis.* **2014**, *20*, 1727–1730. [CrossRef]
72. Goethert, H.K.; Mather, T.N.; Buchthal, J.; Telford, S.R., III. Retrotransposon-based blood meal analysis of nymphal deer ticks demonstrates spatiotemporal diversity of *Borrelia burgdorferi* and *Babesia microti* reservoirs. *Appl. Environ. Microbiol.* **2021**, *87*, e02370-20. [CrossRef]
73. Barbour, A.G.; Bunikis, J.; Travinsky, B.; Hoen, A.G.; Diuk-Wasser, M.A.; Fish, D.; Tsao, J.I. Niche partitioning of *Borrelia burgdorferi* and *Borrelia miyamotoi* in the same tick vector and mammalian reservoir species. *Am. J. Trop. Med. Hyg.* **2009**, *81*, 1120–1131. [CrossRef] [PubMed]
74. Wagemakers, A.; Jahfari, S.; de Wever, B.; Spanjaard, L.; Starink, M.V.; de Vries, H.J.C.; Sprong, H.; Hovius, J.W. *Borrelia miyamotoi* in vectors and hosts in The Netherlands. *Ticks Tick-Borne Dis.* **2017**, *8*, 370–374. [CrossRef] [PubMed]
75. Gray, E.B.; Herwaldt, B.L. Babesiosis Surveillance-United States, 2011–2015. *MMWR Surveill. Summ.* **2019**, *68*, 1–11. [CrossRef] [PubMed]
76. Xia, L.Y.; Jiang, B.G.; Yuan, T.T.; von Fricken, M.; Jia, N.; Jiang, R.R.; Zhang, Y.; Li, X.L.; Sun, Y.; Ruan, X.D.; et al. Genetic Diversity and Coexistence of *Babesia* in Ticks (Acari: Ixodidae) from Northeastern China. *Vector Borne Zoonotic Dis.* **2020**, *20*, 817–824. [CrossRef] [PubMed]
77. Platonov, A.E.; Karan, L.S.; Kolyasnikova, N.M.; Makhneva, N.A.; Toporkova, M.G.; Maleev, V.V.; Fish, D.; Krause, P.J. Humans infected with relapsing fever spirochete *Borrelia miyamotoi*, Russia. *Emerg. Infect. Dis.* **2011**, *17*, 1816–1823. [CrossRef]
78. Ginsberg, H.S.; Hickling, G.J.; Burke, R.L.; Ogden, N.H.; Beati, L.; LeBrun, R.A.; Arsnoe, I.M.; Gerhold, R.; Han, S.; Jackson, K.; et al. Why Lyme disease is common in the northern US, but rare in the south: The roles of host choice, host-seeking behavior, and tick density. *PLoS Biol.* **2021**, *19*, e3001066. [CrossRef]
79. Cornillot, E.; Hadj-Kaddour, K.; Dassouli, A.; Noel, B.; Ranwez, V.; Vacherie, B.; Augagneur, Y.; Bres, V.; Duclos, A.; Randazzo, S.; et al. Sequencing of the smallest Apicomplexan genome from the human pathogen *Babesia microti*. *Nucleic Acids Res.* **2012**, *40*, 9102–9114. [CrossRef] [PubMed]
80. Silva, J.C.; Cornillot, E.; McCracken, C.; Usmani-Brown, S.; Dwivedi, A.; Ifeonu, O.O.; Crabtree, J.; Gotia, H.T.; Virji, A.Z.; Reynes, C.; et al. Genome-wide diversity and gene expression profiling of *Babesia microti* isolates identify polymorphic genes that mediate host-pathogen interactions. *Sci. Rep.* **2016**, *6*, 35284. [CrossRef] [PubMed]
81. Lemieux, J.E.; Tran, A.D.; Freimark, L.; Schaffner, S.F.; Goethert, H.; Andersen, K.G.; Bazner, S.; Li, A.; McGrath, G.; Sloan, L.; et al. A global map of genetic diversity in *Babesia microti* reveals strong population structure and identifies variants associated with clinical relapse. *Nat. Microbiol.* **2016**, *1*, 16079. [CrossRef] [PubMed]
82. Goethert, H.K.; Telford, S.R., III. Not "out of Nantucket": *Babesia microti* in southern New England comprises at least two major populations. *Parasit. Vectors* **2014**, *7*, 546. [CrossRef] [PubMed]
83. Skrip, L.A.; Townsend, J.P. Modeling Approaches Toward Understanding Infectious Disease Transmission. In *Immunoepidemiology*; Krause, P.J., Kavathas, P.B., Ruddle, N.H., Eds.; Springer International Publishing: Cham, Switzerland, 2019; pp. 227–243. [CrossRef]
84. Garner, M.G.; Hamilton, S.A. Principles of epidemiological modelling. *Rev. Sci. Tech.* **2011**, *30*, 407–416. [CrossRef]
85. Hersh, M.H.; Tibbetts, M.; Strauss, M.; Ostfeld, R.S.; Keesing, F. Reservoir competence of wildlife host species for *Babesia microti*. *Emerg. Infect. Dis.* **2012**, *18*, 1951–1957. [CrossRef]
86. Tufts, D.M.; Diuk-Wasser, M.A. Vertical Transmission: A Vector-Independent Transmission Pathway of *Babesia microti* in the Natural Reservoir Host *Peromyscus leucopus*. *J. Infect. Dis.* **2021**, *223*, 1787–1795. [CrossRef]
87. Herwaldt, B.L.; Linden, J.V.; Bosserman, E.; Young, C.; Olkowska, D.; Wilson, M. Transfusion-associated babesiosis in the United States: A description of cases. *Ann. Intern. Med.* **2011**, *155*, 509–519. [CrossRef] [PubMed]
88. Cornett, J.K.; Malhotra, A.; Hart, D. Vertical Transmission of Babesiosis From a Pregnant, Splenectomized Mother to Her Neonate. *Infect. Dis. Clin. Pract.* **2012**, *20*, 408–410. [CrossRef]
89. Brennan, M.B.; Herwaldt, B.L.; Kazmierczak, J.J.; Weiss, J.W.; Klein, C.L.; Leith, C.P.; He, R.; Oberley, M.J.; Tonnetti, L.; Wilkins, P.P.; et al. Transmission of *Babesia microti* Parasites by Solid Organ Transplantation. *Emerg. Infect. Dis.* **2016**, *22*, 1869–1876. [CrossRef]
90. Bloch, E.M.; Krause, P.J.; Tonnetti, L. Preventing Transfusion-Transmitted Babesiosis. *Pathogens* **2021**, *10*, 1176. [CrossRef] [PubMed]

91. Young, C.; Chawla, A.; Berardi, V.; Padbury, J.; Skowron, G.; Krause, P.J. Preventing transfusion-transmitted babesiosis: Preliminary experience of the first laboratory-based blood donor screening program. *Transfusion* **2012**, *52*, 1523–1529. [CrossRef] [PubMed]
92. Moritz, E.D.; Winton, C.S.; Tonnetti, L.; Townsend, R.L.; Berardi, V.P.; Hewins, M.E.; Weeks, K.E.; Dodd, R.Y.; Stramer, S.L. Screening for *Babesia microti* in the U.S. blood supply. *N. Engl. J. Med.* **2016**, *375*, 2236–2245. [CrossRef] [PubMed]
93. Saetre, K.; Godhwani, N.; Maria, M.; Patel, D.; Wang, G.; Li, K.I.; Wormser, G.P.; Nolan, S.M. Congenital babesiosis after maternal infection with *Borrelia burgdorferi* and *Babesia microti*. *J. Pediatric. Infect. Dis. Soc.* **2018**, *7*, e1–e5. [CrossRef] [PubMed]
94. Krause, P.J.; Telford, S.R., III; Pollack, R.J.; Ryan, R.; Brassard, P.; Zemel, L.; Spielman, A. Babesiosis: An underdiagnosed disease of children. *Pediatrics* **1992**, *89*, 1045–1048. [PubMed]
95. Notifiable Diseases and Mortality Tables. *MMWR Morb. Mortal. Wkly. Rep.* **2016**, *65*, Nd-38.
96. Joseph, J.T.; Roy, S.S.; Shams, N.; Visintainer, P.; Nadelman, R.B.; Hosur, S.; Nelson, J.; Wormser, G.P. Babesiosis in Lower Hudson Valley, New York, USA. *Emerg. Infect. Dis.* **2011**, *17*, 843–847. [CrossRef]
97. Rodgers, S.E.; Mather, T.N. Human *Babesia microti* incidence and *Ixodes scapularis* distribution, Rhode Island, 1998–2004. *Emerg. Infect. Dis.* **2007**, *13*, 633–635. [CrossRef] [PubMed]
98. Fida, M.; Challener, D.; Hamdi, A.; O'Horo, J.; Abu Saleh, O. Babesiosis: A Retrospective Review of 38 Cases in the Upper Midwest. *Open Forum Infect. Dis.* **2019**, *6*, ofz311. [CrossRef] [PubMed]
99. Mareedu, N.; Schotthoefer, A.M.; Tompkins, J.; Hall, M.C.; Fritsche, T.R.; Frost, H.M. Risk Factors for Severe Infection, Hospitalization, and Prolonged Antimicrobial Therapy in Patients with Babesiosis. *Am. J. Trop. Med. Hyg.* **2017**, *97*, 1218–1225. [CrossRef] [PubMed]
100. White, D.J.; Talarico, J.; Chang, H.G.; Birkhead, G.S.; Heimberger, T.; Morse, D.L. Human babesiosis in New York State: Review of 139 hospitalized cases and analysis of prognostic factors. *Arch. Intern. Med.* **1998**, *158*, 2149–2154. [CrossRef] [PubMed]
101. Krause, P.J.; Telford, S.R., III; Ryan, R.; Hurta, A.B.; Kwasnik, I.; Luger, S.; Niederman, J.; Gerber, M.; Spielman, A. Geographical and temporal distribution of babesial infection in Connecticut. *J. Clin. Microbiol.* **1991**, *29*, 1–4. [CrossRef] [PubMed]
102. Rand, P.W.; Lubelczyk, C.; Holman, M.S.; Lacombe, E.H.; Smith, R.P., Jr. Abundance of *Ixodes scapularis* (Acari: Ixodidae) after the complete removal of deer from an isolated offshore island, endemic for Lyme Disease. *J. Med. Entomol.* **2004**, *41*, 779–784. [CrossRef] [PubMed]
103. Kilpatrick, H.J.; LaBonte, A.M.; Stafford, K.C. The relationship between deer density, tick abundance, and human cases of Lyme disease in a residential community. *J. Med. Entomol.* **2014**, *51*, 777–784. [CrossRef]
104. Wilson, M.L.; Telford, S.R., III; Piesman, J.; Spielman, A. Reduced abundance of immature *Ixodes dammini* (Acari: Ixodidae) following elimination of deer. *J. Med. Entomol.* **1988**, *25*, 224–228. [CrossRef] [PubMed]
105. Kulkarni, M.A.; Berrang-Ford, L.; Buck, P.A.; Drebot, M.A.; Lindsay, L.R.; Ogden, N.H. Major emerging vector-borne zoonotic diseases of public health importance in Canada. *Emerg. Microbes Infect.* **2015**, *4*, e33. [CrossRef] [PubMed]
106. Ogden, N.H.; AbdelMalik, P.; Pulliam, J. Emerging infectious diseases: Prediction and detection. *Can. Commun. Dis. Rep.* **2017**, *43*, 206–211. [CrossRef] [PubMed]
107. Hatcher, J.C.; Greenberg, P.D.; Antique, J.; Jimenez-Lucho, V.E. Severe babesiosis in Long Island: Review of 34 cases and their complications. *Clin. Infect. Dis.* **2001**, *32*, 1117–1125. [CrossRef] [PubMed]
108. Vannier, E.G.; Diuk-Wasser, M.A.; Ben Mamoun, C.; Krause, P.J. Babesiosis. *Infect. Dis. Clin. N. Am.* **2015**, *29*, 357–370. [CrossRef] [PubMed]
109. Bloch, E.M.; Kumar, S.; Krause, P.J. Persistence of *Babesia microti* Infection in Humans. *Pathogens* **2019**, *8*, 102. [CrossRef] [PubMed]
110. Raffalli, J.; Wormser, G.P. Persistence of babesiosis for >2 years in a patient on rituximab for rheumatoid arthritis. *Diagn. Microbiol. Infect. Dis.* **2016**, *85*, 231–232. [CrossRef] [PubMed]
111. Simon, M.S.; Westblade, L.F.; Dziedziech, A.; Visone, J.E.; Furman, R.R.; Jenkins, S.G.; Schuetz, A.N.; Kirkman, L.A. Clinical and Molecular Evidence of Atovaquone and Azithromycin Resistance in Relapsed *Babesia microti* Infection Associated with Rituximab and Chronic Lymphocytic Leukemia. *Clin. Infect. Dis.* **2017**, *65*, 1222–1225. [CrossRef] [PubMed]
112. Wormser, G.P.; Prasad, A.; Neuhaus, E.; Joshi, S.; Nowakowski, J.; Nelson, J.; Mittleman, A.; Aguero-Rosenfeld, M.; Topal, J.; Krause, P.J. Emergence of resistance to azithromycin-atovaquone in immunocompromised patients with *Babesia microti* infection. *Clin. Infect. Dis.* **2010**, *50*, 381–386. [CrossRef] [PubMed]
113. Swei, A.; O'Connor, K.E.; Couper, L.I.; Thekkiniath, J.; Conrad, P.A.; Padgett, K.A.; Burns, J.; Yoshimizu, M.H.; Gonzales, B.; Munk, B.; et al. Evidence for transmission of the zoonotic apicomplexan parasite *Babesia duncani* by the tick *Dermacentor albipictus*. *Int. J. Parasitol.* **2019**, *49*, 95–103. [CrossRef] [PubMed]
114. Wozniak, E.J.; Lowenstine, L.J.; Hemmer, R.; Robinson, T.; Conrad, P.A. Comparative pathogenesis of human WA1 and *Babesia microti* isolates in a Syrian hamster model. *Lab. Anim. Sci.* **1996**, *46*, 507–515.
115. Hemmer, R.M.; Wozniak, E.J.; Lowenstine, L.J.; Plopper, C.G.; Wong, V.; Conrad, P.A. Endothelial cell changes are associated with pulmonary edema and respiratory distress in mice infected with the WA1 human *Babesia* parasite. *J. Parasitol.* **1999**, *85*, 479–489. [CrossRef] [PubMed]
116. Caulfield, A.J.; Pritt, B.S. Lyme Disease Coinfections in the United States. *Clin. Lab. Med.* **2015**, *35*, 827–846. [CrossRef] [PubMed]
117. Dos Santos, C.C.; Kain, K.C. Two tick-borne diseases in one: A case report of concurrent babesiosis and Lyme disease in Ontario. *Cmaj* **1999**, *160*, 1851–1853.

118. Scott, J.D.; Sajid, M.S.; Pascoe, E.L.; Foley, J.E. Detection of *Babesia odocoilei* in humans with babesiosis symptoms. *Diagnostics* **2021**, *11*, 947. [CrossRef]
119. Gonzalez, J.; Echaide, I.; Pabón, A.; Gabriel Piñeros, J.J.; Blair, S.; Tobón-Castaño, A. Babesiosis prevalence in malaria-endemic regions of Colombia. *J. Vector Borne Dis.* **2018**, *55*, 222–229. [CrossRef] [PubMed]
120. Garnham, P.C. Human babesiosis: European aspects. *Trans. R. Soci. Trop. Med. Hyg.* **1980**, *74*, 153–155. [CrossRef]
121. Gray, J.; Zintl, A.; Hildebrandt, A.; Hunfeld, K.P.; Weiss, L. Zoonotic babesiosis: Overview of the disease and novel aspects of pathogen identity. *Ticks Tick-Borne Dis.* **2010**, *1*, 3–10. [CrossRef] [PubMed]
122. Hildebrandt, A.; Gray, J.S.; Hunfeld, K.P. Human babesiosis in Europe: What clinicians need to know. *Infection* **2013**, *41*, 1057–1072. [CrossRef] [PubMed]
123. Martinot, M.; Zadeh, M.M.; Hansmann, Y.; Grawey, I.; Christmann, D.; Aguillon, S.; Jouglin, M.; Chauvin, A.; De Briel, D. Babesiosis in immunocompetent patients, Europe. *Emerg. Infect. Dis.* **2011**, *17*, 114–116. [CrossRef]
124. Häselbarth, K.; Tenter, A.M.; Brade, V.; Krieger, G.; Hunfeld, K.P. First case of human babesiosis in Germany-Clinical presentation and molecular characterisation of the pathogen. *Int. J. Med. Microbiol.* **2007**, *297*, 197–204. [CrossRef] [PubMed]
125. Hildebrandt, A.; Hunfeld, K.P.; Baier, M.; Krumbholz, A.; Sachse, S.; Lorenzen, T.; Kiehntopf, M.; Fricke, H.J.; Straube, E. First confirmed autochthonous case of human *Babesia microti* infection in Europe. *Eur. J. Clin. Microbiol. Infect. Dis.* **2007**, *26*, 595–601. [CrossRef] [PubMed]
126. Zintl, A.; Mulcahy, G.; Skerrett, H.E.; Taylor, S.M.; Gray, J.S. *Babesia divergens*, a bovine blood parasite of veterinary and zoonotic importance. *Clin. Microbiol. Rev.* **2003**, *16*, 622–636. [CrossRef] [PubMed]
127. Tomassone, L.; Berriatua, E.; De Sousa, R.; Duscher, G.G.; Mihalca, A.D.; Silaghi, C.; Sprong, H.; Zintl, A. Neglected vector-borne zoonoses in Europe: Into the wild. *Vet. Parasitol.* **2018**, *251*, 17–26. [CrossRef] [PubMed]
128. González, L.M.; Estrada, K.; Grande, R.; Jiménez-Jacinto, V.; Vega-Alvarado, L.; Sevilla, E.; Barrera, J.; Cuesta, I.; Zaballos, Á.; Bautista, J.M.; et al. Comparative and functional genomics of the protozoan parasite *Babesia divergens* highlighting the invasion and egress processes. *PLoS Negl. Trop. Dis.* **2019**, *13*, e0007680. [CrossRef]
129. Gray, J.S. Identity of the causal agents of human babesiosis in Europe. *Int. J. Med. Microbiol.* **2006**, *296* (Suppl. 40), 131–136. [CrossRef]
130. Haapasalo, K.; Suomalainen, P.; Sukura, A.; Siikamaki, H.; Jokiranta, T.S. Fatal babesiosis in man, Finland, 2004. *Emerg. Infect. Dis.* **2010**, *16*, 1116–1118. [CrossRef] [PubMed]
131. Mørch, K.; Holmaas, G.; Frolander, P.S.; Kristoffersen, E.K. Severe human *Babesia divergens* infection in Norway. *Int. J. Infect. Dis.* **2015**, *33*, 37–38. [CrossRef]
132. Centeno-Lima, S.; do Rosário, V.; Parreira, R.; Maia, A.J.; Freudenthal, A.M.; Nijhof, A.M.; Jongejan, F. A fatal case of human babesiosis in Portugal: Molecular and phylogenetic analysis. *Trop. Med. Int. Health* **2003**, *8*, 760–764. [CrossRef] [PubMed]
133. Kukina, I.V.; Zelya, O.P.; Guzeeva, T.M.; Karan, L.S.; Perkovskaya, I.A.; Tymoshenko, N.I.; Guzeeva, M.V. Severe babesiosis caused by *Babesia divergens* in a host with intact spleen, Russia, 2018. *Ticks Tick-Borne Dis.* **2019**, *10*, 101262. [CrossRef]
134. Mysterud, A.; Jore, S.; Østerås, O.; Viljugrein, H. Emergence of tick-borne diseases at northern latitudes in Europe: A comparative approach. *Sci. Rep.* **2017**, *7*, 16316. [CrossRef]
135. Onyiche, T.E.; Răileanu, C.; Fischer, S.; Silaghi, C. Global Distribution of Babesia Species in Questing Ticks: A Systematic Review and Meta-Analysis Based on Published Literature. *Pathogens* **2021**, *10*, 230. [CrossRef] [PubMed]
136. Fanelli, A. A historical review of *Babesia* spp. associated with deer in Europe: *Babesia divergens*/*Babesia divergens*-like, *Babesia capreoli*, *Babesia venatorum*, *Babesia* cf. *odocoilei*. *Vet. Parasitol.* **2021**, *294*, 109433. [CrossRef] [PubMed]
137. Vannier, E.; Krause, P.J. Update on babesiosis. *Interdiscip. Perspect. Infect. Dis.* **2009**, *2009*, 984568. [CrossRef]
138. Gonzalez, L.M.; Rojo, S.; Gonzalez-Camacho, F.; Luque, D.; Lobo, C.A.; Montero, E. Severe babesiosis in immunocompetent man, Spain, 2011. *Emerg. Infect. Dis.* **2014**, *20*, 724–726. [CrossRef]
139. Hunfeld, K.P.; Lambert, A.; Kampen, H.; Albert, S.; Epe, C.; Brade, V.; Tenter, A.M. Seroprevalence of Babesia infections in humans exposed to ticks in midwestern Germany. *J. Clin. Microbiol.* **2002**, *40*, 2431–2436. [CrossRef] [PubMed]
140. Langton, C.; Gray, J.S.; Waters, P.F.; Holman, P.J. Naturally acquired babesiosis in a reindeer (*Rangifer tarandus tarandus*) herd in Great Britain. *Parasitol. Res.* **2003**, *89*, 194–198. [CrossRef] [PubMed]
141. Malandrin, L.; Jouglin, M.; Sun, Y.; Brisseau, N.; Chauvin, A. Redescription of Babesia capreoli (Enigk and Friedhoff, 1962) from roe deer (*Capreolus capreolus*): Isolation, cultivation, host specificity, molecular characterisation and differentiation from *Babesia divergens*. *Int. J. Parasitol.* **2010**, *40*, 277–284. [CrossRef] [PubMed]
142. Wiegmann, L.; Silaghi, C.; Obiegala, A.; Karnath, C.; Langer, S.; Ternes, K.; Kämmerling, J.; Osmann, C.; Pfeffer, M. Occurrence of Babesia species in captive reindeer (*Rangifer tarandus*) in Germany. *Vet. Parasitol.* **2015**, *211*, 16–22. [CrossRef] [PubMed]
143. Welc-Falęciak, R.; Pawełczyk, A.; Radkowski, M.; Pancewicz, S.A.; Zajkowska, J.; Siński, E. First report of two asymptomatic cases of human infection with *Babesia microti* (Franca, 1910) in Poland. *Ann. Agric. Environ. Med.* **2015**, *22*, 51–54. [CrossRef]
144. Moniuszko-Malinowska, A.; Swiecicka, I.; Dunaj, J.; Zajkowska, J.; Czupryna, P.; Zambrowski, G.; Chmielewska-Badora, J.; Żukiewicz-Sobczak, W.; Swierzbinska, R.; Rutkowski, K.; et al. Infection with *Babesia microti* in humans with non-specific symptoms in North East Poland. *Infect. Dis.* **2016**, *48*, 537–543. [CrossRef]
145. Arsuaga, M.; Gonzalez, L.M.; Lobo, C.A.; de la Calle, F.; Bautista, J.M.; Azcárate, I.G.; Puente, S.; Montero, E. First Report of *Babesia microti*-Caused Babesiosis in Spain. *Vector Borne Zoonotic Dis.* **2016**, *16*, 677–679. [CrossRef] [PubMed]

146. Meer-Scherrer, L.; Adelson, M.; Mordechai, E.; Lottaz, B.; Tilton, R. *Babesia microti* infection in Europe. *Curr. Microbiol.* **2004**, *48*, 435–437. [CrossRef] [PubMed]
147. Foppa, I.M.; Krause, P.J.; Spielman, A.; Goethert, H.; Gern, L.; Brand, B.; Telford, S.R., III. Entomologic and serologic evidence of zoonotic transmission of *Babesia microti*, eastern Switzerland. *Emerg. Infect. Dis.* **2002**, *8*, 722–726. [CrossRef] [PubMed]
148. Pancewicz, S.; Moniuszko, A.; Bieniarz, E.; Puciło, K.; Grygorczuk, S.; Zajkowska, J.; Czupryna, P.; Kondrusik, M.; Swierzbińska-Pijanowska, R. Anti-*Babesia microti* antibodies in foresters highly exposed to tick bites in Poland. *Scand. J. Infect. Dis.* **2011**, *43*, 197–201. [CrossRef] [PubMed]
149. Gabrielli, S.; Calderini, P.; Cassini, R.; Galuppi, R.; Tampieri, M.P.; Pietrobelli, M.; Cancrini, G. Human exposure to piroplasms in central and northern Italy. *Vet. Ital.* **2014**, *50*, 41–47. [CrossRef] [PubMed]
150. Rigaud, E.; Jaulhac, B.; Garcia-Bonnet, N.; Hunfeld, K.P.; Féménia, F.; Huet, D.; Goulvestre, C.; Vaillant, V.; Deffontaines, G.; Abadia-Benoist, G. Seroprevalence of seven pathogens transmitted by the *Ixodes ricinus* tick in forestry workers in France. *Clin. Microbiol. Infect.* **2016**, *22*, 735.e1–735.e9. [CrossRef] [PubMed]
151. Svensson, J.; Hunfeld, K.P.; Persson, K.E.M. High seroprevalence of *Babesia* antibodies among *Borrelia burgdorferi*-infected humans in Sweden. *Ticks Tick-Borne Dis.* **2019**, *10*, 186–190. [CrossRef] [PubMed]
152. Lempereur, L.; Shiels, B.; Heyman, P.; Moreau, E.; Saegerman, C.; Losson, B.; Malandrin, L. A retrospective serological survey on human babesiosis in Belgium. *Clin. Microbiol. Infect.* **2015**, *21*, 96.e1–96.e7. [CrossRef] [PubMed]
153. Wilhelmsson, P.; Lövmar, M.; Krogfelt, K.A.; Nielsen, H.V.; Forsberg, P.; Lindgren, P.E. Clinical/serological outcome in humans bitten by *Babesia* species positive *Ixodes ricinus* ticks in Sweden and on the Åland Islands. *Ticks Tick-Borne Dis.* **2020**, *11*, 101455. [CrossRef] [PubMed]
154. Schnittger, L.; Yin, H.; Gubbels, M.J.; Beyer, D.; Niemann, S.; Jongejan, F.; Ahmed, J.S. Phylogeny of sheep and goat *Theileria* and *Babesia* parasites. *Parasitol. Res.* **2003**, *91*, 398–406. [CrossRef]
155. Strasek-Smrdel, K.; Korva, M.; Pal, E.; Rajter, M.; Skvarc, M.; Avsic-Zupanc, T. Case of *Babesia crassa*-like infection, Slovenia, 2014. *Emerg. Infect. Dis.* **2020**, *26*, 1038–1040. [CrossRef] [PubMed]
156. Man, S.Q.; Qiao, K.; Cui, J.; Feng, M.; Fu, Y.F.; Cheng, X.J. A case of human infection with a novel *Babesia* species in China. *Infect. Dis. Poverty* **2016**, *5*, 28. [CrossRef] [PubMed]
157. Vannier, E.; Krause, P.J. Babesiosis in China, an emerging threat. *Lancet Infect. Dis.* **2015**, *15*, 137–139. [CrossRef]
158. Chen, Z.; Li, H.; Gao, X.; Bian, A.; Yan, H.; Kong, D.; Liu, X. Human babesiosis in China: A systematic review. *Parasitol. Res.* **2019**, *118*, 1103–1112. [CrossRef] [PubMed]
159. Zhou, X.; Xia, S.; Yin, S.Q.; Zhou, X.N. Emergence of babesiosis in China-Myanmar border areas. *Parasit. Vectors* **2015**, *8*, 390. [CrossRef] [PubMed]
160. Huang, S.; Zhang, L.; Yao, L.; Li, J.; Chen, H.; Ni, Q.; Pan, C.; Jin, L. Human babesiosis in southeast China: A case report. *Int. J. Infect. Dis.* **2018**, *68*, 36–38. [CrossRef]
161. Bloch, E.M.; Kasubi, M.; Levin, A.; Mrango, Z.; Weaver, J.; Munoz, B.; West, S.K. *Babesia microti* and malaria infection in Africa: A pilot serosurvey in Kilosa district, Tanzania. *Am. J. Trop. Med. Hyg.* **2018**, *99*, 51–56. [CrossRef]
162. Qi, C.; Zhou, D.; Liu, J.; Cheng, Z.; Zhang, L.; Wang, L.; Wang, Z.; Yang, D.; Wang, S.; Chai, T. Detection of *Babesia divergens* using molecular methods in anemic patients in Shandong Province, China. *Parasitol. Res.* **2011**, *109*, 241–245. [CrossRef]
163. Wang, J.; Zhang, S.; Yang, J.; Liu, J.; Zhang, D.; Li, Y.; Luo, J.; Guan, G.; Yin, H. *Babesia divergens* in human in Gansu province, China. *Emerg. Microb. Infect.* **2019**, *8*, 959–961. [CrossRef] [PubMed]
164. Sun, Y.; Li, S.G.; Jiang, J.F.; Wang, X.; Zhang, Y.; Wang, H.; Cao, W.C. *Babesia venatorum* infection in child, China. *Emerg. Infect. Dis.* **2014**, *20*, 896–897. [CrossRef] [PubMed]
165. Zhou, X.; Li, S.G.; Chen, S.B.; Wang, J.Z.; Xu, B.; Zhou, H.J.; Ge, H.X.; Chen, J.H.; Hu, W. Co-infections with *Babesia microti* and *Plasmodium* parasites along the China-Myanmar border. *Infect. Dis. Poverty* **2013**, *2*, 24. [CrossRef] [PubMed]
166. Piccaluga, P.P.; Poletti, G.; Martinelli, G.; Gherlinzoni, F. *Babesia* infection in Italy. *Lancet Infect. Dis.* **2004**, *4*, 212. [CrossRef]
167. Blum, S.; Gattringer, R.; Haschke, E.; Walochnik, J.; Tschurtschenthaler, G.; Lang, F.; Oberbauer, R. The case: Hemolysis and acute renal failure. Babesiosis. *Kidney Int.* **2011**, *80*, 681–683. [CrossRef]
168. Hashemi-Fesharki, R. Tick-borne diseases of sheep and goats and their related vectors in Iran. *Parassitologia* **1997**, *39*, 115–117. [PubMed]
169. Chen, Y.; Yan, D.; Zhang, Y.C. Transfusion-associated babesiosis in China: A case report. *Transfus. Apher. Sci.* **2020**, *59*, 102902. [CrossRef] [PubMed]
170. Johnson, S.T.; Cable, R.G.; Tonnetti, L.; Spencer, B.; Rios, J.; Leiby, D.A. Seroprevalence of *Babesia microti* in blood donors from *Babesia*-endemic areas of the northeastern United States: 2000 through 2007. *Transfusion* **2009**, *49*, 2574–2582. [CrossRef] [PubMed]
171. Chen, X.R.; Ye, L.I.; Fan, J.W.; Li, C.; Tang, F.; Liu, W.; Ren, L.Z.; Bai, J.Y. Detection of Kobe-type and Otsu-type *Babesia microti* in wild rodents in China's Yunnan province. *Epidemiol. Infect.* **2017**, *145*, 2704–2710. [CrossRef] [PubMed]
172. Shiota, T.; Kurimoto, H.; Haguma, N.; Yoshida, Y. Studies on babesia first found in murine in Japan: Epidemiology, morphology and experimental infection. *Zentralblatt Bakteriol. Mikrobiol. Hyg. Ser. A Med. Microbiol. Infect. Dis. Virol. Parasitol.* **1984**, *256*, 347–355. [CrossRef]
173. Wei, Q.; Tsuji, M.; Zamoto, A.; Kohsaki, M.; Matsui, T.; Shiota, T.; Telford, S.R., III; Ishihara, C. Human babesiosis in Japan: Isolation of *Babesia microti*-like parasites from an asymptomatic transfusion donor and from a rodent from an area where babesiosis is endemic. *J. Clin. Microbiol.* **2001**, *39*, 2178–2183. [CrossRef]

174. Sayama, Y.; Zamoto-Niikura, A.; Matsumoto, C.; Saijo, M.; Ishihara, C.; Matsubayashi, K.; Nagai, T.; Satake, M. Analysis of antigen-antibody cross-reactivity among lineages and sublineages of *Babesia microti* parasites using human babesiosis specimens. *Transfusion* **2018**, *58*, 1234–1244. [CrossRef] [PubMed]
175. Zamoto-Niikura, A.; Tsuji, M.; Imaoka, K.; Kimura, M.; Morikawa, S.; Holman, P.J.; Hirata, H.; Ishihara, C. Sika deer carrying *Babesia* parasites closely related to *B. divergens*, Japan. *Emerg. Infect. Dis.* **2014**, *20*, 1398–1400. [CrossRef] [PubMed]
176. Elbaz, E.; Moustafa, M.A.M.; Lee, K.; Ching, A.L.C.; Shimozuru, M.; Sashika, M.; Nakao, R.; El-Khodery, S.A.; Tsubota, T. Utilizing attached hard ticks as pointers to the risk of infection by *Babesia* and *Theileria* species in sika deer (*Cervus nippon yesoensis*), in Japan. *Exp. Appl. Acarol.* **2020**, *82*, 411–429. [CrossRef]
177. Hong, S.H.; Lee, S.E.; Jeong, Y.I.; Kim, H.C.; Chong, S.T.; Klein, T.A.; Song, J.W.; Gu, S.H.; Cho, S.H.; Lee, W.J. Prevalence and molecular characterizations of *Toxoplasma gondii* and *Babesia microti* from small mammals captured in Gyeonggi and Gangwon Provinces, Republic of Korea. *Vet. Parasitol.* **2014**, *205*, 512–517. [CrossRef] [PubMed]
178. Tuvshintulga, B.; Sivakumar, T.; Battsetseg, B.; Narantsatsaral, S.O.; Enkhtaivan, B.; Battur, B.; Hayashida, K.; Okubo, K.; Ishizaki, T.; Inoue, N.; et al. The PCR detection and phylogenetic characterization of *Babesia microti* in questing ticks in Mongolia. *Parasitol. Int.* **2015**, *64*, 527–532. [CrossRef] [PubMed]
179. Arsuaga, M.; González, L.M.; Padial, E.S.; Dinkessa, A.W.; Sevilla, E.; Trigo, E.; Puente, S.; Gray, J.; Montero, E. Misdiagnosis of babesiosis as malaria, Equatorial Guinea, 2014. *Emerg. Infect. Dis.* **2018**, *24*, 1588–1589. [CrossRef] [PubMed]
180. Fuller, A.; Manitta, J.; Marks, R.; Tencic, S.; Gordon, C.L. First reported case of imported human *Babesia microti* infection in Australia. *Pathology* **2012**, *44*, 580–582. [CrossRef]
181. Faddy, H.M.; Rooks, K.M.; Irwin, P.J.; Viennet, E.; Paparini, A.; Seed, C.R.; Stramer, S.L.; Harley, R.J.; Chan, H.T.; Dennington, P.M.; et al. No evidence for widespread *Babesia microti* transmission in Australia. *Transfusion* **2019**, *59*, 2368–2374. [CrossRef]
182. Bock, R.; Jackson, L.; de Vos, A.; Jorgensen, W. Babesiosis of cattle. *Parasitology* **2004**, *129*, S247–S269. [CrossRef]
183. Jefferies, R.; Ryan, U.M.; Irwin, P.J. PCR-RFLP for the detection and differentiation of the canine piroplasm species and its use with filter paper-based technologies. *Vet. Parasitol.* **2007**, *144*, 20–27. [CrossRef]

pathogens MDPI

Review
Ticks, Human Babesiosis and Climate Change

Jeremy S. Gray [1,*] and Nicholas H. Ogden [2,3]

1 UCD School of Biology and Environmental Science, University College Dublin, D04 N2E5 Dublin, Ireland
2 Public Health Risk Sciences Division, National Microbiology Laboratory, Public Health Agency of Canada, St-Hyacinthe, QC J2S 2M2, Canada; nicholas.ogden@canada.ca
3 Groupe de Recherche en Épidémiologie des Zoonoses et Santé Publique (GREZOSP), Faculté de Medicine, Vétérinaire, Université de Montréal, St-Hyacinthe, QC J2S 2M2, Canada
* Correspondence: jeremy.gray@ucd.ie

Abstract: The effects of current and future global warming on the distribution and activity of the primary ixodid vectors of human babesiosis (caused by *Babesia divergens*, *B. venatorum* and *B. microti*) are discussed. There is clear evidence that the distributions of both *Ixodes ricinus*, the vector in Europe, and *I. scapularis* in North America have been impacted by the changing climate, with increasing temperatures resulting in the northwards expansion of tick populations and the occurrence of *I. ricinus* at higher altitudes. *Ixodes persulcatus*, which replaces *I. ricinus* in Eurasia and temperate Asia, is presumed to be the babesiosis vector in China and Japan, but this tick species has not yet been confirmed as the vector of either human or animal babesiosis. There is no definite evidence, as yet, of global warming having an effect on the occurrence of human babesiosis, but models suggest that it is only a matter of time before cases occur further north than they do at present.

Keywords: *Ixodes ricinus*; *Ixodes scapularis*; *Babesia microti*; *Babesia divergens*; climate; global warming

Citation: Gray, J.S.; Ogden, N.H. Ticks, Human Babesiosis and Climate Change. *Pathogens* **2021**, *10*, 1430. https://doi.org/10.3390/pathogens10111430

Academic Editors: Estrella Montero, Cheryl Ann Lobo, Luis Miguel González and Lawrence S. Young

Received: 26 September 2021
Accepted: 1 November 2021
Published: 4 November 2021

1. Introduction

According to the 6th IPPC report, published in August 2021, global temperatures over the next 20 years are expected to "reach or exceed an average of 1.5 °C, unless there are immediate, rapid and large-scale reductions in greenhouse gas emissions". Given that similar predictions were made, though with longer time scales, in each of the previous five reports, it now seems that such a global temperature increase is highly likely. This will result in an increasing number of heat waves, longer warm seasons and fundamental changes in rainfall patterns. Indeed, the first signs of these changes are already evident, most obviously in the natural world and relevant here in relation to arthropod vectors of disease [1]. It has been suggested that complex effects of climate change on both host communities and arthropod vectors could result in unanticipated spillover of pathogens from reservoir hosts into domesticated animals or humans resulting in disease emergence, depending on the host range of the pathogen [2], but the risk of emergence of novel *Babesia* spp. is unknown.

The risk of human babesiosis can be affected by climate change in at least three different ways. Firstly, as poikilothermic organisms, the ixodid tick vectors of human babesiosis and the babesia pathogens within them can respond directly to changes in ambient conditions; secondly and more indirectly, both ticks and the vertebrate reservoirs of the pathogens can be affected by the impact of climate change on vegetation, resulting in changes to habitats (e.g., beech woods [3]), and to host food sources (e.g., masting events [4,5]), thirdly anthropogenic responses to climate change, notably human behaviour, but also the management of livestock reservoirs of infection, will affect exposure to the vectors and therefore the risk of disease (Figure 1).

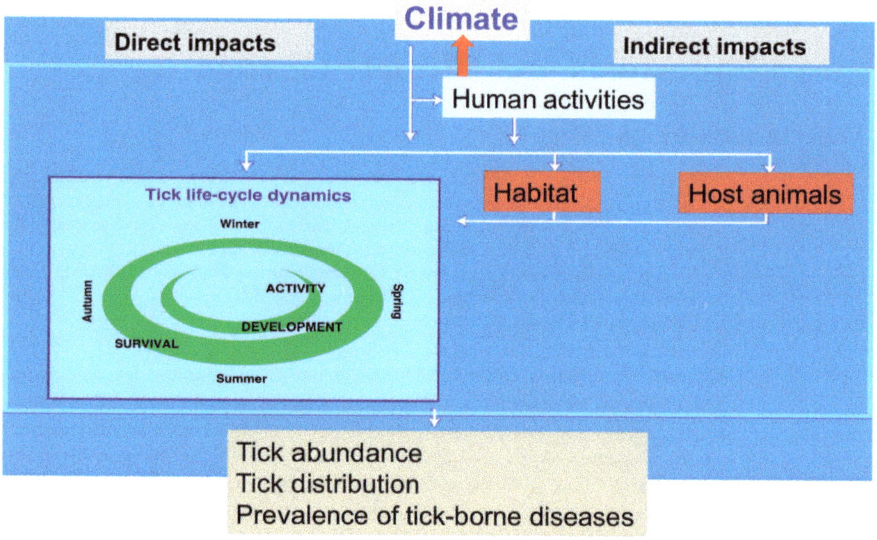

Figure 1. Factors determining the abundance and spread of *Ixodes* spp. Modified from Lindgren et al., 2000 [6].

The predominant vectors of human babesiosis are *Ixodes scapularis* transmitting *Babesia microti* in the USA, and *Ixodes ricinus*, transmitting *Babesia divergens* and *Babesia venatorum* in Europe [7]. *Babesia microti* also occurs in Europe, but human cases are extremely rare [8].

Several cases of *B. divergens* [9], *B. venatorum* [10] and *B. microti* [11], have been reported from China, and the vector, based on DNA detection, is suspected to be *Ixodes persulcatus* [11]. The same tick species is thought to be the vector of *B. microti* and an Asian lineage *B. divergens* in Japan [12,13]. Curiously, *I. persulcatus* has not been associated with either human or bovine babesiosis in Russia or Eastern Europe. Several other *Babesia* species in addition to *B. divergens*, *B. microti* and *B. venatorum* occasionally infect humans, but in most cases the identity of the vectors is unknown. The exceptions are *Babesia duncani*, which recent evidence suggests is transmitted by *Dermacentor albipictus* [14], a *Babesia crassa*-like parasite, probably transmitted by *I. persulcatus* or *Haemaphysalis concinna* [15], and an unnamed *Babesia* species in the USA, closely related to *B. divergens* and probably transmitted by *Ixodes dentatus*, a rabbit tick [16]. Since cases caused by these three *Babesia* species are rare, they will not be considered further here.

2. Life Cycles and Ecology of the Human Babesiosis Vectors

The three tick species responsible for most cases of human babesiosis, *Ixodes persulcatus*, *I. scapularis* and *I. ricinus* belong to the *Ixodes ricinus* species complex, consisting of at least another 15 species. They are three-host ticks, using separate hosts for each of the active stages, larva, nymph and adult, all of which engorge except for the male, which is probably not significantly involved in disease transmission. They are generalist species and feed on a very wide range of hosts, but there is some host selection, with larvae tending to feed preferentially on small mammals, nymphs on medium-sized mammals and birds, and adult females mainly on large mammals, such as deer and domestic livestock. However, there is a great deal of flexibility in these host preferences and large hosts can be heavily parasitised by the immature stages. Unlike most *Ixodes* species, which utilise hosts in nests and burrows, *I. persulcatus*, *I. ricinus* and *I. scapularis* attach to hosts in the open, using vegetation as ambush vantage points. When they have fed to repletion on their hosts over a few days, they drop off back into the vegetation, locate in the litter layer and commence development to the next stage, or commence egg development and then oviposition in the case of the female.

The life cycles of all three tick species are characterised by distinct seasonal activity of questing ticks, partly regulated by ambient conditions, so that little or no questing behaviour occurs at very high or very low temperatures, however, diapause is also a significant regulating mechanism. Diapause can be defined as a form of hormonally controlled arrested development or delayed behaviour that occurs prior to seasonally unfavourable environmental conditions. Conditioning of the ticks results from entrainment by certain environmental stimuli, particularly day length, and usually lasts for a set period. Laboratory studies have shown that temperature can affect diapause directly [17], but temperature may be more important in determining rates of tick development in relation to the seasonally-determined diapause conditioning periods. The role of diapause in regulating the life cycles of *I. persulcatus*, *I. ricinus* and *I. scapularis* has been reviewed recently [18].

The three *Ixodes* vectors of human babesiosis have very wide distributions encompassing several climate zones, for example *I. ricinus* occurs from the western seaboard of Europe to as far eastwards as the Ural Mountains and from the Atlas Mountains in North Africa to Northern Norway, though it is scarce in arid regions of southern Europe. The range of *I. persulcatus* is even greater, extending from Eastern Europe to the temperate Far East, and *I. scapularis* occurs from the southern states of the USA through the eastern seaboard as far north as southern Canada. Despite such wide ranges, the distribution of these tick species is limited by their susceptibility to desiccation when off the host. During development and especially when host-seeking (questing) they are exposed to ambient conditions and therefore confined to habitats that include humid microclimates (>80% RH) at the base of the vegetation, where the ticks obtain water by secreting a hygroscopic fluid onto their mouthparts and then ingesting it. Since questing may continue for several weeks, the ticks must make several journeys from the surface vegetation to soil level to replenish their water supply. The drier the atmosphere the more such trips, all costing energy, so that in hot, dry conditions survival may be limited. *I. persulcatus* differs from the other two species in that the immature stages are more reluctant to climb the vegetation and tend to quest in the litter layer [19], and southern strains of *I. scapularis* show similar behaviour relative to those from more northern regions in the USA [20], which may be a heritable adaptation to the drier conditions in the south. The consequence of the requirement of these ticks for humid microclimates when off the host is that their typical habitats tend to be woodlands with a substantial layer of vegetation litter. Deciduous and mixed forests offer the most favourable conditions, but coniferous forests may also harbour substantial numbers of ticks. Additionally, open habitats of rough vegetation such as the sheep-grazed uplands of north-western Europe, where maritime climates maintain mild winters and high humidity due to frequent rainfall, can maintain large numbers of ticks [21].

Another factor determining distribution and survival is temperature, which affects both development and questing, the lower thresholds of which probably vary with species, with regional differences occurring within tick species [22]. Cold air temperatures seem to have a limited effect on actual survival. For example, *I. scapularis* placed at −20 °C in the laboratory die rapidly, but engorged ticks placed in the litter layer in suitable woodland habitats in Canada over the winter (where air temperatures can often fall to less than −30 °C) have daily mortality rates no greater than those in summer, probably due to the insulating capacity of the litter layer (reviewed in Ogden et al. [23]). Similarly, it has been observed in Germany that *I. ricinus* populations are adversely affected by air temperatures of less than −15 °C only when the insulating snow cover is absent [24]. In the context of global warming, high temperatures are obviously important as drivers of desiccation in limiting tick survival, but laboratory studies suggest that even in the presence of high humidity, *I. ricinus* may suffer much higher mortality when temperatures exceed 30 °C [25].

The third vital component ensuring establishment and survival of tick populations is the availability of adequate numbers of appropriate hosts. In most habitats of the *Ixodes* species considered here, deer are essential hosts for the maintenance of the tick populations, because they are the only animals that feed significant numbers of adult female ticks, although in agricultural settings *I. ricinus* is also maintained by livestock, especially sheep and cattle [21]. Large hosts can feed all tick stages, but in woodland habitats small mammals and birds are important hosts of the immature stages, and many are essential components of tick-borne diseases, such as Lyme borreliosis, tick-borne encephalitis, several rickettsioses and human babesiosis caused by *B. microti*.

It is notable that ticks are increasingly recorded in urban areas and in such settings hedgehogs (*Erinaceus* spp.), another host that can feed all tick stages and thus maintain small populations of *I. ricinus*, could theoretically maintain zoonotic *B. microti* in the absence of large hosts [26,27]. As yet there are no reports of such foci, partly no doubt because zoonotic *B. microti* genotypes are rare in Europe [8].

3. The Roles of Reservoir Hosts of Human Babesiosis

Babesia microti is considered to be the most important cause of human babesiosis since it is responsible for the vast majority of cases, particularly in the USA. However, a study published in 2003 by Goethert and Telford [28], revealed that this is not a single species but consists of a complex belonging to three distinct clades utilizing a wide range of hosts, mostly rodents, but also shrews, dogs, foxes and raccoons. In the USA, some bird species were implicated in a single study as reservoirs of a *B. microti*-like organism [29]. However, the genotype involved is not known, and the distribution pattern of endemic areas of *B. microti*-babesiosis in the USA does not support long-distance distribution of the pathogen by birds. At present there is no evidence for significant bird involvement in the transmission of zoonotic *B. microti* genotypes, but this topic needs further study. In the Goethert and Telford study [28], most of the zoonotic genotypes turned out to belong to a single clade prevalent in the USA (though not confined to that country) and often referred to as the US-type or *B. microti* sensu stricto (s.s.), found in woodland mice, shrews and chipmunks. In Europe, very few cases of human babesiosis have been described despite widespread infection of rodents [8] and transmission by *I. ricinus* [30]. Although these cases appear to have been caused by rodent parasites, their rarity suggests that zoonotic genotypes are uncommon in Europe. In many regions the parasite is transmitted by *Ixodes trianguliceps*, which rarely bites humans, further reducing the risk of zoonotic babesiosis [8].

B. venatorum is a relatively recently described European zoonotic species [31], which has since been reported to have caused many more cases in China [10]. In Europe, good evidence now exists that the reservoir host of *B. venatorum* is roe deer (*Capreolus capreolus*) [32,33]. Sika deer (*Cervus nippon*) probably fulfils this role in China. Thus, two zoonotic *Babesia* spp. (*B. microti* s.s. and *B. venatorum*) are firmly associated with woodland. The third species, *B. divergens*, has until recently been considered to be an exclusive cattle parasite. With the advent of molecular taxonomy this parasite has also been reported from red deer (*Cervus elaphus*) and roe deer (*C. capreolus*) [34], but there is no evidence for wild deer as a source of infection for cattle or vice versa, although splenectomised red and roe deer can evidently be infected with *B. divergens* from cattle [35]. Current data suggest that almost all isolates from human cases closely match bovine babesia sequences, only two with less than 99.9% 18S rRNA gene homology, and having little identity with babesia sequences from deer [8]. The host origins of these babesias are unknown. It must be concluded that at present there is no evidence for deer as a source of *B. divergens* infection of humans and that human cases are predominantly associated with cattle and thus with agricultural rather than woodland habitats.

4. Expected Impacts of Climate Change on the Vectors

While in general, warming temperatures are likely to make northern regions more hospitable for ticks, and possibly less so closer to the equator, direct effects on tick survival of increasing temperatures and changes in rainfall patterns on tick survival in many regions of the northern hemisphere may be limited, because of the protection afforded by the typical woodland habitats and also by their ability to undergo developmental and behavioural diapause to avoid unfavourable conditions [18].

Of greater impact on tick population survival is the expected effect of warming temperatures on rates of development from one life stage to the next, and on host-seeking activity. Because the duration of development from one life stage to the next is mostly temperature-dependent (within the constraints of diapause), warmer temperatures will probably mean shorter tick life cycles, and shorter development times will probably be coupled with extended periods of the year when temperatures are suitable for tick activity [36]. Laboratory experiments by Gilbert et al. [22] also suggest that a greater proportion of *I. ricinus* in the questing phase will become active as temperatures increase, and the interaction of temperature with humidity, driving the saturation deficit, also directly impacts host-seeking activity [37]. The success of host seeking can therefore be influenced directly by temperature effects on the ticks, but is also determined by the abundance and activity of hosts, which will be affected by the temperature-dependent availability of forage.

5. Projected Effects of Climate Change on Tick and *Babesia* spp. Distributions

With the future temperatures projected by climate models, it is expected that the northern limit of the range of *I. scapularis* will expand northwards [38,39] and the leading edge of this expansion is now north of the Canadian border (Figure 2).

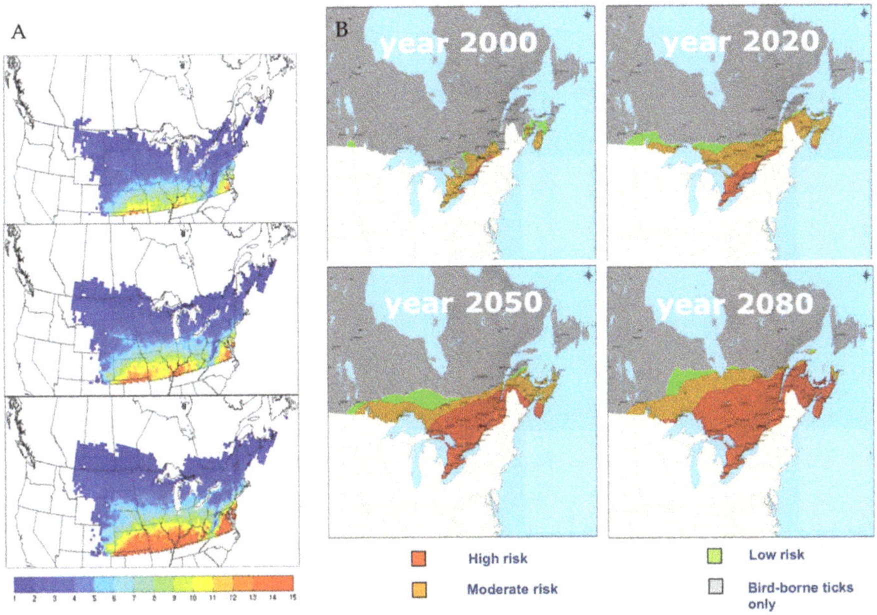

Figure 2. (**A**) Maps of values of the basic reproduction number (R_0) of *Ixodes scapularis* in North America, estimated from ANUSPLIN observed temperature (1971–2000: upper panel), and projected climate obtained from the climate model CRCM4.2.3 following the SRES A2 greenhouse gas emission scenario for 2011–2040 (middle panel) and 2041–2070 (bottom panel). The colour scale indicates R_0 values. Temperature conditions that result in an R_0 of >1 permit survival of *I. scapularis* populations. Reproduced from Ogden et al., 2014 [38]. (**B**) Risk maps for the occurrence of *Ixodes scapularis* in Canada in response to increasing temperatures associated with climate change. The methods used to generate these maps are described by Ogden et al., 2008 [40].

Several studies in Europe have predicted a northwards expansion of the geographic range of *I. ricinus* [41–43], (for example see Figure 3).

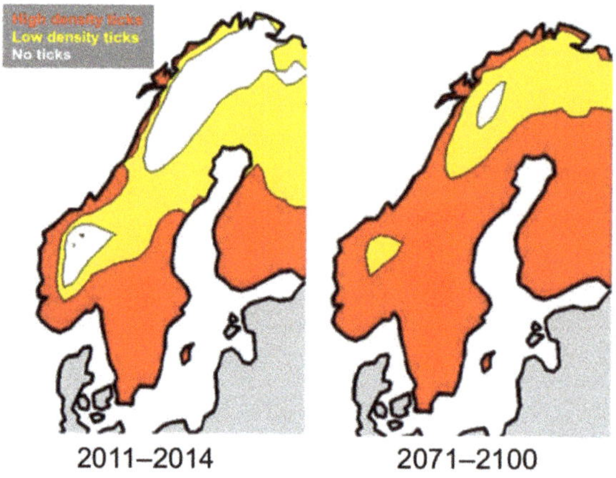

Figure 3. Climate change prediction of *Ixodes ricinus* distribution in Scandinavia based on the length of the vegetation growth period, IPCC 2000 high emission scenario. Modified with permission from Jaenson and Lindgren, 2011 [41].

The models of Porretta et al. [42] and Alkishe et al. [43] also suggest that the distribution of *I. ricinus* is likely to extend eastwards, into habitat currently occupied by *I. persulcatus*. Additionally, *I. ricinus* is predicted to occur at increasingly higher altitudes in mountainous regions [44]. For the main tick vectors of *Babesia* spp. from the northern hemisphere, range expansion driven by climate would only be possible where suitable habitats occur. However, these tick species are, for the most part, woodland habitat generalists and as long as woodland habitats occur, it is likely that the ticks will survive in at least some of them, providing the woodlands also support host densities that are high enough. Some studies have suggested that southern range limits of ticks may contract northwards as more southern regions become too hot for ticks, particularly due to high temperatures inhibiting host-seeking tick activity [25,45]. Increased climate variability and extreme weather events (extreme heat and rainfall) may have relatively limited positive or negative impact on the ticks (compared to dipteran vectors) because of their relatively long multi-year life cycles and the capacity of their woodland habitats to provide an environment that protects the ticks from extreme weather [46]. Impacts of climate change on geographic ranges of hosts such as the white-footed mouse, *Peromyscus leucopus*, will likely have impacts on the geographic ranges and level of entomological risk of *B. microti* in current endemic areas [47]. It is possible that efficient host-to-tick transmission only occurs for a short period after initial infection [48] and if so, locations where there is seasonally synchronous activity of nymphal ticks (that infect the mice) and larval ticks (that acquire infection from mice), may pose a high risk. Effects of climate change on tick development and activity may cause changes to tick seasonality, resulting in locations where synchronous seasonal immature tick activity produce *B. microti* hot spots [23]. In addition to effects on synchrony, increased temperatures may result in changes in the proportions of the tick population feeding at different times of the year. Such an effect was observed in 1976 and 1977 in Ireland when an unusually hot summer in 1976 caused early activity of summer larvae, resulting in a marked increase in the proportion of nymphs active in the late autumn that year and the following spring [49], providing an indication of possible future effects of global warming.

Ticks themselves have very limited capacity for dispersal, and for any change in geographic range to occur, ticks and tick-borne pathogens including *Babesia* spp. need to be dispersed by ticks. Evidence suggests that two processes may be at play [50]—local dispersal that is likely by terrestrial hosts and breeding birds [51], and long-range dispersal by ticks carried on passerines that carry ticks northward in spring [40]. Some of these ticks may be infected with *B. microti*, but it is likely that dispersal by migratory birds is inefficient for *B. microti*, because this pathogen is not transmitted vertically by ticks (transovarial transmission) [30], and birds have, as yet, not been confirmed as reservoirs. As any larvae feeding on migratory birds would not be infected before or during their dispersal by birds, the only infected ticks that birds might carry would be nymphs infected as larvae on small mammal reservoir hosts, as demonstrated by the study of Wilhelmsson et al. [52]. Adult female ticks arising from such nymphs are likely to feed on deer rather than *B. microti* reservoir hosts and would pose little zoonotic risk since they would probably be free of infection following their second moult [30].

6. Observed Effects of Climate Changes

6.1. Climate Effects on Ticks

Studies in Canada suggest that the northern extent of the range of *I. scapularis* is determined by the limit of temperature conditions that allow ticks to complete their life cycles; i.e., when it is probable that an engorged, mated female tick gives rise to at least one other engorged, mated female tick (using the definition of Anderson and May [53] for a macroparasite, when the basic reproduction number of the tick is $\geq$1).

Combinations of data from active field surveillance for ticks, passive tick surveillance (involving detection of ticks at medical and veterinary clinics and by the public), and by inference from surveillance for human cases of tick-borne disease, such as Lyme borreliosis, have detected northern expansion of the range of *I. scapularis* [54–56] (Figure 4).

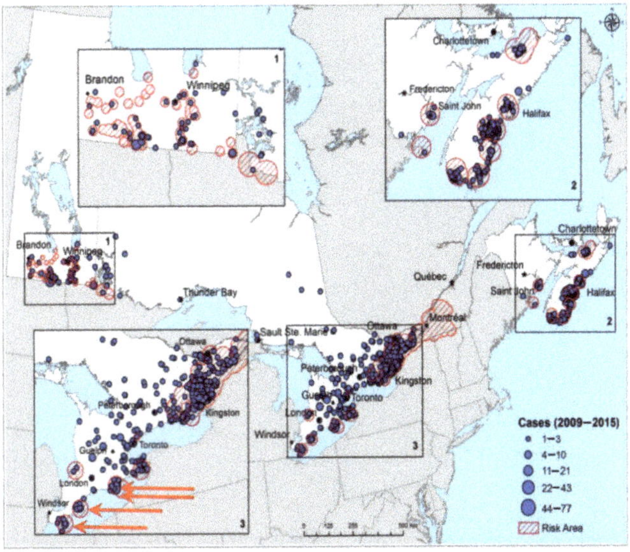

Figure 4. Surveillance for *Ixodes scapularis* populations in central and eastern Canada conducted from 2009 to 2015. Regions where *I. scapularis* populations have been identified by field surveillance are shown as red hatched areas. In 2004 there were only four known *I. scapularis* populations in locations shown by the red arrows. Tick populations have been identified in surveillance programs for Lyme disease (blue circles show municipalities where human Lyme disease cases have been identified). Infections due to *Babesia microti* are not yet nationally notifiable (reproduced with permission from Gasmi et al., 2017 [57]).

Figure 4 shows that *I. scapularis* was only detected at four locations in 2004 (red arrows), but that between 2009 and 2015 ticks and Lyme borreliosis cases had emerged in many other places. Surveillance data have detected a spatio-temporal pattern of range expansion of *I. scapularis* that is consistent with a warmer climate being a key determinant of range spread, and that support the accuracy of model-derived temperature thresholds for *I. scapularis* population survival (reviewed in Ogden et al. [23]). Furthermore, expansion of the tick range has occurred during a period of warming that is now considered a climate anomaly associated with anthropogenic climate change.

Similar trends have been observed for *I. ricinus*, particularly in Scandinavia [6,58,59], but also in Russia [60]. Additionally, the predicted altitudinal changes [23] in *I. ricinus* distribution have already been reported. In 1979 ticks were found up to 700 m a.s.l. in mountainous regions of the Czech Republic, but in 2002 were collected at 1100 m [61,62], and more recently (2020) have been found higher still at 1700 m in the Italian Alps [63]. An earlier study in 1993 had shown that *I. ricinus* was unable to complete its life cycle at such altitudes in the Czech Republic [64].

In Norway, Hvidsten et al. conducted one of the few surveys based on direct observation of *I. ricinus* occurrence at the northern limits of its distribution, collecting specimens by drag-sampling, small mammal trapping, from domestic animals, mainly dogs, and by mailed submissions [59]. Attempts were made to differentiate locations where *I. ricinus* populations were established from those where a few adventitious ticks had been observed or no ticks were detected. The criteria for tick establishment in a local region were the presence of all three life cycle stages in two successive years [65]. Estimates of the vegetation growing season length (VGSL), defined as the number of days when the mean temperature exceeds 5 °C, suggest that established tick populations occurred where the VGSL exceeded 170 days (Figure 5).

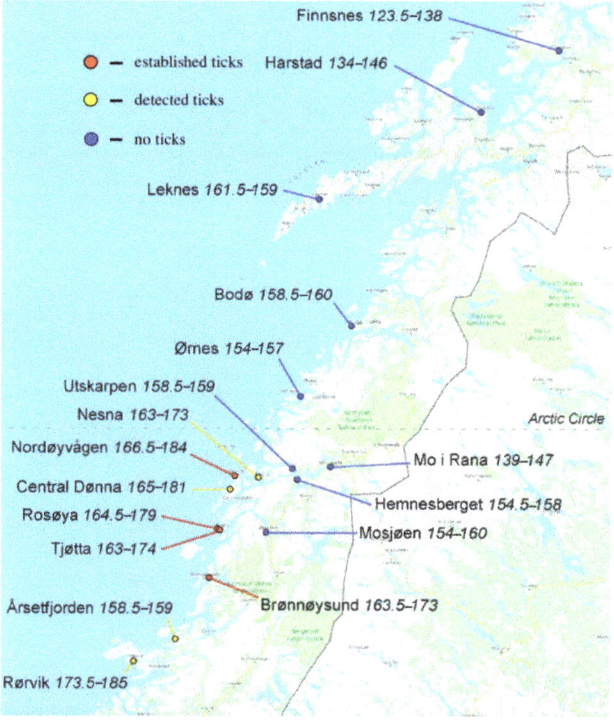

Figure 5. Vegetation growing season length (VGSL) in days in 1961–1990 and 1991–2015 correlated with the presence of *Ixodes ricinus* in northern Norway. The VGSL threshold for tick establishment was estimated to be approximately 170 days. Modified with permission from Hvidsten et al., 2020 [59].

The period of 170 days VGSL is the same minimum value for tick establishment estimated for Scandinavia by Jaenson and Lindgren [41] and was the basis for their projections of tick distribution changes over the next few decades (Figure 3). When the average VGSL values in the Hvidsten et al. study for the period 1961–1990 are compared with those for 1991–2015, an increase in VGSL is evident at all locations, clearly associating the expanding tick distribution with rising temperatures. The most likely mechanism for this temperature effect is the time required for each tick stage to complete development within a season, as demonstrated by Daniel [64] in his altitude study, but low temperatures will also limit questing activity, and Gilbert et al. [22] have shown that *I. ricinus* nymphs from higher latitudes can quest at lower temperatures than those from more southerly regions.

6.2. Climate Effects on Reservoir Hosts

In addition to direct effects on ticks, rising temperatures will also affect their hosts, which is particularly important when these hosts serve as reservoir hosts for tick-borne pathogens. In the case of *B. divergens*, the pathogen's distribution is closely associated with that of cattle. Infections appear to result from local transmission by established tick populations [66], and since tick populations are expanding northwards, it is not surprising that there is some evidence, though indirect, for bovine babesiosis in more northern locations than in previous decades [67]. Since *B. divergens* is transmitted transovarially, infected larval or nymphal ticks could be deposited by birds far to the north of established tick populations. However, there is very little evidence for infections transmitted to cattle by such adventitious ticks, with only one suspected case in the far north of Norway occurring in the last 20 years [66]. A more definite climate effect on bovine babesiosis, though on a local scale, occurred recently in the south of England in February 2019, when temperatures exceeded the average for the time of year by more than 10 °C, causing very early tick activity and an outbreak of bovine babesiosis involving 20 cattle [68]. *Babesia venatorum* is also transmitted transovarially and is associated with roe deer, so presumably the distribution of this pathogen has been affected by the northward range expansion of its host [58]. It can also be distributed by birds carrying infected ticks, which led to speculation that its detection in sheep in Scotland may have resulted from the deposition of ticks by migratory birds from Norway [69]. At present there are insufficient data on the distribution of *B. venatorum* to associate it with any climate change effect.

Genotypes of *B. microti* have been detected in many vertebrate species but those that cause human babesiosis in north-eastern North America appear to be limited to the white-footed mouse, *Peromyscus leucopus*, short tailed shrews, *Blarina* spp., and chipmunks, *Tamia striatus*. Since, in the absence of transovarial transmission, neither birds nor deer can play a significant part in the introduction of the parasite to new reservoir host populations, and it appears that migration of infected small mammals is the main means by which the pathogen can emerge in new areas. *B. microti* infections therefore lag well behind the spread of other *I. scapularis*-borne diseases such as Lyme borreliosis and human granulocytic anaplasmosis [70], both of which can infect birds, though *B. microti* infections are spreading within the northeast and upper midwest endemic regions [50,71]. While the tick vector has spread north into Canada, human babesiosis remains exceedingly rare and to date only three cases of autochthonous infection have been recorded there [72].

There is little information on the effects of climate change on the small mammal reservoir hosts of *B. microti*, but intuitively one might expect milder winters to result in their improved survival, driving expansion of their populations. In *P. leucopus*, one of the main reservoir hosts, tick transmission is relatively inefficient, but appears to be facilitated by the agent of Lyme disease, *B. burgdorferi* sensu stricto [73], which is now prevalent in southern Canada and for which *P. leucopus* is also an important reservoir host. Furthermore, the persistence of *B. microti* in its rodent hosts, *Microtus* spp. and *P. leucopus*, is enhanced by vertical transmission [74,75], so range expansion of these rodents is likely to be fundamental to the spread of *B. microti*. Roy-Dufresne et al. [76] used an ecological niche factor analysis to study the potential effect of global warming on the distribution of *P. leucopus* and concluded that by 2050 the range of this rodent species could have expanded northwards by 3° latitude. Considering that the upper midwest *B. microti* endemic area is only just across the US border, it seems likely that significant numbers of cases will eventually occur in Canada. Indeed, the three recorded autochthonous Canadian *B. microti* infections were apparently all acquired in southern Manitoba not very far from the endemic region in Minnesota [72], although unfortunately it is not known whether the same genotypes responsible for *B. microti* human babesiosis in the US were involved in these Canadian cases. An alternative explanation for the appearance of human babesiosis in new areas, is that zoonotic genotypes of *B. microti* occur in the absence of *I. scapularis*, being transmitted by tick species that generally do not bite humans, for example *Ixodes angustus*. While such cryptic cycles exist [77], there is little evidence so far that they have played a part in the spread of zoonotic babesiosis caused by *B. microti*, although they might have had a role in the establishment of the two separate foci in the northeast and upper midwest of the US, in which the *B. microti* genotypes show distinct differences from each other [78]. *Ixodes scapularis* (or *I. dammini*) is thought to have spread from coastal refugia in the 1950s as a result of reforestation and the growing deer population [79], and it is possible that in the upper midwest *B. microti* genotypes maintained in cryptic cycles were then able to infect this newly arrived bridge vector and thus establish a new focus of human babesiosis.

7. Conclusions

While observations suggest that tick populations have been responding to increasing temperatures with a northwards expansion for some years, it is not possible at present to be certain that the occurrence of human babesiosis has been affected by climate change. This is partly because of lack of data, particularly in Europe, where human babesiosis is much rarer than in North America, but also because the distributions of the pathogens involved depend on infected reservoir hosts, in addition to ticks, and the factors affecting the movements of these animals (small mammals, deer and domestic cattle) are influenced by other factors in addition to climate, notably landscape changes resulting from anthropocentric activity. Nevertheless, observations and models suggest that it is only a matter of time before human babesiosis cases occur more frequently, out of season and further north than at present as a result of climate change.

Author Contributions: Conceptualization, J.S.G.; writing—original draft preparation, J.S.G. and N.H.O.; writing—review and editing, J.S.G. and N.H.O. All authors have read and agreed to the published version of the manuscript.

Funding: This research received no external funding.

Institutional Review Board Statement: Not applicable.

Informed Consent Statement: Not applicable.

Data Availability Statement: Not applicable.

Conflicts of Interest: The authors declare no conflict of interest.

References

1. Rocklöv, J.; Dubrow, R. Climate change: An enduring challenge for vector-borne disease prevention and control. *Nat. Immunol.* **2020**, *21*, 479–483. [CrossRef] [PubMed]
2. Brooks, D.R.; Hoberg, E.P.; Boeger, W.A. *The Stockholm Paradigm: Climate Change and Emerging Disease*; University of Chicago Press: Chicago, IL, USA, 2019; p. 400.
3. Kramer, K.; Degen, B.; Buschbom, J.; Hickler, T.; Thuiller, W.; Sykes, M.T.; Winter, W. Modelling exploration of the future of European beech (*Fagus sylvatica* L.) under climate change—Range, abundance, genetic diversity and adaptive response. *For. Ecol. Manag.* **2010**, *259*, 2213–2222. [CrossRef]
4. Ostfeld, R.S.; Levi, T.; Keesing, F.; Oggenfuss, K.; Canham, C.D. Tick-borne disease risk in a forest food web. *Ecology* **2018**, *99*, 1562–1573. [CrossRef]
5. Bregnard, C.; Rais, O.; Voordouw, M.J. Climate and tree seed production predict the abundance of the European Lyme disease vector over a 15-year period. *Parasit. Vectors* **2020**, *13*, 408. [CrossRef] [PubMed]
6. Lindgren, E.; Tälleklint, L.; Polfeldt, T. Impact of climatic change on the northern latitude limit and population density of the disease-transmitting European tick *Ixodes ricinus*. *Environ. Health Perspect.* **2000**, *108*, 119–123. [CrossRef] [PubMed]
7. Lobo, C.A.; Singh, M.; Rodriguez, M. Human babesiosis: Recent advances and future challenges. *Curr. Opin. Hematol.* **2020**, *27*, 399–405. [CrossRef] [PubMed]

8. Hildebrandt, A.; Zintl, A.; Montero, E.; Hunfeld, K.-P.; Gray, J. Human babesiosis in Europe. *Pathogens* **2021**, *10*, 1165. [CrossRef] [PubMed]
9. Qi, C.; Zhou, D.; Liu, J.; Cheng, Z.; Zhang, L.; Wang, L.; Wang, Z.; Yang, D.; Wang, S.; Chai, T. Detection of *Babesia divergens* using molecular methods in anemic patients in Shandong Province, China. *Parasitol. Res.* **2011**, *109*, 241–245. [CrossRef] [PubMed]
10. Jiang, J.F.; Zheng, Y.C.; Jiang, R.R.; Li, H.; Huo, Q.B.; Jiang, B.G.; Sun, Y.; Jia, N.; Wang, Y.W.; Ma, L.; et al. Epidemiological, clinical, and laboratory characteristics of 48 cases of "*Babesia venatorum*" infection in China: A descriptive study. *Lancet Infect. Dis.* **2015**, *15*, 196–203. [CrossRef]
11. Zhou, X.; Xia, S.; Yin, S.Q.; Zhou, X.N. Emergence of babesiosis in China-Myanmar border areas. *Parasit. Vectors* **2015**, *8*, 390. [CrossRef] [PubMed]
12. Zamoto-Niikura, A.; Morikawa, S.; Hanaki, K.I.; Holman, P.J.; Ishihara, C. *Ixodes persulcatus* ticks as vectors for the *Babesia microti* U.S. lineage in Japan. *Appl. Environ. Microbiol.* **2016**, *82*, 6624–6632. [CrossRef]
13. Zamoto-Niikura, A.; Tsuji, M.; Qiang, W.; Morikawa, S.; Hanaki, K.I.; Holman, P.J.; Ishihara, C. The *Babesia divergens* Asia lineage is maintained through enzootic cycles between *Ixodes persulcatus* and sika deer in Hokkaido, Japan. *Appl. Environ. Microbiol.* **2018**, *84*, e02491-17. [CrossRef] [PubMed]
14. Swei, A.; O'Connor, K.E.; Couper, L.I.; Thekkiniath, J.; Conrad, P.A.; Padgett, K.A.; Burns, J.; Yoshimizu, M.H.; Gonzales, B.; Munk, B.; et al. Evidence for transmission of the zoonotic apicomplexan parasite *Babesia duncani* by the tick *Dermacentor albipictus*. *Int. J. Parasitol.* **2019**, *49*, 95–103. [CrossRef] [PubMed]
15. Jia, N.; Zheng, Y.C.; Jiang, J.F.; Jiang, R.R.; Jiang, B.G.; Wei, R.; Liu, H.B.; Huo, Q.B.; Sun, Y.; Chu, Y.L.; et al. Human babesiosis caused by a *Babesia crassa*-like pathogen: A case series. *Clin. Infect. Dis.* **2018**, *167*, 1110–1119. [CrossRef]
16. Goethert, H.K.; Telford, S.R., III. Enzootic transmission of *Babesia divergens* among cottontail rabbits on Nantucket Island, Massachusetts. *Am. J. Trop. Med. Hyg.* **2003**, *69*, 455–460. [CrossRef]
17. Belozerov, V.N. Diapause and biological rhythms in ticks. In *Physiology of Ticks*; Obenchain, F.D., Galun, R., Eds.; Pergamon Press: Oxford, UK, 1982; pp. 469–500.
18. Gray, J.S.; Kahl, O.; Lane, R.S.; Levin, M.L.; Tsao, J.I. Diapause in ticks of the medically important *Ixodes ricinus* species complex. *Ticks Tick Borne Dis.* **2016**, *7*, 992–1003. [CrossRef]
19. Korenberg, E.I. Comparative ecology and epidemiology of Lyme disease and tick-borne encephalitis in the former Soviet Union. *Parasitol. Today* **1994**, *10*, 157–160. [CrossRef]
20. Arsnoe, I.; Tsao, J.I.; Hickling, G.J. Nymphal *Ixodes scapularis* questing behavior explains geographic variation in Lyme borreliosis risk in the eastern United States. *Ticks Tick Borne Dis.* **2019**, *10*, 553–563. [CrossRef] [PubMed]
21. Gray, J.S. The ecology of Lyme borreliosis vectors. *Exp. Appl. Acarol.* **1998**, *22*, 249–258. [CrossRef]
22. Gilbert, L.; Aungier, J.; Tomkins, J.L. Climate of origin affects tick (*Ixodes ricinus*) host-seeking behavior in response to temperature: Implications for resilience to climate change? *Ecol. Evol.* **2014**, *4*, 1186–1198. [CrossRef]
23. Ogden, N.H.; Beard, C.B.; Ginsberg, H.; Tsao, J. Possible effects of climate change on ixodid ticks and the pathogens they transmit: What has been projected and what has been observed. *J. Med. Entomol.* **2020**, *58*, 1536–1545. [CrossRef]
24. Dautel, H.; Kämmer, D.; Kahl, O. How an extreme weather spell in winter can influence vector tick abundance and tick-borne disease incidence. In *Ecology and Prevention of Lyme Borreliosis*; Braks, M.A.H., Van Wierer, S.E., Takken, W., Sprong, H., Eds.; Wageningen Academic Publishers: Wageningen, The Netherlands, 2016; pp. 335–350.
25. MacLeod, J. *Ixodes ricinus* in relation to its physical environment. II. The factors governing survival and activity. *Parasitology* **1935**, *27*, 123–144. [CrossRef]
26. Földvári, G.; Rigó, K.; Jablonszky, M.; Biró, N.; Majoros, G.; Molnár, V.; Tóth, M. Ticks and the city: Ectoparasites of the Northern white-breasted hedgehog (*Erinaceus roumanicus*) in an urban park. *Ticks Tick Borne Dis.* **2011**, *2*, 231–234. [CrossRef]
27. Rizzoli, A.; Silaghi, C.; Obiegala, A.; Rudolf, I.; Hubálek, Z.; Földvári, G.; Plantard, O.; Vayssier-Taussat, M.; Bonnet, S.; Špitalská, E.; et al. *Ixodes ricinus* and its transmitted pathogens in urban and peri-urban areas in Europe: New hazards and relevance for public health. *Front. Public Health* **2014**, *2*, 251. [CrossRef] [PubMed]
28. Goethert, H.K.; Telford, S.R., III. What is *Babesia microti*? *Parasitology* **2003**, *127*, 301–309. [CrossRef] [PubMed]
29. Hersh, M.H.; Tibbetts, M.; Strauss, M.; Ostfeld, R.S.; Keesing, F. Reservoir competence of wildlife host species for *Babesia microti*. *Emerg. Infect. Dis.* **2012**, *18*, 1951–1957. [CrossRef]
30. Gray, J.S.; von Stedingk, L.-V.; Gürtelschmid, M.; Granström, M. Transmission studies on *Babesia microti* in *Ixodes ricinus* ticks and gerbils. *J. Clin. Microbiol.* **2002**, *40*, 1258–1263. [CrossRef]
31. Herwaldt, B.L.; Cacció, S.; Gherlinzoni, F.; Aspöck, H.; Slemenda, S.B.; Piccaluga, P.; Martinelli, G.; Edelhofer, R.; Hollenstein, U.; Poletti, G.; et al. Molecular characterization of a non-*Babesia divergens* organism causing zoonotic babesiosis in Europe. *Emerg. Infect. Dis.* **2003**, *9*, 942–948. [CrossRef]
32. Bonnet, S.; Jouglin, M.; L'Hostis, M.; Chauvin, A. *Babesia* sp. EU1 from roe deer and transmission within *Ixodes ricinus*. *Emerg. Infect. Dis.* **2007**, *13*, 1208–1210. [CrossRef]
33. Bonnet, S.; Brisseau, N.; Hermouet, A.; Jouglin, M.; Chauvin, A. Experimental in vitro transmission of *Babesia* sp. (EU1) by *Ixodes ricinus*. *Vet. Res.* **2009**, *40*, 21. [CrossRef]
34. Fanelli, A. A historical review of *Babesia* spp. associated with deer in Europe: *Babesia divergens*/*Babesia divergens*-like, *Babesia capreoli*, *Babesia venatorum*, *Babesia* cf. *odocoilei*. *Vet. Parasitol.* **2021**, *294*, 109433. [CrossRef] [PubMed]

35. Zintl, A.; Mulcahy, G.; Skerrett, H.E.; Taylor, S.M.; Gray, J.S. *Babesia divergens*, a bovine blood parasite of veterinary and zoonotic importance. *Clin. Microbiol. Rev.* **2003**, *16*, 622–636. [CrossRef] [PubMed]
36. Monaghan, A.J.; Moore, S.M.; Sampson, K.M.; Beard, C.B.; Eisen, R.J. Climate change influences on the annual onset of Lyme disease in the United States. *Ticks Tick Borne Dis.* **2015**, *6*, 615–622. [CrossRef] [PubMed]
37. Perret, J.L.; Guigoz, E.; Rais, O.; Gern, L. Influence of saturation deficit and temperature on *Ixodes ricinus* tick questing activity in a Lyme borreliosis-endemic area (Switzerland). *Parasitol. Res.* **2000**, *86*, 554–557. [CrossRef] [PubMed]
38. Ogden, N.H.; Radojevic, M.; Wu, X.; Duvvuri, V.R.; Leighton, P.A.; Wu, J. Estimated effects of projected climate change on the basic reproductive number of the tick vector of Lyme disease *Ixodes scapularis*. *Environ. Health Perspect.* **2014**, *122*, 631–638. [CrossRef] [PubMed]
39. McPherson, M.; García-García, A.; Cuesta-Valero, F.J.; Belltrami, H.; Hansen-Ketchum, P.; MacDougall, D.; Ogden, N.H. Expansion of the Lyme disease vector *Ixodes scapularis* in Canada inferred from CMIP5 climate projections. *Environ. Health Perspect.* **2017**, *125*, 057008. [CrossRef] [PubMed]
40. Ogden, N.H.; Lindsay, R.L.; Hanincová, K.; Barker, I.K.; Bigras-Poulin, M.; Charron, D.F.; Heagy, A.; Francis, C.M.; O'Callaghan, C.J.; Schwartz, I.; et al. The role of migratory birds in introduction and range expansion of *Ixodes scapularis* ticks, and *Borrelia burgdorferi* and *Anaplasma phagocytophilum* in Canada. *Appl. Environ. Microbiol.* **2008**, *74*, 1780–1790. [CrossRef]
41. Jaenson, T.G.; Lindgren, E. The range of *Ixodes ricinus* and the risk of contracting Lyme borreliosis will increase northwards when the vegetation period becomes longer. *Ticks Tick Borne Dis.* **2011**, *2*, 44–49. [CrossRef] [PubMed]
42. Porretta, D.; Mastrantonio, V.; Amendolia, S.; Gaiarsa, S.; Epis, S.; Genchi, C.; Bandi, C.; Otranto, D.; Urbanelli, S. Effects of global changes on the climatic niche of the tick *Ixodes ricinus* inferred by species distribution modelling. *Parasit. Vectors* **2013**, *6*, 271. [CrossRef] [PubMed]
43. Alkishe, A.A.; Peterson, A.T.; Samy, A.M. Climate change influences on the potential geographic distribution of the disease vector tick *Ixodes ricinus*. *PLoS ONE* **2017**, *12*, e0189092. [CrossRef] [PubMed]
44. Gilbert, L. Altitudinal patterns of tick and host abundance: A potential role for climate change in regulating tick-borne diseases? *Oecologia* **2010**, *162*, 217–225. [CrossRef] [PubMed]
45. Brownstein, J.S.; Holford, T.R.; Fish, D. Effect of climate change on Lyme disease risk in North America. *EcoHealth* **2005**, *2*, 38–46. [CrossRef]
46. Ogden, N.H.; Linday, L.R. Effects of climate and climate change on vectors and vector-borne diseases: Ticks are different. *Trends Parasitol.* **2016**, *32*, 646–656. [CrossRef]
47. Simon, J.A.; Marrotte, R.R.; Desrosiers, N.; Fiset, J.; Gaitan, J.; Gonzalez, A.; Koffi, J.K.; Lapointe, F.-J.; Leighton, P.A.; Lindsay, L.R.; et al. Climate change, habitat fragmentation, ticks and the white-footed mouse drive occurrence of *B. burgdorferi*, the agent of Lyme disease, at the northern limit of its distribution. *Evol. Appl.* **2014**, *7*, 750–764. [CrossRef]
48. Dunn, J.M.; Krause, P.J.; Davis, S.; Vannier, E.G.; Fitzpatrick, M.C.; Rollend, L.; Belperron, A.A.; States, S.L.; Stacey, A.; Bockenstedt, L.K.; et al. *Borrelia burgdorferi* promotes the establishment of *Babesia microti* in the northeastern United States. *PLoS ONE* **2014**, *9*, e115494. [CrossRef]
49. Gray, J.S. *Ixodes ricinus* seasonal activity: Implications of global warming indicated by revisiting tick and weather data. *Int. J. Med. Microbiol.* **2008**, *298* (Suppl. 1), 19–24. [CrossRef]
50. Walter, K.S.; Pepin, K.M.; Webb, C.T.; Gaff, H.D.; Krause, P.J.; Pitzer, V.E.; Diuk-Wasser, M.A. Invasion of two tick-borne diseases across New England: Harnessing human surveillance data to capture underlying ecological invasion processes. *Proc. R. Soc. B* **2016**, *283*, 20160834. [CrossRef] [PubMed]
51. Madhav, N.K.; Brownstein, J.S.; Tsao, J.I.; Fish, D. A dispersal model for the range expansion of blacklegged tick (Acari: *Ixodidae*). *J. Med. Entomol.* **2004**, *41*, 842–852. [CrossRef] [PubMed]
52. Wilhelmsson, P.; Pawełczyk, O.; Jaenson, T.G.T.; Waldenström, J.; Olsen, B.; Forsberg, P.; Lindgren, P.E. Three *Babesia* species in *Ixodes ricinus* ticks from migratory birds in Sweden. *Parasit. Vectors* **2021**, *14*, 183. [CrossRef] [PubMed]
53. Anderson, R.M.; May, R.M. *Infectious Diseases of Humans*; Oxford University Press: Oxford, UK, 1992; p. 768.
54. Leighton, P.; Koffi, J.; Pelcat, Y.; Lindsay, L.R.; Ogden, N.H. Predicting the speed of tick invasion: An empirical model of range expansion for the Lyme disease vector *Ixodes scapularis* in Canada. *J. Appl. Ecol.* **2012**, *49*, 457–464. [CrossRef]
55. Clow, K.; Ogden, N.H.; Lindsay, L.R.; Michel, P.; Pearl, D.; Jardine, C. The influence of abiotic and biotic factors on the invasion of *Ixodes scapularis* in Ontario, Canada. *Ticks Tick Borne Dis.* **2017**, *8*, 554–563. [CrossRef] [PubMed]
56. Clow, K.; Leighton, P.A.; Ogden, N.H.; Lindsay, L.R.; Michel, P.; Pearl, D.; Jardine, C. Northward range expansion of *Ixodes scapularis* evident over a short timescale in Ontario, Canada. *PLoS ONE* **2017**, *12*, e0189393. [CrossRef] [PubMed]
57. Gasmi, S.; Ogden, N.H.; Lindsay, L.R.; Burns, S.; Fleming, S.; Badcock, J.; Hanan, S.; Gaulin, C.; Leblanc, M.A.; Russell, C.; et al. Surveillance for Lyme disease in Canada: 2009–2015. *Can. Commun. Dis. Rep.* **2017**, *43*, 194–199. [CrossRef] [PubMed]
58. Jaenson, T.G.; Jaenson, D.G.; Eisen, L.; Petersson, E.; Lindgren, E. Changes in the geographical distribution and abundance of the tick *Ixodes ricinus* during the past 30 years in Sweden. *Parasit. Vectors* **2012**, *5*, 8. [CrossRef] [PubMed]
59. Hvidsten, D.; Frafjord, K.; Gray, J.S.; Henningsson, A.J.; Jenkins, A.; Kristiansen, B.E.; Lager, M.; Rognerud, B.; Slåtsve, A.M.; Stordal, F.; et al. The distribution limit of the common tick, *Ixodes ricinus*, and some associated pathogens in north-western Europe. *Ticks Tick Borne Dis.* **2020**, *11*, 101388. [CrossRef] [PubMed]
60. Korotkov, Y.; Kozlova, T.; Kozlovskaya, L. Observations on changes in abundance of questing *Ixodes ricinus*, castor bean tick, over a 35-year period in the eastern part of its range (Russia, Tula region). *Med. Vet. Entomol.* **2015**, *29*, 129–136. [CrossRef] [PubMed]

61. Daniel, M.; Danielová, V.; Kríz, B.; Jirsa, A.; Nozicka, J. Shift of the tick *Ixodes ricinus* and tick-borne encephalitis to higher altitudes in central Europe. *Eur. J. Clin. Microbiol. Infect. Dis.* **2003**, *22*, 327–328. [CrossRef] [PubMed]
62. Daniel, M.; Materna, J.; Honig, V.; Metelka, L.; Danielová, V.; Harcarik, J.; Kliegrová, S.; Grubhoffer, L. Vertical distribution of the tick *Ixodes ricinus* and tick-borne pathogens in the northern Moravian mountains correlated with climate warming (Jeseniky Mts., Czech Republic). *Cent. Eur. J. Public Health* **2009**, *17*, 139–145. [CrossRef]
63. Garcia-Vozmediano, A.; Krawczyk, A.I.; Sprong, H.; Rossi, L.; Ramassa, E.; Tomassone, L. Ticks climb the mountains: Ixodid tick infestation and infection by tick-borne pathogens in the Western Alps. *Ticks Tick Borne Dis.* **2020**, *11*, 101489. [CrossRef] [PubMed]
64. Daniel, M. Influence of the microclimate on the vertical distribution of the tick *Ixodes ricinus* (L) in Central Europe. *Acarologia* **1993**, *34*, 105–113.
65. Anonymous. Consensus conference on Lyme disease. *Can. J. Infect. Dis.* **1991**, *2*, 49–54.
66. Mysterud, A.; Jore, S.; Østerås, O.; Viljugrein, H. Emergence of tick-borne diseases at northern latitudes in Europe: A comparative approach. *Sci. Rep.* **2017**, *7*, 16316. [CrossRef] [PubMed]
67. Jore, S.; Viljugrein, H.; Hofshagen, M.; Brun-Hansen, H.; Kristoffersen, A.B.; Nygård, K.; Brun, E.; Ottesen, P.; Sævik, B.K.; Ytrehus, B. Multi-source analysis reveals latitudinal and altitudinal shifts in range of *Ixodes ricinus* at its northern distribution limit. *Parasit. Vectors* **2011**, *4*, 84. [CrossRef] [PubMed]
68. Johnson, N.; Phipps, L.; McFadzean, H.; Barlow, A.M. An outbreak of bovine babesiosis in February, 2019, triggered by above average winter temperatures in southern England and co-infection with *Babesia divergens* and *Anaplasma phagocytophilum*. *Parasit. Vectors* **2020**, *13*, 305. [CrossRef] [PubMed]
69. Gray, A.; Capewell, P.; Loney, C.; Katzer, F.; Shiels, B.R.; Weir, W. Sheep as host species for zoonotic *Babesia venatorum*, United Kingdom. *Emerg. Infect. Dis.* **2019**, *25*, 2257–2260. [CrossRef]
70. O'Brien, S.F.; Drews, S.J.; Yi, Q.L.; Bloch, E.M.; Ogden, N.H.; Koffi, J.K.; Lindsay, L.R.; Gregoire, Y.; Delage, G. Risk of transfusion-transmitted *Babesia microti* in Canada. *Transfusion* **2021**, *61*, 2958–2968. [CrossRef]
71. Stein, E.; Elbadawi, L.I.; Kazmierczak, J.; Davis, J.P. Babesiosis surveillance, Wisconsin, 2001–2015. *MMWR Morb. Mortal. Wkly. Rep.* **2017**, *66*, 687. [CrossRef]
72. Drews, S.J.; Van Caeseele, P.; Bullard, J.; Lindsay, L.R.; Gaziano, T.; Zeller, M.P.; Lane, D.; Ndao, M.; Allen, V.G.; Boggild, A.K.; et al. *Babesia microti* in a Canadian blood donor and lookback in a red blood cell recipient. *Vox Sang.* **2021**, in press. [CrossRef]
73. Diuk-Wasser, M.A.; Vannier, E.; Krause, P.J. Coinfection by *Ixodes* tick-borne pathogens: Ecological, epidemiological, and clinical consequences. *Trends Parasitol.* **2016**, *32*, 30–42. [CrossRef] [PubMed]
74. Tolkacz, K.; Bednarska, M.; Alsarraf, M.; Dwuznik, D.; Grzybek, M.; Welc-Faleciak, R.; Behnke, J.M.; Bajer, A. Prevalence, genetic identity and vertical transmission of *Babesia microti* in three naturally infected species of vole, *Microtus* spp. (Cricetidae). *Parasit. Vectors* **2017**, *10*, 66. [CrossRef] [PubMed]
75. Tufts, D.M.; Diuk-Wasser, M.A. Transplacental transmission of tick-borne *Babesia microti* in its natural host *Peromyscus leucopus*. *Parasit. Vectors* **2018**, *11*, 286. [CrossRef] [PubMed]
76. Roy-Dufresne, E.; Logan, T.; Simon, J.A.; Chmura, G.L.; Millien, V. Poleward expansion of the white-footed mouse (*Peromyscus leucopus*) under climate change: Implications for the spread of Lyme disease. *PLoS ONE* **2013**, *8*, e80724. [CrossRef] [PubMed]
77. Goethert, H.K.; Lubelcyzk, C.; LaCombe, E.; Holman, M.; Rand, P.; Smith, R.P., Jr.; Telford, S.R., III. Enzootic *Babesia microti* in Maine. *J. Parasitol.* **2003**, *89*, 1069–1071. [CrossRef] [PubMed]
78. Lemieux, J.E.; Tran, A.D.; Freimark, L.; Schaffner, S.F.; Goethert, H.; Andersen, K.G.; Bazner, S.; Li, A.; McGrath, G.; Sloan, L.; et al. A global map of genetic diversity in *Babesia microti* reveals strong population structure and identifies variants associated with clinical relapse. *Nat. Microbiol.* **2016**, *1*, 16079. [CrossRef]
79. Matuschka, F.R.; Spielman, A. The emergence of Lyme disease in a changing environment in North America and central Europe. *Exp. Appl. Acarol.* **1986**, *2*, 337–353. [CrossRef]

pathogens MDPI

Review

Human Babesiosis in Europe

Anke Hildebrandt [1,2], Annetta Zintl [3], Estrella Montero [4], Klaus-Peter Hunfeld [5,6,7] and Jeremy Gray [8,*]

1 St. Vincenz Hospital Datteln, Department of Internal Medicine I, 45711 Datteln, Germany; a.hildebrandt@vincenz-datteln.de
2 Institute of Medical Microbiology, University Hospital Münster, 48149 Münster, Germany
3 UCD School of Veterinary Sciences, University College Dublin, D04 W6F6 Dublin, Ireland; annetta.zintl@ucd.ie
4 Parasitology Reference and Research Laboratory, Centro Nacional de Microbiología, Instituto de Salud Carlos III, Majadahonda, 28220 Madrid, Spain; estrella.montero@isciii.es
5 Institute of Laboratory Medicine, Microbiology & Infection Control, Northwest Medical Center, Medical Faculty Goethe University Frankfurt, Steinbacher Hohl 2-26, 60488 Frankfurt am Main, Germany; K.Hunfeld@em.uni-frankfurt.de
6 Society for Promoting Quality Assurance in Medical Laboratories (INSTAND, e.v.), Ubierstraße 20, 40223 Düsseldorf, Germany
7 ESGBOR Study Group of the European Society for Clinical Microbiology & Infectious Diseases (ESCMID), ESCMID Executive Office, P.O. Box 214, 4010 Basel, Switzerland
8 UCD School of Biology and Environmental Science, University College Dublin, D04 N2E5 Dublin, Ireland
* Correspondence: jeremy.gray@ucd.ie

Abstract: Babesiosis is attracting increasing attention as a worldwide emerging zoonosis. The first case of human babesiosis in Europe was described in the late 1950s and since then more than 60 cases have been reported in Europe. While the disease is relatively rare in Europe, it is significant because the majority of cases present as life-threatening fulminant infections, mainly in immunocompromised patients. Although appearing clinically similar to human babesiosis elsewhere, particularly in the USA, most European forms of the disease are distinct entities, especially concerning epidemiology, human susceptibility to infection and clinical management. This paper describes the history of the disease and reviews all published cases that have occurred in Europe with regard to the identity and genetic characteristics of the etiological agents, pathogenesis, aspects of epidemiology including the eco-epidemiology of the vectors, the clinical courses of infection, diagnostic tools and clinical management and treatment.

Keywords: European babesiosis; *Babesia divergens*; *Babesia venatorum*; *Babesia microti*; *Ixodes ricinus*; parasite identity; epidemiology; clinical cases; diagnosis; treatment

Citation: Hildebrandt, A.; Zintl, A.; Montero, E.; Hunfeld, K.-P.; Gray, J. Human Babesiosis in Europe. *Pathogens* **2021**, *10*, 1165. https://doi.org/10.3390/pathogens10091165

Academic Editor: Cheryl Ann Lobo

Received: 1 August 2021
Accepted: 3 September 2021
Published: 9 September 2021

Publisher's Note: MDPI stays neutral with regard to jurisdictional claims in published maps and institutional affiliations.

1. History

The first reported case of human babesiosis in Europe, and indeed in the world, occurred in 1956 in the former Yugoslavia, now Croatia, in a 33-year-old tailor and part-time farmer who had been splenectomized following a traffic accident 11 years earlier [1]. He presented with fever and severe hemoglobinuria eight days after first feeling unwell and died two days later. The parasites detected in blood smears were identified as *Babesia bovis*. However, *B. bovis* is not known to be zoonotic, and the photomicrographs in the published case report show divergent piroplasms that are characteristic of *Babesia divergens*, as well as a cattle parasite and first described by M'Fadyean and Stockman in 1911 [2]. The second recorded case, another *B. divergens* infection, which also ended fatally, occurred in 1967 in a splenectomized man who had apparently contracted the infection on holiday in the west of Ireland [3]. Further cases then followed in the 1970s in the UK and France, and to date, cases have been recorded in at least 19 European countries, almost always fulminant in splenectomized patients and attributed to *B. divergens*.

A second zoonotic species emerged in 2003 in Italy and Austria [4], initially designated EU1, but now named *Babesia venatorum*. To date, infections with *B. venatorum* have been reported from Germany [5], Austria [6] and Sweden [7], all in splenectomized patients who survived, which possibly indicates a milder course of infection than *B. divergens*, though treatment has improved markedly since the first appearance of zoonotic babesiosis.

The most recent addition to the list of autochthonous zoonotic European *Babesia* spp. is *Babesia microti*, the first confirmed case of which occurred in Germany [8], and caused moderate illness in a spleen-intact but immunocompromised patient. A few mild or asymptomatic other cases have since been recorded, but it is very clear that the strains of *B. microti* present in Europe, where it is common in rodents and ticks, are not as infectious or pathogenic to humans as those in the USA, where *B. microti* infections give rise to approximately 2000 zoonotic babesiosis cases annually [9].

2. Parasite Identity

Two of the three *Babesia* species that infect humans in Europe, *B. divergens* and *B. venatorum*, belong to the *Babesia* sensu stricto (s.s.) group and are closely related, (Clade X; [10]), while the third species, *B. microti*, is phylogenetically distinct, belonging to *Babesia* sensu lato (s.l.) (Clade I; [10]). The three parasites are distinguishable morphologically in Giemsa-stained blood smears, but only by experienced diagnostic microscopists because they share important features. For example, divergent paired pyriforms are characteristic of both *B. divergens* and *B. venatorum*, while pyriform tetrads occur in both *B. divergens* and *B. microti*. The much more frequently observed single round trophozoite ('ring' stage) occurs in infections of all three species (Figure 1).

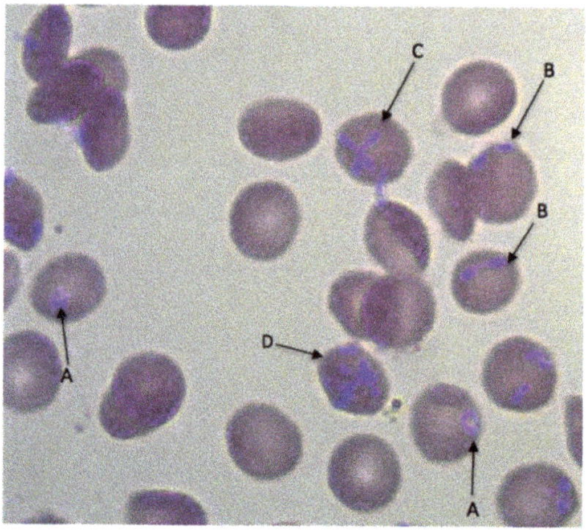

Figure 1. *Babesia divergens* in a Giemsa-stained thin blood smear. Round (**A**), paired pyriform (**B**), tetrad (Maltese cross) (**C**) and multiple parasite (**D**) forms are indicated. Similar round and paired pyriform forms have been observed in infections of *B. venatorum*, and round and tetrad forms occur in *B. microti* infections. Multiple parasite-infected erythrocytes are often seen in high parasitemias. © Estrella Montero, Luis Miguel Gonzalez.

Babesia microti can be distinguished serologically from *B. divergens* and *B. venatorum*, but the latter two are antigenically similar [4]. Serology is further limited by the time required for an antibody response to develop, which may be several weeks in immunocompromised patients [5]. DNA sequence discrimination is not only relatively swift, but can also be used to identify *Babesia* species, and it is now the method of choice for determining parasite identity. The 18S rRNA gene is by far the most commonly used locus for *Babesia* identification. There are several well-established and sensitive nested PCR protocols targeting this gene, as it is easy to amplify and there is much sequence information in the GenBank database.

It has long been accepted that cattle are the main, if not only, reservoir hosts for human *B. divergens* infections in Europe and sequencing of the 18S rRNA gene strongly supports this. Additionally, 5 of the 10 human *B. divergens* isolates for which sequence information is available are 100% identical with bovine isolate GenBank: U16370 (Figure 2), widely used as a reference sequence for *B. divergens* [11]. Another three isolates showed more than 99.9% homology with this bovine isolate reference, but a further two human isolates probably did not have a bovine origin, showing homologies of only 99.7% (GenBank: AF435415) and 99.2% (GenBank: AJ439713). The first of these cases occurred in a 34-year-old asplenic male Canary Island resident with typical clinical signs of acute babesiosis [12]. The patient reported having removed several unidentified ticks two weeks prior to being admitted to hospital. Since *I. ricinus* is apparently absent in the Canary Islands and the patient had no history of travel, the authors suggested the protozoan may have been transmitted by *Ixodes ventalloi*, an endophilic tick species that is common in the islands and primarily infects lagomorphs, carnivores and rodents [13]. However, this tick has never been confirmed as a vector for *B. divergens* or any other zoonotic *Babesia* species. The second case was reported in a 66-year-old acutely ill splenectomized patient in Portugal [14]. As the patient had travelled to Florida, the USA and the UK six weeks prior to his illness, it was not possible to ascertain where he had been infected.

There are several reports of the detection of *B. divergens* DNA in red deer (*Cervus elaphus*), roe deer (*Capreolus capreolus*) and reindeer (*Rangifer tarandus*) [15], and it has been suggested that these host species, especially red and roe deer, may serve as a source for infection for both humans and cattle. However, none of the deer isolates show 18S rRNA homologies of more than 99.9% with the bovine reference strain, and so far there is no evidence that deer '*Babesia divergens*' have ever caused either human or bovine babesiosis.

It is important to point out, that although useful for diagnostics, the 18S rRNA gene probably cannot unequivocally distinguish between *Babesia* species or strains. The reason for this is its highly conserved nature across the genus, on the one hand, combined with considerable intraspecific sequence diversity, on the other hand, particularly for *B. divergens* and *B. microti*. The cytochrome c oxidase subunit I (COI) gene locus has greater genetic diversity than the 18S rRNA gene and is therefore a more useful tool to distinguish between different species but, unfortunately, it has a lower amplification efficiency [16]. However, when examining the role of potential reservoir species, attempts should be made where possible to sequence sizeable fragments of both the COI and 18S rRNA genes [17]. Other loci such as the beta-tubulin, heat shock protein and merozoite surface protein genes have been used to distinguish *Babesia* isolates; however, until more information for these loci is available in the database, they are unlikely to be used more widely.

The clinical presentation of *B. venatorum* infections can closely resemble that of *B. divergens* [4], but this species is clearly distinct, showing only 98.2% homology with the bovine *B. divergens* reference sequence, U16370. Of the six infections reported in Europe so far, four 18S rRNA sequences are available, including the original two with identical sequences GenBank AY046575 [4], one showing 99.7% [5] and one showing 99.6% (asymptomatic–GenBank: KP072001) homology with AY046575. Almost all 18S rRNA sequences of *B. venatorum* from roe deer (*C. capreolus*) are identical to the first human isolates, with the few exceptions differing by one or two nucleotides, and there can be little doubt that roe deer is the main reservoir host of *B. venatorum* in Europe. It is also interesting to note that *B. venatorum* is not restricted to Europe and approximately 50 cases have been diagnosed in China [18], with the available 18S rRNA sequences being identical to the original European isolates or differing by only one or two nucleotides. The suspected but unconfirmed vector and reservoir hosts are *Ixodes persulcatus* and sika deer, or *Cervus nippon*, respectively [19].

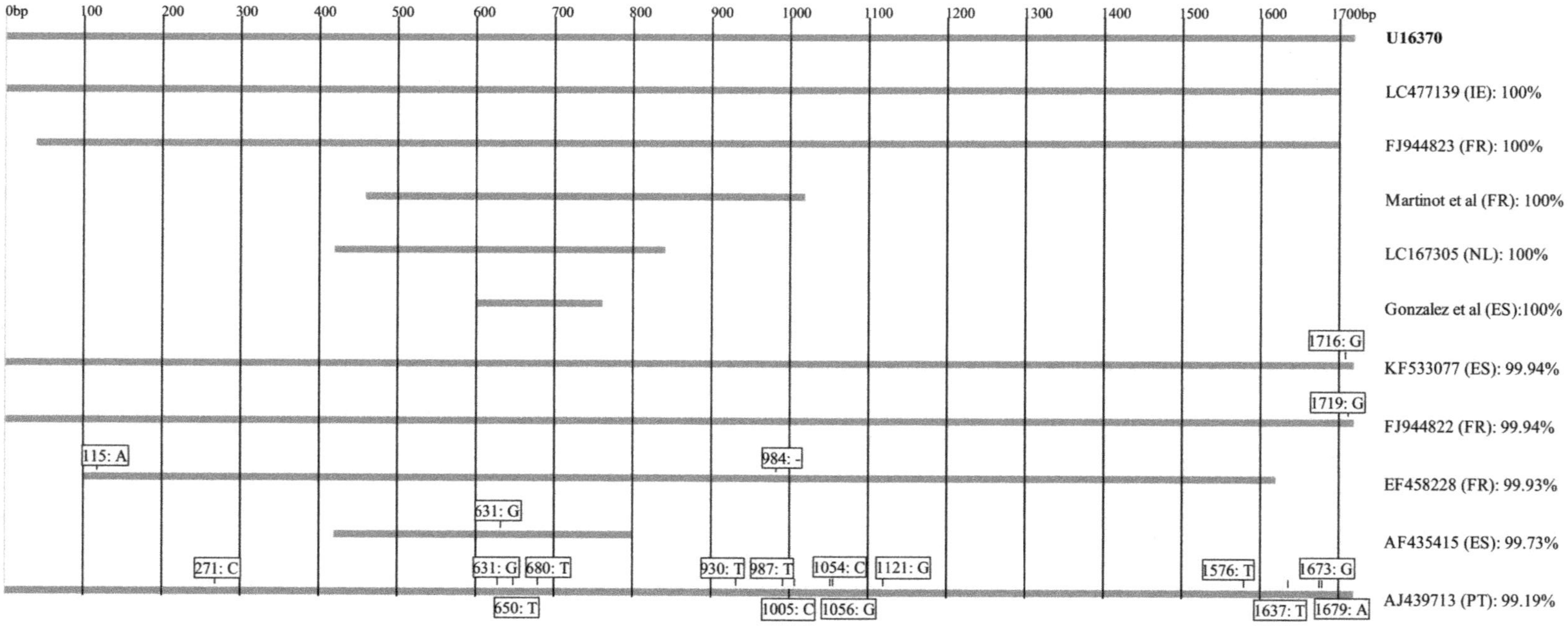

Figure 2. The relative length, positions and heterologies of 18S rRNA sequences of *Babesia* species isolates from human cases compared to the reference sequence U16370. Numbers refer to positions in the reference sequence. Identity scores are according to Clustal Omega. '-' indicates that the base was missing.

Babesia microti is considered to be a species complex, mainly infecting small mammals. Goethert and Telford [20] assigned the parasites in the group to three clades based on analysis of the 18S rRNA and beta tubulin genes, with most of the zoonotic genotypes within Clade 1, which also includes the 'U.S. genotype' (e.g., GenBank: AY693840), responsible for the vast majority of human babesiosis cases. Human *B. microti* infections have expanded across the northeast of the USA over the last few decades [21], and several cases in Europe have been associated with travel from that country. In contrast, very few autochthonous cases have occurred in Europe, the first authenticated one was in Germany in an immunocompromised patient and caused by a strain (Jena–GenBank: EF413181) closely related to the USA genotype [8]. Welc-Faleciak et al. reported the detection of DNA of the same genotype in two other individuals, both asymptomatic, who were participating in a survey of forest workers in Poland [22]. Another *B. microti* strain, the 'Munich' type (GenBank: AB071177) is widely distributed in Europe and was originally presumed to be non-zoonotic [23]. However, DNA of this strain has reportedly been detected in seven patients in Europe, six of whom presented with various symptoms following a tick-bite in Poland (GenBank: KT429729; [24]), and one who presented with non-specific symptoms in Spain (GenBank: KT271759; [25]). A 157 nucleotide DNA fragment of the Munich strain was detected in an eighth patient, originally thought to be suffering from a prolonged bout of malaria while living in Equatorial Guinea. However, the patient made several visits to Spain during that period [26], and it is difficult to determine whether this *B. microti* infection, successfully treated with antibabesials, was contracted in Spain or Africa. All patients infected with the Munich strain were immunocompetent and only this latter patient had detectable parasites (at a very low level) in thin blood smears. These isolated reports indicate that two European genotypes of *B. microti* can infect humans, but that they are considerably less pathogenic than those in the USA. All cases that were imported into Europe appear to have an American origin (mainly North America), and although only three 18S rRNA sequences are available at present (showing 100% identity to the original American isolate GenBank: AY693840), it is probable that they were all caused by parasites closely related to this widespread U.S. genotype.

3. Pathogenesis

Most what is known to date on babesiosis pathobiology has resulted from in vitro experiments and animal studies (mainly in mice and cattle) on *B. microti*, *B. bovis* and *B. divergens* [27–31]. In many human infections, no isolates have been obtained for further investigations, and little information is available on the pathogenesis of *B. venatorum*. Babesia parasites occur within erythrocytes and as extracellular forms in the blood. They multiply within the erythrocytes by a form of budding to produce two or occasionally four daughter cells (merozoites). In fulminant human infections and in highly infected in vitro cultures, multiple parasites may occur within individual erythrocytes (Figure 1). The release of merozoites and eventual erythrocyte lysis is associated with fever and other clinical symptoms including hemolytic anemia, jaundice, hemoglobinuria, obstruction of renal arterioles and renal failure [32]. In vitro observations suggest that erythrocytes are not necessarily completely destroyed when the parasites leave them, but they are damaged. Their optical density decreases, they are reduced in size and are probably removed by the spleen soon afterwards [27–31]. While intermittent episodes of fever have been reported in cases of human babesiosis [32], they typically do not have the same regularity as febrile episodes in malaria, probably because of the asynchronous nature of babesia multiplication and egress from the erythrocytes [33]. In addition to erythrocyte lysis and metabolic alterations, excessive proinflammatory cytokine production contributes to clinical complications [34,35], potentially resulting in vascular leakage, adult respiratory distress syndrome, hypotension and shock [35,36].

Both innate and adaptive immune mechanisms limit the severity of babesial infection [34,37,38]. The spleen plays a central role in host defense by clearing infected erythrocytes from the bloodstream and mounting the protective immune response. The heavily vascularized organ consists of red-pulp and white-pulp zones surrounded by a trabecula and an outer capsule. The marginal zone contains macrophages and neutrophils that recognize and ingest babesia-infected erythrocytes and circulating free parasites as the blood travels through the spleen (in humans, erythrocytes pass through the spleen approximately every 20 min [39]). The red-pulp infected erythrocytes are captured in sieve-like slits in the sinuses as they return to the main circulation and are ingested by macrophages [40,41]. The white pulp of the spleen contains T-cells that produce cytokines, for example gamma interferon (IFNγ), which activate macrophages to phagocytose and destroy parasites, as well as B-cells to secrete babesia-specific antibodies [41]. Antibodies neutralize pathogens, thereby preventing them from entering erythrocytes, and also enhance phagocytosis by macrophages and neutrophils through opsonization and eradicate pathogens through antibody-dependent cytotoxicity by natural killer cells and through the activation of complements [41]. The importance of cellular immunity in controlling parasitemia is demonstrated by the fact that both laboratory mice and humans with depressed cellular immunity have difficulties in controlling infections [5,28,31]. Similarly, the depletion of host macrophages and natural killer cells in mice increases susceptibility to infection [30], while an impaired antibody response due to hematological malignancies and/or rituximab therapy can also lead to difficulties in clearing infection in humans, despite adequate antibabesial therapy [5,42].

In general, factors responsible for severe infections following splenectomy include the delayed and impaired production of immunoglobulin and lack of splenic macrophages, resulting in a reduction in the numbers of infected erythrocytes removed [43]. Consequently, asplenia or hyposplenism often results in fulminant illness and death [1,44–47].

Babesia parasites possess a number of evasive measures to avoid immune attack, which can lead to persistent infections, even in the presence of an intact immune system [41]. Persistent infections (often asymptomatic) are particularly evident in *B. microti* infections of humans, but less so in *B. divergens* and *B. venatorum* infections, which are usually acute, although infection of their natural hosts (cattle and roe deer, respectively) tend to be persistent. The mechanisms for immunoevasion are unclear, although antigenic variation probably occurs to some extent. Capillary sequestration of infected erythrocytes, thus avoiding circulation through the spleen, has only been reported for certain non-zoonotic species (*B. bovis* and *B. canis*) [48].

4. Vector Biology

All zoonotic *Babesia* spp. in Europe are transmitted by the castor bean tick, *Ixodes ricinus*. This three-host tick species spends most of its life (>98%) free living, either host seeking or developing to the next stage. It requires a high humidity at the base of the vegetation (RH >80%), and ideal conditions are to be found in temperate deciduous woodlands with patches of dense vegetation and little air movement. Additionally, *I. ricinus* may be present in appreciable numbers in regions of high rainfall on agricultural land utilized by livestock, such as rough hill land or undergrazed pastures [49]. This tick species occurs in Northern, Western, Central and Eastern regions of Europe, but is sparse in Southern Europe because of its susceptibility to desiccation. In most regions of its distribution, host-seeking activity commences in spring and early summer, with ticks being found on vegetation and animals from late March and peaking in numbers from April to July. In some areas a second, less intense, phase of questing activity occurs in the autumn, and as a result of global warming, tick activity now occurs more frequently in winter [50]. All active stages of larva, nymph and adult ticks ambush their hosts from the vegetation and, with the exception of the male, which generally does not feed, they attach to the skin with specialized mouthparts for several days, the duration depending on the tick life cycle stage.

In infected unfed ticks, babesia parasites occur in the salivary glands, but they are not infective until they have undergone development, which is initiated when the tick starts to feed, and takes about two days to complete. *Ixodes ricinus* was first shown to be the vector of *B. divergens* in transmission experiments using splenectomized calves [51]. It appears that infections are chiefly acquired by adult females while feeding on an infected host and they then pass the infection transovarially to the next generation of ticks, all stages of which (except perhaps for males) are capable of transmitting the infection [52]. While infection acquisition by immature stages has been suggested, this arose out of laboratory studies involving gerbils (*Meriones unguiculatus*) as hosts, and no direct evidence for the implied transstadial transmission that might follow exists [53]. *Ixodes ricinus* was also shown to be the likely vector of *B. venatorum* by Bonnet et al. [54], who demonstrated probable transovarial transmission from adult ticks feeding on roe deer to the next generation larvae. *Ixodes ricinus* as a vector of *B. venatorum* was validated in a subsequent in vitro study, in which both nymphs and females were shown to acquire infections and to transmit them transstadially and transovarially [55]. One of the consequences of transovarial transmission and transstadial persistence in *B. divergens* and *B. venatorum* is that theoretically infected ticks could occur in regions where infected reservoir hosts are not present, particularly as a result of the deposition of infected larvae by birds. Transstadial transmission of the third species, *B. microti*, involving acquisition by *I. ricinus* larvae from rodent hosts, followed by infection of hosts by nymphs, was reported by Walter and Weber in 1981 [56] and confirmed by Gray et al. in 2002 [57]. Additionally, the latter study showed that transovarial transmission of *B. microti* does not occur, that the parasite does not persist in the tick beyond one moult and that *I. ricinus* can transmit a zoonotic American strain, suggesting that it might be the vector of more than one European strain of the parasite.

Using PCR-based techniques, *Babesia* spp. are detectable in unfed free-living *I. ricinus* ticks. *Babesia divergens* occurs at a very low rate in ticks and is often undetectable even when the ticks have been collected from pastures where bovine babesiosis has occurred recently [58,59]. *Babesia venatorum* occurs at a slightly higher frequency [60], and as a parasite of roe deer, almost is always in ticks from woodlands. Tick infection rates of *B. microti*, also associated with rodents and woodlands, tend to be much higher, sometimes exceeding 10% [61].

Human *B. microti* babesiosis cases are exceedingly rare in Europe, despite the fact that this parasite occurs commonly in rodents and can be readily detected in unfed *I. ricinus* ticks [60], which are proven vectors of at least some Europe strains [57]. However, it should be noted that another tick species, *Ixodes trianguliceps*, is the dominant *B. microti* vector in many regions [62], and this tick species rarely bites humans. Furthermore, the parasites it transmits may not be infective for *I. ricinus*. These factors probably contribute to the low disease rate, but nevertheless, serosurveys indicate considerable exposure of the human population to infection [63].

5. Epidemiology

5.1. Autochthonous Babesiosis Cases

Human babesiosis is very rare in Europe, although the exact number of European cases is difficult to establish. Gorenflot et al. reported 22 cases of human babesiosis caused by *B. divergens* up to 1998 [64]. They occurred in France (10), the British Isles (6), Russia (1), Spain (2), Sweden (1), Switzerland (1) and present-day Croatia (1). Some cases were not published but communicated personally, and not all of them were confirmed using molecular methods [1,46,47,64–68]. From 1998 until the present, at least 13 additional cases were published in France [69–72], Portugal [14], Norway [73], Spain [74–76], Turkey [77], Finland [44], Ireland [78] and the UK [79] (Table 1). Overall, this amounts to more than 50 cases, with 35 attributed to *B. divergens*, 5 to *B. venatorum* and 11 to *B. microti* (excluding imported cases) (Tables 1–3).

Table 1. *Babesia divergens* infections in Europe.

Year	Country	Age, Gender, (Outcome)	Course of Disease *	Co-Morbidities Compl./Unusual Features	Misdiagnosis, Time from Symptoms until Diagnosis: Prior ad./Post ad.	Parasitemia	Antibabesial Therapy	References
1957–1998 22 cases		10× in France (8 cured, 2 died) 6× British Isles (2 cured, 4 died) 1× Russia (died) 2× Spain (1 cured, 1 died) 1× Sweden (cured) 1× Switzerland (cured) ** 1× Ex-Yugoslavia (died)	mild to lethal	Co-morbidities: Hodgkin's disease, splenectomy, hypertension, diabetes; Compl: ARF, ARDS, shock, HLH, cardio-respiratory arrest, cardiac effusion	malaria, 3 days/10 days or diagnosis post mortem	2–80%	Drugs used: QN + CLI, QN +CHQ PNT + CTM QN + CLI + PNT QN + DOX CH + CLI CH + DOX + MEF ET	[64]
1999–2021 Asplenic and Hyposplenic Patients								
1999	France	44, M, splenecto-mized (cured)	mild to moderate	NI	3 days/1 day	1%	QN + CLI	[69]
2003	Portugal	66, M, splenecto-mized (died)	severe to lethal	Co-morbidities: MI 1984, subtotal gastrectomy; Compl: ARDS, ARF	malaria, 1 week/4 days	30%	QN + CLI + VI	[14]
2004	Finland	53, M, rudimentary spleen (died)	severe to lethal	Co-morbidities: severe alcohol-induced pancraetitis, diabetes type 1; Compl: Septic shock, multiple organ failure, pulmonary aspergillosis, UF: ECM	1 week/2 days	10%	QN + CLI + CFX, ET	[44]
2005	France	51, M, splenecto-mized (cured)	moderate to severe	Compl: ARF, ARDS	2 days/1 day	60%	QN + CLI	[70]
2015	Norway	58, M, splenecto-mized (cured)	severe	Compl: ARF, ARDS, atrial fibrillation	FUO, 4 days/2 days	30%	QN + CLI, ET	[73]
2015	Spain	37, M, splenecto-mized (cured)	moderate to severe	Co-morbidity: newly diagnosed HIV; Compl: HLH, ARDS	*Mycobacterium* spp., 3 days post ad.	low	QN + CLI, AZM + ATQ	[74]
2015	Turkey	28, F, splenecto-mized (cured)	moderate to severe	NI	malaria, 1 month/2 days	50%	ET, QN + CLI	[77]
2017	Ireland	79, M, hypo-splenism (cured)	moderate to severe	Co-morbidities: adult celiac disease, pulmonary TB; Compl: ARF, HAP	7 days/2 days	20%	ATQ + AZM, CLI + QN	[78]

Table 1. *Cont.*

Year	Country	Age, Gender, (Outcome)	Course of Disease *	Co-Morbidities Compl./Unusual Features	Misdiagnosis, Time from Symptoms until Diagnosis: Prior ad./Post ad.	Parasitemia	Antibabesial Therapy	References
1999–2021 Normosplenic Patients								
2011	France	37, F (cured)	mild	NI	TBD, 3 weeks post ad.	0.29%	DOX	[71]
2011	Spain	46, M (cured)	moderate to severe	Compl: ARF, relapse	3 days/1 day	10%	QN + CLI; relapse: AZM + AP	[75]
2018	Spain	87, F (died)	severe to lethal	Co-morbidities: ovarian tumor, malignant hypertension, transient ischemic attacks, osteoporosis; Compl: ARF, bleeding disorders, cardio-respiratory arrest	3 months/4 days	2.9%	AZM + AP	[76]
2020	France	6 patients, no information about sex and age (cured)	mild to moderate	UF/Compl: 1× unusual cutaneous symptom, 1× K. pneumonia septicemia and hepatic abscesses, 1× acute pneumonia, 1× febrile eosinophilic panniculitis	retrospective analysis	In 2/6 pos.	2 patients: DOX 2 patients: AZM + ATQ 1 patient: CTX + SPI 1 patient: COX + AMC + OFX	[72]
2021	UK	72, F (NI)	moderate to severe	NI	3 days/1 day	20%	NI	[79]

M—male, F—female, ND—not done, NI—no information, pos.—positive, ad.—admission, UF—unusual feature, Compl.—complications, FUO—fever of unknown origin, MI—myocardial infarction, TB—tuberculosis, TBD—bacterial tick-borne disease, ARF—acute renal failure, ARDS—acute respiratory distress syndrome, HAP—hospital-acquired pneumonia, HLH—hemophagocytic lymphohistiocytosis. * Classification of disease severity followed criteria suggested by Vannier and Krause (2009) [80]. ** infection probably acquired in Wales. AZM—azithromycin, ATQ—atovaquone, AP—atovaquone/proguanil, QN—quinine, CLI—clindamycin, VI—vibramycin, CTX—ceftriaxone, COX—cefotaxime, AMC—amikacin, OFX—olfloxacin, CHQ—chloroquine, PNT—pentamidine, CTM—cotrimoxazole, CH—chinin, MEF—mefloquine, ET—exchange transfusio

Table 2. *Babesia venatorum* infections in Europe (all cases with clinical details were splenectomized).

Year	Country	Age, Gender, (Outcome)	Course of Disease *	Co-Morbidities, Compl.	Misdiagnosis, Time from Symptoms until Diagnosis: Prior ad./Post ad.	Parasitemia	Antibabesial Therapy	References
2003	Italy	55, M, (cured)	moderate to severe	Co-morbidities: splenectomized because of Hodgkin's disease, recently started chemotherapy for stage IIIA diffuse large B-cell lymphoma	4 days/6 days	30%	QN + CLI	[4]
	Austria	56, M, (cured)	mild	Co-morbidities: splenectomized, Hodgkin's disease	2 days/1 day	1.3%	CLI	
2007	Germany	63, M, (cured)	moderate to severe	Co-morbidities: splenectomized, Hodgkin's disease, immunosuppressive treatment; Compl.: prolonged, relapse	relapse of Hodgkin's disease, AIHA 3–4 weeks/2 days	4%	QN + CLI, CLI, relapse: AZM + ATQ, ATQ for 5 months	[5]
2011	Austria	68, M (cured)	mild to moderate	Co-morbidities: splenectomized, hairy cell leukemia, immunosuppressive treatment, granular lymphocyte leukemia; Compl.: ARF	AIHA some weeks/3–4 days	30%	QN + CLI	[6]
2015	Poland	NI	asymptomatic	NI	NI	NI	NI	GenBank: KP072001
2017	Sweden	52, M (cured)	moderate to severe	Co-morbidities: splenectomized, T-Cell Lymphoma, immunosuppressive treatment; Compl.: HLH	Hemophagocytic syndrome, 2 months/2 days	4%	QN + CLI, AZM + ATQ	[7]

M—male, F—female, NI—no information, Compl.—complications, AIH—autoimmune hemolytic anemia, ARF—acute renal failure, HLH—hemophagocytic lymphohistiocytosis, ad.—admission * Classification of disease severity followed criteria suggested by Vannier and Krause (2009) [80]. QN—quinine, CLI—clindamycin, ATQ—atovaquone, AZM—azithromycin.

Table 3. *Babesia microti* infections in Europe.

Year	Country	Age, Gender, (Outcome)	Course of Disease *	Co-Morbidities Compl./Unusual Features	Misdiagnosis, Time from Symptoms until Diagnosis: Prior ad./Post ad.	Parasitemia	Antibabesial Therapy	Reference
				Autochthonous *B. microti* Infections				
1981	Belgium	In the 40 s, M, (cured)	moderate	Compl.: prolonged fever	Rickettsiosis, 1 month	NI	T, CHQ	[81]
2007	Germany	42, F, (cured)	moderate	Co-morbidities: AML, immunocompromizing treatment	MI, some weeks/10 days	4.5%	QN + CLI, AZM	[8]
2015	Poland	2 patients >45 (NI)	asymptomatic	NI	NI	ND	no treatment	[22]

Table 3. *Cont.*

Year	Country	Age, Gender, (Outcome)	Course of Disease *	Co-Morbidities Compl./Unusual Features	Misdiagnosis, Time from Symptoms until Diagnosis: Prior ad./Post ad.	Parasitemia	Antibabesial Therapy	Reference
2016	Poland	6 patients (cured)	mild	Co-morbidities: 1 EM, 1 TBE	NI	Neg.	no treatment	[24]
2016	Spain	35, M (cured)	mild	Compl: prolonged parasitemia	several months/few days second ad.	Neg.	ATQ + AZM, AP	[25]
Imported *B. microti* Infections								
1992	Poland	36, M (cured)	moderate	NI	malaria, NI	NI	CLI	[82]
2003	Switzerland	NI	mild	NI	NI	ND	NI	[83]
2003	Czech Rep.	58, M (cured)	mild	NI	28 days/some days	0.14%	QN + DOX	[84]
2010	Austria	63, M (cured)	moderate to severe	Compl.: hemodynamic shock, anuria	malaria, 2 weeks/diagnosis retrospective	high	QN + CLI	[85]
2012	Germany	38, M (cured)	moderate to severe	Co-morbidity: splenectomy after injury, Compl: pneumonia	Borreliosis, 3–4 months	8‰	QN + CLI, AZM + ATQ + DOX	[86]
2013	France	82, M (cured)	moderate	Compl: HLH	5 days/some days	3%	QN + CLI	[87]
2013	Poland	48, F (cured)	moderate	Co-morbidity: neuroborreliosis; Compl.: neck stiffness	10 days/10 days	3%	AP, DOX + AZM + CLI	[88]
2013	Denmark	64, F (cured)	moderate	Co-morbidity: RF; Compl.: erythematous skin changes	Borreliosis, malaria, IE, some days/1 week	4%	AP, AP + AZM	[89]
2015	Spain	66, F (cured)	severe	Compl.: multiorgan failure	2 days/2 days	20%	QN + CLI, ATQ + AZM, ET	[90]
2016	Spain	66, F (cured)	severe	Compl.: ARDS, ARF, multiorgan failure	malaria, 1 week/some days	20%	QN + CLI, AZM + ATQ, ET	[91]
2017	France	69, M (cured)	moderate to severe	Compl.: ARF; UF: diffuse purpura of the lower extremities	malaria, 1–2 days/few days	3%	QN, QN + CLI	[92]
2019	UK	83, M (died)	severe	Co-morbidity: LGLL; Compl.: multiorgan failure	severe sepsis, few days	>20%	Antibabesial therapy, ET	[93]
2020	Spain	72, M (cured)	mild to moderate	Co-morbidity: diabetes	15 days/1 day	0.5%	ATQ + AZM	[94]
Autochthonous or Imported *B. microti* Infection								
2014	Spain	43, F (cured)	moderate	Compl.: prolonged disease	malaria, 8 months	>0.5%	AZM-AP	[26]

M—male, F—female, Rep.—Republic, ND—not done, NI—no information, Neg—negative, ad.—admission, UF—unusual feature, Compl.—complications, MI—myocardial infarction, TB—tuberculosis, ARF—acute renal failure, ARDS—acute respiratory distress syndrome, AML—acute myeloid leukemia, EM—erythema migrans, TBE—tick-borne encephalitis, RF—rheumatic fever, IE—infective endocarditis, HLH—hemophagocytic lymphohistiocytosis, LGLL—low-grade lymphoplasmacytic lymphoma * Classification of disease severity followed criteria suggested by Vannier and Krause (2009) [80]. T—tetracycline, AZM—azithromycin, ATQ—atovaquone, AP—atovaquone/proguanil, QN—quinine, CLI—clindamycin, CHQ—chloroquine, ET—exchange transfusion.

Despite the rarity of the disease in Europe, several serosurveys suggest that infections may be surprisingly frequent. For example, Hunfeld et al. reported positive values of 5.4% and 3.6% for *B. divergens* and *B. microti*, respectively, in a sample of 467 sera collected from the general population in Germany [63], and in Slovenia, IgG titers in 215 samples ranged from 8.4% to 2.8% depending on the IFAT cut-off [95]. However, in contrast to the USA, where transfusion-transmitted infections occur quite frequently, to date, only a single case in Europe (*B. microti* [8]) appears to have resulted from a blood transfusion. At the present time, therefore, and despite the increasing evidence for mild and asymptomatic infections [22,71,72] and the relative frequency of blood transfusions in the population, this form of transmission appears to carry a low risk of babesiosis in Europe.

The two greatest risk factors for zoonotic European babesiosis are exposure to *I. ricinus* ticks (though patients may not be aware of a tick bite) and splenectomy (Tables 1 and 2). Even in the few spleen-intact cases there was usually evidence of splenic dysfunction or other immune incompetence, as discussed below (Section 6.1). In contrast, the few European *B. microti* cases have all been spleen-intact cases. This is also a common feature in the many cases of infection with this parasite in the USA [96]. Considering the numbers of splenectomized individuals in the European population (several hundred thousand in France alone in 1983 [64]), and the abundance of *I. ricinus* throughout Europe, the frequency of babesiosis is surprisingly low, indicating perhaps that additional immunosuppressive conditions are contributing factors in disease occurrence (Table 1), but the low infection rates of ticks, even in habitats frequented by the relevant reservoir hosts, may also be a factor in the rarity of the disease.

Another obvious risk factor for *B. divergens* infection is association with cattle, as indicated by the genetic similarity between cattle isolates and those from human cases where the parasites were sequenced (Figure 2). Although *B. divergens* has been reported in red deer, the parasite genotypes differ from those isolated from cattle or humans (Figure 1, [15]). However, this topic requires further investigation, as discussed in the previous section. Since roe deer have been identified as reservoir hosts of *B. venatorum* [55], it is reasonable to suppose that exposure to ticks in woodland is a risk factor, as discussed in Section 4.

5.2. Imported Babesiosis

To date, 13 cases of human babesiosis have been documented as imported to European countries. All cases were attributed to *B. microti* and were diagnosed in Switzerland [83], the Czech Republic [84], Austria [85], France [87,92], Germany [86], Poland [82,88], Spain [90,91,94], Denmark [89] and the UK [93], having been acquired in the Americas (Table 3).

5.3. Ambiguous Babesiosis Cases

A small number of human babesiosis cases documented from Europe do not fit into any of the categories described above. These include three symptomatic cases with unidentified *Babesia* species reported in France [64,71] and Spain [64]. Additionally, one case of coinfection with *Babesia* spp. and *Borrelia* spp. was reported in Poland. Published sequences showed 98.99% homology to both *B. divergens* and *B. venatorum*, so that exact speciation was not possible [97]. In four more cases of babesia infection, which were detected in a retrospective study in immunocompetent patients in France, species identification was not possible [72]. Finally, one *B. microti* infection, diagnosed in Spain in a 43-year-old woman with an intact spleen, was associated with moderate and prolonged disease, originally diagnosed as malaria. Over an 8-month period, she received six consecutive diagnoses of malaria with different treatment regimens that led to no clear improvement. Because all antimalarial therapies failed, the patient's case was re-evaluated, diagnosed and eventually treated appropriately. It could not be established whether the patient acquired the infection in Europe (autochthonous) or in Equatorial Guinea (imported) [25].

5.4. Reports of Possible Cases with Diagnostic Deficiencies/Lack of Clarity

Of the 22 human cases of *B. divergens* infections that were documented before 1998 and described by Gorenflot et al. [64], and not all fulfill present day diagnostic standards, as some were only diagnosed microscopically without PCR confirmation, sequence analysis or serological testing [1,46,47,65–68,98,99]. Two cases reported as *B. bovis* infections were diagnosed on the basis of their appearance under the microscope only, rendering their identity questionable [1,100]. Even after 1998, at least 26 more cases were published as human babesiosis, despite diagnostic deficiencies or with lack of clarity, including 2 case reports of *B. microti* from Russia [101], 1 case from Spain [102] and 10 cases of unknown *Babesia* spp. from Montenegro [103], which were only diagnosed microscopically. Another case of *B. microti* infection in Switzerland presented doubtful microscopy, negative PCR and borderline serology [104]. A retrospective analysis of cases of babesiosis admitted to Spanish hospitals through data recorded in the minimum basic data set at discharge (MBDS) during the period 2004–2013 found 10 patients diagnosed with human babesiosis [105]. Only two of these were unequivocally identified as *B. divergens* and published [74,75]. Additionally, in a few cases, the co-infection of *Babesia* spp. with other tick-borne pathogens was reported, but unfortunately diagnoses in these cases were only performed on the basis of clinical presentation [105] or had deficiencies in the diagnosis of babesiosis [104,106]. For example, in a case of septic babesiosis reported from Spain [102], the patient presented a widespread exanthema with the presence of well-established annular lesions. Biopsy of one of the annular lesions showed changes compatible with a necrolytic migratory erythema. The patient had clinical symptoms of sepsis, but the diagnosis of human babesiosis was only based on apparent positive microscopy. There are no other reports of babesia infections causing erythema figuratum, and other differential causes have to be considered for this patient such as pancreatic neuroendocrine tumor-like glucagonoma, liver diseases and zinc deficiency [107–109]. Similarly, Strizova et al. reported a case of a 36-year-old man in the Czech Republic who experienced severe polytrauma requiring repetitive blood transfusions. Six months later he presented with possible Reiter's syndrome consisting of arthritis, conjunctivitis and urethritis. The diagnosis of human babesiosis caused by *B. microti* mimicking Reiter's syndrome was performed only based on apparent positive microscopy and the lymphocyte transformation test, which has not been evaluated for its sensitivity and specificity in the diagnosis of babesiosis [110]. Again, it is important to stress that the parasite is difficult to identify using microscopy alone, particularly if parasitemia is low, and confusion with platelets of staining artefacts is common (further discussed in Section 6).

6. Clinical Course of Infections

6.1. Pre-Disposing Factors of Acute Disease

General pre-disposing factors associated with a higher risk of symptomatic human babesia infection and more severe illness are splenectomy, impaired cellular and/or humoral immunity and advanced age [31,32,111]. The latter is explained by the decline in cellular immunity in patients over the age of 50 years [37].

In Europe, most severe cases were either splenectomized [1,4–7,14,45–47,70,73,74,77,86], or they had a rudimentary spleen and hyposplenism [44,78]. Immunosuppressive comorbidities associated with severe babesiosis are hematological malignancies such as Hodgkin's disease [4,5,45], B-cell lymphoma [4], acute myeloid leukemia [8], hairy cell leukemia [6], T-cell lymphoma [7] and HIV [74]. Patients with these malignant diagnoses and moderate-to-severe babesiosis were often on chemotherapeutic drugs with additional immunocompromising effects including prednisone, doxorubicin, cyclophosphamide, methotrexate, bleomycin and rituximab [4–8]. In human infections of *B. microti* in the United States, it has been reported that the severity of the disease increased with increasing parasitemia [112], with severe outcomes or complications of babesiosis associated with parasitemias of >4% [113] or >10% [114,115]. A few exceptions include reports of death in babesiosis patients with parasitemia <3% [116]. This latter observation has also been made in critically ill patients in Europe [76], but in most European cases, parasitemias in patients with complications ranged from 10% up to 80% in *B. divergens* infection [14,44,46,70,75,77–79], 4% to 30% in *B. venatorum* infection [4,5] and 3% to 20% in *B. microti* infection [90–93].

One of the very rare but potentially fatal complications of babesiosis is hemophagocytic lymphohistiocytosis (HLH) [87,117–121]. In HLH, normal downregulation of activated macrophages and lymphocytes does not occur, resulting in excessive inflammation, hypercytokinemia, abnormal immune activation and tissue destruction. Dysregulation is due to the inability of natural killer cells and cytotoxic lymphocytes to eliminate activated macrophages. HLH is classified into a genetically determined primary form and a secondary form that occurs in older people with underlying conditions such as infections, malignancies and autoimmune disorders [122]. In Europe, HLH has been reported in at least four patients with babesiosis caused by *B. divergens* [74,123], *B. venatorum* [7] and *B. microti* [87]. Cofactors for severe disease in these patients were older age [87], and a newly diagnosed HIV infection in one patient [74].

In many European cases, detailed laboratory parameters are frequently not available, so that a retrospective analysis of potential clinical factors that may have rendered patients to be more susceptible is not feasible. Future reports on European cases should consider risk factors for severe disease that have been reported for *B. microti* infection including hemoglobin level <10 g/dL, parasitemia $\geq$10 days, elevated alkaline phosphatase >125 U/L, total white blood cell count >5 $\times$ 10^9/L and prior existing cardiac abnormalities [113,114].

6.2. *Babesia divergens*

This section describes the clinical course of babesiosis cases reported over the last 21 years (2000–2021) in asplenic, hyposplenic and normosplenic patients, who presented with mild-to-severe disease, dependent on age, immune status and co-morbidities (Table 1).

6.2.1. Features of the Disease in Asplenic and Hyposplenic Patients

Since 2000, six patients who had been immunocompromised by splenectomy developed severe infections [14,69,70,73,74,77]. Two other patients had rudimentary spleens probably resulting in functional aspleny [44,78]. The period from onset of symptoms to the diagnosis of babesiosis ranged from one month prior to admission to four days post admission. Before obtaining a correct diagnosis of human babesiosis, patients were misdiagnosed with malaria, fever of unknown origin and *Mycobacterium* spp. infection secondary to HIV. Frequently presented symptoms were a fever up to 40 °C, headache, abdominal and back pain, fatigue, hemolysis with or without anemia and jaundice. Severely ill patients developed acute renal failure, hemophagocytic syndrome, atrial fibrillation, ARDS, hospital-acquired pneumonia, pulmonary aspergillosis, septic shock and multiorgan failure [14,44,69,70,73,74,77,78]. Parasitemias ranged from 1% [69] to 60% [70]. Only two of these eight patients (25.0%), a 66-year-old man [14] and a 53-year-old man [44], succumbed to the infection indicating a significant improvement in survival rates compared to cases reported before 1998 [64].

Interestingly, the two patients who were not splenectomized but were hyposplenic developed very severe disease. One case involved a 79-year-old man in Ireland with a 5-day history of fever, malaise, nausea, generalized pains and dark-colored urine. The patient remembered removing a tick from his arm two weeks prior to the onset of illness. He had been diagnosed with celiac disease several years before admission. A peripheral blood smear revealed babesiosis with 20% parasitemia and the presence of Howell–Jolly bodies. The patient received antibabesial treatment but developed several complications including acute renal failure, ARDS and hospital-acquired pneumonia. Altogether he was hospitalized for 61 days. An MRI scan later revealed an atrophic spleen [78]. Defective splenic function affects more than one-third of adult patients with celiac disease [124]. Eliminating gluten from the diet may improve splenic function [125], but this works inconsistently and apparently not in those patients who have already developed splenic atrophy [125,126].

The second hyposplenic patient was a 53-year-old man from Finland who succumbed to the infection. He showed typical symptoms, but also had dark streaks on his arms and legs, probably caused by massive intravascular hemolysis, and an erythema migrans indicating possible co-infection with *Borrelia burgdorferi* s.l. On post-mortem examination, splenic atrophy was found, probably caused by alcohol consumption and/or by a previous history of alcohol-induced pancreatitis. Unfortunately, no mention was made of any investigation for other possible causes of this case of hyposplenism, such as celiac disease or other autoimmune diseases [44].

6.2.2. Features of the Disease in Normosplenic Patients

Babesia divergens parasitemias in immunocompetent individuals are generally lower than in immunocompromised patients and are often difficult to detect [71]), but at least six cases of infection have been reported in normosplenic patients during the last 21 years [71,72,75,76,79]. The course of disease ranged from mild [71] to severe [75,79] and even lethal [76], and parasitemias ranged from 0.29% [71] to 20% [78,79]. Mild cases presented with fever, chills, headache, arthromyalgia, leukopenia and elevated liver enzymes [71,72]. More severely ill patients had fever, malaise, vomiting, abdominal pain, hemolytic anemia, jaundice, hemoglobinuria and acute renal failure [75,76]. One of these six patients (16.7%) died [76].

One of the cases involved a 46-year-old forest ranger in Spain who was hospitalized after 3 days of fever, severe abdominal pain, jaundice and black and red deposits in his urine. Laboratory parameters indicated hemolytic anemia. CD4+ T cell counts were normal and serologic tests and blood cultures for hepatitis and HIV, as well as *Bartonella*, *Brucella*, *Leishmania*, *Leptospira* and *Borrelia* spp. were negative. Initial parasitemia was 10%, diminished gradually and resolved 10 days after starting a 12-day course of antibabesial therapy of quinine and clindamycin. Interestingly, hemolytic anemia remained severe, as evidenced by low hemoglobin. The patient's illness unexpectedly relapsed on day 18 after treatment. Parasites were again detected in blood samples and he was put on a 7-week course of combined atovaquone/proguanil and azithromycin [75].

In another case, a 72-year-old immunocompetent patient in the UK developed a parasitemia up to 20%. Unfortunately, we have no information about the clinical course of the disease in this patient. Older age was the only known risk factor [79]. Old age was probably also a factor in a fatal *B. divergens* infection in an 87-year-old woman from Spain who was hospitalized after three months of low-grade fever, malaise, vomiting, decreased appetite, jaundice and hemoglobinuria. In her case, parasitemia was low (2.9%). Although she received effective antibabesial treatment that cleared the parasites by day 15 following admission, she developed acute renal failure, nose and mouth bleeding and extensive cutaneous hematomas as result of disseminated intravascular coagulation, which resulted in death [76]. In addition to her advanced age, the patient also had complex cardiovascular co-morbidities, which in *B. microti* infections have been identified as risk factors for severe disease [113].

The first indication that *B. divergens* may cause relatively mild infections was reported by Martinot et al. in 2011 in France [72]. They detected intraerythrocytic parasites and *B. divergens* DNA in a 37-year-old woman with an unremarkable medical history, who presented with fever, headache and arthromyalgia two weeks after a tick bite and who recovered without specific antibabesial medication. Infected erythrocytes were also observed in a 35-year-old man showing similar symptoms, who also recovered uneventfully, but it was not possible to speciate this parasite using PCR. More recently (2018), also in France, Paleau and others detected *Babesia* spp. infection in six patients with flu-like symptoms, using a combination of tests that included PCR [72]. *Babesia divergens* was definitively identified in two of the cases. Interestingly, one patient was additionally diagnosed with *K. pneumonia* septicemia and hepatic abscesses, perhaps indicating an unrelated co-infection or a superinfection of acute or chronic human babesiosis. Another patient was diagnosed additionally with hemolytic anemia and acute pneumonia. Although pulmonary symptoms have been described in relation to human babesiosis, an unrelated co-infection could not be ruled out. Finally, babesiosis was diagnosed in a patient presenting with febrile eosinophilic panniculitis, which is an unusual cutaneous symptom in babesiosis. Unfortunately, there is no information on the patient's history, medication or co-morbidities [72].

6.3. *Babesia venatorum*

Altogether, five cases of *B. venatorum* have been described in Europe to date, in Austria [4,6], Italy [4], Germany [5] and Sweden [7] (Table 2). An additional unpublished case from Poland, listed in GenBank under accession number KP072001, is not discussed in this section. Interestingly, the five patients were over 50 years of age, splenectomized and diagnosed with hematological malignancies including Hodgkin's disease [4,5,7] and hairy cell leukemia in the fifth [6]. One of the Hodgkin's patients also had large B-cell lymphoma [4]. Four patients received immunosuppressive drugs including bleomycin [4], prednisolone + rituximab [5], methotrexate [6] and cyclosporine + prednisolone [5]. One patient developed mild [4], one patient mild-to-moderate [6] and three patients moderate-to-severe [4,5,7] disease. Reported symptoms were recurrent episodes of fever, progressive weakness, shortness of breath, thrombocytopenia, jaundice, abdominal pain, hemolytic anemia with elevated serum lactate dehydrogenase, elevated indirect bilirubin values, low haptoglobin levels and acute renal failure with dark urine as result of hemoglobinuria [4–7]. In two patients, a positive direct Coombs test led to an initial misdiagnosis of autoimmune hemolytic anemia potentially due to ongoing Hodgkin's disease [5] or ongoing hairy cell leukemia [6]. Moreover, elevated C-reactive protein and procalcitonin levels suggested persistent infection in two patients [5,7]. Bone marrow examination of the Swedish patients showed a few phagocytosing macrophages and monocytosis leading to a tentative diagnosis of hemophagocytic lymphohistiocytosis with supporting laboratory evidence including elevated triglycerides, ferritin and soluble interleukin-2- receptor [7]. Parasitemias in the *B. venatorum* infections ranged between 1.3% [4] and 30% [4,6]. While all patients eventually seroconverted [4–7], the German case remained seronegative for specific antibodies for several months and suffered a relapse after the conclusion of the initial treatment. Moreover, retreatment with atovaquone and azithromyin for two months was unsuccessful in clearing the parasite, and low-level parasitemia persisted for several months despite maintenance therapy with atovaquone, possibly due to the previous combined application of rituximab and prednisolone, which have highly immunosuppressive effects. The Swedish patient also had fluctuating parasitemia for several months, although it was not clear whether this was a natural feature of the infection or due to injections with human immunoglobulin [7]. All five patients were cured [4–7]. A study in China on people who sought medical help after a tick bite detected 48 out of 2912 individuals with *B. venatorum* infections [127], suggesting that cases caused by this parasite generally take a milder course than those caused by *B. divergens*, requiring special awareness for detection and appropriate treatment.

6.4. *Babesia microti*

6.4.1. Autochthonous *B. microti* Infections

Babesia microti infections in humans are rarely reported outside the United States. So far, only 11 autochthonous cases have been reported from Europe (Table 3). A marked characteristic of *B. microti* infections, in contrast to those caused by *B. divergens* and *B. venatorum*, is that the vast majority of cases have occurred in normosplenic patients. Moreover, asymptomatic infections appear to be common. However, clinical manifestations in asplenic patients are very similar to those caused by *B. divergens* and *B. venatorum*, often fulminating and resulting in death [32,42,113,114,128,129]. Patients who have recovered from acute babesiosis often maintain persistent asymptomatic parasitemia lasting for several months. In immunocompromised individuals, *B. microti* infections may even persist through multiple courses of treatment [42,130]. Relapse of illness is also more common in immunocompromised than previously healthy adults, but even in this group it may occur as long as 27 months after the initial illness [131,132]. Since many infections are asymptomatic and/or persistent, transmission of *B. microti* through blood transfusion is a serious public health threat in the USA [32,133]. Transfusion-related transmission may arise at any time of the year and incubation periods can be much longer than in tick-transmitted infection [134,135].

The first reported European case of *B. microti* occurred in Belgium in an otherwise healthy man in his 40s in Belgium in 1981 [81]. He suffered from fever and weight loss of 8 kg within one month. His serum was reactive for *R. conori* and *B. microti* and *B. rodhaini*. The patient was cured, but it is not clear whether he was infected with *B. microti* or if antibodies showed cross-reactivity with *Rickettsia* spp. [81]. The first validated case occurred in Germany [8] and is the only one so far in which parasites were observed within erythrocytes. The other nine documented cases occurred within the last six years in Poland [22,24] and Spain [25] and were diagnosed by the detection of parasite DNA. All patients had an intact spleen, and in all but one patient immunocompetence could be assumed. The exception was the German case, who was immunocompromised because of treatment for myeloid leukemia. In this case, a moderate disease developed with fever, heavy chest pain, hypertension, tachycardia and pancytopenia. Microscopy showed an initial parasitemia of 4.5% [8]. However, it is difficult to determine whether pancytopenia resulted from the *B. microti* infection, the underlying disease of acute myeloid leukemia or a combination of both. It is notable that this patient showed acute onset of babesiosis with clinical symptoms of coronary heart disease, probably due to ongoing anemia. Acute disease manifestation was followed by subsequent seroconversion for *B. microti*-specific antibodies six weeks later and points to a newly acquired infection rather than an acute exacerbation of a pre-existing subclinical parasitemia. The specific antibody response disappeared four weeks after seroconversion, probably owing to the start of another cycle of chemotherapy with cytarabine and idarubicin. The source of infection in this case was apparently an infected blood transfusion from an asymptomatic blood donor [8], whereas in the other patients tick-bite transmission is probable. The other patients with *B. microti* infections included two individuals, who were randomly identified as part of a study of forestry workers, employed in the Podlaskie province of Eastern Poland. Both were >45-years-old adults and reported several tick bites while working in forests over the preceding two years [22]. Six patients in Poland and one patient in Spain had a mild disease with nonspecific clinical symptoms such as fever, muscle pain, joint pain, headache, vertigo, fatigue and general malaise [24,25]. The case in Spain is an example of low-grade chronic human babesiosis caused by *B. microti*, with intermittent symptoms for a period of at least four months. Such cases may go undiagnosed in immunocompetent patients [25]. Altogether, four patients seroconverted and all those with symptoms were cured.

6.4.2. Imported *B. microti* Infections

Parasitemias of imported cases ranged up to 20% [90,91,93] (Table 3). Clinical symptoms were similar to those of autochthonous cases characterized by fever, fatigue, malaise, chills and headache, as well as signs of hemolytic anemia, thrombocytopenia, acute renal failure and multiorgan failure in severe cases [90,91,93]. Unusual symptoms were neck stiffness in a patient with additionally diagnosed neuroborreliosis [88], and lower back pain, continuous knee pain and erythematous skin changes without any detected co-infection [89]. Bone marrow aspiration of a patient with severe pancytopenia showed typical hemophagocytosis [87]. Although all 13 patients with imported *B. microti* infections were evidently in good health for travel [82–94], an 83-year-old man diagnosed with low-grade lymphoplasmacytic lymphoma died of the infection [93]. *Babesia microti* infection should definitely be a differential diagnosis in Europe, especially for patients with a travel history to the Americas.

7. Laboratory Diagnostics

As human babesiosis can take a fulminant course of disease, especially in immunocompromised patients infected with *B. divergens*, rapid diagnosis is essential. A study of patients infected with *B. microti* reported that cases where diagnosis was delayed for 7 days or more were significantly associated with more severe disease [115]. In Europe, misdiagnoses (malaria, autoimmune hemolytic anemia with positive Coombs test) and lack of awareness of the existence of *Babesia* spp. as a causative infective agent have occasionally led to delayed diagnosis in the past, resulting in prolonged and potentially life-threatening disease [1,14,25,68,85] (Table 1, Table 2, Table 3). Indeed, in some cases, human babesiosis was only diagnosed post mortem [1,68]. We strongly recommend that diagnostic procedures for babesiosis should be initiated in patients that present with intermittent fever, fever of unknown origin or signs of hemolytic anemia. Patient records should include information on potential immunocompromising conditions, exposure to ticks, having received blood transfusions and travel to the USA or China within the last 6 months.

Clinical laboratory diagnosis of human babesiosis is challenging and it is uncertain whether automated hematology analyzers can reliably detect piroplasms. Where there are typical clinical symptoms, a positive Coombs test in combination with hemolytic anemia and elevated procalcitonine levels is highly suggestive of babesiosis and should prompt further diagnostic testing [5,136].

7.1. Light Microscopy

Ideally, direct pathogen detection is recommended for a definitive diagnosis. The gold standard is microscopic detection in a Giemsa or Romanowsky stained blood smears [111,137]. However, early in the course of infection or because of a low-level parasitemia, parasites may be difficult to find and smears from serial blood collection must be investigated [80,137,138]. Malaria is the most important differential diagnosis because the early stages of *Plasmodium* spp. intraerythrocytic ring forms lack the parasite pigment (hemozoin) that occurs in later stages, and thus resemble the round forms of *Babesia* spp. Hence, reliable *Babesia* spp. identification is not possible microscopically unless paired pyriforms or tetrads (Maltese crosses) are seen [111]. Piroplasms appearing in thin blood smears are ring- or pear-shaped forms with reddish chromatin and slightly bluish cytoplasm (Figure 1). Babesia merozoites arranged as tetrads usually occur in cases where there is a high parasitemia and are mainly observed in Clade 1 *Babesia* spp. (*B. microti, B. duncani*), but also in *B. divergens*. Parasitemias can range from <1% to 80% of infected erythrocytes and are mostly low in immunocompetent patients and at the onset of disease. Therefore, a thorough evaluation of $\geq$300 fields of vision and serial preparation of multiple smears is recommended [111,137]. It is important to stress that for species identification, microscopical detection of parasites in blood smears without additional molecular analysis of the pathogen is not sufficient.

7.2. Molecular Diagnostics

Nucleic acid testing is usually performed as a PCR targeting the 18S rRNA gene. This test is sensitive and specific in detecting *Babesia* spp. from clotted or EDTA blood. Sequencing of the 18S rRNA gene can be used for species identification, which has an epidemiological and therapeutic significance. The detection limit is approx. 1–3 parasites/µL of blood, and thus below that of microscopic methods [139]. There are various modifications of the test format and the molecular target structure including DNA/RNA hybridization (e.g., FISH), and real-time PCR methods [4,139], but there is currently no commercial test or sufficiently validated protocol available in Europe for diagnosis confirmation by a broadly accepted gold standard test [111].

7.3. Culture

Babesia divergens, *B. microti* and *B. duncani* can be cultivated in gerbils, mice and hamsters, respectively, while *B. venatorum* has not yet been adapted to a laboratory animal species. Approximately 0.5–1 mL of EDTA or heparin anticoagulated whole blood are inoculated intraperitoneally, and the animal blood is monitored at least once a week for up to two months. Parasitemia is detectable after one week at the earliest but can be reliably detected after up to four weeks. There are many reasons why xenodiagnosis is impracticable in routine laboratories (e.g., labor-intensive and time-consuming process, availability, ethics and sensitivity). Likewise, the in vitro cultivation of piroplasms, which is possible in principle, requires sophisticated techniques, and is thus labor intensive and costly. Having in mind these practical drawbacks, culturing is reserved for specialized laboratories, although a broader approach to cultivating more isolates both from the veterinarian and the human medical fields is clearly desirable [111,140].

7.4. Infection Serology

The indirect immunofluorescence assay is the most commonly used serological test method. Cut-off titers for IgG antibodies from 1:32 to 1:160 were found to be sensitive (>88%) and specific (>90%) in multicenter studies with *B. microti* and *B. divergens* antigens [63,141]. However, cut-off titers should be adjusted to the local seroepidemiological situation and circulating *Babesia* species [63]. IgG titers of ≥1:1028 occur during the course of infection, which then decrease to titers of 1:64 within months to years. IgG assays do not reliably differentiate between acute, chronic or past infections [63,111,136,141]. On the other hand, IgM antibodies are detectable from approx. two weeks after the onset of symptoms onwards and indicate acute infection [141,142]. However, since false IgM-positive test results are common, particularly as part of untargeted testing in non-endemic areas, a two-step procedure is required in which only IgG-positive samples are further tested for the presence of IgM antibodies [63,140]. Assays that detect anti-*B. microti* antibodies do not detect antibodies against *B. duncani*, *B. divergens* or *B. venatorum* [143]. In contrast, cross-reactivity between *B. divergens* and *B. venatorum* can be exploited diagnostically [5,137].

In addition to the general limitations of immunofluorescence assays (unknown test quality, investigator dependent variability, etc.), false-positive reactions have been described in sera from rheumatic patients and from patients with other, especially closely related infectious diseases such as malaria and toxoplasmosis [63,143]. Furthermore, the antibody response may not yet be present in the early phase as shown in acute European case reports or may be absent in immunocompromised individuals [5,136,140]. Therefore, it is not suitable for acute diagnosis but primarily for epidemiological purposes. Several publications describe other immunoassay formats (e.g., enzyme immunoassays, bead-based assays or immunoblots) that use a wide variety of antigens [140]. However, standardized serological test methods that have been validated by multicenter studies are currently not available in Europe due to low demand and lack of diagnostic evaluation.

Finally, it should be stated that, except for research and surveillance purposes, the practice of generally applying multiplex approaches for molecular diagnostics and/or serology in patients after a tick bite or in individuals with suspected Lyme borreliosis is not recommended, because from a statistical stand point, such diagnostic regimes will end up with many false-positive test results given the generally low incidence of tick-borne infections other than Lyme borreliosis in most European countries.

8. Clinical Management

Several drugs are available for the treatment of human babesiosis (Table 4), but their efficacy is variable, particularly against *B. microti*, which animal studies suggest is less susceptible to classic antibabesials than are *B. divergens* and *B. venatorum* [144]. However, available information on antibabesial susceptibility from case reports and clinical investigations suggests that there is no convincing scientific evidence for any clinically relevant differences in the susceptibilities of the pathogenic *Babesia* spp. to the therapeutic agents commonly used to treat human babesiosis [111,145]. Nevertheless, there is room for improvement in drug efficacy, particularly in relation to side effects, drug resistance and speed of response. In the case of most infections caused by *B. divergens* and *B. venatorum*, as well as severe cases of *B. microti* infection, the speed of response to antibabesial administration is particularly important, and adjunct measures are often necessary. Most of the recent cases of human babesiosis caused by previously unknown *Babesia* spp. have responded to antibabesials used against known species [111,145]. However, until further data become available, treatment of infections caused by unknown *Babesia* spp. should include close monitoring of the course of parasitemia and long-term follow-up of such patients.

Table 4. Commonly and experimentally used drugs for the treatment of human babesiosis (modified from Hildebrandt et al., 2013 [111]).

Drug (Generic Name)	Regular Single Dose	Application	Dosage Regimen
Adults	**Dose—70 kg adult**		
Standard drugs			
Quinine	650 mg	p.o.	3 times daily
Clindamycin	600 mg	p.o., i.v.	3 times daily
Azithromycin	500 mg/1st day, 250 mg thereafter [a]	p.o., i.v.	once daily
Atovaquone	750 mg	p.o.	twice daily
Doxycycline	200 mg	p.o.	once daily
Unlicensed Drugs for Human Babesiosis [g]			
Pentamidine	4 mg/kg/day	i.v.	once daily
Trimethoprim/sulfametoxazole	4/20 mg/kg	p.o., i.v.	twice daily
Proguanil	400 mg/day	p.o.	once daily
Imidocarb dipropionate [h]	0.6 mg/kg	i.m.	12 hourly for 4 doses
Children	**Dose/kg**		
Standard drugs			
Quinine	8 mg [c]	p.o.	3 times daily
Clindamycin	7–10 mg [d]	p.o., i.v.	3 times daily
Azithromycin [b]	10 mg/1st day 5 mg/day thereafter [e]	p.o., i.v.	once daily
Atovaquone	20 mg/day [f]	p.o.	twice daily

[a] In immunocompromised patients, higher initial doses (600–1000 mg/day) may be required. [b] In immunocompromised patients, higher dose may be required. [c] maximum: 650 mg per dose. [d] maximum: 600 mg per dose, [e] maximum: 250 mg per dose. [f] maximum: 750 mg per dose. [g] In addition to standard drugs, alternative substances have been used successfully in some severe adult cases of babesiosis (see also Table 3) (111). [h] Imidocarb dipropionate is not licensed for use in humans. The dosing regimen for treatment of human babesiosis is derived from two successfully treated Irish cases with *B. divergens* infections (146).

8.1. *Babesia divergens*

Although sporadically observed in immunocompetent patients with viral-like illnesses, clinical cases of *B. divergens* have almost always been reported in asplenic or spleen-impaired individuals [71,78,111]. Many *B. divergens* infections in the past ended fatally with general organ failure occurring four to seven days after the initial presentation of hemoglobinuria. Outcome data in severely ill asplenic individuals show a mortality rate of 42% [27,70,71,137,146]. Consequently, the status of asplenic *B. divergens*-infected patients is regarded as a medical emergency, requiring immediate treatment to arrest hemolysis and prevent complications [111,137]. The combination of clindamycin and quinine for 7 to 10 days (Table 5) dramatically improves disease outcome [137,146–149], but in recent years, a more favorable disease course has been increasingly reported for *B. divergens*-infected patients, including those not treated with a full course of clindamycin and quinine because of quinine side effects [70,111,150]. These findings underscore the impact of improved adjunctive measures provided by modern intensive care medicine, including exchange transfusion [111,137]. This measure is usually reserved only for the most extremely ill *B. microti*-infected patients but has also been recommended for all severe *B. divergens* cases [27,111,137,145]. Alternative treatment options for *B. divergens* infections have included clindamycin monotherapy or imidocarb in conjunction with the above-mentioned adjunctive measures (Table 4) [69,102,111,137,151]. Imidocarb, one of the most effective antimicrobials for use in *Babesia*-infected animals, is highly active against this organism in vitro [152]. It was used successfully to treat two Irish patients infected with *B. divergens* but is not licensed for use in humans [153]. Atovaquone proved more effective than imidocarb in an experimental *B. divergens* gerbil model and perhaps should be considered in combination with azithromycin for treatment of *B. divergens* infections and more generally for those caused by any *Babesia* s.s. species [152]. Atovaquone, together with either azithromycin or proguanil, has been used in three recent cases, following problems with toxicity or inadequate efficacy of other drug regimens [74–76], and it resulted in patient recovery in two of them [74,75].

Table 5. Commonly used drug combinations and treatment alternatives for human babesiosis with regard to parasite species and severity of the disease (adapted and modified from Hildebrandt et al., 2013 [111]).

Parasite	Mild Disease [a] (Drug)	Severe Disease [a,b] (Drug)	Adjunctive/Alternative Therapy in Severe Cases [b]
B. divergens	clindamycin	clindamycin *plus* quinine	Exchange transfusion, hemodialysis *consider* atovaquone/azithromycin, atovaquone/proguanil *or* pentamidine/ trimethoprim-sulfametoxazole *as possible alternatives for severe and intractable infections*
B. venatorum	clindamycin	clindamycin *plus* quinine	Exchange transfusion, *Consider alternative treatment with* atovaquone/azithromycin *or* atovaquone/proguanil *in persisting babesiosis*
B. microti	atovaquone *plus* azithromycin	clindamycin *plus* quinine	Exchange transfusion hemodialysis *Consider adding* doxycycline *or* proguanil *in relapsing or persisting babesiosis*

[a] Usual duration of treatment is 7–10 days. Longer treatment (>6 weeks) may be necessary in immunocompromised or relapsed patients. In immunocompromised individuals, reduction of immunosuppressive therapy may be needed if possible for clearing the parasite. [b] Severe illness criteria according to White et al., 1998 [113]: parasitemia > 4%, alkaline phosphatase >125 U/L and white blood cell counts >5 × 10^9/L. Partial or complete exchange transfusion is recommended in case of high parasitemia (>10%), severe anemia (<10 g/dL) and pulmonary or hepatic failure. In severe disease cases i.v. treatment is suggested. Alternative treatments as derived from single case reports or case studies cited in the literature (Hildebrandt et al., 2013 [111]).

Although quinine, clindamycin, atovaquone and azithromycin, and some in combination, are proven antibabesials for the treatment of *B. divergens* infections in humans, there are concerns about rapid efficacy, drug resistance and recrudescent infections. However, cases do not occur frequently enough to justify research in drug discovery and development for human treatment alone. In recent years a significant number of drugs have been tested against this parasite in vitro for veterinary use, for example atranorin [154], cryptolepine [155], fusidic acid [156], hydroxyurea and eflornithine [155], myrrh oil [157] trans-chalcone and chalcone 4 hydrate [158], and the hope is that promising drugs will also prove useful for human infections.

8.2. *Babesia venatorum*

In general clindamycin with or without quinine and with or without subsequent combined atovaquone and azithromycin treatment have been used successfully in European cases of *B. venatorum* infection [5–7]. Problems with speed of response to therapy and parasite persistence occurred in one case [5].

In contrast to the more sporadic occurrence of *B. venatorum* cases in Europe, the disease is endemic in northwestern China with more than 48 reported cases [159–162], all of which were immunocompetent, in contrast to European patients. In these cases, 4 of the 48 Chinese patients received clindamycin alone and no deaths were reported [162]. Although the clinical course of *B. venatorum* generally seems to be milder than that of *B. divergens*, clinicians should be aware that immunocompromised patients might experience relapse and persistence of infection despite antimicrobial treatment. In such cases, it is important to monitor parasitemia by blood smear examination and PCR analysis and provide long-term clinical follow-up [5,111].

8.3. *Babesia microti*

Autochthonous *B. microti* infections in Europe are rare and most cases have been reported in travelers, mainly those returning from the USA. In such cases, treatment should follow American standards [145]. Animal studies showed that regimes of azithromycin in combination with quinine [163], azithromycin with atovaquone [164] and atovaquone with clindamycin [144] were all effective (Tables 4 and 5).

Randomized trials in humans infected with *B. microti* showed that atovaquone plus azithromycin therapy was as effective as the standard quinine/clindamycin combination and there were fewer side effects (15% versus 72%) [165]. In view of the low risk of side effects associated with atovaquone/azithromycin, it has been argued that all patients diagnosed with *B. microti* infection should be treated with this drug combination [111,137]. In severe cases, similar adjunctive measures to those used for *B. divergens* infections may be necessary [111] (Table 5).

Major obstacles to the development of new drugs against *B. microti* are, firstly, that a continuous in vitro culture system is lacking for this parasite despite much research on the topic, and secondly, that although continuous culture systems already exist for *Babesia* s.s. species such as *B. divergens* [152], antibabesials developed against these parasites appear to be relatively ineffective against *B. microti* [144]. However, the recent successful development of continuous in vitro culture systems for *Babesia duncani*, using human or hamster erythrocytes [166,167] promises progress in this area since *B. duncani* is more closely related to *B. microti* than to the *Babesia* s.s. species [10].

8.4. *Exchange Transfusion Management*

Exchange transfusion has been recommended for severe *B. microti* infection characterized by parasitemias of more than 10%, and/or severe anemia (hemoglobin <10 g/dL) and/or evidence of organ dysfunction (hepatic, pulmonary or renal compromise), as well as for all emergency cases involving *B. divergens* [111,137,145]. Such a procedure can contribute to the rapid reduction of parasitemia, correction of anemia and elimination of toxins and harmful metabolites, but it is complex and should take place under the supervision of specialised hematologists, taking into account the status and co-morbidities of the patient. Although erythrocyte exchange transfusion as an adjunct to treatment of severely ill patients can be life-saving in selected cases [168], it requires more research, since there has not yet been a prospective clinical study of outcomes of exchange transfusion combined with antimicrobial agents, compared with antimicrobial agents alone.

9. Conclusions

The spread of infectious diseases among people and animals is a worldwide challenge. The One Health approach provides the opportunity to systematically and comprehensively address emerging zoonoses such as human babesiosis in order to increase awareness of the risk of infection and improve precise diagnostic and seroprevalence tests and treatment protocols. Advances in laboratory methodologies are required to increase our knowledge and understanding of the diversity of zoonotic *Babesia* species and the roles that domestic animals, wildlife and tick populations play in their maintenance. Further development of laboratory tools is necessary for babesia research, including molecular characterization of *Babesia* species and in vitro culture, particularly for testing parasite susceptibility to antibabesial drugs, and the development of screening diagnostics that can be used routinely, for example for the protection of the transfusion blood supply. The improvement of patient care continues to be important, as awareness is raised among health care professionals and the provision of information on disease prevention behavior is considered by local, national and international governmental institutions.

Author Contributions: Conceptualization, J.G., K.-P.H. and E.M.; Investigation A.H., J.G., A.Z., K.-P.H. and E.M.; Writing—original draft preparation, A.H., J.G., A.Z. and K.-P.H.; Writing—review and editing, A.H., J.G., A.Z., K.-P.H. and E.M.; Supervision, K.-P.H. and J.G.; Project administration, E.M. and J.G.; Funding, K.-P.H. Acquisition, K.-P.H. All authors have read and agreed to the published version of the manuscript.

Funding: Funding has been provided by a grant from the Society for Promoting Quality Assurance in Medical Laboratories (INSTAND, e.V. Düsseldorf) and a grant from the Health Institute Carlos III (PI20CIII/00037 to EM and LGM), Spain.

Institutional Review Board Statement: Not applicable.

Informed Consent Statement: Not applicable.

Data Availability Statement: Not applicable.

Conflicts of Interest: The authors declare no conflict of interest.

References

1. Skrabalo, Z.; Deanovic, Z. Piroplasmosis in man; report of a case. *Doc. Med. Geogr. Trop.* **1957**, *9*, 11–16.
2. M'Fadyean, J.; Stockman, S. A new species of piroplasm found in the blood of British cattle. *Comp. Path. Ther.* **1911**, *24*, 340–354. [CrossRef]
3. Fitzpatrick, J.E.; Kennedy, C.C.; McGeown, M.G.; Oreopoulos, D.G.; Robertson, J.H.; Soyannwo, M.A. Human case of piroplasmosis (babesiosis). *Nature* **1968**, *217*, 861–862. [CrossRef]
4. Herwaldt, B.L.; Cacció, S.; Gherlinzoni, F.; Aspöck, H.; Slemenda, S.B.; Piccaluga, P.; Martinelli, G.; Edelhofer, R.; Hollenstein, U.; Poletti, G.; et al. Molecular characterization of a non-*Babesia divergens* organism causing zoonotic babesiosis in Europe. *Emerg. Infect. Dis.* **2003**, *9*, 942–948. [CrossRef]
5. Häselbarth, K.; Tenter, A.M.; Brade, V.; Krieger, G.; Hunfeld, K.P. First case of human babesiosis in Germany—Clinical presentation and molecular characterisation of the pathogen. *Int. J. Med. Microbiol. IJMM* **2007**, *297*, 197–204. [CrossRef]
6. Blum, S.; Gattringer, R.; Haschke, E.; Walochnik, J.; Tschurtschenthaler, G.; Lang, F.; Oberbauer, R. The case: Hemolysis and acute renal failure. Babesiosis. *Kidney Int.* **2011**, *80*, 681–683. [CrossRef]
7. Bläckberg, J.; Lazarevic, V.L.; Hunfeld, K.P.; Persson, K.E.M. Low-virulent *Babesia venatorum* infection masquerading as hemophagocytic syndrome. *Ann. Hematol.* **2018**, *97*, 731–733. [CrossRef]
8. Hildebrandt, A.; Hunfeld, K.P.; Baier, M.; Krumbholz, A.; Sachse, S.; Lorenzen, T.; Kiehntopf, M.; Fricke, H.J.; Straube, E. First confirmed autochthonous case of human *Babesia microti* infection in Europe. *Eur. J. Clin. Microbiol. Infect. Dis. Off. Publ. Eur. Soc. Clin. Microbiol.* **2007**, *26*, 595–601. [CrossRef] [PubMed]
9. Westblade, L.F.; Simon, M.S.; Mathison, B.A.; Kirkman, L.A. *Babesia microti*: From mice to ticks to an increasing number of highly susceptible humans. *J. Clin. Microbiol.* **2017**, *55*, 2903–2912. [CrossRef] [PubMed]
10. Jalovecka, M.; Sojka, D.; Ascencio, M.; Schnittger, L. Babesia life cycle—When phylogeny meets biology. *Trends Parasitol.* **2019**, *35*, 356–368. [CrossRef] [PubMed]
11. Gray, J.; Zintl, A.; Hildebrandt, A.; Hunfeld, K.P.; Weiss, L. Zoonotic babesiosis: Overview of the disease and novel aspects of pathogen identity. *Ticks Tick-Borne Dis.* **2010**, *1*, 3–10. [CrossRef] [PubMed]
12. Olmeda, A.S.; Armstrong, P.M.; Rosenthal, B.M.; Valladares, B.; del Castillo, A.; de Armas, F.; Miguelez, M.; Gonzalez, A.; Rodriguez Rodriguez, J.A.; Spielman, A.; et al. A subtropical case of human babesiosis. *Acta Trop.* **1997**, *67*, 229–234. [CrossRef]
13. Petney, T.N.; Otranto, D.; Dantas-Torres, F.; Pfaffle, M.P. Ixodes ventalloi Gil Collado, 1936. In *Ticks of Europe and North. Africa. A Guide to Species Identification*; Estrada-Peña, A., Mihalca, A.D., Petney, T., Eds.; Springer: Berlin/Heidelberg, Germany, 2017; p. 183.
14. Centeno-Lima, S.; do Rosário, V.; Parreira, R.; Maia, A.J.; Freudenthal, A.M.; Nijhof, A.M.; Jongejan, F. A fatal case of human babesiosis in Portugal: Molecular and phylogenetic analysis. *Trop. Med. Int. Health TMIH* **2003**, *8*, 760–764. [CrossRef]
15. Fanelli, A. A historical review of *Babesia* spp. associated with deer in Europe: *Babesia divergens/Babesia divergens*-like, *Babesia capreoli*, *Babesia venatorum*, *Babesia* cf. *odocoilei*. *Vet. Parasitol.* **2021**, *294*, 109433. [CrossRef] [PubMed]
16. Azagi, T.; Jaarsma, R.I.; Docters van Leeuwen, A.; Fonville, M.; Maas, M.; Franssen, F.F.J.; Kik, M.; Rijks, J.M.; Montizaan, M.G.; Groenevelt, M.; et al. Circulation of *Babesia* species and their exposure to humans through *Ixodes ricinus*. *Pathogens* **2021**, *10*, 386. [CrossRef] [PubMed]
17. Gray, A.; Capewell, P.; Zadoks, R.; Taggart, M.A.; French, A.; Katzer, F.; Shiels, B.R.; William Weir, W. Wild deer in the United Kingdom are a potential reservoir for the livestock parasite *Babesia divergens*. *Curr. Res. Parasitol. Vector-Borne Dis.* **2021**, *1*, 100019. [CrossRef]

18. Yang, Y.; Christie, J.; Koster, L.; Du, A.; Yao, C. Emerging human babesiosis with "Ground Zero" in North America. *Microorganisms* **2021**, *9*, 440. [CrossRef]
19. Zamoto-Niikura, A.; Tsuji, M.; Qiang, W.; Morikawa, S.; Hanaki, K.I.; Holman, P.J.; Ishihara, C. The *Babesia divergens* Asia lineage is maintained through enzootic cycles between *Ixodes persulcatus* and sika deer in Hokkaido, Japan. *Appl. Environ. Microbiol.* **2018**, *84*, e02491-17. [CrossRef]
20. Goethert, H.K.; Telford, S.R. What is *Babesia microti*? *Parasitology* **2003**, *127*, 301–309. [CrossRef]
21. Goethert, H.K.; Molloy, P.; Berardi, V.; Weeks, K.; Telford, S.R. Zoonotic *Babesia microti* in the northeastern U.S.: Evidence for the expansion of a specific parasite lineage. *PLoS ONE* **2018**, *13*, e0193837. [CrossRef] [PubMed]
22. Welc-Faleciak, R.; Pawelczyk, A.; Radkowski, M.; Pancewicz, S.A.; Zajkowska, J.; Sinski, E. First report of two asymptomatic cases of human infection with *Babesia microti* (Franca, 1910) in Poland. *Ann. Agric. Environ. Med. AAEM* **2015**, *22*, 51–54. [CrossRef]
23. Sinski, E.; Bajer, A.; Welc, R.; Pawelczyk, A.; Ogrzewalska, M.; Behnke, J.M. *Babesia microti*: Prevalence in wild rodents and *Ixodes ricinus* ticks from the Mazury Lakes District of North-Eastern Poland. *Int. J. Med. Microbiol. IJMM* **2006**, *296* (Suppl. S40), 137–143. [CrossRef] [PubMed]
24. Moniuszko-Malinowska, A.; Świecicka, I.; Dunaj, J.; Zajkowska, J.; Czupryna, P.; Zambrowski, G.; Chmielewska-Badora, J.; Żukiewicz-Sobczak, W.; Swierzbinska, R.; Rutkowski, K.; et al. Infection with *Babesia microti* in humans with non-specific symptoms in North East Poland. *Infect. Dis.* **2016**, *48*, 537–543. [CrossRef]
25. Arsuaga, M.; Gonzalez, L.M.; Lobo, C.A.; de la Calle, F.; Bautista, J.M.; Azcarate, I.G.; Puente, S.; Montero, E. First report of *Babesia microti*-caused babesiosis in Spain. *Vector Borne Zoonotic Dis.* **2016**, *16*, 677–679. [CrossRef]
26. Arsuaga, M.; Gonzalez, L.M.; Padial, E.S.; Dinkessa, A.W.; Sevilla, E.; Trigo, E.; Puente, S.; Gray, J.; Montero, E. Misdiagnosis of babesiosis as malaria, Equatorial Guinea, 2014. *Emerg. Infect. Dis.* **2018**, *24*, 1588–1589. [CrossRef]
27. Zintl, A.; Mulcahy, G.; Skerrett, H.E.; Taylor, S.M.; Gray, J.S. *Babesia divergens*, a bovine blood parasite of veterinary and zoonotic importance. *Clin. Microbiol. Rev.* **2003**, *16*, 622–636. [CrossRef]
28. Clawson, M.L.; Paciorkowski, N.; Rajan, T.V.; La Vake, C.; Pope, C.; La Vake, M.; Wikel, S.K.; Krause, P.J.; Radolf, J.D. Cellular immunity, but not gamma interferon, is essential for resolution of *Babesia microti* infection in BALB/c mice. *Infect. Immun.* **2002**, *70*, 5304–5306. [CrossRef] [PubMed]
29. Hemmer, R.M.; Ferrick, D.A.; Conrad, P.A. Role of T cells and cytokines in fatal and resolving experimental babesiosis: Protection in TNFRp55-/- mice infected with the human *Babesia* WA1 parasite. *J. Parasitol.* **2000**, *86*, 736–742. [CrossRef] [PubMed]
30. Aguilar-Delfin, I.; Wettstein, P.J.; Persing, D.H. Resistance to acute babesiosis is associated with interleukin-12- and gamma interferon-mediated responses and requires macrophages and natural killer cells. *Infect. Immun.* **2003**, *71*, 2002–2008. [CrossRef] [PubMed]
31. Telford, S.R., III; Maguire, J.H. Babesiosis. In *Tropical Infectious Diseases: Principles, Pathogens, and Practice*, 2nd ed.; Guerrant, R.L., Walker, D.H., Weller, P.F., Eds.; Churchill Livingstone; Elsevier: Amsterdam, The Netherlands, 2006; pp. 1063–1071.
32. Krause, P.J. Human babesiosis. *Int. J. Parasitol.* **2019**, *49*, 165–174. [CrossRef]
33. Krause, P.J.; Daily, J.; Telford, S.R.; Vannier, E.; Lantos, P.; Spielman, A. Shared features in the pathobiology of babesiosis and malaria. *Trends Parasitol.* **2007**, *23*, 605–610. [CrossRef]
34. Hemmer, R.M.; Ferrick, D.A.; Conrad, P.A. Up-regulation of tumor necrosis factor-alpha and interferon-gamma expression in the spleen and lungs of mice infected with the human *Babesia* isolate WA1. *Parasitol. Res.* **2000**, *86*, 121–128. [CrossRef] [PubMed]
35. Shaio, M.F.; Lin, P.R. A case study of cytokine profiles in acute human babesiosis. *Am. J. Trop. Med. Hyg.* **1998**, *58*, 335–337. [CrossRef]
36. Clark, I.A.; Jacobson, L.S. Do babesiosis and malaria share a common disease process? *Ann. Trop. Med. Parasitol.* **1998**, *92*, 483–488. [CrossRef] [PubMed]
37. Vannier, E.; Borggraefe, I.; Telford, S.R., III; Menon, S.; Brauns, T.; Spielman, A.; Gelfand, J.A.; Wortis, H.H. Age-associated decline in resistance to *Babesia microti* is genetically determined. *J. Infect. Dis.* **2004**, *189*, 1721–1728. [CrossRef] [PubMed]
38. Terkawi, M.A.; Cao, S.; Herbas, M.S.; Nishimura, M.; Li, Y.; Moumouni, P.F.; Pyarokhil, A.H.; Kondoh, D.; Kitamura, N.; Nishikawa, Y.; et al. Macrophages are the determinant of resistance to and outcome of nonlethal *Babesia microti* infection in mice. *Infect. Immun.* **2015**, *83*, 8–16. [CrossRef] [PubMed]
39. Mebius, R.E.; Kraal, G. Structure and function of the spleen. *Nat. Rev. Immunol.* **2005**, *5*, 606–616. [CrossRef]
40. Vannier, E.; Krause, P.J. Human babesiosis. *N. Engl. J. Med.* **2012**, *366*, 2397–2407. [CrossRef]
41. Bloch, E.M.; Kumar, S.; Krause, P.J. Persistence of *Babesia microti* infection in humans. *Pathogens* **2019**, *8*, 102. [CrossRef] [PubMed]
42. Krause, P.J.; Gewurz, B.E.; Hill, D.; Marty, F.M.; Vannier, E.; Foppa, I.M.; Furman, R.R.; Neuhaus, E.; Skowron, G.; Gupta, S.; et al. Persistent and relapsing babesiosis in immunocompromised patients. *Clin. Infect. Dis. Off. Publ. Infect. Dis. Soc. Am.* **2008**, *46*, 370–376. [CrossRef]
43. Tahir, F.; Ahmed, J.; Malik, F. Post-splenectomy sepsis: A review of the literature. *Cureus* **2020**, *12*, e6898. [CrossRef] [PubMed]
44. Haapasalo, K.; Suomalainen, P.; Sukura, A.; Siikamaki, H.; Jokiranta, T.S. Fatal babesiosis in man, Finland, 2004. *Emerg. Infect. Dis.* **2010**, *16*, 1116–1118. [CrossRef] [PubMed]
45. Entrican, J.H.; Williams, H.; Cook, I.A.; Lancaster, W.M.; Clark, J.C.; Joyner, L.P.; Lewis, D. Babesiosis in man: A case from Scotland. *Br. Med. J.* **1979**, *2*, 474. [CrossRef]
46. Clarke, C.S.; Rogers, E.T.; Egan, E.L. Babesiosis: Under-reporting or case-clustering? *Postgrad. Med. J.* **1989**, *65*, 591–593. [CrossRef]

47. Fitzpatrick, J.E.; Kennedy, C.C.; McGeown, M.G.; Oreopoulos, D.G.; Robertson, J.H.; Soyannwo, M.A. Further details of third recorded case of redwater (Babesiosis) in man. *Br. Med. J.* **1969**, *4*, 770–772. [CrossRef] [PubMed]
48. Clark, I.A.; Budd, A.C.; Hsue, G.; Haymore, B.R.; Joyce, A.J.; Thorner, R.; Krause, P.J. Absence of erythrocyte sequestration in a case of babesiosis in a splenectomized human patient. *Malar. J.* **2006**, *5*, 69. [CrossRef]
49. Gray, J.S. The development and seasonal activity of the tick, *Ixodes ricinus*: A vector of Lyme borreliosis. *Rev. Med. Vet. Entomol.* **1991**, *79*, 323–333.
50. Gray, J.; Kahl, O.; Zintl, A. What do we still need to know about *Ixodes ricinus*? *Ticks Tick-Borne Dis.* **2021**, *12*, 101682. [CrossRef]
51. Joyner, L.P.; Davies, S.F.; Kendall, S.B. The experimental transmission of *Babesia divergens* by *Ixodes ricinus*. *Exp. Parasitol.* **1963**, *14*, 367–373. [CrossRef]
52. Donnelly, J.; Peirce, M.A. Experiments on the transmission of *Babesia divergens* to cattle by the tick *Ixodes ricinus*. *Int. J. Parasitol.* **1975**, *5*, 363–367. [CrossRef]
53. Mackenstedt, U.; Gauer, M.; Mehlhorn, H.; Schein, E.; Hauschild, S. Sexual cycle of *Babesia divergens* confirmed by DNA measurements. *Parasitol. Res.* **1990**, *76*, 199–206. [CrossRef]
54. Bonnet, S.; Jouglin, M.; L'Hostis, M.; Chauvin, A. *Babesia* sp. EU1 from roe deer and transmission within *Ixodes ricinus*. *Emerg. Infect. Dis.* **2007**, *13*, 1208–1210. [CrossRef] [PubMed]
55. Bonnet, S.; Brisseau, N.; Hermouet, A.; Jouglin, M.; Chauvin, A. Experimental in vitro transmission of *Babesia* sp. (EU1) by *Ixodes ricinus*. *Vet. Res.* **2009**, *40*, 21. [CrossRef] [PubMed]
56. Walter, G.; Weber, G. A study on the transmission (transstadial, transovarial) of *Babesia microti*, strain "Hannover i", in its tick vector, *Ixodes ricinus* (author's transl). *Trop. Parasitol.* **1981**, *32*, 228–230.
57. Gray, J.; von Stedingk, L.V.; Gurtelschmid, M.; Granstrom, M. Transmission studies of *Babesia microti* in *Ixodes ricinus* ticks and gerbils. *J. Clin. Microbiol.* **2002**, *40*, 1259–1263. [CrossRef]
58. Lempereur, L.; Lebrun, M.; Cuvelier, P.; Sepult, G.; Caron, Y.; Saegerman, C.; Shiels, B.; Losson, B. Longitudinal field study on bovine *Babesia* spp. and *Anaplasma phagocytophilum* infections during a grazing season in Belgium. *Parasitol. Res.* **2012**, *110*, 1525–1530. [CrossRef]
59. Springer, A.; Holtershinken, M.; Lienhart, F.; Ermel, S.; Rehage, J.; Hulskotter, K.; Lehmbecker, A.; Wohlsein, P.; Barutzki, D.; Gietl, C.; et al. Emergence and epidemiology of bovine babesiosis due to *Babesia divergens* on a Northern German beef production farm. *Front. Vet. Sci.* **2020**, *7*, 649. [CrossRef]
60. Onyiche, T.E.; Raileanu, C.; Fischer, S.; Silaghi, C. Global distribution of *Babesia* species in questing ticks: A systematic review and meta-analysis based on published literature. *Pathogens* **2021**, *10*, 230. [CrossRef]
61. Asman, M.; Witecka, J.; Korbecki, J.; Solarz, K. The potential risk of exposure to *Borrelia garinii*, *Anaplasma phagocytophilum* and *Babesia microti* in the Wolinski National Park (north-western Poland). *Sci. Rep.* **2021**, *11*, 4860. [CrossRef]
62. Bown, K.J.; Lambin, X.; Telford, G.R.; Ogden, N.H.; Telfer, S.; Woldehiwet, Z.; Birtles, R.J. Relative importance of *Ixodes ricinus* and *Ixodes trianguliceps* as vectors for *Anaplasma phagocytophilum* and *Babesia microti* in field vole (*Microtus agrestis*) populations. *Appl. Environ. Microbiol.* **2008**, *74*, 7118–7125. [CrossRef] [PubMed]
63. Hunfeld, K.P.; Lambert, A.; Kampen, H.; Albert, S.; Epe, C.; Brade, V.; Tenter, A.M. Seroprevalence of *Babesia* infections in humans exposed to ticks in midwestern Germany. *J. Clin. Microbiol.* **2002**, *40*, 2431–2436. [CrossRef]
64. Gorenflot, A.; Moubri, K.; Precigout, E.; Carcy, B.; Schetters, T.P. Human babesiosis. *Ann. Trop. Med. Parasitol.* **1998**, *92*, 489–501. [CrossRef]
65. Uhnoo, I.; Cars, O.; Christensson, D.; Nystrom-Rosander, C. First documented case of human babesiosis in Sweden. *Scand. J. Infect. Dis.* **1992**, *24*, 541–547. [CrossRef]
66. Miguelez, M.; Linares Feria, M.; Gonzalez, A.; Mesa, M.C.; Armas, F.; Laynez, P. Human babesiosis in a patient after splenectomy. *Med. Clin.* **1996**, *106*, 427–429.
67. Loutan, L.; Rossier, J.; Zufferey, G.; Cuenod, D.; Hatz, C.; Marti, H.P.; Gern, L. Imported babesiosis diagnosed as malaria. *Lancet* **1993**, *342*, 749. [CrossRef]
68. Rabinovich, S.A.; Voronina, Z.K.; Stepanova, N.I.; Maruashvili, G.M.; Bakradze, T.L. 1st detection of human babesiasis in the USSR and a short analysis of the cases described in the literature. *Meditsinskaia Parazitol. I Parazit. Bolezn.* **1978**, *47*, 97–107.
69. Denes, E.; Rogez, J.P.; Dardé, M.L.; Weinbreck, P. Management of *Babesia divergens* babesiosis without a complete course of quinine treatment. *Eur. J. Clin. Microbiol. Infect. Dis. Off. Publ. Eur. Soc. Clin. Microbiol.* **1999**, *18*, 672–673. [CrossRef] [PubMed]
70. Corpelet, C.; Vacher, P.; Coudore, F.; Laurichesse, H.; Conort, N.; Souweine, B. Role of quinine in life-threatening *Babesia divergens* infection successfully treated with clindamycin. *Eur. J. Clin. Microbiol. Infect. Dis. Off. Publ. Eur. Soc. Clin. Microbiol.* **2005**, *24*, 74–75. [CrossRef] [PubMed]
71. Martinot, M.; Zadeh, M.M.; Hansmann, Y.; Grawey, I.; Christmann, D.; Aguillon, S.; Jouglin, M.; Chauvin, A.; De Briel, D. Babesiosis in immunocompetent patients, Europe. *Emerg. Infect. Dis.* **2011**, *17*, 114–116. [CrossRef]
72. Paleau, A.; Candolfi, E.; Souply, L.; De Briel, D.; Delarbre, J.M.; Lipsker, D.; Jouglin, M.; Malandrin, L.; Hansmann, Y.; Martinot, M. Human babesiosis in Alsace. *Med. Mal. Infect.* **2020**, *50*, 486–491. [CrossRef] [PubMed]
73. Mørch, K.; Holmaas, G.; Frolander, P.S.; Kristoffersen, E.K. Severe human *Babesia divergens* infection in Norway. *Int. J. Infect. Dis. IJID Off. Publ. Int. Soc. Infect. Dis.* **2015**, *33*, 37–38. [CrossRef]

74. Gonzalez, L.M.; Castro, E.; Lobo, C.A.; Richart, A.; Ramiro, R.; Gonzalez-Camacho, F.; Luque, D.; Velasco, A.C.; Montero, E. First report of *Babesia divergens* infection in an HIV patient. *Int. J. Infect. Dis. IJID Off. Publ. Int. Soc. Infect. Dis.* **2015**, *33*, 202–204. [CrossRef] [PubMed]
75. Gonzalez, L.M.; Rojo, S.; Gonzalez-Camacho, F.; Luque, D.; Lobo, C.A.; Montero, E. Severe babesiosis in immunocompetent man, Spain, 2011. *Emerg. Infect. Dis.* **2014**, *20*, 724–726. [CrossRef]
76. Asensi, V.; Gonzalez, L.M.; Fernandez-Suarez, J.; Sevilla, E.; Navascues, R.A.; Suarez, M.L.; Lauret, M.E.; Bernardo, A.; Carton, J.A.; Montero, E. A fatal case of *Babesia divergens* infection in Northwestern Spain. *Ticks Tick-Borne Dis.* **2018**, *9*, 730–734. [CrossRef] [PubMed]
77. Tanyel, E.; Guler, N.; Hokelek, M.; Ulger, F.; Sunbul, M. A case of severe babesiosis treated successfully with exchange transfusion. *Int. J. Infect. Dis. IJID Off. Publ. Int. Soc. Infect. Dis.* **2015**, *38*, 83–85. [CrossRef] [PubMed]
78. O'Connell, S.; Lyons, C.; Abdou, M.; Patowary, R.; Aslam, S.; Kinsella, N.; Zintl, A.; Hunfeld, K.P.; Wormser, G.P.; Gray, J.; et al. Splenic dysfunction from celiac disease resulting in severe babesiosis. *Ticks Tick-Borne Dis.* **2017**, *8*, 537–539. [CrossRef] [PubMed]
79. Chan, W.Y.; MacDonald, C.; Keenan, A.; Xu, K.; Bain, B.J.; Chiodini, P.L. Severe babesiosis due to *Babesia divergens* acquired in the United Kingdom. *Am. J. Hematol.* **2021**, *96*, 889–890. [CrossRef] [PubMed]
80. Vannier, E.; Krause, P.J. Update on babesiosis. *Interdiscip. Perspect. Infect. Dis.* **2009**, *2009*, 984568. [CrossRef] [PubMed]
81. Jadin, J.B.; Giroud, P. Babèsioses et rickettsioses. In *Parasitolological Topics: A Presentation Volume to P. C. C. Garnham on the Occasion of His Birthday*; Canning, E.U., Ed.; Society of Protozoologists: Utica, NY, USA, 1981; pp. 132–135.
82. Humiczewska, M.; Kuźna-Grygiel, W. A case of imported human babesiosis in Poland. *Wiad. Parazytol.* **1997**, *43*, 227–229. [PubMed]
83. Baumann, D.; Pusterla, N.; Péter, O.; Grimm, F.; Fournier, P.E.; Schar, G.; Bossart, W.; Lutz, H.; Weber, R. Fever after a tick bite: Clinical manifestations and diagnosis of acute tick bite-associated infections in northeastern Switzerland. *Dtsch. Med. Wochenschr.* **2003**, *128*, 1042–1047. [CrossRef]
84. Nohýnková, E.; Kubek, J.; Měst'ánková, O.; Chalupa, P.; Hubálek, Z. A case of *Babesia microti* imported into the Czech Republic from the USA. *Cas. Lek. Ceskych.* **2003**, *142*, 377–381.
85. Ramharter, M.; Walochnik, J.; Lagler, H.; Winkler, S.; Wernsdorfer, W.H.; Stoiser, B.; Graninger, W. Clinical and molecular characterization of a near fatal case of human babesiosis in Austria. *J. Travel Med.* **2010**, *17*, 416–418. [CrossRef] [PubMed]
86. Berens-Riha, N.; Zechmeister, M.; Hirzmann, J.; Draenert, R.; Bogner, J.; Löscher, T. Babesiose Bei Einem Splenektomierten Reisenden Aus Den USA—Nach Deutschland Importierte Infektion Durch Zecken. *Flugmed. Trop. Reisemedizin—FTR* **2012**, *19*, 113–115. [CrossRef]
87. Poisnel, E.; Ebbo, M.; Berda-Haddad, Y.; Faucher, B.; Bernit, E.; Carcy, B.; Piarroux, R.; Harle, J.R.; Schleinitz, N. *Babesia microti*: An unusual travel-related disease. *BMC Infect. Dis.* **2013**, *13*, 99. [CrossRef] [PubMed]
88. Jablonska, J.; Zarnowska-Prymek, H.; Stanczak, J.; Kozlowska, J.; Wiercinska-Drapalo, A. Symptomatic co-infection with *Babesia microti* and *Borrelia burgdorferi* in patient after international exposure; a challenging case in Poland. *Ann. Agric. Environ. Med. AAEM* **2016**, *23*, 387–389. [CrossRef] [PubMed]
89. Holler, J.G.; Roser, D.; Nielsen, H.V.; Eickhardt, S.; Chen, M.; Lester, A.; Bang, D.; Frandsen, C.; David, K.P. A case of human babesiosis in Denmark. *Travel Med. Infect. Dis.* **2013**, *11*, 324–328. [CrossRef] [PubMed]
90. Merino, A. Blood film findings in severe babesiosis. *Br. J. Haematol.* **2016**, *172*, 839. [CrossRef]
91. de Ramon, C.; Cid, J.; Rodriguez-Tajes, S.; Alvarez-Martinez, M.J.; Valls, M.E.; Fernandez, J.; Lozano, M. Severe *Babesia microti* infection in an American immunocompetent patient diagnosed in Spain. *Transfus. Apher. Sci.* **2016**, *55*, 243–244. [CrossRef] [PubMed]
92. Stahl, P.; Poinsignon, Y.; Pouedras, P.; Ciubotaru, V.; Berry, L.; Emu, B.; Krause, P.J.; Ben Mamoun, C.; Cornillot, E. Case report of the patient source of the *Babesia microti* R1 reference strain and implications for travelers. *J. Travel Med.* **2018**, *25*, tax073. [CrossRef] [PubMed]
93. McGregor, A.; Lambert, J.; Bain, B.J.; Chiodini, P. Unexpected babesiosis with dramatic morphological features. *Am. J. Hematol.* **2019**, *94*, 947–948. [CrossRef]
94. Guirao-Arrabal, E.; Gonzalez, L.M.; Garcia-Fogeda, J.L.; Miralles-Adell, C.; Sanchez-Moreno, G.; Chueca, N.; Anguita-Santos, F.; Munoz-Medina, L.; Vinuesa-Garcia, D.; Hernandez-Quero, J.; et al. Imported babesiosis caused by *Babesia microti*-a case report. *Ticks Tick-Borne Dis.* **2020**, *11*, 101435. [CrossRef] [PubMed]
95. Rojko, T.; Duh, D.; Avšič-Zupanc, T.; Strle, F.; Lotric-Furlana, S. Seroprevalence of *Babesia divergens* infection among forestry workers in Slovenia. *Int. J. Med. Microbiol.* **2008**, *298*, 347–350. [CrossRef]
96. Vannier, E.; Gewurz, B.E.; Krause, P.J. Human babesiosis. *Infect. Dis. Clin. N. Am.* **2008**, *22*, 469–488. [CrossRef] [PubMed]
97. Welc-Falęciak, R.; Hildebrandt, A.; Siński, E. Co-infection with *Borrelia* species and other tick-borne pathogens in humans: Two cases from Poland. *Ann. Agric. Environ. Med. AAEM* **2010**, *17*, 309–313. [PubMed]
98. Raoult, D.; Soulayrol, L.; Toga, B.; Dumon, H.; Casanova, P. Babesiosis, pentamidine, and cotrimoxazole. *Ann. Intern. Med.* **1987**, *107*, 944. [CrossRef]
99. Loutan, L.; Rossier, J.; Zufferey, G.; Cuenod, D.; Hatz, C.; Marti, H.P.; Gern, L. Human babesiosis: First case report in Switzerland. *Rev. Med. Suisse Romande* **1994**, *114*, 111–116.
100. Calvo de Mora, A.; Garcia Castellano, J.M.; Herrera, C.; Jimenez-Alonso, J. Human babesiosis: Report of a case with fatal outcome. *Med. Clin.* **1985**, *85*, 515–516.

101. Tokmalaev, A.K.; Chentsov, V.B.; Malov, V.A.; Maleyev, V.V.; Kozhevnikova, G.M.; Polovinkina, N.A.; Golub, V.P.; Konnov, V.V.; Kharlamova, T.V. Human babesiosis: Clinical cases in the european part of the Russian Federation. *Ter. Arkhiv.* **2019**, *91*, 60–65. [CrossRef] [PubMed]
102. Moreno Giménez, J.C.; Jiménez Puya, R.; Galàn Gutiérrez, M.; Ortega Salas, R.; Dueñas Jurado, J.M. Erythema figuratum in septic babesiosis. *J. Eur. Acad. Dermatol. Venereol. JEADV* **2006**, *20*, 726–728. [CrossRef] [PubMed]
103. Andric, B.; Golubovic, M.; Terzic, D.; Dupanovic, B.; Icevic, M. First diagnostic cases of human babesiosis in Montenegro. *Braz. J. Infect. Dis. Off. Publ. Braz. Soc. Infect. Dis.* **2012**, *16*, 498–499. [CrossRef] [PubMed]
104. Meer-Scherrer, L.; Adelson, M.; Mordechai, E.; Lottaz, B.; Tilton, R. *Babesia microti* infection in Europe. *Curr. Microbiol.* **2004**, *48*, 435–437. [CrossRef] [PubMed]
105. Guerrero Espejo, A.; Munoz Parada, C.; Tomas Dols, S. Incidence of human babesiosis in Spain obtained from the diagnoses at hospital discharge. *Med. Clin.* **2017**, *149*, 84–85. [CrossRef]
106. Moniuszko, A.; Dunaj, J.; Swiecicka, I.; Zambrowski, G.; Chmielewska-Badora, J.; Zukiewicz-Sobczak, W.; Zajkowska, J.; Czupryna, P.; Kondrusik, M.; Grygorczuk, S.; et al. Co-infections with *Borrelia* species, *Anaplasma phagocytophilum* and *Babesia* spp. in patients with tick-borne encephalitis. *Eur. J. Clin. Microbiol. Infect. Dis. Off. Publ. Eur. Soc. Clin. Microbiol.* **2014**, *33*, 1835–1841. [CrossRef] [PubMed]
107. Inamadar, A.C.; Shivanna, R.; Ankad, B.S. Necrolytic Acral Erythema: Current Insights. *Clin. Cosmet. Investig. Derm.* **2020**, *13*, 275–281. [CrossRef] [PubMed]
108. Fukushima, H.; Fujii, T.; Sugiura, K. Zinc-responsive necrolytic acral erythema in ovarian cancer. *J. Dermatol.* **2020**, *47*, e266–e267. [CrossRef] [PubMed]
109. Mohrenschlager, M.; Kohler, L.D.; Bruckbauer, H.; Walch, A.; Ring, J. Squamous epithelial carcinoma-associated necrolytic migratory erythema. *Der Hautarzt Z. Fur Dermatol. Venerol. Verwandte Geb.* **1999**, *50*, 198–202. [CrossRef]
110. Strizova, Z.; Havlova, K.; Patek, O.; Smrz, D.; Bartunkova, J. The first human case of babesiosis mimicking Reiter's syndrome. *Folia Parasitol.* **2020**, *67*, 031. [CrossRef] [PubMed]
111. Hildebrandt, A.; Gray, J.S.; Hunfeld, K.P. Human babesiosis in Europe: What clinicians need to know. *Infection* **2013**, *41*, 1057–1072. [CrossRef]
112. O'Bryan, J.; Gokhale, A.; Hendrickson, J.E.; Krause, P.J. Parasite burden and red blood cell exchange transfusion for babesiosis. *J. Clin. Apher.* **2021**, *36*, 127–134. [CrossRef]
113. White, D.J.; Talarico, J.; Chang, H.G.; Birkhead, G.S.; Heimberger, T.; Morse, D.L. Human babesiosis in New York State: Review of 139 hospitalized cases and analysis of prognostic factors. *Arch. Intern. Med.* **1998**, *158*, 2149–2154. [CrossRef]
114. Hatcher, J.C.; Greenberg, P.D.; Antique, J.; Jimenez-Lucho, V.E. Severe babesiosis in Long Island: Review of 34 cases and their complications. *Clin. Infect. Dis. Off. Publ. Infect. Dis. Soc. Am.* **2001**, *32*, 1117–1125. [CrossRef]
115. Mareedu, N.; Schotthoefer, A.M.; Tompkins, J.; Hall, M.C.; Fritsche, T.R.; Frost, H.M. Risk factors for severe infection, hospitalization, and prolonged antimicrobial therapy in patients with babesiosis. *Am. J. Trop. Med. Hyg.* **2017**, *97*, 1218–1225. [CrossRef] [PubMed]
116. Meldrum, S.C.; Birkhead, G.S.; White, D.J.; Benach, J.L.; Morse, D.L. Human babesiosis in New York State: An epidemiological description of 136 cases. *Clin. Infect. Dis. Off. Publ. Infect. Dis. Soc. Am.* **1992**, *15*, 1019–1023. [CrossRef]
117. Akel, T.; Mobarakai, N. Hematologic manifestations of babesiosis. *Ann. Clin. Microbiol. Antimicrob.* **2017**, *16*, 6. [CrossRef] [PubMed]
118. Auerbach, M.; Haubenstock, A.; Soloman, G. Systemic babesiosis. Another cause of the hemophagocytic syndrome. *Am. J. Med.* **1986**, *80*, 301–303. [CrossRef]
119. Slovut, D.P.; Benedetti, E.; Matas, A.J. Babesiosis and hemophagocytic syndrome in an asplenic renal transplant recipient. *Transplantation* **1996**, *62*, 537–539. [CrossRef] [PubMed]
120. Gupta, P.; Hurley, R.W.; Helseth, P.H.; Goodman, J.L.; Hammerschmidt, D.E. Pancytopenia due to hemophagocytic syndrome as the presenting manifestation of babesiosis. *Am. J. Hematol.* **1995**, *50*, 60–62. [CrossRef]
121. Mecchella, J.N.; Rigby, W.F.; Zbehlik, A.J. Pancytopenia and cough in a man with amyopathic dermatomyositis. *Arthritis Care Res.* **2014**, *66*, 1587–1590. [CrossRef] [PubMed]
122. Filipovich, A.H.; Chandrakasan, S. Pathogenesis of hemophagocytic lymphohistiocytosis. *Hematol. Oncol. Clin. N. Am.* **2015**, *29*, 895–902. [CrossRef] [PubMed]
123. Morales, M.M.; Feria, M.L.; Mesa, M.D. Hemophagocytic syndrome due to babesiosis in a splenectomized patient. *Br. J. Haematol.* **1995**, *91*, 1033. [CrossRef]
124. Di Sabatino, A.; Brunetti, L.; Carnevale Maffe, G.; Giuffrida, P.; Corazza, G.R. Is it worth investigating splenic function in patients with celiac disease? *World J. Gastroenterol. WJG* **2013**, *19*, 2313–2318. [CrossRef] [PubMed]
125. Di Sabatino, A.; Rosado, M.M.; Cazzola, P.; Riboni, R.; Biagi, F.; Carsetti, R.; Corazza, G.R. Splenic hypofunction and the spectrum of autoimmune and malignant complications in celiac disease. *Clin. Gastroenterol. Hepatol.* **2006**, *4*, 179–186. [CrossRef]
126. Di Sabatino, A.; Carsetti, R.; Corazza, G.R. Post-splenectomy and hyposplenic states. *Lancet* **2011**, *378*, 86–97. [CrossRef]
127. Chen, Z.; Li, H.; Gao, X.; Bian, A.; Yan, H.; Kong, D.; Liu, X. Human babesiosis in China: A systematic review. *Parasitol. Res.* **2019**, *118*, 1103–1112. [CrossRef] [PubMed]

128. Krause, P.J.; Telford, S.R., III; Spielman, A.; Sikand, V.; Ryan, R.; Christianson, D.; Burke, G.; Brassard, P.; Pollack, R.; Peck, J.; et al. Concurrent Lyme disease and babesiosis. Evidence for increased severity and duration of illness. *JAMA J. Am. Med. Assoc.* **1996**, *275*, 1657–1660. [CrossRef]
129. Joseph, J.T.; Roy, S.S.; Shams, N.; Visintainer, P.; Nadelman, R.B.; Hosur, S.; Nelson, J.; Wormser, G.P. Babesiosis in Lower Hudson Valley, New York, USA. *Emerg. Infect. Dis.* **2011**, *17*, 843–847. [CrossRef] [PubMed]
130. Kjemtrup, A.M.; Conrad, P.A. Human babesiosis: An emerging tick-borne disease. *Int. J. Parasitol.* **2000**, *30*, 1323–1337. [CrossRef]
131. Krause, P.J.; Spielman, A.; Telford, S.R., III; Sikand, V.K.; McKay, K.; Christianson, D.; Pollack, R.J.; Brassard, P.; Magera, J.; Ryan, R.; et al. Persistent parasitemia after acute babesiosis. *N. Engl. J. Med.* **1998**, *339*, 160–165. [CrossRef]
132. Raffalli, J.; Wormser, G.P. Persistence of babesiosis for >2 years in a patient on rituximab for rheumatoid arthritis. *Diagn. Microbiol. Infect. Dis.* **2016**, *85*, 231–232. [CrossRef]
133. Leiby, D.A. Transfusion-transmitted *Babesia* spp.: Bull's-eye on *Babesia microti*. *Clin. Microbiol. Rev.* **2011**, *24*, 14–28. [CrossRef]
134. Pantanowitz, L.; Cannon, M.E. Extracellular *Babesia microti* parasites. *Transfusion* **2001**, *41*, 440. [CrossRef] [PubMed]
135. Gubernot, D.M.; Nakhasi, H.L.; Mied, P.A.; Asher, D.M.; Epstein, J.S.; Kumar, S. Transfusion-transmitted babesiosis in the United States: Summary of a workshop. *Transfusion* **2009**, *49*, 2759–2771. [CrossRef]
136. Hildebrandt, A.; Tenter, A.M.; Straube, E.; Hunfeld, K.P. Human babesiosis in Germany: Just overlooked or truly new? *Int. J. Med. Microbiol.* **2008**, *298*, 336–346. [CrossRef]
137. Hunfeld, K.P.; Hildebrandt, A.; Gray, J.S. Babesiosis: Recent insights into an ancient disease. *Int. J. Parasitol.* **2008**, *38*, 1219–1237. [CrossRef]
138. Krause, P.J.; Telford, S.R., III. Babesiosis. In *Protozoal Diseases*; Gilles, H.M., Ed.; Arnold: London, UK, 1999; pp. 236–248.
139. Wilson, M.; Glaser, K.C.; Adams-Fish, D.; Boley, M.; Mayda, M.; Molestina, R.E. Development of droplet digital PCR for the detection of *Babesia microti* and *Babesia duncani*. *Exp. Parasitol.* **2015**, *149*, 24–31. [CrossRef] [PubMed]
140. Lohr, B.; Hildebrandt, A.; Hunfeld, K.P. Humane Babesiose: Ein kurzer klinisch-mikrobiologischer Steckbrief. *GMS Z Forder Qual. Med. Lab.* **2017**, *8*, Doc04, URN: Urn:nbn:de:0183-lab0000271. [CrossRef]
141. Krause, P.J.; Telford, S.R., III; Ryan, R.; Conrad, P.A.; Wilson, M.; Thomford, J.W.; Spielman, A. Diagnosis of babesiosis: Evaluation of a serologic test for the detection of *Babesia microti* antibody. *J. Infect. Dis.* **1994**, *169*, 923–926. [CrossRef]
142. Krause, P.J.; Ryan, R.; Telford, S., III; Persing, D.; Spielman, A. Efficacy of immunoglobulin M serodiagnostic test for rapid diagnosis of acute babesiosis. *J. Clin. Microbiol.* **1996**, *34*, 2014–2016. [CrossRef] [PubMed]
143. Krause, P.J.; McKay, K.; Thompson, C.A.; Sikand, V.K.; Lentz, R.; Lepore, T.; Closter, L.; Christianson, D.; Telford, S.R.; Persing, D.; et al. Disease-specific diagnosis of coinfecting tickborne zoonoses: Babesiosis, human granulocytic ehrlichiosis, and Lyme disease. *Clin. Infect. Dis. Off. Publ. Infect. Dis. Soc. Am.* **2002**, *34*, 1184–1191. [CrossRef] [PubMed]
144. Gray, J.S.; Pudney, M. Activity of atovaquone against *Babesia microti* in the Mongolian gerbil, *Meriones unguiculatus*. *J. Parasitol.* **1999**, *85*, 723–728. [CrossRef]
145. Smith, R.P.; Hunfeld, K.P.; Krause, P.J. Management strategies for human babesiosis. *Expert Rev. Anti-Infect. Ther.* **2020**, *18*, 625–636. [CrossRef]
146. Gorenflot, A.; Bazin, C.; Ambroise-Thomas, P. Human babesiosis. Treatment of severe forms. *Presse Med.* **1987**, *16*, 1099. [PubMed]
147. Gray, E.B.; Herwaldt, B.L. Babesiosis surveillance—United States, 2011–2015. *MMWR Surveill. Summ.* **2019**, *68*, 1–11. [CrossRef]
148. Marcus, L.C.; Mabray, C.J.; Sturgis, G.H. *Babesia microti* infection in the hamster: Failure of quinine and pyrimethamine in chemotherapeutic trials. *Am. J. Trop. Med. Hyg.* **1984**, *33*, 21–23. [CrossRef]
149. Brasseur, P.; Lecoublet, S.; Kapel, N.; Favennec, L.; Ballet, J.J. Quinine in the treatment of *Babesia divergens* infections in humans. *Eur. J. Clin. Microbiol. Infect. Dis. Off. Publ. Eur. Soc. Clin. Microbiol.* **1996**, *15*, 840–841. [CrossRef]
150. Cervera-Hernandez, M.E.; Zaidi, N.; Sweeney, J.D. Heavy parasitemia in babesiosis treated without adjunctive red cell exchange. *Transfus. Apher. Sci.* **2019**, *58*, 439–441. [CrossRef]
151. Vial, H.J.; Gorenflot, A. Chemotherapy against babesiosis. *Vet. Parasitol.* **2006**, *138*, 147–160. [CrossRef] [PubMed]
152. Pudney, M.; Gray, J.S. Therapeutic efficacy of atovaquone against the bovine intraerythrocytic parasite, *Babesia Divergens*. *J. Parasitol.* **1997**, *83*, 307–310. [CrossRef]
153. Egan, E.L.; Duggan, C. Human babesiosis divergens treated with imidocarb dipropionate with a note on clinical diagnosis. In Proceedings of the International Society of Hematology 23rd Congress and the 32nd Annual Meeting of the American Society of Hematology, Boston, MA, USA, 28 November–4 December 1990; Saunders: Philadelphia, PA, USA, 1991.
154. Beshbishy, A.M.; Batiha, G.E.; Alkazmi, L.; Nadwa, E.; Rashwan, E.; Abdeen, A.; Yokoyama, N.; Igarashi, I. Therapeutic effects of atranorin towards the proliferation of *Babesia* and *Theileria* parasites. *Pathogens* **2020**, *9*, 127. [CrossRef]
155. Batiha, G.E.; Beshbishy, A.M.; Alkazmi, L.M.; Nadwa, E.H.; Rashwan, E.K.; Yokoyama, N.; Igarashi, I. In vitro and in vivo growth inhibitory activities of cryptolepine hydrate against several *Babesia* species and *Theileria equi*. *PLoS Negl. Trop. Dis.* **2020**, *14*, e0008489. [CrossRef]
156. Salama, A.A.; Aboulaila, M.; Moussa, A.A.; Nayel, M.A.; El-Sify, A.; Terkawi, M.A.; Hassan, H.Y.; Yokoyama, N.; Igarashi, I. Evaluation of in vitro and in vivo inhibitory effects of fusidic acid on *Babesia* and *Theileria* parasites. *Vet. Parasitol.* **2013**, *191*, 1–10. [CrossRef]
157. AbouLaila, M.; El-Sayed, S.A.E.; Omar, M.A.; Al-Aboody, M.S.; Aziz, A.R.A.; Abdel-Daim, M.M.; Rizk, M.A.; Igarashi, I. Myrrh oil In Vitro inhibitory growth on bovine and equine piroplasm parasites and *Babesia microti* of mice. *Pathogens* **2020**, *9*, 173. [CrossRef]

158. Batiha, G.E.; Beshbishy, A.M.; Tayebwa, D.S.; Adeyemi, O.S.; Shaheen, H.; Yokoyama, N.; Igarashi, I. The effects of trans-chalcone and chalcone 4 hydrate on the growth of *Babesia* and *Theileria*. *PLoS Negl. Trop. Dis.* **2019**, *13*, e0007030. [CrossRef] [PubMed]
159. Vannier, E.; Krause, P.J. Babesiosis in China, an emerging threat. *Lancet Infect. Dis.* **2015**, *15*, 137–139. [CrossRef]
160. Zhou, X.; Xia, S.; Huang, J.L.; Tambo, E.; Ge, H.X.; Zhou, X.N. Human babesiosis, an emerging tick-borne disease in the people inverted question marks Republic of China. *Parasites Vectors* **2014**, *7*, 509. [CrossRef] [PubMed]
161. Zhou, X.; Xia, S.; Yin, S.Q.; Zhou, X.N. Emergence of babesiosis in China-Myanmar border areas. *Parasites Vectors* **2015**, *8*, 390. [CrossRef]
162. Jiang, J.F.; Zheng, Y.C.; Jiang, R.R.; Li, H.; Huo, Q.B.; Jiang, B.G.; Sun, Y.; Jia, N.; Wang, Y.W.; Ma, L.; et al. Epidemiological, clinical, and laboratory characteristics of 48 cases of "*Babesia venatorum*" infection in China: A descriptive study. *Lancet Infect. Dis.* **2015**, *15*, 196–203. [CrossRef]
163. Weiss, L.M.; Wittner, M.; Wasserman, S.; Oz, H.S.; Retsema, J.; Tanowitz, H.B. Efficacy of azithromycin for treating *Babesia microti* infection in the hamster model. *J. Infect. Dis.* **1993**, *168*, 1289–1292. [CrossRef]
164. Wittner, M.; Lederman, J.; Tanowitz, H.B.; Rosenbaum, G.S.; Weiss, L.M. Atovaquone in the treatment of *Babesia microti* infections in hamsters. *Am. J. Trop. Med. Hyg.* **1996**, *55*, 219–222. [CrossRef]
165. Krause, P.J.; Lepore, T.; Sikand, V.K.; Gadbaw, J., Jr.; Burke, G.; Telford, S.R., III; Brassard, P.; Pearl, D.; Azlanzadeh, J.; Christianson, D.; et al. Atovaquone and azithromycin for the treatment of babesiosis. *N. Engl. J. Med.* **2000**, *343*, 1454–1458. [CrossRef] [PubMed]
166. Abraham, A.; Brasov, I.; Thekkiniath, J.; Kilian, N.; Lawres, L.; Gao, R.; DeBus, K.; He, L.; Yu, X.; Zhu, G.; et al. Establishment of a continuous In Vitro culture of *Babesia duncani* in human erythrocytes reveals unusually high tolerance to recommended therapies. *J. Biol. Chem.* **2018**, *293*, 19974–19981. [CrossRef] [PubMed]
167. McCormack, K.A.; Alhaboubi, A.; Pollard, D.A.; Fuller, L.; Holman, P.J. In Vitro cultivation of *Babesia duncani* (Apicomplexa: Babesiidae), a zoonotic hemoprotozoan, using infected blood from Syrian hamsters (*Mesocricetus auratus*). *Parasitol. Res.* **2019**, *118*, 2409–2417. [CrossRef] [PubMed]
168. Spaete, J.; Patrozou, E.; Rich, J.D.; Sweeney, J.D. Red cell exchange transfusion for babesiosis in Rhode Island. *J. Clin. Apher.* **2009**, *24*, 97–105. [CrossRef] [PubMed]

pathogens

MDPI

Article

Babesia and Theileria Identification in Adult Ixodid Ticks from Tapada Nature Reserve, Portugal

Nélida Fernández [1], Belen Revuelta [2], Irene Aguilar [1], Jorge Francisco Soares [3], Annetta Zintl [4], Jeremy Gray [5], Estrella Montero [2,*] and Luis Miguel Gonzalez [2]

1 Facultad de Veterinaria, Alfonso X el Sabio University, 28691 Madrid, Spain; nfernpat@uax.es (N.F.); i.aguilar.garcia@hotmail.com (I.A.)
2 Parasitology Reference and Research Laboratory, Centro Nacional de Microbiología, Instituto de Salud Carlos III, Majadahonda, 28220 Madrid, Spain; belen.revuelta@isciii.es (B.R.); lmgonzal@isciii.es (L.M.G.)
3 Wild Animal Health, BeWild Conservation Medicine, 1600-646 Lisboa, Portugal; conservationmedicine@be-wild.org
4 UCD School of Veterinary Sciences, University College Dublin, D04 W6F6 Dublin, Ireland; annetta.zintl@ucd.ie
5 UCD School of Biology and Environmental Science, University College Dublin, D04 N2E5 Dublin, Ireland; jeremy.gray@ucd.ie
* Correspondence: estrella.montero@isciii.es

Citation: Fernández, N.; Revuelta, B.; Aguilar, I.; Soares, J.F.; Zintl, A.; Gray, J.; Montero, E.; Gonzalez, L.M. *Babesia* and *Theileria* Identification in Adult Ixodid Ticks from Tapada Nature Reserve, Portugal. *Pathogens* 2022, *11*, 222. https://doi.org/10.3390/pathogens11020222

Academic Editor: Lawrence S. Young

Received: 9 December 2021
Accepted: 4 February 2022
Published: 8 February 2022

Publisher's Note: MDPI stays neutral with regard to jurisdictional claims in published maps and institutional affiliations.

Abstract: This study, conducted in a nature reserve in southern Portugal, investigated the frequency and diversity of tick-borne piroplasms in six species of adult ixodid ticks removed from 71 fallow deer (*Dama dama*) and 12 red deer (*Cervus elaphus*), collected over the period 2012–2019. The majority of 520 ticks were *Ixodes ricinus* (78.5%), followed by *Rhipicephalus sanguineus* sensu lato, *Hyalomma lusitanicum*, *Haemaphysalis punctata*, *Dermacentor marginatus*, and *Ixodes hexagonus*. The *R. sanguineus* ticks collected from the deer were clearly exophilic, in contrast to the endophilic species usually associated with dogs. Four tick-borne piroplasms, including *Theileria* spp., and the zoonotic species, *Babesia divergens* and *Babesia microti*, were detected. *B. divergens* 18S rDNA, identical to that of the bovine reference strain U16370 and to certain strains from red deer, was detected in *I. ricinus* ticks removed from fallow deer. The sporadic detection of infections in ticks removed from the same individual hosts suggests that the piroplasms were present in the ticks rather than the hosts. *Theileria* sp. OT3 was found in *I. ricinus* and, along with *T. capreoli*, was also detected in some of the other tick species. The natural vector and pathogenic significance of this piroplasm are unknown.

Keywords: *Babesia*; host blood analysis; fallow deer; ixodid ticks; piroplasm; red deer; *Theileria*

1. Introduction

The most common tick-borne diseases (TBDs) of humans in Europe (Lyme borreliosis and tick-borne encephalitis) are notifiable to the European Centre for Disease Prevention and Control (ECDC). However, diseases caused by less common tick-borne pathogens (TBPs), such as *Babesia*, *Theileria*, and *Rickettsia* species, although representing potential health risks for humans, domestic animals, or wildlife, are not included in current surveillance schemes. In the absence of relevant surveillance schemes, molecular analysis of ticks collected in areas where humans and animals are exposed to tick bites can detect endemic TBPs; identify new ones; and, alongside reported human cases and serosurveys, contribute to epidemiological information.

The climate, flora, and fauna of Tapada Nacional de Mafra, where the present study was carried out, constitute a potential environment for ixodid ticks and TBPs. From 2012 to 2019, several species of adult ticks were collected from parasitized fallow (*Dama dama*) and red deer (*Cervus elaphus*) during the spring and autumn seasons, when most tick host-seeking activity occurs. The tick species involved can transmit and maintain several viral, bacterial, and protozoan pathogens of public health and veterinary importance [1–6]. In this study, we focused on the detection of piroplasm protozoans of the *Babesia* and *Theileria* genera. These parasites infect erythrocytes (and also lymphocytes in the case of *Theileria* spp.) of a variety of vertebrate hosts, but particularly cervids, which are prominent components of the Tapada Nature Reserve fauna.

Of particular interest were the zoonotic species *Babesia divergens* and *B. venatorum*, which belong to the *Babesia* sensu stricto (s.s.) group (Clade X [7]), and are transmitted by *Ixodes ricinus*, the castor bean tick, the most widespread ixodid species in Europe [8]. While roe deer (*Capreolus capreolus*) are considered the natural hosts of *B. venatorum* [9,10], cattle are the main reservoirs of *B. divergens* and frequently suffer clinical disease (redwater fever) as a consequence of infection [11]. *B. divergens*-like DNA sequences have also been reported in red deer, roe deer, reindeer (*Rangifer tarandus*), and fallow deer [9,12–18], but there is some uncertainty about the precise identity of these parasites and, so far, there is no evidence that *Babesia* isolates from deer are infectious for either humans or cattle [12,19].

Babesia microti, which is also potentially zoonotic, particularly in the USA [20], is distinct from the *Babesia* s.s. group and consists of a species complex divided into five distinct clades, infecting a wide range of vertebrates with the notable exception of ungulates [21]. Those in clade 1, also referred to as *B. microti* sensu stricto (s.s.), cause most of the human babesiosis cases worldwide, and those in clade 3 include the *B. microti* Munich strain, which has an ambiguous zoonotic status [21]. In Europe, both *B. microti* s.s. strains and the *B. microti* Munich strain have been detected in *I. ricinus* and in several mammal species, particularly rodents. On the other hand, few cases of human babesiosis have been reported in Europe so far [22], which appears to be at odds with the frequent occurrence of the parasites in small mammals.

Theileria species are known to be transmitted by ixodid ticks of the genera *Amblyomma*, *Haemaphysalis*, *Hyalomma*, and *Rhipicephalus* [23], and the recent detection of DNA of *Theileria* spp., such as *Theileria* OT3 in *I. ricinus*, suggests that this tick species might also be a *Theileria* vector [4,24]. *Theileria* spp. are not considered zoonotic [25], but some have a major impact on the livestock industry, especially in tropical and sub-tropical countries [26], while others can infect wild animals including red deer [27,28].

This study, focused on a sample of 520 adult ticks collected from fallow and red deer in Tapada Nature Reserve, was conducted to determine the diversity and relative abundance of the tick fauna, and their possible roles in the maintenance and transmission of *Babesia* and *Theileria* parasites by the detection and amplification of the 18S rRNA and cytochrome c oxidase subunit I (COI) genes.

2. Results

2.1. Ticks Removed from Deer

During the period 2012–2019, a total of 520 adult ticks were collected from May to September in Tapada Nacional de Mafra, Portugal (Figure 1).

Of this total, 350 engorged female (67.3%) and 114 male ticks (21.9%) were removed from 71 fallow deer, and 27 engorged female (5.19%) and 29 (5.58%) male ticks from 12 red deer. Most of the identified ticks removed from fallow deer were *I. ricinus* (n = 377, 81.2%, $p < 0.05$), followed by *Rhipicephalus sanguineus* sensu lato (s.l.) (n = 42, 9.0%), *Hyalomma lusitanicum* (n = 22, 4.7%), *Haemaphysalis punctata* (n = 15, 3.2%), *Dermacentor marginatus* (n = 6, 1.3%), and *Ixodes hexagonus* (n = 2, 0.4%). Ticks removed from red deer were identified as *I. ricinus* (n = 31, 55.4%), again the most abundant tick ($p < 0.05$), followed by *R. sanguineus* s.l., (n = 23, 41.1%) and *D. marginatus* (n = 2, 3.6%) (Table 1).

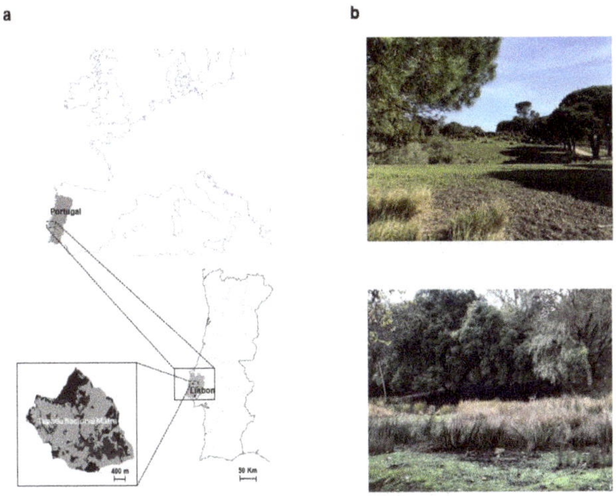

Figure 1. The locations of Tapada Nacional de Mafra and examples of sample sites. (**a**) The location of Tapada Nacional de Mafra in Europe. (**b**) Pictures show different areas of Tapada Nacional de Mafra inhabited by fallow and red deer.

Table 1. Species of ticks removed from fallow deer (*Dama dama*) and red deer (*Cervus elaphus*) in the Tapada Nature Reserve, Portugal.

Hosts	Ticks Species	Common Name	Relative Abundance in Portugal [29]	Zoonotic Pathogens * Transmitted	Tested (n)	Female	Male
Fallow deer	*Ixodes ricinus*	Castor bean tick	Common	*Babesia, Borrelia, Rickettsia, Anaplasma*, TBEV	377	291	86
	Rhipicephalus sanguineus s.l.	Brown dog tick	Common	*Rickettsia*	42	24	18
	Hyalomma lusitanicum	None	Locally common in south	None	22	15	7
	Haemaphysalis punctata	Red sheep tick	Sporadic distribution	None	15	13	2
	Dermacentor marginatus	Ornate sheep tick	Locally common	*Rickettsia*	6	5	1
	Ixodes hexagonus	Hedgehog tick	Common	None	2	2	-
Red deer	*I. ricinus*	As above	As above	As above	31	19	12
	R. sanguineus s.l.	As above	As above	As above	23	7	16
	D. marginatus	As above	As above	As above	2	1	1
Total					520	377	143

s.l.—sensu lato; TBEV—tick-borne encephalitis virus. * Most of these tick species have been implicated as carriers of the agent of Q-fever, *Coxiella burnetii,* but their role as vectors of this pathogen is unclear.

2.2. Piroplasm Infection and Coinfection

Out of the 520 ticks tested, only 75 specimens of *I. ricinus*, *R. sanguineus* s.l., and *H. lusitanicum* were found to be infected with piroplasms. *B. divergens*, *T. capreoli*, and *Theileria* sp. OT3 were detected by real-time polymerase chain reaction (PCR) and sequencing of part of the 18S rRNA gene (408–430 bp) [30,31], with *Theileria* sp. OT3 being the most abundant ($p < 0.05$). In addition, two different *B. microti* 18S rDNA fragments of 157 and

155 bp were detected by using a highly sensitive real-time PCR designed for the diagnosis of *B. microti* human babesiosis [32].

In particular, of the 377 *I. ricinus* samples removed from fallow deer, 8 (2.1%) were positive for *B. divergens* and 25 (6.6%) for *B. microti*. The *B. microti* 18S rDNA fragment of 157 bp was amplified in 7 ticks, while the fragment of 155 bp was amplified in another 18 ticks. *I. ricinus* was also infected with *T. capreoli* (n = 10, 2.7%) and *Theileria* sp. OT3 (n = 31, 8.3%) (Table 2).

Table 2. *Babesia* spp. and *Theileria* spp. DNA detected in ticks collected from fallow deer and red deer.

Host	Tick species	Tested (n)	qPCR Result (n[%])									
			1 pathogen				2 pathogens					3 pathogens
			Babesia divergens	*Babesia microti*	*Theileria sp. OT3*	*Theileria capreoli*	*Babesia Divergens* + *Babesia microti*	*Babesia Divergens* + *Theileria sp. OT3*	*Babesia microti* + *Theileria sp. OT3*	*Babesia microti* + *Theileria capreoli*	*Theileria capreoli* + *Theileria sp. OT3*	*Babesia microti* + *Theileria capreoli* + *Theileria sp. OT3*
Fallow deer	*I. ricinus*	377	5 (1.3)	14 (3.7)	22 (5.8)	6 (1.6)	2 (0.5)	1 (0.3)	6 (1.6)	2 (0.5)	1 (0.3)	1 (0.3)
	R. sanguineus s.l.	42	-	3 (7.1)	2 (4.8)	-	-	-	1 (2.4)	-	-	-
	H. lusitanicum	22	-	2 (9.1)	-	-	-	-	-	-	-	-
Red deer	*I. ricinus*	31	-	-	-	5 (16.1)	-	-	-	-	-	-
	R. sanguineus s.l.	23	-	-	1 (4.3)	1 (4.3)	-	-	-	-	-	-

Co-infections involving *B. microti* with the following species were as follows:

B. divergens (n = 2), *T. capreoli* (n = 2), *Theileria* sp. OT3 (n = 6), and *T. capreoli* / *Theileria* sp. OT3 (n = 1). Coinfections with *B. divergens*/*Theileria* sp.OT3 (n = 1) and *T. capreoli*/*Theileria* sp. OT3 (n = 1) were also detected (Table 2).

Of the 31 *I. ricinus* samples collected from red deer, 5 (16.1%) tested positive for *T. capreoli* (Table 2). Of the 42 *R. sanguineus* s.l. ticks collected from fallow deer, 3 (7.1%) were positive for *B. microti* (155 bp fragment) and 2 (4.8%) for *Theileria* sp. OT3. One *B. microti*/*Theileria* sp. OT3 coinfection was also detected. Of the 23 *R. sanguineus* s.l. ticks collected from red deer, 4.3% were positive for *T. capreoli* (n = 1) and *Theileria* sp. OT3 (n = 1), respectively.

Finally, of the 22 *H. lusitanicum* samples removed from fallow deer, 2 (9.1%) were found to be infected with *B. microti* (155 bp fragment). We did not detect co-infections in ticks collected from red deer or infected *H. lusitanicum* (Table 2).

Of note, in most cases (63%), only one of several ticks removed from the same deer tested positive for any one of the piroplasms (Supplementary Tables S1 and S2).

2.2.1. *Babesia* Spp. Typing

An almost entire sequence (1492 bp) of the *B. divergens* 18S rRNA gene was obtained from four of the eight infected *I. ricinus* ticks that were removed from fallow deer. No nucleotide variations were detected among these sequences, which were 100% identical to several entire human and bovine isolates including the bovine isolate GenBank: U16370, widely used as a reference [33] (Figure 2). The presence of *B. capreoli*, a very closely related species to *B. divergens* commonly associated with deer [12], was ruled out by both the 18S rDNA analysis [19] and also by amplification of part (234 bp) of the COI gene, which confirmed the identity of the piroplasms as *B. divergens*.

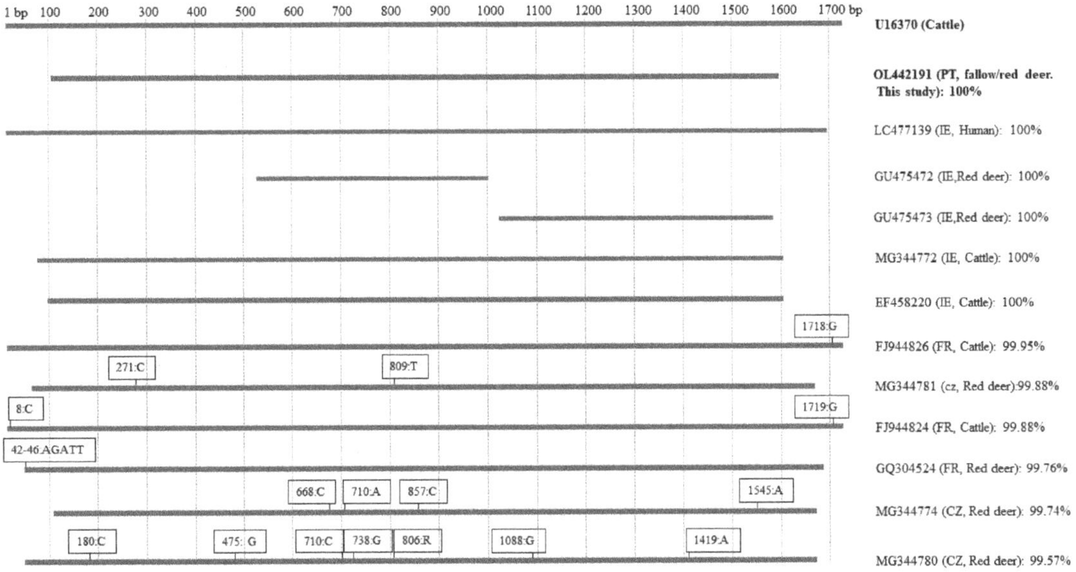

Figure 2. The relative length, positions, and heterologies of 18S rDNA gene sequences of *Babesia divergens* obtained in this work, together with others from cattle, human, and red deer compared to the reference sequence U16370. Of the 13 *B. divergens* isolates used to compare regions of the 18S rRNA gene, the sequences obtained in this work (QL442191) were 100% identical to that of the reference bovine isolate (U16370) and to those of several others from cattle and red deer, and also to one human isolate. However, most other published red deer sequences differed from QL442191 and the bovine *B. divergens* reference strain by up to 7 nucleotides in various positions. The numbers and letters refer to positions and nucleotide bases that are different from the reference sequence. Identity scores are made according to Clustal Omega.

The *B. microti* 157 bp fragment was 100% identical to the *B. microti* 18S rRNA gene of seven different sequences in GenBank, five of which had been identified as the *B. microti* Munich strain. The 155 bp fragment was 100% identical to the *B. microti* 18S rDNA from a number of human and *Ixodes* tick isolates of *B. microti* (n = 47), including the *B. microti* isolate Jena EF413181 responsible for the autochthonous human *B. microti* infection that occurred in Germany [34] (Supplementary Figure S1). To provide phylogenetic analysis of the two *B. microti* isolates, PCR reactions for amplifying larger fragments of the 18S rRNA gene and also part of the COI gene were performed [35], but did not yield any products. The limitation in obtaining large fragments of the gene could be associated with a low number of parasites present in ticks and an inverse correlation between the efficiency of the amplification and the size of the fragment.

2.2.2. *Theileria* Spp. Typing

To obtain more sequence information about the *Theileria* isolates, we amplified and sequenced almost the entire 18S rRNA gene. The 18S rDNA sequence (1230 bp length) obtained from 1 *I. ricinus* of 16 ixodid ticks infected with *T. capreoli* was 100% identical to 3 *T. capreoli* 18S rDNA isolates in the databank, including one associated with the first theileriosis case detected in Spain in a red deer imported from Northern Europe (GenBank: AY421708.1) [36].

The 18S rDNA sequences obtained from 4 *I. ricinus* ticks out of 33 infected with *Theileria* sp. OT3 (1218 bp) were 100% identical to each other and to two *Theileri* sp. 18S rDNA records in GenBank, while one of them was associated with the first report on the occurrence of *Theileria* sp. OT3 in sheep in China (KF470868) [37]. These nucleotide sequences from Tapada and China differed by one or two nucleotides (99.92–99.84%) from *Theileria* sp. OT3 18S rDNA sequences from sheep, chamois, red deer, and roe deer from Spain [28].

3. Discussion

Six different tick species were collected from fallow and red deer in Tapada, Portugal. These tick species occur across the Iberian Peninsula [15,29,38–41] and five of them, *I. ricinus*, *R. sanguineus*, *H. lusitanicum*, *H. punctata*, and *D. marginatus*, have been previously associated with fallow and red deer in Portugal [29]. The finding of the hedgehog tick, *I. hexagonus*, on fallow deer is unusual, though it has been reported previously on roe deer [42].

Some of the tick species collected (e.g., *R. sanguineus* s.l., *D. marginatus*, and *H. lusitanicum*) are regarded as adapted to drier habitats than occur in the reserve. It was, therefore, surprising to find them in the wet habitat and fauna of Tapada where they coexist with *I. ricinus*, which, as the most common species in Atlantic climatic regions [38], was the most abundant, as expected.

B. divergens was detected in 2.1% of *I. ricinus* specimens, which is similar to infection rates for adult ticks elsewhere in Europe [43]. The pathogen's identity was determined by detection of the almost complete 18S rRNA gene, which was identical to the bovine isolate U16370 and differed slightly from the closely related cervine species, *B. capreoli*, [19]. Specific amplification of part of the *B. divergens* cytochrome c oxidase subunit I (COI) gene unequivocally supported the 18S rRNA gene differentiation of these *B. divergens* sequences from *B. capreoli*. The apparent absence of *B. capreoli* is perhaps surprising considering that it is regarded as a cervid *Babesia* species. However, it should be noted that roe deer, possibly its primary host, are not present in this habitat, which also explains the absence of *Babesia venatorum*.

It is curious that the *B. divergens* sequences were only detected in ticks removed from fallow deer, considering that the only previous reports of complete identity of *B. divergens* in deer with U16370 have been in occasional samples from red rather than fallow deer (e.g., [16] and GenBank accession numbers MH697659, KX018019, MT151377, MN563158, and GQ304524). This apparent association of *B. divergens*-infected ticks with fallow deer is difficult to interpret, considering that red deer were also present in the habitat, but did not yield *B. divergens*-infected ticks, though it should be noted that the number of *I. ricinus* obtained from fallow deer was far higher than from red deer (371 versus 31). *B. divergens*-like parasites have rarely been reported from fallow deer, as reports either provide no sequence data [15,44] or only partial sequences [GenBank Accession Numbers KY242395, KY242396] which show low homology with the bovine reference strain U16370. It, therefore, appears probable that the detected pathogen was present in the ticks rather than in the fallow deer on which they were feeding. Since there are no cattle near the study site, red deer remain the most plausible source of these *B. divergens* sequences, which showed 100% identity to two long 18S rDNA sequences of 1639 bp and 1648 bp deposited in GenBank (GQ304524, GQ304525) obtained from red deer spleen. It is notable that the infected ticks were collected from deer that were mostly a source of uninfected ticks, again suggesting that the infections were present in the ticks rather than the deer, having been acquired by the previous tick generation and persisted in the collected ticks.

It is important to point out that there is, in fact, still no unequivocal evidence that *B. divergens*-like piroplasms from deer can cause human babesiosis or, indeed, even infect cattle, and it is interesting that, in a recent study, *B. divergens* was not detected in cattle that were in close proximity to infected deer [45]. The 18S rRNA gene is probably not the optimal choice for discrimination of *B. divergens* genotypes, although sequences of this gene are the most widely available [22]. Cross transmission studies are required to further explore the host specificity of *B. divergens* from deer, including the use of gerbils *(Meriones unguiculatus)* as proxies for humans [46]. So far, transmission experiments have not resulted in established infections, except in deer that had been splenectomized [11].

The other *Babesia* species identified in this study was *B. microti,* DNA fragments of which were detected in *I. ricinus, R. sanguineus* s.l., and *H. lusitanicum* adult ticks. While *I. ricinus* is a recognized vector of *B. microti* [47], *R. sanguineus* s.l. does not transmit the parasite [48]. So far, the uncommon *H. lusitanicum–B. microti* association, although previously detected in Spain, has not been supported by vector competence evidence either [15]. Based on the 18S rRNA gene fragments obtained in this study, two different *B. microti* strains may infect *I. ricinus* ticks in Tapada. One strain is evidently related to clade 1, to which zoonotic North American genotypes belong, and the second to the Munich strain, which belongs to clade 3 [21]. This latter genotype was once thought to be transmitted only by *I. trianguliceps*, which does not bite humans, but it has been detected in the anthropophilic *I. ricinus* [49–51] and has been associated with asymptomatic and moderate human babesiosis in Europe [52,53]. It seems, therefore, that zoonotic forms of *B. microti* might occur in Tapada, and to investigate this further, we are currently validating methods, such as the MinION long-read sequencing technology, to generate full-length nucleotide sequences of different molecular markers.

The detection in *I. ricinus* of DNA of *Theileria* sp OT3 and *T. capreoli,* associated with sheep and red deer, respectively, in China and Spain, supports previous suggestions that this tick species is a vector of certain *Theileria* spp. [14,24,54–56]. No sheep are observed in the immediate vicinity of Tapada and it is probable that deer are the reservoir hosts for the *Theileria* species detected in this study.

The co-existence of different piroplasms within the same tick in Tapada added an additional layer of complexity to the analysis of the tick–host relationships and pathogen transmission. Coinfections could be due to blood feeding on different vertebrate hosts or through co-feeding [3,57], although the latter is less likely to consider the small number of deer that carried several infected ticks at the same time. However, this hypothesis demands a more comprehensive evaluation and robust co-infection models [3,58].

4. Conclusions

This study shows the presence of *Babesia* and *Theileria* DNA in ticks from Tapada and suggests certain associations between infected ticks and susceptible hosts. The finding of *B. divergens* DNA identical to sequences from cattle supports observations made previously for a small proportion of sequences from red deer, and has possible implications for the role of these hosts in bovine and human babesiosis. However, at present, there are no transmission or epidemiological studies which suggest that the *B. divergens* strains detected in deer are infective for humans or cattle. Another interesting outcome of the study is the possible association of *Theileria* spp. with *I. ricinus,* which has not been firmly established as a vector of these piroplasms. The detection of *B. microti* in the ticks is not surprising, since this species complex is very widespread in Europe as a parasite of small mammals, but the fragments of *B. microti* DNA obtained were too small to draw any firm conclusions about the presence of zoonotic strains of this parasite in the reserve. Future studies should focus on alternatives to the 18S rRNA gene for pathogen identification, and should be combined with innovative sensitive and specific blood meal analysis methods, such as the use of retrotransposons in qPCR assays [59] in both fed and unfed ticks, to obtain a more complete picture of tick-borne pathogen epidemiology in complex habitats such as Tapada Nature Reserve.

5. Materials and Methods

5.1. Tick Samples

A total of 520 adult ticks were manually removed from 71 fallow deer (*D. dama*) and 12 red deer (*C. elaphus*) from May to September, during the period of 2012 to 2019 in Tapada Nacional de Mafra (38°57′10′′ N, 9°17′47.68′′ W), district of Lisbon, west coast of Portugal. This nature reserve of 819 hectares is about 7 km from Mafra, Portugal. Mixed forests of eucalyptus (*Eucalyptus globulus*); cork oak (*Quercus suber*); maritime pine (*Pinus pinaster*); stone pine (*Pinus pinea*); and other less common tree species, bushes, and shrubs constitute the main vegetation. Within this habitat, fallow and red deer coexist with medium-sized mammals such as foxes and wild boar, as well as small mammals including shrews, mice, and several species of bats [60]. There are no livestock in the reserve which can be visited by the public on weekends.

The ticks in this study were collected from the deer as part of management of the reserve. Deer immobilization and tick collection were authorized by Tapada Nacional de Mafra-Cooperativa de Interesse Público de Responsabilidade Limitada (CIPRL), following the European Council Directive 97/62/EC of 27.10.1997 on the conservation of natural habitats and of wild fauna and flora, and conducted by qualified veterinarians from the non-profit nature conservation organization BeWild. The collected ticks were then kindly donated to the study by BeWild. Tissue and/or blood samples from these animals for pathogen analysis were not available. Ticks were received in polypropylene tubes containing 70% ethanol. They were then separated by sex and identified to species level following morphological and taxonomic keys [61]. All ticks were individually stored at 4 °C until molecular analysis.

5.2. Genomic DNA Extraction

Ticks were individually rinsed in sterile phosphate buffered saline (PBS) solution, before being disrupted and homogenized with pestles. Genomic DNA was extracted from each homogenized tick using the commercial kit Speedtools® tissue DNA extraction (Biotools, Madrid, Spain) according to the manufacturer's instructions with slight modifications. RNA was removed by RNase digestion (Roche Diagnostic GmbH, Germany). Quantification and purity of the DNA samples were determined by spectrophotometry with a NanoDrop ND-1000 spectrophotometer (Nucliber, Madrid, Spain). DNA samples were eluted in 100 μL of sterile water and stored at −20 °C for further analysis.

5.3. Detection of Piroplasms

Molecular methods for detecting the presence of piroplasms were based on amplification of part of the 18S rRNA gene. All ticks were tested using (i) the piroplasm real-time PCR and primers PIRO-A and PIRO-B [30,31] and (ii) a *B. microti* real-time PCR using the specific set of primers Bab2/Bab3 [32]. To unequivocally distinguish between *B. divergens* and *B. capreoli*, amplification of part of the COI gene was carried out following a previously described protocol [13]. A conventional PCR was optimized to amplify large fragments of the 18S rRNA gene using samples that were previously found positive for *B. divergens* and *Theileria* species. A nested PCR was also performed to amplify large fragments of the 18S rRNA gene using positive *B. microti* samples [35]. The set of primers were: 18SRNABABF1/18SRNABABR1 for *B. divergens*, BABGF2/18SRNABABR1 for *Theileria* spp., and Piro0F2/Piro6R2 and Piro1F2/Piro5R2 for *B. microti*. Table 3 shows all primers and expected sizes of the amplified products.

Each reaction was performed in a final volume of 50 μL containing 200–400 ng of DNA, 2X PrimeStar GXL Buffer (Takara Bio, Shiga, Japan), 800 μM of dNTPs mixture (Takara Bio), 1.25 U of PrimerStar GXL DNA polymerase (Takara Bio), 1 μL (20 mg/mL) of BSA DNAse Free (Roche, Basel Switzerland), and 0.3 μM of each primer.

DNA from *B. divergens* Bd Rouen 1987 and *B. microti* Gray (ATCC® 30221™) were used as positive controls and water as negative control. To minimize contamination, false-positive samples, DNA extraction, PCR master-mix preparation, sample addition, and PCR reactions were performed in different biosafety cabinets in separate laboratories.

5.4. DNA Sequencing and Analysis

All positives qPCR and PCR products were separated on 1% and 2% agarose gels (Conda, Spain) stained with Pronasafe nucleic acid staining solution (10 mg/mL) (Conda, Spain) and visualized under UV illumination. The DNA bands were cut out of agarose gels under UV exposure, and purified using the mi-Gel Extraction Kit (Metabion international AG, Steinkirchen Germany). Both strands of DNA fragments were sequenced using an ABI

PRISM 3730XL DNA Analyzer (Applied Biosystems, San Francisco, CA, USA). Primers and internal walking primers were used for sequencing *B. divergens*, *T. capreoli*, and *Theileria* sp. OT3 18S rRNA and cyt b genes. The subsequent electropherograms of the nucleotide sequences were manually inspected, corrected, and edited using ChromasPro program (McCarthy, Queensland, Australia) and LaserGene 12.1 program (DNAStar, Madison, WI, USA). All nucleotide sequences were compared to those deposited in the NCBI GenBank database using the BLAST algorithm (http://www.ncbi.nlm.nih.gov/BLAST, 27 November 2012). Nucleotide sequences longer than 200 bp were deposited in the NCBI GenBank under the following accession numbers: OL442188, OL442187, and OL442191.

Table 3. Targets, oligonucleotide primers, size of amplicons, and melting temperature of the primers used for the PCR detection of piroplasms in ticks removed from fallow deer and red deer.

Target Gene *	Primer Name	Nucleotide Sequence (5′-3′)	Product Size (bp)	Tm (°C)	Reference
18S rRNA	PIROA	AATACCCAATCCTGACACAGGG	408–430	62	[30,31]
	PIROB	TTAAATACGAATGCCCCCAAC			
	Bab2	GTTATAGTTTATTTGATGTTCGTTT	155–157	54	[32]
	Bab3	AAGCCATGCGATTCGCTAAT			
COI	Bdiv-F165	AGTGGAACTGGGTGGACATTGTAC	234	60	[13]
	Bdiv-R398	TACCGGCAATGACAAAAGTAG			
	BcapF165	AGTGGAACAGGATGGACGCTATAT	443	60	[13]
	Bcap-R607	GTCTGATTACCGAACACTTCC			
18S rRNA	18SRNABABF1	GCATGTCTAAGTACAAACTTTTTAC	1610	60	This study
	18SRNABABR1	AAGGTTCACAAGACTTCCCTAGGC			
	BABGF2	GTCTTGTAATTGGAATGATGG	1192	55	This study
	18SRNABABR1	AAGGTTCACAAGACTTCCCTAGGC			
	Piro0F2	GCCAGTAGTCATATGCTTGTCTTA	1702	60	[35]
	Piro6R2	CTCCTTCCTTTAAGTGATAAGGTTCAC			
	Piro1F2	CCATGCATGTCTTAGTATAAGCTTTTA	1670	60	[35]
	Piro5R2	CCTTTAAGTGATAAGGTTCACAAAACTT			
COI	Cox1F133	GGAGAGCTAGGTAGTAGTGGAGATAGG	1023	56	[35]
	Cox1R1130	GTGGAAGTGAGCTACCACATACGCTG			

18S rRNA- 18S ribosomal RNA, COI- cytochrome c oxidase subunit I, Tm- melting temperature.

5.5. Statistical Analysis

Statistical analyses were performed using the ABI-Prism 9 software. The level of significance was set at $p < 0.05$.

Supplementary Materials: The following are available online at https://www.mdpi.com/article/10.3390/pathogens11020222/s1, Figure S1: *Babesia microti* detection by PCR and DNA sequencing. Table S1: Tick species removed from fallow deer, showing distribution of piroplasm-infected ticks. Table S2: Tick species removed from red deer, showing distribution of piroplasm-infected ticks.

Author Contributions: Conceptualization, L.M.G. and E.M.; Investigation, L.M.G., E.M., N.F., I.A., B.R., J.F.S., A.Z. and J.G.; Writing—original draft preparation, E.M. and J.G.; Writing—review and editing, E.M., L.M.G., A.Z. and J.G.; Funding, L.M.G., E.M. and N.F.; Acquisition, E.M and L.M.G. All authors have read and agreed to the published version of the manuscript.

Funding: Funding was provided by a grant from the Health Institute Carlos III (PI20CIII/00037 to E.M. and L.G.M.), Spain and a grant from Alfonso X el Sabio Foundation (1.010.911 to N.F.), Spain.

Institutional Review Board Statement: Not applicable.

Informed Consent Statement: Not applicable.

Data Availability Statement: Not applicable.

Conflicts of Interest: The authors declare no conflict of interest.

References

1. Estrada-Peña, A.; Jongejan, F. Ticks feeding on humans: A review of records on human-biting Ixodoidea with special reference to pathogen transmission. *Exp. Appl. Acarol.* **1999**, *23*, 685–715. [CrossRef] [PubMed]
2. Rizzoli, A.; Silaghi, C.; Obiegala, A.; Rudolf, I.; Hubálek, Z.; Földvári, G.; Plantard, O.; Vayssier-Taussat, M.; Bonnet, S.; Spitalská, E.; et al. *Ixodes ricinus* and its transmitted pathogens in urban and peri-urban areas in Europe: New hazards and relevance for Public Health. *Front. Public Health* **2014**, *2*, 251. [CrossRef] [PubMed]
3. Cutler, S.J.; Vayssier-Taussat, M.; Estrada-Peña, A.; Potkonjak, A.; Mihalca, A.D.; Zeller, H. Tick-borne diseases and co-infection: Current considerations. *Ticks Tick Borne Dis.* **2021**, *12*, 101607. [CrossRef] [PubMed]
4. Remesar, S.; Díaz, P.; Prieto, A.; García-Dios, D.; Panadero, R.; Fernández, G.; Brianti, E.; Díez-Baños, P.; Morrondo, P.; López, C.M. Molecular detection and identification of piroplasms (*Babesia* spp. and *Theileria* spp.) and *Anaplasma phagocytophilum* in questing ticks from northwest Spain. *Med. Vet. Entomol.* **2021**, *35*, 51–58. [CrossRef] [PubMed]
5. Kumar, B.; Manjunathachar, H.V.; Ghosh, S. A Review on *Hyalomma* species infestations on human and animals and progress on management strategies. *Heliyon* **2020**, *6*, e05675. [CrossRef]
6. Bakheit, M.A.; Latif, A.A.; Vatansever, Z.; Seitzer, U.; Ahmed, J. The huge risks due to *Hyalomma* ticks. In *Arthropods as Vectors of Emerging Diseases*; Mehlhorn, A., Ed.; Springer: Berlin/Heidelberg, Germany, 2012; pp. 167–194.
7. Jalovecka, M.; Sojka, D.; Ascencio, M.; Schnittger, L. *Babesia* life cycle-when phylogeny meets biology. *Trends Parasitol.* **2019**, *35*, 356–368. [CrossRef]
8. Hildebrandt, A.; Gray, J.S.; Hunfeld, K.-P. Human babesiosis in Europe: What clinicians need to know. *Infection* **2013**, *41*, 1057–1072. [CrossRef]
9. Duh, D.; Petrovec, M.; Bidovec, A.; Avsic-Zupanc, T. Cervids as Babesiae hosts, Slovenia. *Emerg. Infect. Dis.* **2005**, *11*, 1121–1123. [CrossRef]
10. Bonnet, S.; Jougli, M.; L'Hostis, M.; Chauvin, A. *Babesia* sp. EU1 from roe deer and transmission within *Ixodes ricinus*. *Emerg. Infect. Dis.* **2007**, *13*, 1208. [CrossRef]
11. Zintl, A.; Mulcahy, G.; Skerrett, H.E.; Taylor, S.M.; Gray, J.S. *Babesia divergens*, a bovine blood parasite of veterinary and zoonotic importance. *Clin. Microbiol. Rev.* **2003**, *16*, 622–636. [CrossRef]
12. Fanelli, A. A historical review of *Babesia* spp. associated with deer in Europe: *Babesia divergens*/*Babesia divergens*-like, *Babesia capreoli*, *Babesia venatorum*, *Babesia* cf. *odocoilei*. *Vet. Parasitol.* **2021**, *294*, 109433. [CrossRef] [PubMed]
13. Azagi, T.; Jaarsma, R.I.; Docters van Leeuwen, A.; Fonville, M.; Maas, M.; Franssen, F.F.J.; Kik, M.; Rijks, J.M.; Montizaan, M.G.; Groenevelt, M.; et al. Circulation of *Babesia* species and their exposure to humans through *Ixodes ricinus*. *Pathogens* **2021**, *10*, 386. [CrossRef] [PubMed]
14. Remesar, S.; Díaz, P.; Prieto, A.; Markina, F.; Díaz Cao, J.M.; López-Lorenzo, G.; Fernández, G.; López, C.M.; Panadero, R.; Díez-Baños, P.; et al. Prevalence and distribution of *Babesia* and *Theileria* species in roe deer from Spain. *Int. J. Parasitol. Parasites Wildl.* **2019**, *9*, 195–201. [CrossRef] [PubMed]
15. Díaz-Cao, J.M.; Adaszek, Ł.; Dzięgiel, B.; Paniagua, J.; Caballero-Gómez, J.; Winiarczyk, S.; Winiarczyk, D.; Cano-Terriza, D.; García-Bocanegra, I. Prevalence of selected tick-borne pathogens in wild ungulates and ticks in southern Spain. *Transbound. Emerg. Dis.* **2021**. Online ahead of print. [CrossRef]
16. Zintl, A.; Finnerty, E.J.; Murphy, T.M.; de Waal, T.; Gray, J.S. Babesias of red deer (*Cervus elaphus*) in Ireland. *Vet. Res.* **2011**, *42*, 7. [CrossRef]
17. Ebani, V.V.; Rocchigiani, G.; Bertelloni, F.; Nardoni, S.; Leoni, A.; Nicoloso, S.; Mancianti, F. Molecular survey on the presence of zoonotic arthropod-borne pathogens in wild red deer (*Cervus elaphus*). *Comp. Immunol. Microbiol. Infect. Dis.* **2016**, *47*, 77–80. [CrossRef]
18. Michel, A.O.; Mathis, A.; Ryser-Degiorgis, M.-P. *Babesia* spp. in European wild ruminant species: Parasite diversity and risk factors for infection. *Vet. Res.* **2014**, *45*, 65. [CrossRef]
19. Malandrin, L.; Jouglin, M.; Sun, Y.; Brisseau, N.; Chauvin, A. Redescription of *Babesia capreoli* (Enigk and Friedhoff, 1962) from roe deer (*Capreolus capreolus*): Isolation, cultivation, host specificity, molecular characterisation and differentiation from *Babesia divergens*. *Int. J. Parasitol.* **2010**, *40*, 277–284. [CrossRef]
20. Kumar, A.; O'Bryan, J.; Krause, P.J. The global emergence of human babesiosis. *Pathogens* **2021**, *10*, 1447. [CrossRef]
21. Goethert, H.K. What *Babesia microti* is now. *Pathogens* **2021**, *10*, 1168. [CrossRef]
22. Hildebrandt, A.; Zintl, A.; Montero, E.; Hunfeld, K.-P.; Gray, J. Human babesiosis in Europe. *Pathogens* **2021**, *10*, 1165. [CrossRef] [PubMed]
23. Mans, B.J.; Pienaar, R.; Latif, A.A. A review of *Theileria* diagnostics and epidemiology. *Int. J. Parasitol. Parasites Wildl.* **2015**, *4*, 104–118. [CrossRef] [PubMed]
24. Zanet, S.; Battisti, E.; Pepe, P.; Ciuca, L.; Colombo, L.; Trisciuoglio, A.; Ferroglio, E.; Cringoli, G.; Rinaldi, L.; Maurelli, M.P. Tick-borne pathogens in Ixodidae ticks collected from privately-owned dogs in Italy: A country-wide molecular survey. *BMC Vet. Res.* **2020**, *16*, 46. [CrossRef] [PubMed]
25. Lempereur, L.; Beck, R.; Fonseca, I.; Marques, C.; Duarte, A.; Santos, M.; Zúquete, S.; Gomes, J.; Walder, G.; Domingos, A.; et al. Guidelines for the detection of *Babesia* and *Theileria* parasites. *Vector Borne Zoonotic Dis.* **2017**, *17*, 51–65. [CrossRef]
26. Agina, O.A.; Shaari, M.R.; Isa, N.M.M.; Ajat, M.; Zamri-Saad, M.; Hamzah, H. Clinical pathology, immunopathology and advanced vaccine technology in bovine theileriosis: A review. *Pathogens* **2020**, *9*, 697. [CrossRef]

27. Zanet, S.; Trisciuoglio, A.; Bottero, E.; de Mera, I.G.; Gortazar, C.; Carpignano, M.; Ferroglio, E. Piroplasmosis in wildlife: *Babesia* and *Theileria* affecting free-ranging ungulates and carnivores in the Italian Alps. *Parasit. Vectors* **2014**, *7*, 70. [CrossRef]
28. García-Sanmartía, J.; Aurtenetxe, O.; Barral, M.; Marco, I.; Lavin, S.; García-Pérez, A.L.; Hurtado, A. Molecular detection and characterization of piroplasms infecting cervids and chamois in northern Spain. *Parasitology* **2007**, *134*, 391. [CrossRef]
29. Santos-Silva, M.M.; Beati, L.; Santos, A.S.; De Sousa, R.; Núncio, M.S.; Melo, P.; Santos-Reis, M.; Fonseca, C.; Formosinho, P.; Vilela, C.; et al. The hard-tick fauna of mainland Portugal (Acari: Ixodidae): An update on geographical distribution and known associations with hosts and pathogens. *Exp. Appl. Acarol.* **2011**, *55*, 85–121. [CrossRef]
30. Armstrong, P.M.; Katavolos, P.; Caporale, D.A.; Smith, R.P.; Spielman, A.; Telford, S.R. Diversity of *Babesia* infecting deer ticks (*Ixodes dammini*). *Am. J. Trop. Med. Hyg.* **1998**, *58*, 739–742. [CrossRef]
31. De Marco, M.D.M.F.; Hernández-Triana, L.M.; Phipps, L.P.; Hansford, K.; Mitchell, E.S.; Cull, B.; Swainsbury, C.S.; Fooks, A.R.; Medlock, J.M.; Johnson, N. Emergence of *Babesia canis* in southern England. *Parasit. Vectors* **2017**, *10*, 241. [CrossRef]
32. Bloch, E.M.; Lee, T.-H.; Krause, P.J.; Telford, S.R.; Montalvo, L.; Chafets, D.; Usmani-Brown, S.; Lepore, T.J.; Busch, M.P. Development of a real-time polymerase chain reaction assay for sensitive detection and quantitation of *Babesia microti* infection. *Transfus. Paris* **2013**, *53*, 2299–2306. [CrossRef]
33. Gray, J.; Zintl, A.; Hildebrandt, A.; Hunfeld, K.-P.; Weiss, L. Zoonotic babesiosis: Overview of the disease and novel Aspects of pathogen identity. *Ticks Tick Borne Dis.* **2010**, *1*, 3–10. [CrossRef] [PubMed]
34. Hildebrandt, A.; Hunfeld, K.-P.; Baier, M.; Krumbholz, A.; Sachse, S.; Lorenzen, T.; Kiehntopf, M.; Fricke, H.-J.; Straube, E. First confirmed autochthonous case of human *Babesia microti* infection in Europe. *Eur. J. Clin. Microbiol. Infect. Dis.* **2007**, *26*, 595–601. [CrossRef] [PubMed]
35. Tuvshintulga, B.; Sivakumar, T.; Battsetseg, B.; Narantsatsaral, S.; Enkhtaivan, B.; Battur, B.; Hayashida, K.; Okubo, K.; Ishizaki, T.; Inoue, N.; et al. The PCR detection and phylogenetic characterization of *Babesia microti* in questing ticks in Mongolia. *Parasitol. Int.* **2015**, *64*, 527–532. [CrossRef] [PubMed]
36. Höfle, U.; Vicente, J.; Nagore, D.; Hurtado, A.; Peña, A.; de la Fuente, J.; Gortazar, C. The risks of translocating wildlife. *Vet. Parasitol.* **2004**, *126*, 387–395. [CrossRef] [PubMed]
37. Tian, Z.; Liu, G.; Yin, H.; Xie, J.; Wang, S.; Yuan, X.; Wang, F.; Luo, J. First report on the occurrence of *Theileria* sp. OT3 in China. *Parasitol. Int.* **2014**, *63*, 403–407. [CrossRef] [PubMed]
38. Ruiz-Fons, F.; Fernández-de-Mera, I.G.; Acevedo, P.; Höfle, U.; Vicente, J.; de la Fuente, J.; Gortazár, C. Ixodid ticks parasitizing Iberian red deer (*Cervus elaphus hispanicus*) and European wild boar (*Sus scrofa*) from Spain: Geographical and temporal distribution. *Vet. Parasitol.* **2006**, *140*, 133–142. [CrossRef]
39. Norte, A.C.; de Carvalho, I.L.; Ramos, J.A.; Gonçalves, M.; Gern, L.; Núncio, M.S. Diversity and seasonal patterns of ticks parasitizing wild birds in western Portugal. *Exp. Appl. Acarol.* **2012**, *58*, 327–339. [CrossRef]
40. Orden Ixodida: Las Garrapatas. Available online: https://docplayer.es/44688524-Orden-ixodida-las-garrapatas.html (accessed on 26 October 2021).
41. Pereira, A.; Parreira, R.; Cotão, A.J.; Nunes, M.; Vieira, M.L.; Azevedo, F.; Campino, L.; Maia, C. Tick-borne bacteria and protozoa detected in ticks collected from domestic animals and wildlife in central and southern Portugal. *Ticks Tick Borne Dis.* **2018**, *9*, 225–234. [CrossRef]
42. Opalińska, P.; Wierzbicka, A.; Asman, M.; Rączka, G.; Dyderski, M.K.; Nowak-Chmura, M. Fivefold higher abundance of ticks (Acari: Ixodida) on the European roe deer (*Capreolus capreolus* L.) forest than field ecotypes. *Sci. Rep.* **2021**, *11*, 10649. [CrossRef]
43. Radzijevskaja, J.; Paulauskas, A.; Rosef, O. Prevalence of *Anaplasma phagocytophilum* and *Babesia divergens* in *Ixodes ricinus* ticks from Lithuania and Norway. *Int. J. Med. Microbiol.* **2008**, *298*, 218–221. [CrossRef]
44. Silaghi, C.; Fröhlich, J.; Reindl, H.; Hamel, D.; Rehbein, S. *Anaplasma phagocytophilum* and *Babesia* species of sympatric roe deer (*Capreolus capreolus*), fallow deer (*Dama dama*), sika deer (*Cervus nippon*) and red deer (*Cervus elaphus*) in Germany. *Pathogens* **2020**, *9*, 968. [CrossRef] [PubMed]
45. Hrazdilová, K.; Rybářová, M.; Široký, P.; Votýpka, J.; Zintl, A.; Burgess, H.; Steinbauer, V.; Žákovčík, V.; Modrý, D. Diversity of *Babesia* spp. in cervid ungulates based on the 18S rDNA and cytochrome c oxidase subunit I phylogenies. *Infect. Genet. Evol.* **2020**, *77*, 104060. [CrossRef] [PubMed]
46. Langton, C.; Gray, J.; Waters, P.; Holman, P. Naturally acquired babesiosis in a reindeer (*Rangifer tarandus tarandus*) herd in Great Britain. *Parasitol. Res.* **2003**, *89*, 194–198. [CrossRef] [PubMed]
47. Walter, G.; Weber, G. A study on the transmission (transstadial, transovarial) of *Babesia microti*, strain "Hannover i", in its tick vector, *Ixodes ricinus* (in German, author's transl). *Trop. Parasitol.* **1981**, *32*, 228–230.
48. Walter, G. Transmission of *Babesia microti* by nymphs of *Dermacentor marginatus, D. reticulatus, Haemaphysalis punctata, Rhipicephalus sanguineus* and *Ixodes hexagonus*. *Z. Parasitenkd.* **1982**, *66*, 353–354. [CrossRef]
49. Pieniążek, N.; Sawczuk, M.; Skotarczak, B. Molecular identification of *Babesia* parasites isolated from *Ixodes ricinus* ticks collected in northwestern Poland. *J. Parasitol.* **2006**, *92*, 32–35. [CrossRef]
50. Welc-Falęciak, R.; Werszko, J.; Cydzik, K.; Bajer, A.; Michalik, J.; Behnke, J.M. Co-infection and genetic diversity of tick-borne pathogens in roe deer from Poland. *Vector Borne Zoonotic Dis.* **2013**, *13*, 277–288. [CrossRef]
51. Welc-Falęciak, R.; Bajer, A.; Paziewska-Harris, A.; Baumann-Popczyk, A.; Siński, E. Diversity of *Babesia* in *Ixodes ricinus* ticks in Poland. *Adv. Med. Sci.* **2012**, *57*, 364–369. [CrossRef]

52. Moniuszko-Malinowska, A.; Swiecicka, I.; Dunaj, J.; Zajkowska, J.; Czupryna, P.; Zambrowski, G.; Chmielewska-Badora, J.; Żukiewicz-Sobczak, W.; Swierzbinska, R.; Rutkowski, K.; et al. Infection with *Babesia microti* in humans with non-specific symptoms in north east Poland. *Infect. Dis.* **2016**, *48*, 537–543. [CrossRef]
53. Arsuaga, M.; Gonzalez, L.M.; Lobo, C.A.; de la Calle, F.; Bautista, J.M.; Azcárate, I.G.; Puente, S.; Montero, E. First report of *Babesia microti* -caused babesiosis in Spain. *Vector Borne Zoonotic Dis.* **2016**, *16*, 677–679. [CrossRef] [PubMed]
54. García-Sanmartía, J.; Barandika, J.F.; Juste, R.A.; García-Pérez, A.L.; Hurtado, A. Distribution and molecular detection of *Theileria* and *Babesia* in questing ticks from northern Spain. *Med. Vet. Entomol.* **2008**, *22*, 318–325. [CrossRef] [PubMed]
55. Giangaspero, A.; Marangi, M.; Papini, R.; Paoletti, B.; Wijnveld, M.; Jongejan, F. *Theileria* sp. OT3 and other tick-borne pathogens in sheep and ticks in Italy: Molecular characterization and phylogeny. *Ticks Tick Borne Dis.* **2015**, *6*, 75–83. [CrossRef]
56. Galuppi, R.; Aureli, S.; Bonoli, C.; Caffara, M.; Tampieri, M.P. Detection and molecular characterization of *Theileria* sp. in fallow deer (*Dama dama*) and ticks from an Italian natural preserve. *Res. Vet. Sci.* **2011**, *91*, 110–115. [CrossRef] [PubMed]
57. Voordouw, M.J. Co-feeding transmission in Lyme disease pathogens. *Parasitology* **2015**, *142*, 290–302. [CrossRef] [PubMed]
58. Eisen, L. Vector Competence studies with hard ticks and *Borrelia burgdorferi* sensu lato spirochetes: A review. *Ticks Tick Borne Dis.* **2020**, *11*, 101359. [CrossRef] [PubMed]
59. Goethert, H.K.; Mather, T.N.; Buchthal, J.; Telford, S.R. Retrotransposon-based blood meal analysis of nymphal deer ticks demonstrates spatiotemporal diversity of *Borrelia burgdorferi* and *Babesia microti* reservoirs. *Appl. Environ. Microbiol.* **2021**, *87*, e02370-20. [CrossRef]
60. BNP-Tapada de Mafra. Available online: http://bibliografia.bnportugal.gov.pt/bnp/bnp.exe/registo?1687264 (accessed on 21 June 2021).
61. Estrada-Peña, A.; Pfäffle, M.; Baneth, G.; Kleinerman, G.; Petney, T.N. Ixodoidea of the Western Palaearctic: A review of available literature for identification of species. *Ticks Tick-Borne Dis.* **2017**, *8*, 512–525. [CrossRef]

pathogens

MDPI

Review

Semicentennial of Human Babesiosis, Nantucket Island

Sam R. Telford III [1,*], Heidi K. Goethert [1] and Timothy J. Lepore [2]

[1] Department of Infectious Disease and Global Health, Tufts University, 200 Westboro Road, North Grafton, MA 01536, USA; heidi.goethert@tufts.edu
[2] Nantucket Cottage Hospital, Nantucket, MA 02554, USA; tjalepore@me.com
* Correspondence: sam.telford@tufts.edu

Abstract: Fifty years ago, the index case of human babesiosis due to *Babesia microti* was diagnosed in a summer resident of Nantucket Island. Human babesiosis, once called "Nantucket fever" due to its seeming restriction to Nantucket and the terminal moraine islands of southern New England, has emerged across the northeastern United States to commonly infect people wherever Lyme disease is endemic. We review the history of babesiosis on Nantucket, analyze its epidemiology and ecology there, provide summaries of the first case histories, and comment on its future public health burden.

Keywords: *Babesia microti*; human babesiosis; Nantucket Island; epidemiology; ecology; human risk

Citation: Telford, S.R., III; Goethert, H.K.; Lepore, T.J. Semicentennial of Human Babesiosis, Nantucket Island. *Pathogens* **2021**, *10*, 1159. https://doi.org/10.3390/pathogens10091159

Academic Editors: Estrella Montero, Jeremy Gray, Cheryl Ann Lobo and Luis Miguel González

Received: 6 August 2021
Accepted: 28 August 2021
Published: 9 September 2021

1. Introduction

Fifty years ago, a New England Journal of Medicine [1] case report summarized the index case of human babesiosis due to *Babesia microti*. Babesiosis had previously been reported in 4 patients (1 from Yugoslavia, 2 from Ireland, 1 from California), all of whom had been splenectomized; the Yugoslavian and Irish cases were due to *B. divergens*, a cattle parasite, and the California case was due to an unidentified *Babesia* sp. (likely *B. duncani*). The new case was in a spleen-intact person. Through 1976, 14 cases of symptomatic *B. microti* babesiosis had been identified on Nantucket and the infection was given the popular name "Nantucket fever" [2], even though sporadic cases were reported from nearby Martha's Vineyard, Shelter Island, NY and Montauk, NY by 1977. From 2011–2015, 27 states reported 7612 cases of babesiosis, but only 7 states accounted for 95% of these (Massachusetts, New York, Connecticut, New Jersey, Rhode Island, Wisconsin and Minnesota [3]. Nantucket County still reports more cases of babesiosis than any other in the U.S., with annual incidence of >100 per 100,000 (compared to about 1 per 100,000 nationally). We revisit the early investigations of Nantucket fever in the 1970s and highlight the major findings that defined the epidemiology and ecology of this infection.

2. The Grey Lady

Nantucket Island is a 120 sq km island (land area; another 670 sq km is coastal waters) 50 km south of Cape Cod, Massachusetts (Figure 1). It was formed by the deposition of moraine from the retreat of the Laurentide ice sheet 15,000–18,000 years ago; the moraine and outwash deposits became an island due to rising sea levels 5000–6000 years ago. Due to the influence of strong winds containing oceanic salt spray, trees were limited to species that were relatively small and salt tolerant. European settlers were established by 1660, bringing cattle, horses, sheep and pigs. By the late 1700s, the island had become essentially treeless pasture, with a peak sheep herd of 15,000 (125/sq km). From the late 1600s to 1850, Nantucket's economy was a function of whaling; Nantucket figures prominently in Melville's Moby Dick. After the Civil War, a tourism industry developed, with an intensification by the 1920s.

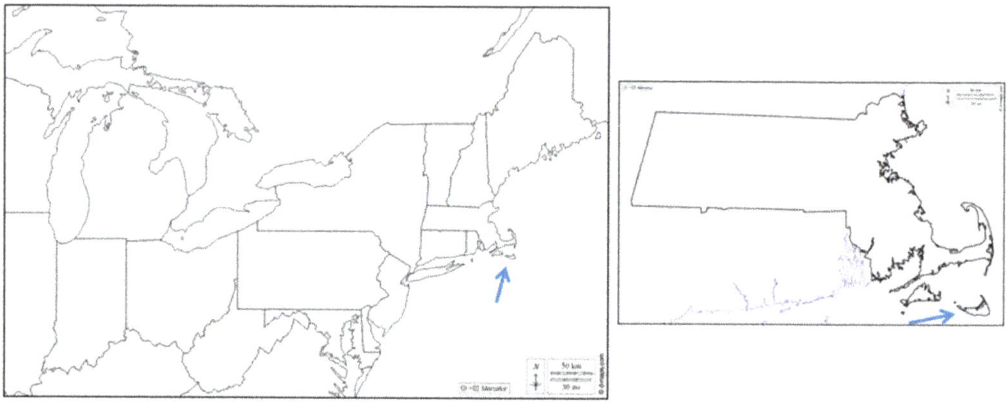

Figure 1. Nantucket Island, Massachusetts. Left panel, northeastern United States with arrow pointing to Nantucket Island. Right panel, Massachusetts with the location of Nantucket (arrow). Map from https://d-maps.com, accessed on 30 July 2021.

The end of sheep pasturing allowed for successional growth of shrubs. The landscape is dominated by patches of thick scrub comprising bayberry (*Myrica pensylvanica*), saltspray rose (*Rosa rugosa*), poison ivy (*Rhus rhadicans*), black huckleberry (*Gaylussacia baccata*), highbush blueberry (*Vaccinium corymbosum*), sweet pepperbush (*Clethra alnifolia*), sumac (*Rhus glabra*), and scrub oak (*Quercus ilicifolia*). These patches are interspersed with grassland, although in most places scrub patches have expanded over the years (Figure 2). A pitch pine forest comprises 47 hectares in the center of the island. The climate is moderated by the Atlantic Ocean, with an average annual temperature of 10.5 °C (range of −3 °C in January to 23.9 °C in July) and 33.3 mm of rainfall. The island is often covered with a dense fog (hence the name "Grey Lady").

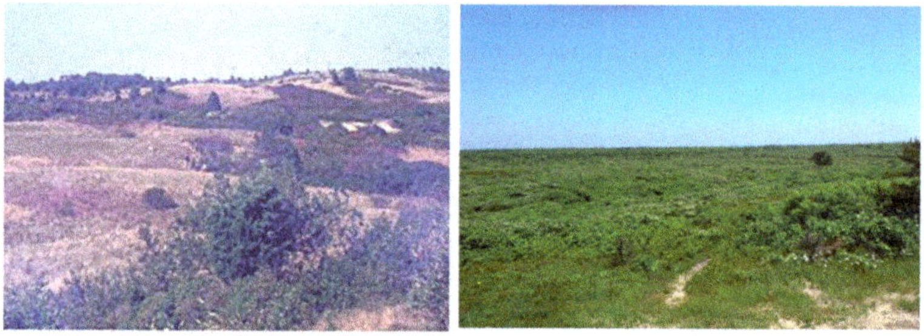

Figure 2. Changes in the landscape. Left panel, middle moors near Altar Rock, mid 1980s. "Heath" patches comprising grasses and low-lying shrubs, with interspersed thickets. Right panel, similar vantage point, 2021, demonstrating expansion of brush thicket into the heath.

Nantucket Island is accessible only by ferry or other boat, or by airplane. There are currently 17,200 year round residents, with as many as an additional 11,000 living there for 2 or more weeks during the tourist summer season (Memorial Day to Labor Day). There were 6600 seasonal workers in July 2017, and 500,000 visitor trips, 100,000 in August alone (www.nantucketdataplatform.com/projects, accessed on 30 July 2021). The median home value was $2.55 million and the average was $3.37 million at the end of 2020 and there are 12,675 housing units, 70.5% of which are owner occupied. There were 3713 households recorded in 2015–2019, with a median household income of $107,717.

The mammalian fauna includes no mesomammals (raccoons, skunks, weasels, fox, coyote, opossum) but has rodents and shrews typical for southern New England, with the exception of the red backed vole, *Myodes gapperi*. Norway rats (*Rattus norvegicus*) may be found in all habitats. There are large numbers of eastern cottontail rabbits (*Sylvilagus floridanus*). White tailed deer (*Odocoileus virginianus*) may be as dense as 56–65 per sq km. Besides the deer tick (*Ixodes dammini*, the junior subjective synonym for *I. scapularis*), there are American dog ticks, *Dermacentor variabilis* (increasingly scarce due to the use of preventives on domestic dogs; there are no other reproductive hosts for this tick there); rabbit ticks *I. dentatus* and *Haemaphysalis leporispalustris*, and an emerging infestation of Lone Star ticks, *Amblyomma americanum*.

None of these physical or socioeconomic characteristics, except perhaps the moderate climate, help explain why Nantucket was first recognized as and still is the most intensely zoonotic site for babesiosis due to *Babesia microti*.

3. Index and Other Early Cases

The first cases of Nantucket fever provided the general details of the course of illness and its management, as well as parasite strains that have been widely used in laboratory studies of the pathobiology of *B. microti* babesiosis. CDC investigations provided a good knowledge of the epidemiology and the asymptomatic to symptomatic ratio. CDC and Harvard studies outlined the general ecology of the parasite.

On 4 July 1969, a 59 year old woman who was a summer resident of Nantucket Island became ill and during the following 9 days sustained intermittent fever. The diagnosis remained elusive on Nantucket, but the critical observation, that she might have malaria, was made at St. Peter's Hospital (SPH) in New Jersey. Diverse accounts (including [1,4]) have been provided about the connection between the Nantucket patient and New Jersey, but the true story appears in [5]: a friend of the index patient had asked a colorectal surgeon from SPH, Benjamin Glasser, who had treated members of the family, to come to Nantucket to see the "dying" patient, who was transported by private plane to SPH and admitted on 13 July. Malaria parasites were found by a microscopist examining a routine blood smear at the clinical lab at SPH. Gordon Benson, a gastroenterologist at SPH was asked for his opinion on the slides because "someone thought I knew something about malaria". Benson, after encountering no interest from the Massachusetts Department of Public Health, called the CDC on 16 July about a possible autochthonous malaria case. The key people in the story of the index case were thus a concerned family friend, an excellent clinical lab microscopist, and a phone call from someone who knew that malaria cases needed to be reported.

On 18 July, the CDC chief of malaria surveillance, Karl Western, and Arthur Dover, an Epidemic Intelligence Service (EIS) officer, left for New Jersey. The blood smears that prompted Dr. Benson's call, arrived at CDC on 18 July. Mike Schultz, who was director of the parasitic diseases division of the CDC at the time, argued with their expert parasitology microscopist, Neva Gleason, about the identity of the infection, insisting that it was not malaria (M.G. Schultz, personal communication). Gleason found tetrads on her third reexamination of the slides and Schultz, who had earned both DVM and MD degrees and had trained at the London School of Hygiene and Tropical Medicine with the eminent malariologist Leonard Bruce-Chwatt, immediately knew this was a case of babesiosis. The internal National Communicable Disease Center memo, dated 18 July, was titled "Cryptic parasitemia—New Jersey" (Figure 3). The investigation and case report conducted by Western and Dover was published in the NEJM [1] almost verbatim from the internal 5 December 1969 CDC report, although Dover was surprisingly not included as an author.

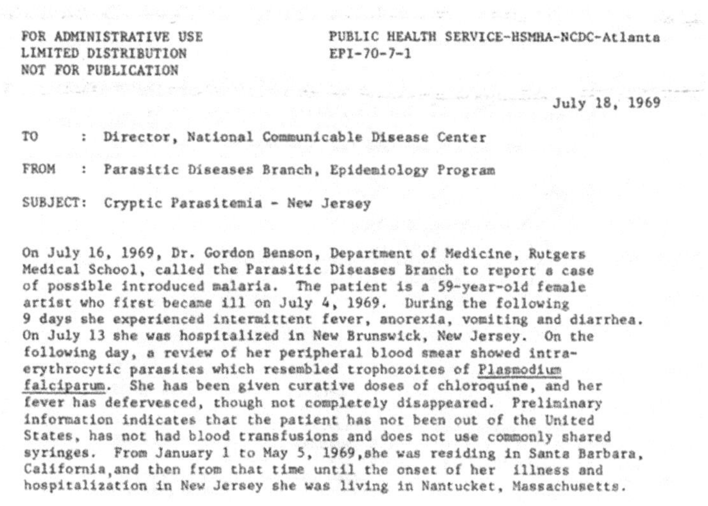

FOR ADMINISTRATIVE USE
LIMITED DISTRIBUTION
NOT FOR PUBLICATION

PUBLIC HEALTH SERVICE-HSMHA-NCDC-Atlanta
EPI-70-7-1

July 18, 1969

TO : Director, National Communicable Disease Center

FROM : Parasitic Diseases Branch, Epidemiology Program

SUBJECT: Cryptic Parasitemia - New Jersey

On July 16, 1969, Dr. Gordon Benson, Department of Medicine, Rutgers Medical School, called the Parasitic Diseases Branch to report a case of possible introduced malaria. The patient is a 59-year-old female artist who first became ill on July 4, 1969. During the following 9 days she experienced intermittent fever, anorexia, vomiting and diarrhea. On July 13 she was hospitalized in New Brunswick, New Jersey. On the following day, a review of her peripheral blood smear showed intra-erythrocytic parasites which resembled trophozoites of Plasmodium falciparum. She has been given curative doses of chloroquine, and her fever has defervesced, though not completely disappeared. Preliminary information indicates that the patient has not been out of the United States, has not had blood transfusions and does not use commonly shared syringes. From January 1 to May 5, 1969,she was residing in Santa Barbara, California,and then from that time until the onset of her illness and hospitalization in New Jersey she was living in Nantucket, Massachusetts.

Figure 3. Internal CDC memorandum reporting the index case of babesiosis on Nantucket.

Blood from the patient received on 19 July was subinoculated by George Healy, chief of the parasitology laboratory at CDC into hamsters and other experimental animals and propagated by subinoculation of hamsters [6]. The identity of the parasite was inferred from its morphology and infection kinetics in a prairie vole (*Microtus ochrogaster*) model and its comparison with *B. rodhaini* and "*B. microti*" from California rodents [7]. As was convention at the time (no longer done due to patient confidentiality), the parasite isolate was designated the Gray strain. Ristic et al. [8] also report isolation of *B. microti* from a blood sample taken from the index patient on August 4, with parasites passed into hamsters as well as a splenectomized monkey. The Gray strain was deposited at ATCC by the malariologist Julius Kreier at Ohio State. The provenance of the material that Kreier deposited (as outlined in the ATCC specification sheet) was "Western-Holbrook-Kreier" (presumably A. Holbrook of USDA, an expert on the ruminant babesias) and not from his frequent collaborator Miodrag Ristic (expert on diverse hemotropic infections, University of Illinois). As far as we know, the Gray strain has not been replenished from other sources in the interim, and what is available from ATCC (catalog number 30221) has been serially passaged between hamsters countless times from the original Kreier material. The ATCC material has been confirmed to have a Nantucket origin by variable nucleotide tandem repeat genotyping and by whole genome analysis [9,10].

The index case would have remained just the 5th sporadic case of babesiosis but in September of 1973, another case was diagnosed, this time at the Nantucket Cottage Hospital (NCH). A 50 year old female was admitted for fever and chills 25 days after she removed a tick; she had started having daily fevers 11 days afterwards but had symptomatic relief by the use of aspirin. The dates for these events and some details of her course of illness differ between the hospital discharge report and the case report [11], but the main features of the case are (1) the patient sustained daily or intermittent fevers to 104 °F that led her to seek medical attention; (2) that tetracycline (no dose indicated) was started because Rocky Mountain Spotted Fever was endemic on Cape Cod and the islands at that time; (3) that a blood smear was examined when the patient failed to improve on tetracycline; (4) that chloroquine phosphate 1.5 grams was provided in the first 24 hours after finding parasites on blood smear, then at 0.5 gram daily, presumably by mouth; (5) that she defervesced and felt better within 3 days of starting the chloroquine, despite parasites continuing to be found at low level in her blood smear; (6) Her hematocrit dropped to 23% on the sixth day of admission and she required two units of blood; (7) She was discharged on September 22 with no fever and was maintained on chloroquine twice weekly for

6 months. Interestingly, the case report mentions subinoculating two gerbils ("dictated by the availability of such animals in the local pet store") with blood from the patient on the day parasites were found on blood smear, presumably by Dr. Anderson of Cape Cod Hospital, who was the consulting pathologist for NCH. Both gerbils became infected, and a second sample of blood, retained for 5 days in the refrigerator, infected hamsters at the CDC, which maintained the strain. This is the origin of the Peabody-mjr strain (ATCC PRA-99), which was adapted to inbred mice [12] by serial passage. C3H mice were found to be most susceptible in the first experiments trying to adapt hamster origin parasites. Subsequent work using the Peabody strain in balb/c mice confirmed earlier work with the British *B. microti* King's strain [13] that the protective effect of adoptive transfer of immune splenocytes or lymph node cells was abrogated when the infected donor mouse had been depleted of T cells [14], suggesting a requirement for both T and B cells in controlling parasitemia.

Rodent subinoculation, as done by the CDC parasitologists and by Dr. Anderson, became the gold standard for confirming a case of *B. microti* babesiosis until the advent of polymerase chain reaction assays. Hamsters required only 300 parasites to become infected [15], which provided great sensitivity for confirming a diagnosis because one could intraperitoneally inoculate as much as 1 mL of blood (depending on the size of the hamster); the theoretical sensitivity was thus 0.3 parasites per microliter of blood, which is the same as a typical PCR assay using agarose gel detection of amplicons [16]. In practice, hamster inoculation could be complicated by transient parasitemias being missed or the hamster not being monitored a full month after subinoculation, and some parasites "preferred" splenectomized or immune-deficient mice and thus infection never became patent in hamsters (unpublished).

No cases were identified in 1974, but in 1975, an additional 6 cases were diagnosed on Nantucket, prompting another EIS investigation, this time headed by Trenton Ruebush II. The EIS report dated 9 January 1976 provided details on 6 cases, but the published report included only 5 of these [17]. The omitted case was a 86 year old male with fever, shaking chills, drenching sweats, myalgia/arthralgia, fatigue, splenomegaly, and hepatomegaly. A parasitemia of 25% was recorded on admission, but a blood smear taken 2 weeks previously was positive when retrospectively examined. The patient improved with chloroquine treatment, as did the other 5 cases, but he was parasitemic for another 10 weeks after discharge. This case was likely that alluded to in the first paper on reservoir hosts on Nantucket [18] as having been diagnosed in October. All but one of these first 8 cases from Nantucket were in people aged 50 years or older, establishing the fact that clinically apparent disease was associated with age.

A particularly interesting observation is that none of the early clinical reports [1,2,11,19] alluded to erythema migrans or other rash, although the first two cases sustained "tick bite" reactions, one of which resolved when the site of the bite was excised. About a fifth of babesiosis cases have evidence of concurrent Lyme disease [20] and a similar proportion of host seeking ticks on Nantucket infected by *B. microti* also contain *B. burgdorferi* [21]. However, an "insect bite" was reported in the first case from Shelter Island [22] and although the swelling that was reported is not typical for erythema migrans, the lesion abated with ampicillin treatment. Nonetheless, cases of odd rashes were not noted during the intensive EIS investigations of 1969 and 1975–1976, suggesting that *B. burgdorferi* was not commonly infecting people there at the time. This is a paradox, given that the agent had been enzootic in the area since the late 1890s [23] and certainly must have been co-transmitted by *I. dammini* long before human risk was apparent.

The early cases had been treated with chloroquine due to clinical similarity with malaria, but the efficacy of chloroquine had been questioned even for the index and subsequent cases. Parasitological cure was not demonstrated, and the drug had no effect whatever in reducing parasitemia in experimental hamster infections [24]. It should be noted, though, that in all of the early cases, prompt symptomatic relief was noted when chloroquine was provided, certainly well within the range of the week that was observed for symptomatic relief when current drug regimens (quinine/clindamycin or atovaquone/azithromycin) are used. Excess production of pro-inflammatory cytokines appears to be the basis for the signs and symptoms of acute babesiosis [25]. Chloroquine is immunomodulatory, inhibiting immune activation, including cytokine production [26] and would be expected to provide symptomatic relief. Although babesiacidal therapy is the standard, there may be benefits to immunomodulation in the treatment of babesiosis, and its possible role in combination therapy should be reexamined.

4. Epidemiology and Ecology of *B. microti* Babesiosis

Ruebush's comprehensive epidemiologic investigation in 1975 included a home visit and telephone survey of the frequency of tick bites and febrile illnesses and a cross-sectional serosurvey. The results were published in 3 remarkable papers [17,19,27]. Complementary studies of potential reservoir hosts and vectors were done at the same time by his CDC colleague George Healy (who had undertaken the hamster subinoculation studies of the 1969 and 1973 cases) and Andrew Spielman of the Harvard School of Public Health [18,28]. The main findings were that 8.3% of 687 Nantucket residents (seasonal and full time) had sustained a tick bite in the 4 months preceding the survey; that asymptomatic infection was common (21 of 673 Nantucket residents were identified as seropositive, and of the 19 that could be followed up, 13 denied any febrile illness within 6 months of providing the blood sample). Ruebush et al. [19] made the prescient remark "Although transfusion-induced babesiosis has never been reported in man, the prolonged parasitemia noted in Case 3 suggests that transmission by this route may occur". Babesiosis is now the most common protozoal hazard associated with blood transfusionin the United States [29].

On the ecology aspects, the team determined that 80% of white-footed mice (*Peromyscus leucopus*) trapped on Nantucket were infected. Spielman, using larval "*I. scapularis*" derived from engorged females removed from hunter killed deer on Nantucket, demonstrated vector competence by transmitting the Gray strain between hamsters. The ecology of babesiosis on Nantucket became the focus of Spielman's graduate student, Joe Piesman, who developed methods of detecting *B. microti* in ticks (with the key finding that the parasites needed to be reactivated with the formation of sporozoites in order to be detected by microscopy), experimental challenge of deer (which were not susceptible), and seasonality of transmission [30].

Spielman and Piesman noted morphologic differences between the Nantucket "*I. scapularis*" and those from elsewhere in the eastern U.S., and described it as a new species, *Ixodes dammini*, with Nantucket as the type locality [31]. Although the name *I. dammini* was synonymized with *I. scapularis* in the early 1990s and few now use the junior subjective synonym, there are epidemiological reasons to continue to make the distinction, viz., the northern form bites people in the nymphal stage [32]. The main argument for synonymy was that ticks from southern sites (*I. scapularis*) would form fertile F1 hybrids with ticks from Massachusetts sites (*I. dammini*), but we now know that this is not a useful criterion to test for conspecificity in *Ixodes* ticks [33]. There are well defined genetic lineages of "*I. scapularis*" (likely a species complex) across the eastern U.S. [34] and it is likely that future analyses will reject the hypothesis that all the lineages have public health significance.

Gustave J. Dammin, after whom the tick was named, was pathologist in chief at the Peter Bent Brigham Hospital and part of the team undertaking the first successful kidney transplantation that won its surgeon, Francis Moore, a Nobel Prize in 1990. Dammin had married Anita Coffin, whose family were descended from the colonial founders of Nantucket in 1659, and frequently summered on Nantucket and nearby Tuckernuck Island. Dammin, who had made numerous notable contributions to tropical medicine and pathology, was keenly interested in the new infection, particularly after 1983 when he sustained an erythema migrans (perhaps the first well documented case on Nantucket) and made the rounds at the hospital whenever possible to tabulate babesiosis cases. He provided logistical assistance, funding, advice, and encouragement for Spielman's early studies.

5. Has Risk Changed over 50 Years?

With confounding due to changes in the population at risk and enhanced awareness by local physicians, one might argue that it is difficult to test the hypothesis that risk has changed. The number of cases on Nantucket over the years fluctuates, ranging from none to a couple dozen, with a median of 13 from 1991–1999 (data collected by S.R.T.III and T.J.L.). One might argue that the sensitivity of identifying cases was probably great in the early years, when the infection was new and then as novelty waned, so did physician and laboratorian interest. However, the late Patricia Snow MT was the main microscopist at the Cottage Hospital from 1973 until the mid 1990s and indeed she was the microscopist for the second case [11]. Snow kept a log of all babesiosis cases, and with the arrival of T.J.L. in 1982, as well as Dr. Dammin's efforts suggests reasonably good consistency in the level of effort taken to diagnosing babesiosis at NCH. Spielman gave S.R.T.III the responsibility of confirming cases by hamster inoculation, and reviewing all blood smears sent to him by Snow and this provided additional consistency to the data and thus comparable between years. The graph of annual babesiosis cases detected at NCH from 1969–1999 (Figure 4), then, is at least a consistent effort among years by the same people. The increase in cases detected from 1992–1997 does not reflect the advent of PCR or a change in risk. Snow had recently purchased a Coulter counter to perform complete blood counts and differential cells counts, and from her experience knew that babesiosis was accompanied by low platelet counts and leukopenia. She had the machine flag any such sample from a febrile case, and then spent 30 min on the microscope with the blood smear instead of the typical 10 min. This doubled the number of confirmed cases (with positive blood smear as the gold standard).

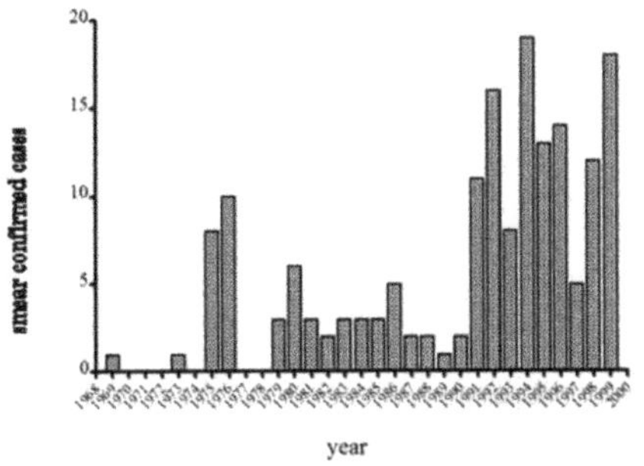

Figure 4. Nantucket cases identified from 1969-1999. All cases were blood smear positive. Cases from 1969–1986 compiled from the literature, or from Dr. G.J. Dammin's notes. 1987–1999, compiled by T.J.L./S.R.T.III.

After 1999, the hospital changed from in house detection to a commercial laboratory (Imugen, Inc., which is no longer in existence) and thus estimates of case numbers are elusive. Massachusetts started mandatory reporting for babesiosis in 2006, with automatic electronic submission directly from commercial laboratories. Thus, the reports from 2009 onwards (oddly, fewer than 5 cases were reported from Nantucket during 2007 and 2008; the Nantucket Board of Health counted vastly more cases, personal communication to S.R.T.III and T.J.L.) are likely to be comparable between years (Figure 5). A median of 23 was reported from 2009–2019, suggesting a doubling in annual incidence from earlier years. Such a doubling likely reflects increased human exposure and susceptibility, not changes in the force of enzootic and zoonotic transmission: the population has doubled (Figure 6) and there has been a 12% increase in the number of Nantucket residents older than 65 years. Then, too, even though 40% of Nantucket land is held in perpetuity for conservation, thanks to the Nantucket Conservation, Land Bank, Massachusetts Audubon, and other organizations, the pace of development has greatly increased. The density of homes in buildable plots of land has increased over time; developers buy up older homes and subdivide the properties (Figure 7).

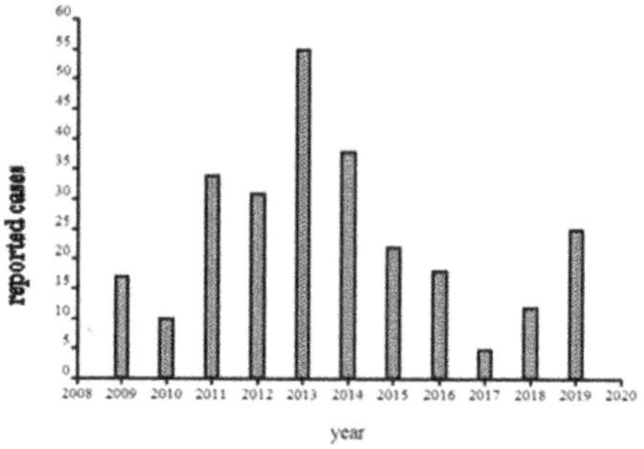

Figure 5. Nantucket cases reported to and by the Massachusetts Department of Public Health following mandatory direct laboratory reporting instituted in 2007. Data courtesy of Susan Soliva, MADPH Bureau of Infectious Disease and Laboratory Sciences.

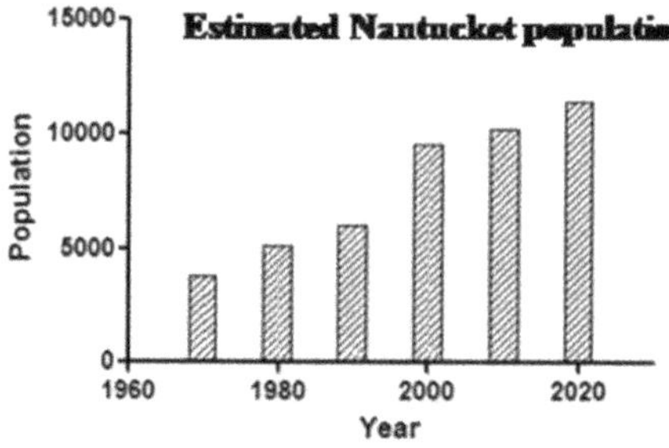

Figure 6. Doubling of Nantucket population 1970–2020. (Data from the Town of Nantucket; also available from www.nantucketdataplatform.com/projects, accessed on 30 July 2021).

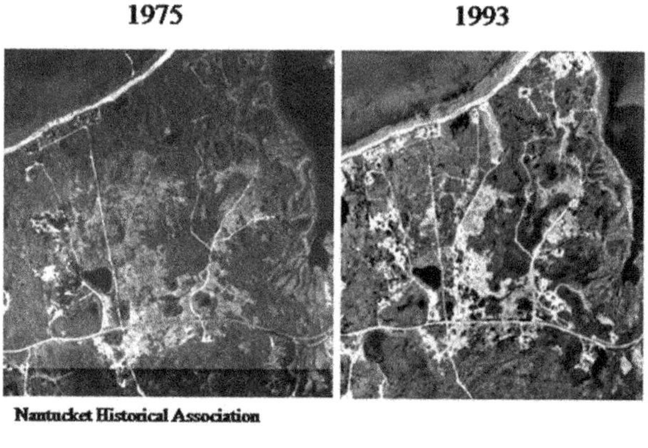

Figure 7. Increased development on Nantucket. Nantucket Historical Association, Aerial views of the Quaise/Polpis area demonstrating an increase in access roads and cleared spaces for new or larger houses; many older homes were purchased, razed, and new megamansion compounds built on the site. Source: https://www.nha.org/digitalexhibits/aerialviews/AP1975Web/index.htm; https://www.nha.org/digitalexhibits/aerialviews/AP1993Web/index.htm, accessed on 30 July 2021.

There is no evidence for an increased force of enzootic or zoonotic *B. microti* transmission. The comprehensive studies in 1975–1976 by Ruebush and colleagues reported 3.1% (95% confidence interval, 2.0–4.8) seroprevalence in a cross-sectional serosurvey using NCH discard sera (samples taken for routine blood work). T.J.L. and S.R.T.III determined that 4.3% of 4524 (95% CI, 3.7–4.9) NCH discard sera from 1991–1997 were seropositive, using the identical indirect immunofluorescence assay [35] used by Ruebush, with the same cut-off (1:64 IgG). There was a median annual prevalence of 10% *B. microti* infection in host-seeking nymphal *I. dammini* from 1984–1991, estimated by dissection of salivary glands and Feulgen staining [21,36]; Telford unpublished, and the same median annual prevalence was observed from the same sampling sites during 2016–2021 using PCR (Goethert unpublished). The tick population was at equilibrium from 1985–2004 (Figure 8), as measured by indices of infestation of white footed mice. More recent trapping studies in the same Nantucket field sites (since 2005, trapped only during June and September, to provide annual indices of nymphal and larval *I. dammini*) do not indicate any differences in mouse infestation. Even though the force of transmission has not appreciably changed, there is evidence that genetic diversity of *B. microti* in ticks and mice has increased from 1987–2013, with more diversity of minor variable number tandem repeat (VNTR) genotypes in later years; samples from 1986–1988 were dominated by the 49e haplotype [37].

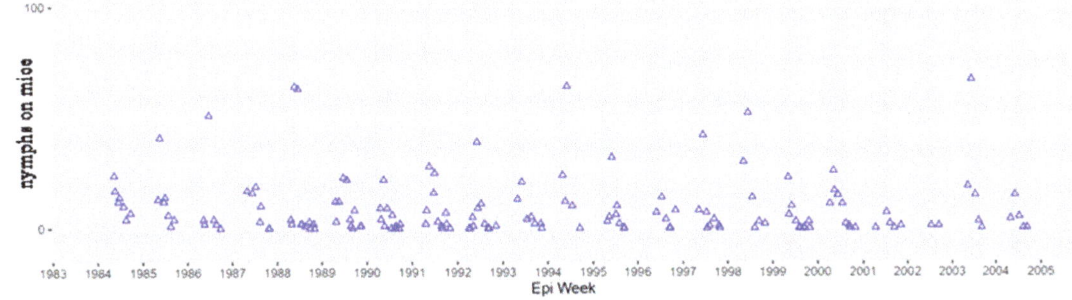

Figure 8. Nymphal *I. dammini* infestations on the UMass Field Station. Each datapoint represents the burden of an individual mouse. An intensive capture-mark-release study of *P. leucopus* was undertaken from 1984–2004, with monthly sampling from May to September of each year. No general trend (increasing or decreasing) is apparent, suggesting that the population has been at ecological equilibrium for 20 years.

Nantucket was not the original source of American *B. microti* and did not seed the remainder of southern New England, despite all the cases of "Nantucket Fever". There are 3 major lineages of *B. microti* across its range in the northeastern U.S. [37] suggesting that there were relict, epidemiologically silent enzootic foci across southern New England and that parasite range expansion was driven by local intensification and expansion into nearby areas. *B. microti* had been reported from rodents on nearby Martha's Vineyard in 1937 [38], and cases of human babesiosis were identified from that island and eastern Long Island very quickly after the few Nantucket fever cases [22,24]. The peculiar focus in early zoonotic *B. microti* to the terminal moraine sites from Long Island to Cape Cod suggested that these were the first sites after the retreat of the Wisconsin glacier to be reinvaded from refugia farther south, serving as relict longstanding foci [39]. Consistent with this hypothesis, the upper midwestern zoonotic *B. microti* foci in Wisconsin and Minnesota are north of a prominent glacial refuge ("driftless zone").

6. The Deer Tick Microbial Guild

Nantucket recorded its first cases of Lyme disease in the early 1980s, and the foundational babesiosis studies done by Spielman and Piesman on *I. dammini* and its ecology were immediately relevant to understanding risk for that bacterial zoonosis. *B. burgdorferi* was immediately incorporated into the existing babesiosis ecology and epidemiology program at Harvard. When human granulocytic ehrlichiosis (now "human anaplasmosis") due to *Anaplasma phagocytophilum* was identified in northern Wisconsin [40], a prospective search was made by T.J.L. for febrile patients with elevated liver function tests, headache, and inclusions in their neutrophils. Pat Snow's microscopy clinched the diagnosis of the index case for the northeastern U.S. [41] and led to the description of the agent's natural history [42]. A focus on infections of cottontail rabbits identified a *Babesia divergens*-like parasite that was genetically identical to that causing MO-1 babesiosis, and the detailed ecological work [43] provides a basis for explaining its apparent rarity as a zoonosis; the vector is *I. dentatus*, which rarely bites humans. It remains a puzzle as to why MO-1 parasites have never been detected in febrile Nantucket residents despite determined efforts by T.J.L., S.R.T.III and H.K.G. When deer tick virus (Powassan lineage II) was discovered in 1995 [44], a virus isolate (NFS001) was quickly made from Nantucket ticks and evidence of *P. leucopus* exposure there demonstrated [45]. Again, it is a puzzle why a deer tick virus encephalitis case has never been detected from Nantucket given its regular detection in host seeking *I. dammini* there over the years, despite intensive efforts by T.J.L. and S.R.T.III.

7. Control and Prevention

From the very beginning, CDC and Harvard investigators attempted to make recommendations for risk reduction. In the 9 January 1976 EIS report, the concluding paragraph made points that are still germane today. "Temporary and permanent residents of the island and medical personnel should be alerted to the risk of a tick bite and the characteristic symptoms of babesiosis ... Before control programs directed against vectors or reservoir hosts of babesiosis can even be considered, studies are needed to identify and define: (a) other possible tick vectors; (b) additional reservoir hosts in wild and domestic animals; (c) the distribution and fluctuation in the vector and reservoir host populations, and (d) the prevalence of infection in vector and reservoir hosts. Finally the risk of infection for man must be determined so that a cost-benefit analysis can be made of proposed control measures". The Nantucket Board of Selectmen was more to the point; Andy Spielman spoke of a grizzled seaman with tattooed arms asking him "so, doc, what do we spray?" Even though we know the main aspects of *B. microti* perpetuation, its reservoirs, prevalence of animal and tick infection, and the risk of infection, no cost-benefit analysis has been done and no sustained public health effort has been made to reduce the risk of babesiosis or Lyme disease.

Nantucket served as the control site for the seminal Great Island deer reduction experiment [46] and deer reduction has been strongly advocated for Nantucket, first by Spielman and subsequently by S.R.T.III and T.J.L. However, reducing the deer herd is hindered by sociopolitical factors that include a public reluctance to kill Bambi (the embodiment of charismatic megafauna). Habitat management is difficult: an attempt by S.R.T.III to convince Nantucket landscapers to propose to homeowners that vegetation be eliminated around their homes (thereby removing microhabitat needed for the tick to survive) was met with derision. "People want that thick stuff there for privacy". Damminix tick tubes [47] remain available but few homes regularly and consistently use them. "Spraying" is effectively prohibited as a mode of intervention due to the fact that all of Nantucket's freshwater comes from a freshwater "lens" 40–500 meters below the ground surface and people are concerned about chemicals contaminating it. Personal protection remains the best preventive method, which comprises promoting awareness, using repellents, permethrin treated clothing, and doing tick checks. The late Jim Lentowski, director of the Nantucket Conservation Foundation for 40 years, was the island leader in promoting awareness, having suffered from 3 of the 5 deer tick-transmitted infections.

The hopes for vaccination remain doubtful, particularly given the general failures (even with tremendous effort and funding) for effective vaccination against the related malarial parasites. Even if an effective and safe vaccine were developed, market analysis by pharmaceutical companies would not support the investment of $150 million or more to acquire the data for U.S. Food and Drug Administration approval. Indeed, Nantucket was one of the sites for Phase II and Phase III trials of Lymerix [the human Lyme disease vaccine developed by SmithKline Beecham (King of Prussia, PA, USA) and approved by the Food and Drug Administration], a safe and effective product that was sold for 5 years and then withdrawn from the market because sufficient cost recovery was not apparent in the face of anti-vaccine activism. Even an effective vaccine has no guarantee of financial and public health success. It is discouraging that after 50 years of research, we seem to have done little to reduce the risk for acquiring babesiosis on Nantucket.

One success in developing interventions in the last 50 years is that of therapy for babesiosis. Nantucket was the main site for the pivotal prospective randomized clinical trial of atovaquone and azithromycin (AA) [48]. Clindamycin and quinine (CQ), which had been demonstrated effective for parasitological cure in hamster infections [49] had been the treatment of choice for *B. microti* babesiosis since 1983 [50]. In the clinical trial, AA induced a more rapid parasitological response than did CQ, and did so with only 15% of the subjects reporting adverse reactions to treatment, compared with 72% for CQ. However, azithromycin, clindamycin, and quinine have failed to clear parasitemia in mouse models of *B. microti* infection [51], and treatment failures are not unusual, particularly in immunocompromised patients. Additional drug regimens for treating babesiosis are needed, particularly for those who are immunocompromised [52].

8. What Can We Predict for Nantucket Fever at Its Centennial?

In the ideal future world, a common sense approach will be taken on environmental modification with combinations of habitat management, environmentally friendly, targeted insecticides, robotic vector control, and deer reduction. The landscape is successional; humans have influenced every inch of Nantucket land and there should be no protected worship of poison ivy and invasive plant-dominated habitat. A return to pasture and heathlands would reduce habitat for deer ticks and white footed mice. Deer reduction must be strongly pursued, even if an effective and economical sterilization method was available (reduce the herd, then control their reproduction). Mechanical means of removing host-seeking deer ticks might be accomplished by advances in robotics; future generation insecticides might be developed with less impact on non-target species or more degradable to preempt suggestions of drinking water contamination.

In 2069, genetic modification of reservoir hosts and ticks and replacement of their populations with those genetically modified to be less competent to maintain enzootic transmission will no longer be considered science fiction nor evoke suspicion. Indeed, efforts are underway to modify *P. leucopus* so that they constitutively and heritably express anti-OspA, rendering them less reservoir competent for *B. burgdorferi*. Nantucket is a candidate site for larger field trials to release such mice, once small scale proof of concept regulatory studies have been completed [53]. *B. microti* antigens that appear to induce some degree of transmission blocking immunity could easily be incorporated in such a platform.

Anti-tick vaccines, which would reduce the risk for the transmission of all 5 of the deer tick transmitted zoonoses (in the northeastern U.S.; a sixth, *Ehrlichia muris*, is present in the upper midwestern states) by interfering with tick feeding, may become available and could be commercially successful. When Lymerix was deployed, there was debate on its merit because the vaccine only protected against Lyme disease and people would still have to take all required precautions to avoid infection with the other deer tick-transmitted pathogens. Accordingly, an anti-tick vaccine could be more widely acceptable. The current situation with COVID-19, however, demonstrates that even when an effective vaccine is available, people may not avail themselves of its benefits; accordingly, environmental approaches remain critical to develop and implement.

Personal protection remains the only prevention method that could greatly reduce risk at the individual level if consistently practiced. Permethrin treated clothing is now readily available from online retailers at prices that should not deter their routine use. Joe Piesman, who saw the beginnings of the zoonotic situation that has intensified across the eastern

U.S., frequently said in his role as Lyme disease vector studies chief at CDC, "we know what we have to do, we just can't get people to do it". Alas, the same may be said about any public health issue, from smoking to heart disease to sexually transmitted infections.

Even if a new Nantucket fever appears in the next 50 years (*ex Nantucket semper aliquid novi*) we remain optimistic that the technological advances that will have taken place by 2069 will provide the great public health benefits for Nantucket residents and visitors that unfortunately have eluded us in the last 50 years despite a strong evidence basis for diverse interventions.

Author Contributions: Conceptualization, S.R.T.III, H.K.G., T.J.L.; Methodology, S.R.T.III; Formal Analysis, S.R.T.III; Investigation, S.R.T.III, H.K.G., T.J.L.; Resources, S.R.T.III, H.K.G., T.J.L.; Data Curation, S.R.T.III; Writing—Original Draft Preparation, S.R.T.III; Writing-Review & Editing, S.R.T.III, H.K.G., T.J.L.; Project Administration, S.R.T.III; Funding Acquisition, S.R.T.III, T.J.L. All authors have read and agreed to the published version of the manuscript.

Funding: S.R.T.III and H.K.G.'s Nantucket research has been supported over the years by grants from the National Institutes of Health (R01 AI 19693 and R01 AI39002) and currently by R01 AI 137424 and R01 AI 130105 as well as by The Rainwater Foundation, the Gordon and Llura Gund Foundation, and the Dorothy Harrison Egan Foundation.

Institutional Review Board Statement: Not applicable.

Informed Consent Statement: Not applicable.

Data Availability Statement: Not applicable.

Acknowledgments: The NantucketConservation Foundation and the late Jim Lentowski in particular provided logistical support and access to study sites. Heather Champoux and Alexandra Weld performed the serological assays for the 1991–1997 samples; Tucker Taylor generated Figure 8. We thank these agencies, organizations, and people for their support and help. This is a contribution of the University of Massachusetts Nantucket Field Station, and of the Tufts Lyme Disease Initiative.

Conflicts of Interest: The authors declare no conflict of interest.

References

1. Western, K.A.; Benson, G.D.; Gleason, N.N.; Healy, G.R.; Schultz, M.G. Babesiosis in a Massachusetts resident. *N. Engl. J. Med.* **1970**, *283*, 854–856. [CrossRef]
2. Scharfman, W.B.; Taft, E.G. Nantucket fever: An additional case of babesiosis. *J. Am. Med. Assoc.* **1977**, *238*, 1281–1282. [CrossRef]
3. Gray, E.B.; Herwaldt, B.L. Babesiosis surveillance—United States, 2011–2015. *MMWR Surveill. Summ.* **2019**, *68*, 1–11. [CrossRef]
4. Desowitz, R.S. *New Guinea Tapeworms and Jewish Grandmothers*; WW Norton: New York, NY, USA, 1981.
5. Moss, S. Long odyssey of babesiosis. *N. J. Med.* **1990**, *87*, 291–294.
6. Gleason, N.N.; Healy, G.R.; Western, K.A.; Benson, G.D.; Schultz, M.G. The Gray strain of *Babesia microti* established in laboratory animals. *J. Parasitol.* **1970**, *56*, 1256–1257. [CrossRef]
7. Van Peenen, P.F.D.; Healy, G.R. Infection of Microtus ochrogaster with piroplasms isolated from man. *J. Parasitol.* **1971**, *56*, 1029–1031. [CrossRef]
8. Ristic, M.; Conroy, J.D.; Siwe, S.; Healy, G.R.; Smith, A.R.; Huxsoll, D.L. Babesia species isolated from a woman with clinical babesiosis. *Am. J. Trop. Med. Hyg.* **1971**, *20*, 14–22. [CrossRef] [PubMed]
9. Goethert, H.K.; Molloy, P.J.; Berardi, V.P.; Weeks, K.; Telford, S.R. Zoonotic *Babesia microti* in the northeastern United States: Evidence for expansion of a specific parasite lineage. *PLoS ONE* **2018**, *13*, e0193837. [CrossRef] [PubMed]
10. Lemieux, J.E.; Tran, A.D.; Freimark, L.; Schaffner, S.F.; Goethert, H.; Andersen, K.G.; Bazner, S.; Lisa, F.; McGrath, G.; Sloan, L.; et al. A global map of genetic diversity in *Babesia microti* reveals strong population structure and identifies variants associated with clinical relapse. *Nat. Microbiol.* **2016**, *1*, 1–7. [CrossRef]
11. Anderson, A.E.; Cassaday, P.B.; Healy, G.R. Babesiosis in man: Sixth documented case. *Am. J. Clin. Pathol.* **1974**, *62*, 612–615. [CrossRef] [PubMed]
12. Ruebush, M.J.; Hanson, W.L. Susceptibility of five strains of laboratory mice to *Babesia microti* of human origin. *J. Parasitol.* **1979**, *65*, 430–433. [CrossRef] [PubMed]
13. Clark, I.A. Immunity to Intra-Erythrocytic Protozoa in Mice, with Special Reference to *Babesia* sp. Ph.D. Thesis, University of London, London, UK, 1976.
14. Ruebush, M.J.; Hanson, W.L. Transfer of immunity to *Babesia microti* of human origin using T lymphocytes in mice. *Cell. Immunol.* **1980**, *52*, 255–265. [CrossRef]

15. Piesman, J.; Spielman, A. Human babesiosis on Nantucket Island: Prevalence of *Babesia microti* in ticks. *Am. J. Trop. Med. Hyg.* **1980**, *29*, 742–746. [CrossRef]
16. Persing, D.H.; Mathieson, D.; Marshall, W.F.; Telford, S.R., III; Spielman, A.; Thomford, J.; Conrad, P.A. Detection of *Babesia microti* by polymerase chain reaction. *J. Clin. Microbiol.* **1992**, *30*, 2097–2103. [CrossRef]
17. Ruebush, T.K.; Cassaday, P.B.; Marsh, H.J.; Lisker, S.A.; Voorhees, D.B.; Mahoney, E.B.; Healy, G.R. Human babesiosis on Nantucket Island: Clinical characteristics. *Ann. Intern. Med.* **1977**, *86*, 6–9. [CrossRef]
18. Healy, G.R.; Spielman, A.; Gleason, N. Human babesiosis: Reservoir of infection on Nantucket Island. *Science* **1976**, *192*, 479–480. [CrossRef]
19. Ruebush, T.K., II; Juranek, D.D.; Chisholm, E.S.; Snow, P.C.; Healy, G.R.; Sulzer, A.J. Human babesiosis on Nantucket Island. Evidence for self-limited and subclinical infections. *N. Engl. J. Med.* **1977**, *297*, 825–827. [CrossRef] [PubMed]
20. Meldrum, S.C.; Birkhead, G.S.; White, D.J.; Benach, J.L.; Morse, D.L. Human babesiosis in New York State: An epidemiological description of 136 cases. *Clin. Infect. Dis.* **1992**, *15*, 1019–1023. [CrossRef] [PubMed]
21. Piesman, J.; Mather, T.N.; Telford, S.R., III; Spielman, A. Concurrent *Borrelia burgdorferi* and *Babesia microti* infection in nymphal *Ixodes dammini*. *J. Clin. Microbiol.* **1986**, *24*, 446–447. [CrossRef]
22. Grunwaldt, E. Babesiosis on Shelter Island. *N. Y. State J. Med.* **1977**, *77*, 1320–1321.
23. Marshall, W.F.; Telford, S.R., III; Rhys, P.N.; Rutledge, B.J.; Mathiesen, D.; Spielman, A.; Persing, D.H. Detection of *Borrelia burgdorferi* DNA in museum specimens of *Peromyscus leucopus*. *J. Infect. Dis.* **1994**, *170*, 1027–1032. [CrossRef] [PubMed]
24. Miller, L.H.; Neva, F.A.; Gill, F. Failure of chloroquine in human babesiosis (*Babesia microti*). *Ann. Intern. Med.* **1978**, *88*, 200–202. [CrossRef] [PubMed]
25. Krause, P.J.; Daily, J.; Telford, S.R.; Vannier, E.; Lantos, P.; Spielman, A. Shared features in the pathobiology of babesiosis and malaria. *Trends Parasitol.* **2007**, *23*, 605–610. [CrossRef] [PubMed]
26. Schrezenmeier, E.; Dorner, T. Mechanisms of action of hydroxychloroquine and chloroquine: Implications for rheumatology. *Nat. Rev. Rheumatol.* **2020**, *16*, 155–166. [CrossRef]
27. Ruebush, T.K.; Juranek, D.D.; Spielman, A.; Piesman, J.; Healy, G.R. Epidemiology of human babesiosis on Nantucket Island. *Am. J. Trop. Med. Hyg.* **1981**, *30*, 937–941. [CrossRef]
28. Spielman, A. Human babesiosis on Nantucket Island: Transmission by nymphal Ixodes ticks. *Am. J. Trop. Med. Hyg.* **1976**, *25*, 784–787. [CrossRef]
29. Moritz, E.D.; Winton, C.S.; Tonnetti, L.; Townsend, R.L.; Berardi, V.P.; Hewins, M.E.; Weeks, K.E.; Dodd, R.Y.; Stramer, S.L. Screening for *Babesia microti* in the US blood supply. *N. Engl. J. Med.* **2016**, *375*, 2236–2245. [CrossRef] [PubMed]
30. Piesman, J. *Ixodes Dammini*: Its Role in Transmitting *Babesia microti* to Man. Ph.D. Thesis, Harvard School of Public Health, Boston, MA, USA, 1980.
31. Spielman, A.; Clifford, C.M.; Piesman, J.; Corwin, M.D. Human babesiosis on Nantucket Island, USA: Description of the vector, *Ixodes* (Ixodes) *dammini*, n. sp. (Acarina: Ixodidae). *J. Med. Entomol.* **1979**, *15*, 218–234. [CrossRef]
32. Telford, S.R., III. The name *Ixodes dammini* epidemiologically justified. *Emerg. Infect. Dis.* **1998**, *4*, 132–134. [CrossRef] [PubMed]
33. Kovalev, S.Y.; Mikhaylishcheva, M.S.; Mukhacheva, T.A. Natural hybridization of the ticks *Ixodes persulcatus* and *Ixodes pavlovskyi* in their sympatric populations in Western Siberia. *Infect. Genet. Evol.* **2015**, *32*, 388–395. [CrossRef]
34. Sakamoto, J.M.; Goddard, J.; Rasgon, J. Population and demographic structure of *Ixodes scapularis* Say in the Eastern United States. *PLoS ONE* **2014**, *9*, e101389. [CrossRef] [PubMed]
35. Chisholm, E.S.; Ruebush, T.K.; Sulzer, A.J.; Healy, G.R. *Babesia microti* infection in man: Evaluation of an indirect immu nofluorescent antibody test. *Am. J. Trop. Med. Hyg.* **1978**, *27*, 14–19. [CrossRef] [PubMed]
36. Piesman, J.; Mather, T.N.; Dammin, G.J.; Telford, S.R., III; Lastavica, C.C.; Spielman, A. Seasonal variation of transmission risk of Lyme disease and human babesiosis. *Am. J. Epidemiol.* **1987**, *126*, 1187–1189. [CrossRef] [PubMed]
37. Goethert, H.K.; Telford, S.R., III. Not "out of Nantucket": *Babesia microti* in southern New England comprises at least two major populations. *Parasits Vectors* **2014**, *7*, 1–11. [CrossRef] [PubMed]
38. Tyzzer, E.E. *Cytoecetes microti*, n.g., n.sp., a parasite developing in granulocytes and infective for small rodents. *Parasitology* **1938**, *30*, 242–257. [CrossRef]
39. Telford, S.R., III; Gorenflot, A.; Brasseur, P.; Spielman, A. Babesial infections of humans and wildlife. In *Parasitic Protozoa*, 2nd ed.; Kreier, J.P., Baker, J.R., Eds.; Academic Press: New York, NY, USA, 1993; Volume 5, pp. 1–47.
40. Bakken, J.S.; Dumler, J.S.; Chen, S.M.; Eckman, M.R.; Van Etta, L.L.; Walker, D.H. Human granulocytic ehrlichiosis in the upper Midwest United States. A new species emerging? *JAMA* **1994**, *272*, 212–218. [CrossRef]
41. Telford, S.R., III; Lepore, T.J.; Snow, P.; Warner, C.K.; Dawson, J.E. Human granulocytic ehrlichiosis in Massachusetts. *Ann. Int. Med.* **1995**, *123*, 277–279. [CrossRef]
42. Telford, S.R., III; Dawson, J.E.; Katavolos, P.; Warner, C.K.; Kolbert, C.P.; Persing, D.H. Perpetuation of the agent of human granulocytic ehrlichiosis in a deer tick-rodent cycle. *Proc. Nat. Acad. Sci. USA* **1996**, *93*, 6209–6214. [CrossRef]
43. Goethert, H.K.; Telford, S.R., III. Enzootic transmission of *Babesia divergens* among cottontail rabbits on Nantucket Island, Massachusetts. *Am. J. Trop. Med. Hyg.* **2003**, *69*, 455–460. [CrossRef]
44. Telford, S.R., III; Armstrong, P.M.; Katavolos, P.; Foppa, I.; Garcia, A.S.; Wilson, M.L.; Spielman, A. A new tick-borne encephalitis-like virus infecting deer ticks, *Ixodes dammini*. *Emerg. Infect. Dis.* **1997**, *3*, 165–170. [CrossRef]

45. Ebel, G.D.; Campbell, E.N.; Goethert, H.K.; Spielman, A.; Telford, S.R., III. Enzootic transmission of deer tick virus in New England and Wisconsin sites. *Am. J. Trop. Med. Hyg.* **2000**, *63*, 36–42. [CrossRef]
46. Wilson, M.L.; Telford, S.R.; Piesman, J.; Spielman, A. Reduced abundance of immature *Ixodes dammini* (Acari: Ixodidae) following elimination of deer. *J. Med. Èntomol.* **1988**, *25*, 224–228. [CrossRef] [PubMed]
47. Mather, T.N.; Ribeiro, J.M.; Spielman, A. Lyme disease and babesiosis: Acaricide focused on potentially infected ticks. *Am. J. Trop. Med. Hyg.* **1987**, *36*, 609–614. [CrossRef] [PubMed]
48. Krause, P.J.; Lepore, T.; Sikand, V.K.; Gadbaw, J., Jr.; Burke, G.; Telford, S.R., III; Brassard, P.; Pearl, D.; Azlanzadeh, J.; Christianson, D.; et al. Atovaquone and azithromycin for the treatment of babesiosis. *N. Engl. J. Med.* **2000**, *343*, 1454–1458. [CrossRef] [PubMed]
49. Rowin, K.S.; Tanowitz, H.B.; Wittner, M. Therapy of experimental babesiosis. *Ann. Intern. Med.* **1982**, *97*, 556–558. [CrossRef]
50. Dammin, G.J.; Spielman, A.; Mahoney, E.B.; Bracker, E.F.; Kaplan, K. Epidemiologic notes and reports: Clindamycin and quinine treatment for *Babesia microti* infections. *MMWR* **1983**, *32*, 65–66.
51. Lawres, L.A.; Garg, A.; Kumar, V.; Bruzual, I.; Forquer, I.P.; Renard, I.; Virji, A.Z.; Boulard, P.; Rodriguez, E.X.; Allen, A.J.; et al. Radical cure of experimental babesiosis in immunodeficient mice using a combination of an endochin-like quinolone and atovaquone. *J. Exp. Med.* **2016**, *213*, 1307–1318. [CrossRef]
52. Krause, P.J.; Gewurz, B.E.; Hill, D.; Marty, F.M.; Vannier, E.; Foppa, I.M.; Furman, R.R.; Neuhaus, E.; Skowron, G.; Gupta, S.; et al. Persistent and relapsing babesiosis in immunocompromised patients. *Clin. Infect. Dis.* **2008**, *46*, 370–376. [CrossRef]
53. Buchthal, J.; Evans, S.W.; Lunshof, J.; Telford, S.R.; Esvelt, K.M. Mice against ticks: An experimental community-guided effort to prevent tick-borne disease by altering the shared environment. *Philos. Trans. R. Soc. B Biol. Sci.* **2019**, *374*, 20180105. [CrossRef] [PubMed]

pathogens

Review

What *Babesia microti* Is Now

Heidi K. Goethert

Cummings School of Veterinary Medicine, Tufts University, Grafton, MA 01536, USA; Heidi.goethert@tufts.edu

Abstract: Parasites from diverse hosts morphologically identified as *Babesia microti* have previously been shown to belong to a paraphyletic species complex. With a growing number of reports of *B. microti*-like parasites from across the world, this paper seeks to report on the current knowledge of the diversity of this species complex. Phylogenetic analysis of 18S rDNA sequences obtained from GenBank shows that the diversity of the *B. microti* species complex has markedly increased and now encompasses at least five distinct clades. This cryptic diversity calls into question much of our current knowledge of the life cycle of these parasites, as many biological studies were conducted before DNA sequencing technology was available. In many cases, it is uncertain which *B. microti*-like parasite was studied because parasites from different clades may occur sympatrically and even share the same host. Progress can only be made if future studies are conducted with careful attention to parasite identification and PCR primer specificity.

Keywords: *Babesia microti*; *Babesia*; diversity; phylogenetic analysis

Citation: Goethert, H.K. What *Babesia microti* Is Now. *Pathogens* **2021**, *10*, 1168. https://doi.org/10.3390/pathogens10091168

Academic Editors: Estrella Montero, Jeremy Gray, Cheryl Ann Lobo and Luis Miguel González

Received: 11 August 2021
Accepted: 2 September 2021
Published: 10 September 2021

Babesia microti has historically been identified by the intra-erythrocytic morphology of the parasites, typically appearing in infected cells as small (1–2.0 μm in diameter) basket-shaped rings with extended chromatin. Relying solely on this morphology for identification, parasites from diverse hosts, such as shrews, mice, rats, raccoons, and dogs, are all referred to as *B. microti* or *B. microti*-like [1–4]. In 2003, a phylogenetic study was published demonstrating that such parasites are not a single organism. Sequences from both the 18S ribosomal and the beta-tubulin genes were paraphyletic, demonstrating that *B. microti* is, in fact, a species complex comprised of three genetically distinct clades [5]. Furthermore, parasites from only one of the clades are responsible for most human babesiosis cases. Indeed, cryptic diversity is common among parasites with few morphological traits that can be used for differentiation [6]. In the intervening 20 years, there has been a growing number of reports of *B. microti*-like parasites from diverse hosts worldwide. It is now clear that this species complex is even more diverse than originally described. This paper seeks to report the current knowledge of the species diversity and clarify, once again, what *Babesia microti* is.

To this aim, all the 18S ribosomal DNA sequences >800 bp currently in GenBank that are either named *Babesia microti* in the database or appear on a Blast search with a sequence similarity of >95% to the *B. microti* human strains from the United States were downloaded. Although the 18S gene may not be the best target for describing diversity because of its highly conserved nature, it is the only gene that is reliably sequenced from the majority of studies. Limiting this analysis to large pieces of the gene maximizes the amount of diversity obtained from this conserved gene. From the large list of sequences available, a sample was chosen that attempted to encompass the genetic diversity of the entire database while removing large numbers of highly similar sequences that make the trees difficult to interpret. Thirty-nine sequences were aligned using Geneious (GenBank numbers are in the figure) and then trimmed so that they were all the same length, corresponding to bases 478–1350 from the Gray strain (GenBank #AY693840). A neighbor-joining tree was constructed with MEGA X [7] using *B. divergens* and *B. leo* as outgroups (Figure 1). This new analysis reveals that the three originally described clades remain, but they are joined by at least 2 additional clades.

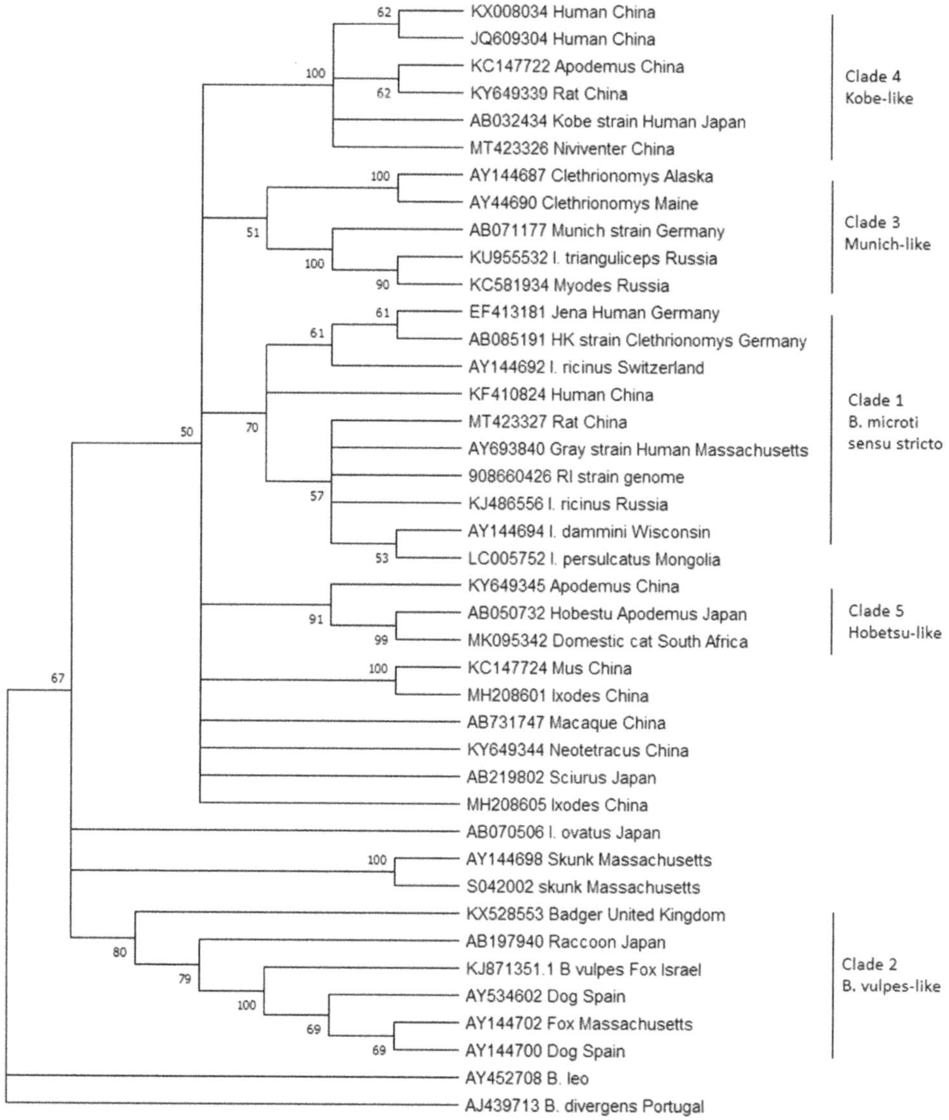

Figure 1. Phylogenetic analysis of the 18S rDNA gene of *B. microti*-like piroplasms. A neighbor-joining tree was constructed using MEGA X with 500 bootstrap replicates. Evolutionary distances were calculated using the Kimera-2 parameter method with *B. divergens* and B. leo as outgroups. Branches with less than 50% bootstrap support were consolidated. GenBank accession numbers are listed on the tree.

Clade 1: Clade 1 has also been referred to as *B. microti sensu stricto* (or the US-type), as the parasites from this clade are arguably the most important because of their public health impact as the major cause of human babesiosis worldwide. This parasite is also the most studied. Clade 1 parasites are remarkably conserved, with virtually identical 18S rDNA sequences described across the globe: North America, Europe, and Asia. Despite this, human cases are only common in the United States. There, people are readily exposed because of the highly anthropophilic tick *Ixodes dammini* (the northern clade of *Ixodes scapularis*) that serves as its main vector [8,9]. In Europe, *B. microti ss* is thought to be maintained by *I. trianguliceps*, a host-specific tick that does not attack people, which would explain the lack of human disease. However, much of the work with *I. trianculiceps* was conducted before molecular methods were available, and it is uncertain whether the parasite under study belonged to this clade or clade 3 (For example see [3,10,11]). To date, no definitive molecular sequencing of field-derived *I. trianguliceps* has shown *B. microti* ss in these ticks. *I. ricinus*, an anthropophilic tick that serves as the vector for Lyme disease, is often sympatric, feeds on similar rodent reservoir hosts, and has been shown to be capable of transmitting piroplasms in the laboratory [12]. Indeed, *B. microti* ss is regularly detected in this vector, as well as *I. persulcatus* in Eurasia [13–15]. Therefore, the zoonotic potential should exist throughout the range of these ticks in Europe and Asia. Serosurveys show that tick-exposed people are indeed exposed to the parasite, but few cases of illness have been detected [16,17]. Whether the parasites are less virulent in the rest of the world compared to those in North America or whether physicians fail to diagnosis this disease because of lack of physician awareness and diagnostic capabilities has not been determined [18].

Clade 2: Clade 2 includes *Babesia spp.* that are known to infect carnivores, including raccoons, foxes, and badgers across the world. Also included in this clade is the parasite originally described from sick domestic dogs from Spain, which has been called by many names: *B. microti*-like, *Babesia* c.f. *microti, Theileria annae*, and *Babesia annae* [2,19]. Recently, it has been proposed that this parasite be designated a new species called *Babesia vulpes* [20,21]. The phylogenetic trees published by Baneth et al. in 2015 suggest that they propose the name *B. vulpes* only be applied to the *Babesia* in wild foxes, which also causes disease in domestic dogs, but not to the closely related *Babesia* found in other carnivores. The current phylogenetic analysis clearly shows that other sequences from raccoons and badgers group with *B. vulpes* in a strongly supported clade to the exclusion of the other *B. microti*-like parasites. If the name *B. vulpes* is indeed adopted, it seems unduly confusing to continue to refer to the other carnivore *Babesia* as *B. microti*-like. The vectors for the parasites in this clade have not been definitively established but are likely to be *Ixodid* ticks that feed primarily on carnivores, such as *I. texanus* in North America. In Europe, *I. hexagonus* and *Dermacentor reticulatus* have both been suggested as possible vectors [22,23]. It may also be transmitted by other routes that do not involve a vector, such as direct transmission through bites [24].

Not included within Clade 2 are the sequences from skunks originally described from Massachusetts [6]. The phylogenetic position of these skunk sequences is unstable, as they either cluster with the *B. vulpes* group, with the *B. microti* ss group, or, as is the case in this analysis, separated from both, depending on the type of algorithm used (see [6]). To date, no other similar sequences have been described, despite recent work in the U.S. characterizing small *Babesia* in medium-sized mammals [25–27], leaving our knowledge of this parasite limited and their placement among the *B. microti* clade uncertain. It is clear, however, that these piroplasms are distinct from the previously described *Babesia* from skunks, *B. mephitis* [28].

Clade 3: Clade 3 includes *B. microti* similar to the Munich strain that have been primarily detected from voles. These piroplasms occur in Europe and North America but have not been found in Asia. There is distinct separation in this clade between the sequences originating from the two continents. The *Babesia* from this clade are not known to cause human infection. In fact, they have been detected from areas of the US where human babesiosis has not been described and the anthropophilic vector, *I. dammini*, is not present [29,30]. Instead, *I. angustus* is known to occur in these areas, suggesting that this host-specific tick that rarely bites humans is the major vector in North America and the reason that this piroplasm is not known to infect humans. In Europe, the Munich type appears to be present only in areas where *I. trianguliceps* occurs, and it has been suggested that this tick is the primary vector [31]. However, throughout much of its range, either *I. ricinus* or *I. persulcatus* also occur, and as mentioned above, many ecological studies could not discern between the Munich-type and US-type parasites. Rar et al. [32] showed that in an area with sympatric *I. trianguliceps* and *I. persulcatus*, Munich-type *B. microti* was only detected in *I. trianguliceps* [32] and concluded that *I. persulcatus* was not the vector. However, others have detected sequences consistent with the Munich-type in *I. ricinus* [33–35], thus leaving the zoonotic potential for this piroplasm and the enzoonotic cycle in nature uncertain.

Clades 4 and 5: Clades 4 and 5 comprise *Babesia* that have only been detected in Asia. Clade 4 includes the Kobe strain from Japan together with sequences derived from China. Clade 5 comprises the Hobetsu and Otsu types, along with other sequences from voles from China. Although often referred to as if they are different parasites, these are actually the same and have 100% sequence similarity in the 18S rDNA gene (only Hobetsu is shown on the tree in Figure 1). None of the parasites from either clade have been detected in Europe or North America, though the US-type occurs sympatrically with both these parasites in Asia. Hobetsu parasites have been found primarily in Japan, with one report in rodents from mainland China [36,37], but Kobe appears to be more widespread in Japan, mainland China, and other parts of southeastern Asia and has been detected in more diverse rodent hosts [38–40]. In Japan, parasites from these two clades are often sympatric, but only the Kobe clade has been shown to infect humans. The Hobetsu strain has been detected in I. ovatus, and laboratory studies have confirmed the competence of this vector [37]. However, the vector for the Kobe strain remains undescribed; to date, it has never been detected in field-collected ticks. There is an odd report from a sick domestic cat in South Africa, which appeared to be coinfected with *B. felis* and *B. microti*-like parasites with 100% similarity to the Hobetsu strain [41]. This lone report remains an anomaly, as cats are not otherwise known to become infected with *B. microti*-like parasites, though they do harbor other small *Babesia* that are more closely related to *B. rodhaini*, *B. leo*, and *B. felis* [42].

Finally, there are a number of sequences from GenBank which fall within the *B. microti* species complex but do not group with other previously described parasites to create well-defined clades. The vast majority of these new sequences originate from rodents or ticks collected primarily in China but also Japan. Most remain as single reports or unpublished sequences deposited in GenBank, so little is known about their life cycles or their zoonotic potential. Interestingly, similar sequences were detected in squirrels collected in Japan and macaques from China [43,44]. Further investigations are necessary to characterize these parasites as well as create isolates. In the future, there will likely be 4 additional clades added to the *B. microti* species complex.

As this analysis shows, the parasites that are part of the *B. microti* species complex are a diverse group with unique life cycles. However, the understanding of the ecology of these parasites has been muddled because of the lack of precision in many studies and the confusion between similar parasites. As pointed out above, much of the basic biology of *B. microti*, both in the US and Europe, was conducted before molecular methods were available to distinguish between parasites. It is virtually impossible to know for certain which parasite, Clade 1 *B. microti ss* or Clade 3 Munich-type, was being studied in the older literature (for example, [45,46]), but also in more recent work (for example, [11,47,48]). In the United States in particular, researchers have focused their efforts on *B. microti* ss because of its public health importance there. Indeed, most studies are conducted in areas of the country where human cases are detected and presume the presence of that single parasite. This is likely to be an accurate assumption when surveying ticks. To date, *B. microti* ss is the only *B. microti*-like parasite found in the zoonotic vectors *I. dammini* and *I. scapularis*. Other *Ixodes* ticks that are more host-specific, such as *I. cookei* and *I. angustus*, are rarely studied. Surprisingly few studies in the U.S. have actually sequenced PCR amplicons obtained from wildlife sources to confirm the identity of *B. microti* unless the host is from an area where human babesiosis has not been detected. Unexpected results can arise when performing due diligence to confirm the identity of parasites (see [29,30] and the descriptions of *B. conradae* [49] and *B. duncani* [50]). Therefore, it is imperative at the start of any new study to confirm the identity of parasites by sequencing using a sufficiently informative gene segment (such as [30,51]). Once the specific clade of *B. microti* has been confirmed, it is not necessary to sequence every positive PCR given that the primers used are specific enough to amplify only the intended target. The use of non-specific PCR primers that are capable of amplifying other *B. microti*-like parasites can call into question the conclusions of a paper. Many different primer sets have been used in the literature, and a quick search using PrimerBlast from NCBI is useful to give a reader an estimate of their specificity. This issue becomes even more crucial with the use of real-time PCR, which usually amplifies small pieces of DNA that cannot be confirmed subsequently by sequencing.

It is clear from this analysis that there is much still unknown about the basic biology of the many parasites that make up the *B. microti* species complex. However, progress will only be obtained with well-designed studies that are careful to identify which *B. microti*-like parasite is being studied.

Funding: The author is supported by National Institutes of Health grants R01 AI 130105 and R01 AI 137424.

Institutional Review Board Statement: Not applicable.

Informed Consent Statement: Not applicable.

Data Availability Statement: All data used in the study is publicly available from GenBank. Accession numbers are included in the figure.

Conflicts of Interest: The author declares no conflict of interest.

References

1. Spielman, A.; Etkind, P.; Piesman, J.; Ruebush, T.K.; Juranek, D.D.; Jacobs, M.S. Reservoir Hosts of Human Babesiosis on Nantucket Island. *Am. J. Trop. Med. Hyg.* **1981**, *30*, 560–565. [CrossRef] [PubMed]
2. Camacho, A.T.; Guitián, F.J.; Pallas, E.; Gestal, J.J.; Olmeda, A.S.; Goethert, H.K.; Telford, S.R. Infection of Dogs in North-West Spain with a *Babesia Microti*-like Agent. *Vet. Rec.* **2001**, *149*, 552–555. [CrossRef]
3. Young, A.S. Investigations on the Epidemiology of Blood Parasites of Small Mammals with Special Reference to Piroplasms. Ph.D. Thesis, King's College, London, UK, 1970.
4. Healing, T.D. Infections with Blood Parasites in the Small British Rodents Apodemus Sylvaticus, Clethrionomys Glareolus and Microtus Agrestis. *Parasitology* **1981**, *83*, 179–189. [CrossRef]
5. Goethert, H.K.; Telford III, S. What Is Babesia Microti? *Parasitology* **2003**, *127*, 301–309. [CrossRef] [PubMed]
6. Perkins, S.L.; Martinsen, E.S.; Falk, B.G. Do Molecules Matter More than Morphology? Promises and Pitfalls in Parasites. *Parasitology* **2011**, *138*, 1664–1674. [CrossRef]
7. Kumar, S.; Stecher, G.; Li, M.; Knyaz, C.; Tamura, K. MEGA X: Molecular Evolutionary Genetics Analysis across Computing Platforms. *Mol. Biol. Evol.* **2018**, *35*, 1547–1549. [CrossRef]
8. Spielman, A. Human Babesiosis on Nantucket Island: Transmission by Nymphal Ixodes Ticks. *Am. J. Trop. Med. Hyg.* **1976**, *25*, 784–787. [CrossRef]
9. Spielman, A.; Wilson, M.L.; Levine, J.F.; Piesman, J. Ecology of *Ixodes Dammini*-Borne Human Babesiosis and Lyme Disease. *Ann. Rev. Ent.* **1985**, *30*, 439–460. [CrossRef]
10. Krampitz, H.E. *Babesia Microti*: Morphology, Distribution and Host Relationship in Germany. *Zentralbl. Bakteriol. Orig. A* **1979**, *244*, 411–415.
11. Randolph, S.E. The Effect of *Babesia Microti* on Feeding and Survival in Its Tick Vector, Ixodes Trianguliceps. *Parasitology* **1991**, *102*, 9–16. [CrossRef]
12. Gray, J.; von Stedingk, L.V.; Gürtelschmid, M.; Granström, M. Transmission Studies of *Babesia Microti* in Ixodes Ricinus Ticks and Gerbils. *J. Clin. Microbiol.* **2002**, *40*, 1259–1263. [CrossRef]
13. Duh, D.; Petrovec, M.; Avsic-Zupanc, T. Diversity of *Babesia* Infecting European Sheep Ticks (Ixodes Ricinus). *J. Clin. Microbiol.* **2001**, *39*, 3395–3397. [CrossRef] [PubMed]
14. Foppa, I.M.; Krause, P.J.; Spielman, A.; Goethert, H.; Gern, L.; Brand, B.; Telford, S.R. Entomologic and Serologic Evidence of Zoonotic Transmission of *Babesia Microti*, Eastern Switzerland. *Emerg. Infect. Dis.* **2002**, *8*, 722–726. [CrossRef]
15. Rar, V.A.; Epikhina, T.I.; Livanova, N.N.; Panov, V.V. Genetic Diversity of *Babesia* in Ixodes Persulcatus and Small Mammals from North Ural and West Siberia, Russia. *Parasitology* **2011**, *138*, 175–182. [CrossRef] [PubMed]
16. Hunfeld, K.-P.; Lambert, A.; Kampen, H.; Albert, S.; Epe, C.; Brade, V.; Tenter, A.M. Seroprevalence of *Babesia* Infections in Humans Exposed to Ticks in Midwestern Germany. *J. Clin. Microbiol.* **2002**, *40*, 2431–2436. [CrossRef]
17. Wilhelmsson, P.; Lovmar, M.; Krogfelt, K.A.; Nielsen, H.V.; Forsberg, P.; Lindgren, P.E. Clinical/Serological Outcome in Humans Bitten by *Babesia* Species Positive Ixodes Ricinus Ticks in Sweden and on the Aland Islands. *Ticks Tick Borne Dis.* **2020**, *11*, 101455. [CrossRef]

18. Hunfeld, K.-P.; Brade, V. Zoonotic *Babesia*: Possibly Emerging Pathogens to Be Considered for Tick-Infested Humans in Central Europe. *Int. J. Med. Microbiol. Suppl.* **2004**, *293*, 93–103. [CrossRef]
19. Zahler, M.; Rinder, H.; Schein, E.; Gothe, R. Detection of a New Pathogenic *Babesia Microti*-like Species in Dogs. *Vet. Parasitol.* **2000**, *89*, 241–248. [CrossRef]
20. Baneth, G.; Florin-Christensen, M.; Cardoso, L.; Schnittger, L. Reclassification of Theileria Annae as *Babesia* Vulpes Sp. Nov. *Parasites Vectors* **2015**, *8*, 207. [CrossRef]
21. Baneth, G.; Cardoso, L.; Brilhante-Simões, P.; Schnittger, L. Establishment of *Babesia* Vulpes n. Sp. (Apicomplexa: Babesiidae), a Piroplasmid Species Pathogenic for Domestic Dogs. *Parasites Vectors* **2019**, *12*, 129. [CrossRef] [PubMed]
22. Camacho, A.T.; Pallas, E.; Gestal, J.J.; Guitián, F.J.; Olmeda, A.S.; Telford, S.R.; Spielman, A. Ixodes Hexagonus Is the Main Candidate as Vector of Theileria Annae in Northwest Spain. *Vet. Parasitol.* **2003**, *112*, 157–163. [CrossRef]
23. Hodžić, A.; Zörer, J.; Duscher, G.G. Dermacentor Reticulatus, a Putative Vector of *Babesia* Cf. *Microti* (Syn. Theileria Annae) Piroplasm. *Parasitol. Res.* **2017**, *116*, 1075–1077. [CrossRef] [PubMed]
24. Yeagley, T.J.; Reichard, M.V.; Hempstead, J.E.; Allen, K.E.; Parsons, L.M.; White, M.A.; Little, S.E.; Meinkoth, J.H. Detection of *Babesia Gibsoni* and the Canine Small *Babesia* 'Spanish Isolate' in Blood Samples Obtained from Dogs Confiscated from Dog Fighting Operations. *J. Am. Vet. Med. Assoc.* **2009**, *235*, 535–539. [CrossRef] [PubMed]
25. Clark, K.; Savick, K.; Butler, J. *Babesia Microti* in Rodents and Raccoons from Northeast Florida. *J. Parasitol.* **2012**, *98*, 1117–1121. [CrossRef] [PubMed]
26. Garrett, K.B.; Hernandez, S.M.; Balsamo, G.; Barron, H.; Beasley, J.C.; Brown, J.D.; Cloherty, E.; Farid, H.; Gabriel, M.; Groves, B.; et al. Prevalence, Distribution, and Diversity of Cryptic Piroplasm Infections in Raccoons from Selected Areas of the United States and Canada. *Int. J. Parasitol. Parasites Wildl.* **2019**, *9*, 224–233. [CrossRef]
27. Modarelli, J.J.; Westrich, B.J.; Milholland, M.; Tietjen, M.; Castro-Arellano, I.; Medina, R.F.; Esteve-Gasent, M.D. Prevalence of Protozoan Parasites in Small and Medium Mammals in Texas, USA. *Int. J. Parasitol. Parasites Wildl.* **2020**, *11*, 229–234. [CrossRef] [PubMed]
28. Holbrook, A.A.; Frerichs, W.M. *Babesia* Mephitis Sp. n. (Protozoa: Piroplasmida), a Hematozoan Parasite of the Striped Skunk, Mephitis Mephitis. *J. Parasitol.* **1970**, *56*, 930–931. [CrossRef]
29. Goethert, H.K.; Cook, J.A.; Lance, E.W.; Telford, S.R. Fay and Rausch 1969 Revisited: *Babesia Microti* in Alaskan Small Mammals. *J. Parasitol.* **2006**, *92*, 826–831. [CrossRef]
30. Goethert, H.K.; Lubelcyzk, C.; LaCombe, E.; Holman, M.; Rand, P.; Smith, R.P., Jr.; Telford, S.R., III. Enzootic *Babesia Microti* in Maine. *J. Parasitol.* **2003**, *89*, 1069–1071. [CrossRef]
31. Bown, K.J.; Lambin, X.; Telford, G.R.; Ogden, N.H.; Telfer, S.; Woldehiwet, Z.; Birtles, R.J. Relative Importance of *Ixodes Ricinus* and *Ixodes Trianguliceps* as Vectors for *Anaplasma Phagocytophilum* and *Babesia Microti* in Field Vole (Microtus Agrestis) Populations. *Appl. Environ. Microbiol.* **2008**, *74*, 7118–7125. [CrossRef]
32. Rar, V.; Yakimenko, V.; Makenov, M.; Tikunov, A.; Epikhina, T.; Tancev, A.; Bobrova, O.; Tikunova, N. High Prevalence of *Babesia Microti* "Munich" Type in Small Mammals from an Ixodes Persulcatus/Ixodes Trianguliceps Sympatric Area in the Omsk Region, Russia. *Parasitol. Res.* **2016**, *115*, 3619–3629. [CrossRef]
33. Pieniążek, N.; Sawczuk, M.; Skotarczak, B. Molecular Identification of *Babesia* Parasities Isolated from Ixodes Ricinus Ticks Collected in Northwestern Poland. *Parasitology* **2006**, *92*, 32–35. [CrossRef]
34. Siński, E.; Bajer, A.; Welc, R.; Pawełczyk, A.; Ogrzewalska, M.; Behnke, J.M. *Babesia Microti*: Prevalence in Wild Rodents and Ixodes Ricinus Ticks from the Mazury Lakes District of North-Eastern Poland. *Int. J. Med. Microbiol.* **2006**, *296*, 137–143. [CrossRef]
35. Welc-Falęciak, R.; Bajer, A.; Paziewska-Harris, A.; Baumann-Popczyk, A.; Siński, E. Diversity of *Babesia* in *Ixodes Ricinus* Ticks in Poland. *Adv. Med. Sci.* **2012**, *57*, 364–369. [CrossRef] [PubMed]
36. Chen, X.-R.; Ye, L.I.; Fan, J.-W.; Li, C.; Tang, F.; Liu, W.; Ren, L.-Z.; Bai, J.-Y. Detection of Kobe-Type and Otsu-Type *Babesia Microti* in Wild Rodents in China's Yunnan Province. *Epidemiol. Infect.* **2017**, *145*, 2704–2710. [CrossRef] [PubMed]
37. Zamoto-Niikura, A.; Tsuji, M.; Qiang, W.; Nakao, M.; Hirata, H.; Ishihara, C. Detection of Two Zoonotic *Babesia Microti* Lineages, the Hobetsu and U.S. Lineages, in Two Sympatric Tick Species, Ixodes Ovatus and Ixodes Persulcatus, Respectively, in Japan. *Appl. Environ. Microbiol.* **2012**, *78*, 3424–3430. [CrossRef]
38. Saito-Ito, A.; Takada, N.; Ishiguro, F.; Fujita, H.; Yano, Y.; Ma, X.-H.; Chen, E.-R. Detection of Kobe-Type *Babesia Microti* Associated with Japanese Human Babesiosis in Field Rodents in Central Taiwan and Southeastern Mainland China. *Parasitology* **2008**, *135*, 691–699. [CrossRef] [PubMed]
39. Saito-Ito, A.; Kasahara, M.; Kasai, M.; Dantrakool, A.; Kawai, A.; Fujita, H.; Yano, Y.; Kawabata, H.; Takada, N. Survey of *Babesia Microti* Infection in Field Rodents in Japan: Records of the Kobe-Type in New Foci and Findings of a New Type Related to the Otsu-Type. *Microbiol. Immunol.* **2007**, *51*, 15–24. [CrossRef]
40. Tsuji, M.; Wei, Q.; Zamoto, A.; Morita, C.; Arai, S.; Shiota, T.; Fujimagari, M.; Itagaki, A.; Fujita, H.; Ishihara, C. Human Babesiosis in Japan: Epizootiologic Survey of Rodent Reservoir and Isolation of New Type of *Babesia Microti*-Like Parasite. *J. Clin. Microbiol.* **2001**, *39*, 4316–4322. [CrossRef]
41. Bosman, A.-M.; Penzhorn, B.L.; Brayton, K.A.; Schoeman, T.; Oosthuizen, M.C. A Novel *Babesia* Sp. Associated with Clinical Signs of Babesiosis in Domestic Cats in South Africa. *Parasites Vectors* **2019**, *12*, 138. [CrossRef]
42. Penzhorn, B.L.; Oosthuizen, M.C. *Babesia* Species of Domestic Cats: Molecular Characterization Has Opened Pandora's Box. *Front. Vet. Sci.* **2020**, *7*, 134. [CrossRef]

43. Tsuji, M.; Zamoto, A.; Kawabuchi, T.; Kataoka, T.; Nakajima, R.; Asakawa, M.; Ishihara, C. *Babesia Microti*-Like Parasites Detected in Eurasian Red Squirrels (*Sciurus Vulgaris OriEnt.is*) in Hokkaido, Japan. *J. Vet. Med. Sci.* **2006**, *68*, 643–646. [CrossRef]
44. Voorberg-vd Wel, A.; Kocken, C.H.M.; Zeeman, A.-M.; Thomas, A.W. Detection of New *Babesia Microti*-like Parasites in a Rhesus Monkey (Macaca Mulatta) with a Suppressed Plasmodium Cynomolgi Infection. *Am. J. Trop. Med. Hyg.* **2008**, *78*, 643–645.
45. Coles, A. Blood Parasites Found in Mammals, Birds and Fishes in England. *Parasitology* **1914**, *7*, 17–61. [CrossRef]
46. Franca, C. Sur Une Piroplasme Nouvelle Chez Une Mangouste. *Bull. Soc. Pathol. Exot.* **1908**, *1*, 410.
47. Anderson, J.F.; Johnson, R.C.; Magnarelli, L.A.; Hyde, F.W.; Myers, J.E. Peromyscus Leucopus and Microtus Pennsylvanicus Simultaneously Infected with Borrelia Burgdorferi and *Babesia Microti*. *J. Clin. Microbiol.* **1986**, *23*, 135–137. [CrossRef]
48. Anderson, J.F.; Magnarelli, L.A.; Kurz, J. Intraerythrocytic Parasites in Rodent Populations of Connecticut: *Babesia* and *Grahamella Species*. *J. Parasitol.* **1979**, *65*, 599–604. [CrossRef]
49. Kjemtrup, A.M.; Wainwright, K.; Miller, M.; Penzhorn, B.L.; Carreno, R.A. *Babesia* Conradae, Sp. Nov., a Small Canine *Babesia* Identified in California. *Vet. Parasitol.* **2006**, *138*, 103–111. [CrossRef] [PubMed]
50. Conrad, P.A.; Kjemtrup, A.M.; Carreno, R.A.; Thomford, J.; Wainwright, K.; Eberhard, M.; Quick, R.; Telford III, S.R.; Herwaldt, B.L. Description of *Babesia* Duncani n.Sp. (Apicomplexa: Babesiidae) from Humans and Its Differentiation from Other Piroplasms. *Int. J. Parasitol.* **2006**, *36*, 779–789. [CrossRef] [PubMed]
51. Armstrong, P.M.; Katavolos, P.; Caporale, D.A.; Smith, R.P.; Spielman, A.; Telford, S.R. Diversity of *Babesia* Infecting Deer Ticks (*Ixodes Dammini*). *Am. J. Trop. Med. Hyg.* **1998**, *58*, 739–742. [CrossRef] [PubMed]

pathogens

Article

The New Human *Babesia* sp. FR1 Is a European Member of the *Babesia* sp. MO1 Clade

Claire Bonsergent [1,*], Marie-Charlotte de Carné [2], Nathalie de la Cotte [1], François Moussel [3], Véronique Perronne [2] and Laurence Malandrin [1,*]

1 BIOEPAR, INRAE, Oniris, 44300 Nantes, France; nathalie.delacotte@oniris-nantes.fr
2 Service de Maladies Infectieuses et Tropicales, Hôpital F. Quesnay, 78200 Mantes-la Jolie, France; mcdecarne@ch-versailles.fr (M.-C.d.C.); veronique.perronne@aphp.fr (V.P.)
3 Laboratoire de Biologie Médicale, Hôpital F. Quesnay, 78200 Mantes-la-Jolie, France; f.moussel@ch-mantes-la-jolie.fr
* Correspondence: claire.bonsergent-guillou@inrae.fr (C.B.); laurence.malandrin@inrae.fr (L.M.)

Abstract: In Europe, *Babesia divergens* is responsible for most of the severe cases of human babesiosis. In the present study, we describe a case of babesiosis in a splenectomized patient in France and report a detailed molecular characterization of the etiological agent, named *Babesia* sp. FR1, as well as of closely related *Babesia divergens*, *Babesia capreoli* and *Babesia* sp. MO1-like parasites. The analysis of the conserved 18S rRNA gene was supplemented with the analysis of more discriminant markers involved in the red blood cell invasion process: *rap-1a* (rhoptry-associated-protein 1) and *ama-1* (apical-membrane-antigen 1). The *rap-1a* and *ama-1* phylogenetic analyses were congruent, placing *Babesia* sp. FR1, the new European etiological agent, in the American cluster of *Babesia* sp. MO1-like parasites. Based on two additional markers, our analysis confirms the clear separation of *B. divergens* and *B. capreoli*. *Babesia* sp. MO1-like parasites should also be considered as a separate species, with the rabbit as its natural host, differing from those of *B. divergens* (cattle) and *B. capreoli* (roe deer). The natural host of *Babesia* sp. FR1 remains to be discovered.

Keywords: *Babesia divergens*; *Babesia* sp. MO1; *Babesia capreoli*; *rap-1a*; *ama-1*; phylogeny

Citation: Bonsergent, C.; de Carné, M.-C.; de la Cotte, N.; Moussel, F.; Perronne, V.; Malandrin, L. The New Human *Babesia* sp. FR1 Is a European Member of the *Babesia* sp. MO1 Clade. *Pathogens* **2021**, *10*, 1433. https://doi.org/10.3390/pathogens10111433

Academic Editors: Estrella Montero, Jeremy Gray, Cheryl Ann Lobo and Luis Miguel González

Received: 1 October 2021
Accepted: 30 October 2021
Published: 4 November 2021

1. Introduction

Babesiosis is a tick-borne disease affecting a wide range of vertebrates worldwide. Symptoms of this disease are caused by the intraerythrocytic development of Protozoa of the genus *Babesia*, causing fever, jaundice, hemoglobinuria and anemia, possibly leading to death, depending on the *Babesia* species and the host. About one hundred species of *Babesia* have been described and transmission of the parasite between hosts occurs almost exclusively through Ixodid tick bites [1].

Even though humans are not natural hosts of *Babesia*, human infections caused by several different species of *Babesia* have been reported worldwide. *Babesia microti*, *B. duncani* (WA1) [2] and to a lesser extent *B. divergens*-like (*Babesia* sp. MO1 clade) [3] have been reported to cause disease in humans in the USA. The most prevalent species is *B. microti* responsible of infections that follow a relatively benign course [4]. In Asia, a few cases have recently been reported, caused by *B. divergens*-, *B. venatorum*- or *B. crassa*-like strains [5–7].

In Europe, the first case of human babesiosis was described in 1957 in Croatia [8,9]. In 1997, a review on human babesiosis in Europe reported 24 cases in splenectomized (20/24) and non-splenectomized (4/24) patients, 46% of which were fatal even in non-splenectomized patients (2/4) [10]. At that time, the molecular diagnosis of the parasite species was lacking and cases were attributed to *B. divergens* based on morphological and/or serological grounds. A few years later, molecular analysis revealed a new etiological babesiosis agent, *Babesia* sp. EU1, which was found to be responsible for human cases in Austria, Italy [11], Germany [12] and Sweden [13]. Human babesiosis cases due to *B.*

microti have been reported in Europe but usually they are imported cases from the USA [14], with only one autochtonous case reported to date in Germany [15]. Severe sporadic cases are usually attributed to *B. divergens* [16–24]. However, molecular confirmation of the species is not always undertaken [25–27]. Serological analysis and morphology on smears are not sufficient to ascertain *B. divergens* as the etiological agent. Even for specialists, the morphological distinction of *B. divergens* from *Babesia* sp. EU1 on smears is impossible [11,12]. Confirmed cases of babesiosis due to *B. divergens* can remain serologically negative [28–30], and serology can be confusing due to dot-like reactivity patterns of most human positive sera, concentrated at the apical pole of the parasite [31]. This reactivity pattern was confirmed with a serum from a clinically and molecularly confirmed human *B. divergens* case in Finland [18,31].

The phylogenetic group including *B. divergens* gathers different named or as yet unnamed species that are very closely related, and we will refer to this group as *B. divergens*-like. *B. divergens* is indeed closely related and can be confused with *B. capreoli*, a parasite frequently found in roe deer in Europe, due to their high 18S rRNA sequence relatedness [32,33]. However, the conservation of three base differences in this gene between isolates of *B. divergens* (pathogen of cattle/humans) and isolates of *B. capreoli* (pathogen of roe deer), linked to different in vitro host ranges, allowed the delineation of these two species [33]. *Babesia* sp. MO1 also belongs to this phylogenetic group, and is responsible for a small number of severe or fatal human babesiosis in splenectomized patients in the USA [3,34–36]. Cottontail rabbits are the natural hosts of *Babesia* sp. MO1 [37,38]. In vitro cultivation features as well as in vivo experimental infections demonstrated the incapacity of this genetic variant to infect cattle, and, combined with 18S rRNA sequence differences, led to its species differentiation from *B. divergens* and the provisional name *Babesia* sp. MO1 [39–41].

In splenectomized patients, babesiosis due to *B. divergens* is fulminant with symptoms that appear within 1–3 weeks post infection, with persistent high fevers and headaches, followed by severe intravascular hemolysis, hemoglobinuria, and jaundice. Babesiosis in splenectomized patients is often fatal in Europe, as diagnosis and therefore adequate treatment are often delayed due to uncharacteristic flu-like symptoms and the infrequency of cases [42,43]. Severe symptoms and fatal cases also occur in non-splenectomized patients with known or unknown predispositions such as splenic dysfunction or a rudimentary spleen [18,19]. In immunocompetent patients, *B. divergens* infection is associated with flu-like symptoms shortly after a tick bite [29] or may remain asymptomatic [44].

In the present study, we describe an unusually mild babesiosis in an asplenic patient in France, originally suspected to be caused by *B. divergens*. Intrigued by the unusual course of infection, we carried out the molecular characterization of the responsible agent. As the 18S rRNA gene is rather conserved within the *B. divergens* taxonomic group, and therefore not sufficiently informative, we supplemented the molecular description with two additional and more variable markers: the apical membrane antigen 1 (*ama-1*) and the rhoptry-associated-protein-1a (*rap-1a*) genes. Molecular characterization and polymorphism of these two genes were also analyzed for different members of the *Babesia divergens*-like phylogenetic group, including the phylogenetically closely related *B. capreoli* and *Babesia* sp. AR1 identical to *Babesia* sp. MO1 but from a patient in Arkansas [35], and compared to available sequences of these genes for *B. divergens*.

2. Results

2.1. *Babesia* sp. *FR1: Report of the Clinical Case*

A 56-year-old man came into the emergency room with a suspected meningitidis syndrome. He was Caucasian and his only notable antecedent was a splenectomy in 2001 following a skiing accident (pneumococcal vaccine administered in November 2016, no *Haemophilus* nor meningococcal vaccines).

The patient stayed on the Île de Ré from 4 August 2017 to 24 August, then from 29 August to 3 September, at a house located at the edge of a forest. He also stayed in Béthune from 25 August to 28 August. He had a fever for 2 weeks associated with headaches. He then developed severe asthenia, sweats, tachypnea, myalgia, and elbow, shoulder, and knee arthralgia.

The first blood test (5 September) revealed thrombopenia: 99 giga/L, CRP 65.6 mg/L, ASAT 82U/L, ALAT 73U/L. On 9 September 2017, he developed vomiting, photophobia and a stiff neck, which led to the patient being transferred to hospital (11 September). Nothing specific was revealed by non-injected brain CT. Lumbar puncture was normal, and culture was sterile. Blood tests revealed the following: platelets 71 giga/L, leukocytes 8.40 giga/L (PNN 7.056 giga/L, lymphocytes 0.670 giga/L), hemoglobin 14.4g/dL, ASAT 57 U/L, ALAT 61 U/L, GGT 128 U/L, PAL 188 U/L, normal kidney function.

On 12 September, when admitted to the infectious disease unit, clinical examination showed fever, asthenia, and non-significant axillary lymph nodes. The same day, a blood smear showed red blood cells with *Babesia* corpuscles inside, reaching a parasitemia of 3.7% (Figure 1). Blood analysis revealed thrombopenia (60 giga/L) and hemolysis signs without anemia (Hb 14.4 g/dL, LDH 890 U/L). Lyme, HCV and HBV serologies were all negative, and protein electrophoresis was normal.

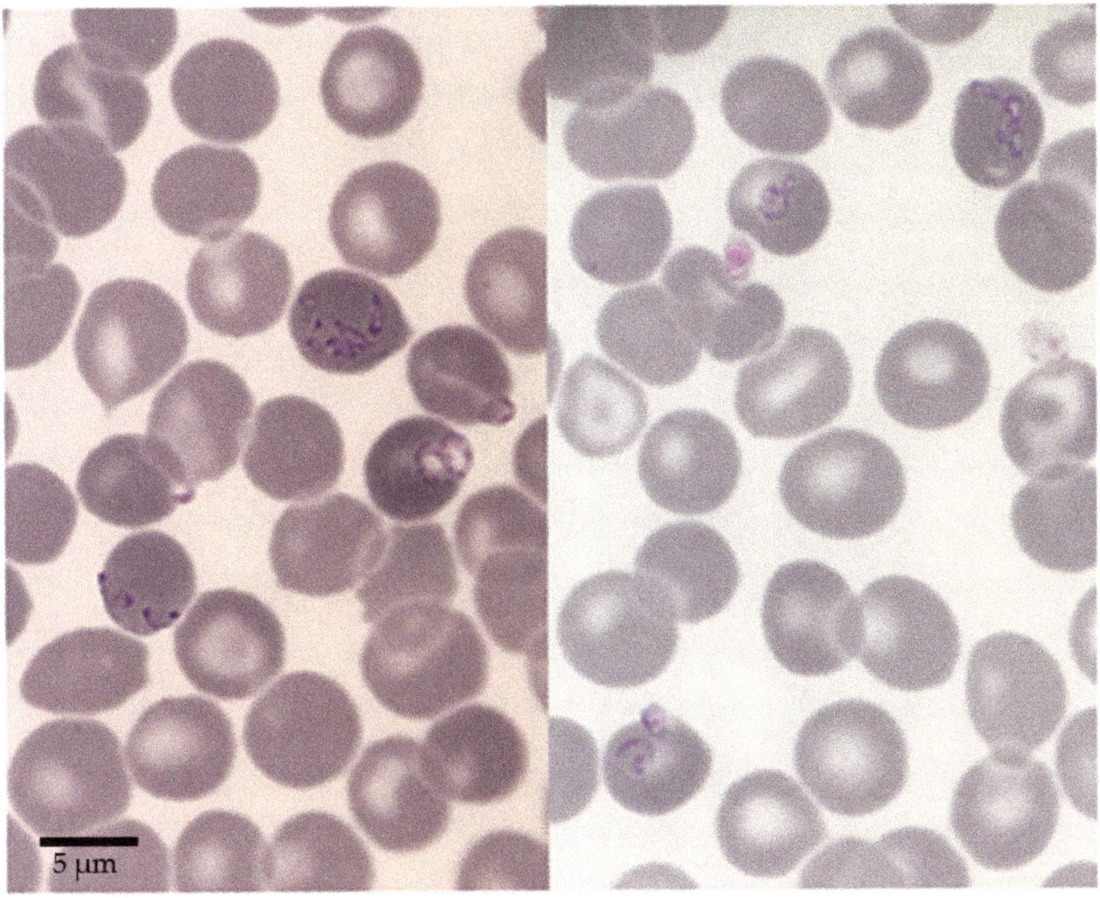

Figure 1. Blood smears of *Babesia* sp. FR1 used to diagnose the *Babesia divergens*-like infection of the patient. Human red blood cells infected with dividing pear shaped merozoites are visible, as well as rounded trophozoites. Bar = 5 µm.

Antimicrobial therapy was undertaken on the same day with Atovaquone (750 mg/12h) and Azithromycine (500 mg on day 1 then 250 mg per day). The patient rapidly felt better with apyrexia and disappearance of all symptoms. On 14 September, parasites were still detected on the blood smear and cytolysis was persistent.

Diagnosis of a *B. divergens*-like infection was confirmed by serology (IFAT with *B. divergens* antigen) with a titer of 1:1024 and by PCR on the 18S rRNA gene as described in materials and methods. Sequencing of the amplified 18S rRNA gene portion confirmed that the responsible agent was closely related to *B. divergens*, the most commonly responsible agent of human babesiosis in France, but different.

Control of the patient's infectious status was performed 16 months later. Serology using the same antigen remained positive with a titer reduced to 1:128. PCR was negative.

2.2. Analysis of 18S rRNA Sequences and Position of Babesia sp. FR1 within the B. Divergens-Like Phylogenetic Group

A 1641 bp sequence was obtained for *Babesia* sp. FR1, covering the positions that are discriminant among members of the *B. divergens*-like phylogenetic group: nucleotide positions 631, 663, 819, and 1637. The sequence is highly similar (99.95%) to published *Babesia* sp. MO1-like and *B. capreoli* sequences, with only one nucleotide modification at position 819 and 663 respectively. It is also related to *B. divergens* (99.9%) with two nucleotide substitutions at positions 631 and 1637 (Table 1).

Table 1. Biological and molecular features of the *Babesia* belonging to the *B. divergens*-like phylogenetic group.

Organism	Natural Host	Human Infection	Geographical Occurence	Vector	18S rRNA Sequence Differences at Nucleotide Position [b]			
					631	663	819	1637
B. divergens	Cattle	+	Europe	*I. ricinus*	A	A	T	C
B. capreoli	Roe deer	−	Europe	*I. ricinus*	G	T	T	T
Babesia sp. MO1/AR1	Cottontail rabbit	+	USA	*I. dentatus* [a]	G	A	A	T
Babesia sp. FR1	nd [c]	+	France	nd [c]	G	A	T	T

[a] likely vector according to [36]. [b] corresponding to position described in [33]. [c] not determined.

The sequence of 1643 bp from the Arkansas case [35] obtained in this study (named *Babesia* sp. AR1) was 100% identical to the first *Babesia* sp. MO1 case from Missouri (GenBank AY048113) [3], to the Kentucky case (GenBank AY887131) [34] and to the cottontail rabbit isolates [38]. They differ from *B. divergens* by three mutations at positions 631, 819 and 1637 (99.8% identity), and from *B. capreoli* by two mutations at positions 663 and 819 (99.9% identity) (Table 1).

2.3. Major Differences in Ama-1 and Rap-1a Genes within the B. divergens-Like Phylogenetic Group

Before analyzing the detailed sequence polymorphism of *ama-1* and *rap-1a* genes between the *B. divergens*-like phylogenetic group members, some major differences in gene sequences appeared on the alignment (Figure 2).

Complete *ama-1* sequences (sizes between 1803 and 1857 bp) were obtained in this study for four clonal lines of *B. capreoli*, for *Babesia* sp. FR1 and for *Babesia* sp. AR1, and were compared to *B. divergens ama-1* sequences [45]. An 18 bp sequence located between bases 553 and 570 was absent only in *Babesia* sp. AR1, corresponding probably to a deletion, which did not modify the translation frame (Supplementary Figure S1). *Babesia* sp. FR1 *ama-1* sequence differs from all the others by an insertion of a 36 bp sequence located between bases 1496 and 1531. The inserted sequence is highly similar to an upstream 36 bp sequence (differing by two nucleotides) and seems therefore to correspond to a gene conversion event of this small gene portion.

Gene		*B. divergens*	*B. capreoli*	*Babesia* sp. AR1	*Babesia* sp. FR1
ama-1	18 bp deletion	N	N	Y	N
	36 bp duplication	N	N	N	Y
rap-1a	Copy number	1	2 (id 95.9-96.4%)	1	1
	3 bp deletion	N	N	Y	N
	33 bp deletion	Y	Y and N	N	N

(a)

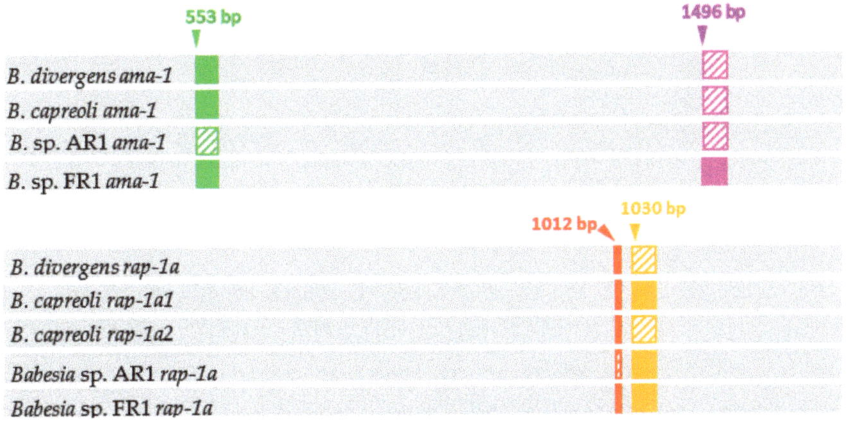

(b)

Figure 2. Major differences in *ama-1* and *rap-1a* genes between members of the *B. divergens*-like phylogenetic group. (**a**) Copy number, and presence (Y) or absence (N) of insertion/deletion in *ama-1* and *rap-1a* genes; (**b**) Schematic representation of the major differences and their positions in gene sequence. The colors used in the part (**a**) correspond to the colors used in the graphical representation of the corresponding deletions/insertions in the part (**b**). The deleted or absent regions are dashed.

Regarding the *rap-1a* gene, partial sequences (sizes between 1203 and 1236 bp) were obtained for four clonal lines of *B. capreoli*, for *Babesia* sp. FR1 and for *Babesia* sp. AR1, and were compared to *B. divergens rap-1a* sequences [46]. Comparison of *rap-1a* sequences from *B. divergens*, *Babesia* sp. AR1, and *Babesia* sp. FR1 highlighted a 3 bp deletion (nucleotides 1012 to 1014) in *Babesia* sp. AR1 only and a 33 bp deletion located between bases 1034 and 1066 in the 12 *rap-1a B. divergens* sequences performed, which did not modify the translation frame. As superposed chromatograms were observed for *B. capreoli* at the 3′ end of the *rap-1a* gene, the presence of multiple copies of this gene was suspected and confirmed by cloning/sequencing and subsequent specific amplifications of each gene copy from each of the four isolates. Two *rap-1a* gene copies were observed, which we named *rap-1a1* and *rap-1a2*. The *rap-1a1* copy was characterized by the absence of the two deletions, as found for *Babesia* sp. FR1. The *rap-1a2* copy contained the 33 bp deletion only and therefore resembled *B. divergens rap-1a*.

These major deletions/insertions were not included in the sequence identity calculations, nor in the phylogenetic analyses, as they represent one-time, usually non-reversible events, with different evolutionary tempo and mode compared to substitutions.

2.4. Intraspecific Sequence Diversity of Rap-1a and Ama-1 within B. divergens and B. capreoli

The genetic variability within the *B. divergens* and *B. capreoli* strains have been analyzed previously for the 18S rRNA gene and no variations were found [33].

Intraspecific genetic variability of *B. divergens ama-1* and *rap-1a* genes was previously analyzed in studies performed at our lab and was found to be very low [45,46]. Sequence identities higher than 99.5% were highlighted for both genes, when comparing sequences of the same set of nine and twelve French isolates, for *ama-1* and *rap-1a* respectively (Table 2 and Table S1). The *ama-1* sequences showed between 99.9 to 100% conserved sites; two similar nucleotide substitutions were noted in *ama-1* sequences of 1505B F14, 3601B E2 and Rouen87 F5 isolates, compared to *ama-1* sequences of the other six clonal lines. The *rap-1a* sequences showed sequence identities between 99.6 and 100%, corresponding to a pairwise maximum of six nucleotide substitutions.

Table 2. Genetic variability of 18S rRNA, *ama-1* and *rap-1a* genes within *B. divergens* and *B. capreoli*.

***Babesia* Species**	**Gene**	**Number of Isolates**	**Nucleotide Differences**	**Identities**
B. divergens	18S rRNA	12	None	100% [33]
	rap-1a	12	0–6 nt/1242 bp	99.6–100% [46]
	ama-1	9	0–2 nt/1821 bp	99.9–100% [45]
B. capreoli	18S rRNA	9	None	100% [33]
	rap-1a1	4	0–7 nt/1236 bp	99.5–100%
	rap-1a2	4	0–5 nt/1203 bp	99.6–100%
	ama-1	4	0–6 nt/1821 bp	99.7–100%

In the case of *B. capreoli*, we analyzed the genetic polymorphism of *ama-1* and *rap-1a* for four isolates collected and cultivated at our laboratory from previous studies [33,47]. The *ama-1* sequences showed sequence identities between 99.7 to 100%. The 2770 F6 and CVD08 005 *ama-1* sequences were identical and up to nine polymorphic sites were identified resulting in six different nucleotide substitutions between *ama-1* sequences of 2704C and 2801 F10 isolates, and were compared to the other two identical *ama-1* sequences.

The two copies of the *rap-1a* gene (*rap-1a1* and *rap-1a2*) were identified in all four *B. capreoli* isolates. Sequence variability of each gene copy was low (less than seven nucleotide substitutions), and identities ranged between 99.5–100% and between 99.6–100% among the *rap-1a1* and the *rap-1a2* sequences, respectively. Sequence identities between *rap-1a1* and *rap-1a2* copies ranged between 96.1 and 96.5%. Most substitutions specific to each gene copy (39 positions) were non silent (39 substitutions resulting in 28 amino acid modifications), with a majority of substitutions on the first (nine substitutions) and/or second codon position (16 substitutions).

2.5. Genetic Variability within the *B. divergens*-Like Phylogenetic Group

As explained above, sequence identities were calculated without the regions corresponding to deletions/insertions and are presented as a contingency table including all three analyzed genes (Table 3). In general, the *ama-1* gene seemed to be more conserved than the *rap-1a* gene as the percentage of sequence identities ranged between 94.3 to 98.7% for *ama-1* and between 86.6 to 98.7% for *rap-1a*. For both genes, the lowest sequence identities were evidenced between *B. divergens* and all other analyzed *Babesia* within the group. The highest sequence identities for *ama-1* and *rap-1a* were obtained between *Babesia* sp. FR1 and *Babesia* sp. AR1 sequences (98.7% identities for both genes). *B. capreoli* was found to be more closely related to *Babesia* sp. AR1 and *Babesia* sp. FR1 than to *B. divergens*.

It was not possible to determine if one of the two copies of *B. capreoli rap-1a* was more related to the unique *rap-1a* gene sequence of other members of the phylogenetic group, as sequence identity values were highly similar.

Table 3. Contingency table for 18S rRNA, *rap-1a* (partial cds) and *ama-1* genes. For the 18S rRNA sequences, the number of nucleotide differences between 18S rRNA gene sequences are indicated in red, instead of the identity percentages. For *ama-1* and *rap-1a* genes, percentage of identities are indicated in green and blue, respectively. Sequence identities with each *rap-1a* copy (*rap-1a1* and *rap-1a2*) are indicated. The identities are calculated excluding the deletions and duplication indicated in Figure 2. Accession numbers of sequences used to perform the analysis are indicated in supplementary Table S1.

Organism	*B. divergens*	*B. capreoli*	*Babesia* sp. AR1	*Babesia* sp. FR1
B. divergens	0 99.9–100% 99.6–100%			
B. capreoli	3 95–95.3% (rap-1a1) 86.6–89.1% (rap1-a2) 88.6–89.1%	0 99.7–100% (rap-1a1) 99.5–100% (rap1-a2) 99.6–100%		
Babesia sp. AR1	3 94.3% 89.5–89.8%	2 97.2–97.3% (rap-1a1) 95.1–95.4% (rap1-a2) 95.3–95.7%	0 100% 100%	
Babesia sp. FR1	2 94.5% 89.8–90%	1 97.3–97.4% (rap-1a1) 95.2–95.5% (rap1-a2) 95.7–96.1%	1 98.7% 98.7%	0 100% 100%

2.6. Phylogenetic Analysis

The phylogenetic analyses based on 18S rRNA, *ama-1* and *rap-1a* genes were concordant and confirmed the placement of the *Babesia* sp. FR1 into the *B. divergens*-like phylogenetic group, with strong bootstrap values of 100 (Figures 3–5). According to the 18S rRNA phylogenetic analysis, and despite the high level of conservation of this marker, two sister groups were supported by good bootstrap values, and *Babesia* sp. FR1 clustered with *B. capreoli*, *Babesia* sp. AR1 and *Babesia* sp. MO1 (bootstrap of 73), and not with *B. divergens* (forming the second cluster supported by a bootstrap value of 89) (Figure 3). The separation of these two clusters was also well supported in the phylogenetic analysis with *ama-1* and *rap-1a* as markers (Figures 4 and 5). The *B. divergens* clade was supported by bootstrap values of 99 and 100 (*ama-1* and *rap-1a* respectively). The *B. capreoli*/*Babesia* sp. AR1/*Babesia* sp. FR1 clade was also well supported by bootstrap values of 100 (*ama-1* and *rap-1a*), but splits on the one hand into a subclade with *B. capreoli* (bootstraps of 100 and 83) and on the other hand into a second subclade with *Babesia* sp. FR1 and *Babesia* sp. AR1 (bootstraps of 100 and 99). The two *Babesia capreoli rap-1a* copies clustered into two sister groups with strong support (100).

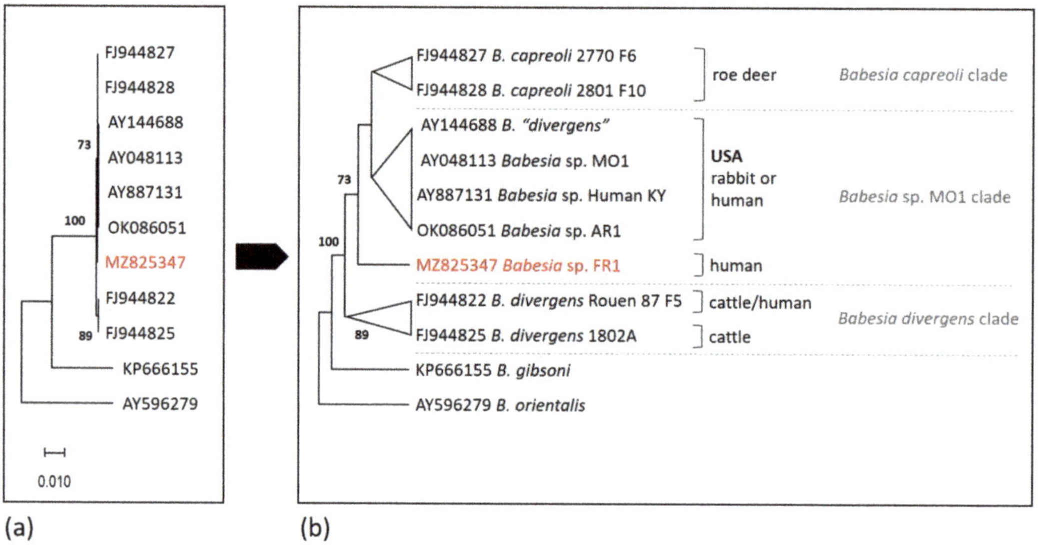

Figure 3. Maximum likelihood unrooted phylogenetic tree of *Babesia* from the *Babesia divergens*-like phylogenetic group based on partial 18S rRNA sequences (1189 bp in the final data set). Branch support/bootstrap values are indicated at each node. *Babesia* sp. FR1 sequence obtained in this study is emphasized in red. (**a**) Scale bar indicates nucleotide substitution rate per site. (**b**) Topology of the tree allowing a better visualization of the bootstrap values; hosts of *Babesia* isolates are indicated.

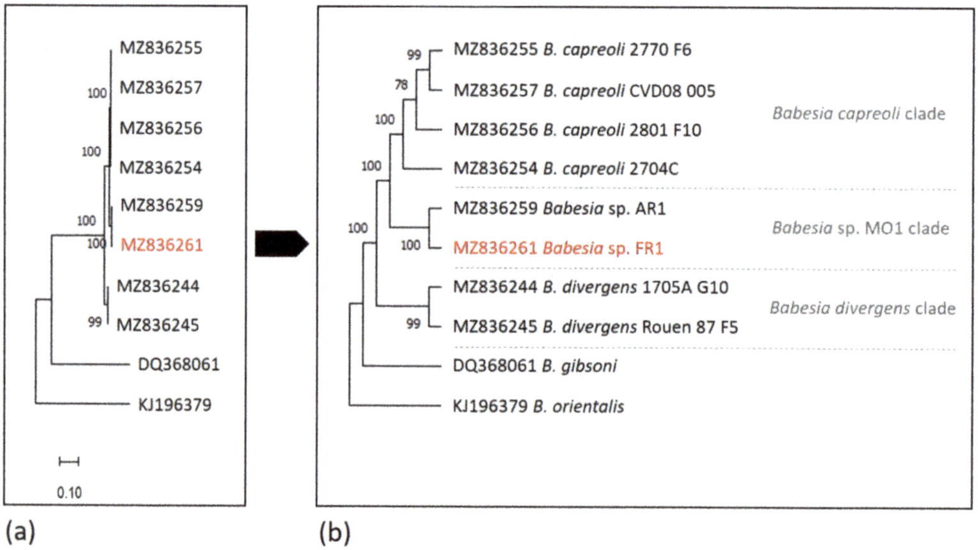

Figure 4. Maximum likelihood unrooted phylogenetic tree of *Babesia* from the *Babesia divergens*-like phylogenetic group based on partial *ama-1* gene sequences (1728 bp in the final data set). Branch support/bootstrap values are indicated at each node. *Babesia* sp. FR1 sequence obtained in this study is emphasized in red. (**a**) Scale bar indicates nucleotide substitution rate per site. (**b**) Topology of the tree allowing a better visualization of the bootstrap values.

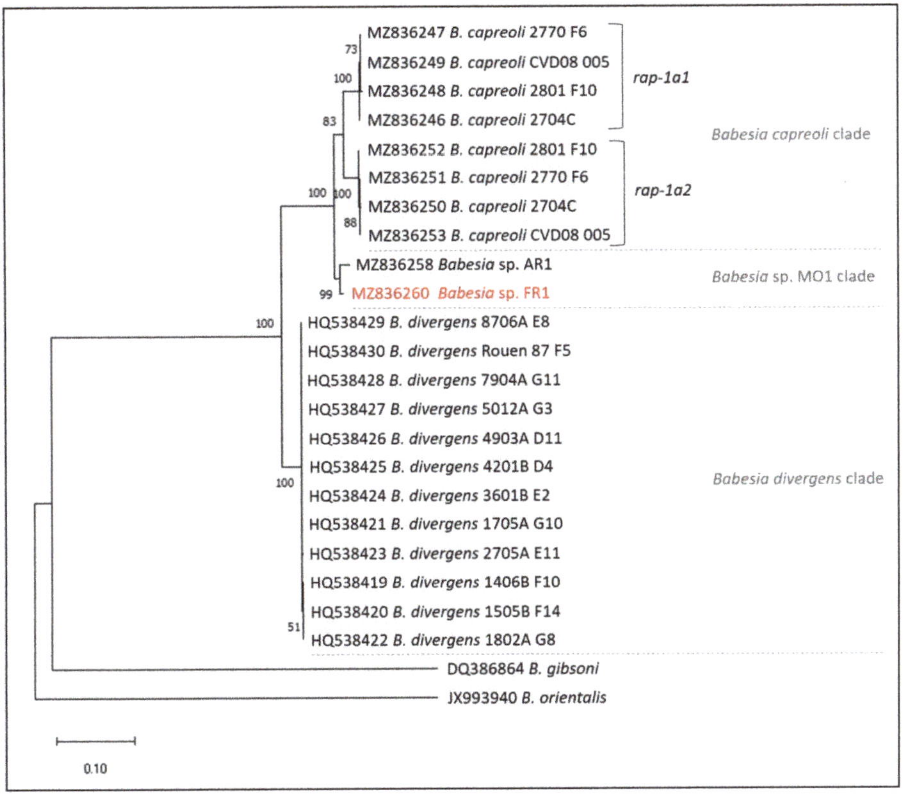

Figure 5. Maximum likelihood unrooted phylogenetic tree of *Babesia* from the *Babesia divergens*-like phylogenetic group based on partial *rap-1a* gene sequences (1138 bp in the final data set). Branch support/bootstrap values are indicated at each node. *Babesia* sp. FR1 sequence obtained in this study is emphasized in red. Scale bar indicates nucleotide substitution rate per site.

3. Discussion

Most human babesiosis cases are recorded in North America and are mainly due to *Babesia microti*, sporadically to *B. duncani* (*Babesia* sp. WA1) and to *Babesia* sp. MO1-like parasites. Sporadic cases were reported in Asia, Africa, and South America, with diverse and often partially characterized etiological agents [48]. In Europe, human babesiosis is rare and *B. divergens* is the main causal agent [43,49]. The most impacted countries are France, Ireland and Great Britain, and in France, Western regions and Normandy are most affected [10], due to substantial farming of bovines, the natural host of *B. divergens* [50].

The patient was most probably bitten by a tick on the Île de Ré, even if he had no recollection of a tick bite. This is the most probable place of tick acquisition by the patient, as it is close to a forest, where the abundance of the potential vector *I. ricinus* is high, increasing the risk of contracting tick-borne pathogens [51]. The patient was asplenic, which is also a major risk factor for severe or fatal babesiosis [10,43,49]. However, the symptoms in this patient developed slowly (two to three weeks between the onset of symptoms and admission to hospital) despite aspleny, while *B. divergens'* course of infection in such cases is usually fulminant [42]. Biological diagnosis of the provisionally named *Babesia* sp. FR1 was based on a blood smear, which led to the administration of antibabesial therapy (Atovaquone and Azithromycine) as soon as practicable. This treatment was effective, as symptoms rapidly disappeared, and parasite clearance was attested 16 months later by a negative PCR, correlated with a reduction of the serology titer.

Molecular characterization of *Babesia* sp. FR1 required a deeper analysis. Sequence and phylogenetic analysis of 18S rRNA revealed that it was genetically close but different from typical *B. divergens* isolates infecting cattle or humans (two polymorphic sites at positions 831 and 1637) [33], but that it closely resembled the American *B. divergens*-like parasite *Babesia* sp. MO1. Despite the genetic difference with *B. divergens*, the infection could be diagnosed using *B. divergens*-specific serological tools (IFAT), confirming anyway a close relationship with *B. divergens*.

We decided to explore new markers to improve knowledge on the *B. divergens*-like phylogenetic clade and to correctly position this new isolate within this species complex. We chose *rap-1a* and *ama-1* for two reasons. First, both genes code for proteins involved in the process of red blood cell invasion by the parasite [52], and as host range/specificity is an important biological feature in the description of this intra-erythrocytic obligatory parasite, they represent markers of interest. Second, we know from previous studies that both genes were well conserved among *B. divergens* isolates from cattle or humans [45,46]. Their interspecies divergence remained to be determined.

Regardless of the marker used, the sequences of *B. divergens* (cattle as a natural host) are grouped in a cluster well-separated from the other two clusters corresponding to *B. capreoli* and *Babesia* sp. MO1/AR1/FR1. Phylogenies based on more discriminant markers (*rap-1a* or *ama-1*) placed *Babesia* sp. FR1 in the cluster formed by isolates responsible for cases of human babesiosis in the USA represented by *Babesia* sp. AR1. This cluster is separated from the cluster of *B. capreoli* sequences, and from the cluster of *B. divergens* sequences. We can therefore conclude that *Babesia* sp. FR1 is not a *B. divergens*.

The phylogenetic group containing *Babesia* sp. MO1 is sometimes referred to as the *B. divergens* US lineage [53,54]. However, *Babesia* sp. FR1, which clusters with *Babesia* sp. MO1 and *Babesia* sp. AR1, was clearly acquired locally and is an autochthonous case as the patient did not travel to the USA in the months before the onset of the symptoms. Therefore, we not only confirm in the present study that *Babesia* sp. MO1-like sequences form a well-supported taxon, but we also highlight that the geographical distribution of this group is not restricted to the USA, but extends to Europe as it includes *Babesia* sp. FR1. The three clusters within *Babesia divergens*-like, i.e., *B. divergens*, *B. capreoli*, and *Babesia* sp. MO1-like might be associated with their natural host rather than with geographic distribution. Humans are only incidental hosts for parasites belonging to the *B. divergens*-like group, the natural hosts being cattle for *B. divergens*, roe deer for *B. capreoli* and rabbits for *Babesia* sp. MO1. The natural host for *Babesia* sp. FR1 has not been characterized but could also well be a Laporidae, especially in the Île de Ré context, a highly touristic and populated island where cattle and cervids are rare or absent, due to limited forested areas dominated by resinous trees (mainly maritime pine trees) and typical local productions (vineyards and salt marshes). The European rabbit (*Oryctolagus cuniculus*) is highly abundant on this island where it has been pullulating since the 2000s, and could therefore be the potential natural host for *Babesia* sp. FR1.

In this study, we did not include isolates described as *B. divergens* in sika deer described in Japan or in humans in China [6,53,54]. Our goal in this study was to characterize and correctly place the new *Babesia* sp. FR1 isolate in the phylogenetic group of *Babesia divergens*-like, among biologically well-characterized isolates, i.e., whose host range has been studied and whose parasites have been cultured [33,38–41,55]. The isolates described in Japan from sika deer and named *B. divergens* are not included in the *B. divergens*-like phylogenetic group because they differ at the 18S rRNA sequence from all other members of this group by at least six conserved substitutions all of which are different from those described within this group. These isolates form a sister group to *B. divergens*-like. The name *B. divergens* should be reserved for isolates from cattle or humans whose 18S rRNA sequences match the many descriptions already published [18–23,29,30,33,49]. There is no evidence that isolates from sika deer are capable of infecting either cattle, gerbils (*B. divergens* experimental host), or humans.

The sequences named as "*B. divergens*" and described in humans in China [6] actually match those described for *B. capreoli*, with the characteristic differences at positions 631 and 663 [33]. This information raises the possibility of human infections by *B. capreoli*, a species that has never been molecularly characterized as responsible for symptomatic cases of human babesiosis in Europe and described as not growing in vitro in human red blood cells [33]. However, short-term asymptomatic carriage of parasites could occur in humans in geographic areas with high parasite and vector prevalences. We unsuccessfully attempted to obtain DNA from these parasites to include them in our study.

In the present study, we characterized *rap-1a* genes in the *B. divergens*-like phylogenetic group. The *rap-1a* genes belong to a multigene family, and multiple copies have already been demonstrated in a few *Babesia* species: two copies in *B. bovis* and *B. canis*, four to five in *B. ovis*, at least seven copies in *Babesia* sp. Xinjiang, eleven in *B. bigemina* and twelve in the *B. motasi*-like group members [52,56–61]. The multiple copies of *rap-1a* are usually different, allowing their differentiation, except in the case of *B. divergens* where the presence of two identical copies was highlighted when its genome was sequenced [52]. It is highly probable that two identical and therefore undistinguishable copies of *rap-1a* exist in all the *B. divergens* isolates characterized. We cannot exclude the presence of two identical copies also for members of the *Babesia* sp. MO1-like clade. In all *B. capreoli* isolates analyzed, two different but closely related *rap-1a* copies, named *rap-1a1* and *rap-1a2* (sequence identities of about 96%) were identified. Each copy is equally different from either *B. divergens*, *Babesia* sp. FR1 or *Babesia* sp. AR1 *rap-1a* genes, and the two copies place as sister groups to each other, indicating a gene duplication that occurred after *B. capreoli* speciation. While genetic divergence occurred between the two *rap-1a* copies of *B. capreoli*, it was not the case between *B. divergens rap-1a* copies. *B. divergens rap-1a* gene has been previously characterized and its genetic variability among cattle and human isolates was found to be limited [51,62,63]. A greater sequence diversity among *B. capreoli* isolates compared to *B. divergens* was also highlighted in the case of the merozoite surface antigen *Bc37/41* compared to *Bd37*, and a greater selection pressure was hypothesized [64]. This could also explain the sequence divergence between the two copies of *rap-1a* in *B. capreoli* and not between the two *B. divergens* copies of *rap-1*. But a more recent event of the *rap-1a* gene duplication in *B. divergens* could also explain the difference in sequence divergence between the two copies. Whether the last common ancestor of members of the *B. divergens*-like group possesses one or two copies of *rap-1a*, or when and how many times *rap-1a* gene duplication occurred in the speciation process is difficult to evaluate. Despite the presence of all motives that characterized RAP-1 family members, *rap-1b* sequence identity with the other two copies of *rap-1a* in the *B. divergens* genome is extremely low (45%) and was not amplified with the primers used.

In conclusion, we describe here a case of human babesiosis in Europe (France) due to a *Babesia* isolate more closely related to the American *Babesia* sp. MO1 and AR1 than to *B. divergens*. Using two discriminant molecular markers, our study confirms the existence of three phylogenetic clades within the *B. divergens*-like group that would deserve the rank of species as their phylogenetic classification corresponds with their natural hosts; *B. divergens* natural host is cattle, *B. capreoli* infects mainly roe deer, and *Babesia* sp. MO1-like parasites probably infect Laporidae.

In Europe, diagnosis of human babesiosis is complicated due to its infrequency which often leads to a delayed detection and treatment. This delayed treatment promotes the development of a fulminant manifestation of this parasitic disease, in particular for asplenic or immunocompromised patients. Thus, the infection results often in the death of the patient, which could probably have been avoided by a more precocious diagnosis and treatment [23,26]. In Europe, the serological and molecular tools developed to diagnose *B. divergens* infections should principally be adequate to detect *Babesia* sp. FR1 infections. However, it needs to be taken into account that atypical immunofluorescence patterns (dots and weak fluorescence of the parasite surface) may lead to a negative conclusion when carrying out an immunofluorescence test. Prophylactic treatments are advised, such as wearing long clothes and performing skin examination for tick detection after exposure to high-risk environments.

4. Materials and Methods

4.1. Babesia Isolates and DNA Origins

A preliminary identification of *Babesia* sp. FR1 responsible for the mild form of babesiosis was performed on blood smears stained with May-Grünwald Giemsa. Further diagnosis was carried out by serology (IFAT with *B. divergens* antigen) [31], as well as 18S rRNA gene amplification [33] and sequencing from blood DNA extracted using the Nucleospin Blood kit according to the manufacturer's instructions (Macherey-Nagel, Düren, Germany).

B. capreoli isolates were collected and characterized in previous studies performed at our lab [33,47]. We included in our analysis four in vitro cultivated isolates from roe deer blood samples or spleen, from three different regions of France (Supplementary Table S1). *B. divergens* isolates were also cultivated in vitro from acute piroplasmosis cases in cows (11 isolates) or in humans (one isolate) [55].

DNA from cultured *B. capreoli* clonal lines (2704C, 2770 F6, 2801 F10 and CVD08 005) was extracted as previously mentioned.

DNA from one American case of human babesiosis was kindly provided by Mayo Medical Laboratory, Rochester, USA. This fatal case occurred in an asplenic patient, in Arkansas in 2015, with a possible acquisition through transfusion [35]. Due to its geographical origin, we named this isolate *Babesia* sp. AR1. It was characterized as a *Babesia* sp. MO1-like babesiosis etiological agent.

As all these isolates are very closely related to *B. divergens*, we have used throughout the manuscript the terminology *B. divergens*-like phylogenetic group to qualify the following isolates, species or clades: *B. divergens*, *B. capreoli*, *Babesia* sp. MO1, *Babesia* sp. AR1, and the new *Babesia* isolate, named *Babesia* sp. FR1.

4.2. Comparison of 18S rDNA Sequences within the B. divergens Taxonomic Group

Babesia sp. AR1 18S rRNA sequences (560 bp) from the previously mentioned isolates were kindly provided by Mayo Medical Laboratory, Rochester, USA. Published *B. capreoli* as well as *B. divergens* 18S rRNA sequences were used as a comparison [33]. Their origin and accession numbers are described in Supplementary Table S1. The partial 18S rRNA sequence of *Babesia* sp. FR1 was obtained using the same primers [33] (Table 4). With the aim of obtaining sequences of comparable sizes, the 18S rRNA partial sequence of *Babesia* sp. AR1 was also amplified with these primers and sequenced. The alignment was done using the ClustalW program as implemented in the Geneious R6 software (https://www.geneious.com accessed on 1 October 2021).

4.3. Amplification of Ama-1 (Apical Membrane Antigen-1) and Rap-1a (Rhoptry Associated protein-1) Genes for B. capreoli, Babesia sp. *AR1, and Babesia* sp. *FR1*

PCR was performed to amplify the *ama-1* and *rap-1a* genes of *B. capreoli*, *Babesia sp.* AR1, and *Babesia* sp. FR1 isolates using ama1-S1/ama1-R3 and rap1-fw/rap1-rev primers respectively (Table 4). Reactions were carried out in 30 µL reaction mixtures containing 1 X GoTaq buffer, 4 mM $MgCl_2$, 0.2 mM of each dNTP (Eurobio Scientific, Les Ulis, France), 1 unit GoTaq G2 Flexi DNA Polymerase (Promega, Madison, WI, USA), 0.5 µM of each primer and 1 µL of DNA template. The amplification conditions comprised 5 min at 95 °C followed by 40 cycles of 30 s at 95 °C, 30 s at the temperatures indicated in Table 4, 1 min 30 s at 72 °C, and a final extension at 72 °C for 5 min. The amplified fragments were purified with the ExoSAP-IT reagent according to the manufacturer's instructions (Affymetrix, Santa Clara, CA, USA) and sequencing was performed on both strands (Eurofins Genomics, Ebersberg, Germany) using the same primers for *rap-1a* gene, or using primers distributed along the sequence for *ama-1* gene (Table 4). Sequences were then assembled using the Geneious R6 software.

Table 4. Description of the primers used in this study for gene amplification as well as sequencing.

Target Gene	Primer Name	Sequence (5′–3′)	Tm (°C)	PCR	Amplicon Length (bp)	Sequencing	References
18S rRNA	CRYPTOF	AACCTGGTTGATCCTGCCAGTAGTCAT	63	×	1728	×	[33]
	CRYPTOR	TGATCCTTCTGCAGGTTCACCTA		×		×	
	BAB-GF2	GTCTTGTAATTGGAATGATGG	61	×	560	×	[11]
	BAB-GR2	CCAAAGACTTTGATTTCTCT		×		×	
ama-1	ama1-S1	TGACTGCCATATCGACGAAG	61	×	≈2000	×	this study
	ama1-R3	CTCTAGTGAATTACGATAGC		×		×	[50]
	ama1-As1	GGCGGATATTCGGTTGAGG				×	this study
	ama1-S2	CATGGCCAAGTTTGACCTTG				×	this study
	ama1-As2	CTGCGTCACGCGTGAATTC				×	this study
	ama1-S3	CTCCTGTGTATGGAGCCGA				×	this study
	ama1-As3	GTGAAAGCGCGGTTGTGAC				×	this study
	ama1-S4	AGCAGTTGGATCGCCTCTC				×	this study
rap-1a	rap1-fw	AATGTCCTACTGGGAAACGC	58	×	≈1300	×	this study
	rap1-rev	GCGGAGTCCATGCCTGTACC		×		×	this study
rap-1a1 (5′)	rap1-fw	see above	58	×	1146	×	
	rap1-a1-rev	GCTTAGTAGCATGCATCTTC		×		×	this study
rap-1a1 (3′)	rap1-a1-fw	GGACTCCGAGAAAAAAGGATG	58	×	261	×	this study
	rap1-rev	see above		×		×	
rap-1a2 (5′)	rap1-fw	see above	58	×	1123	×	
	rap1-a2-rev	TGGAACAACTTCTTCATAGG		×		×	this study
rap-1a2 (3′)	rap1-a2-fw	GGGCTTCTGGAAAAAGAAGG	58	×	228	×	this study
	rap1-rev	see above		×		×	

For the four isolates of *B. capreoli* (2704C, 2770 F6, 2801 F10 and CVD08 005), preliminary sequencing results of *rap-1a* gene highlighted superposed chromatograms at the gene 3′ end, suggesting the presence of multiple copies of this gene, a frequent feature for this gene. The PCR products were therefore cloned in the pGEM-T easy vector according to the manufacturer's instructions (Promega, Madison, WI, USA), to determine the number and sequences of the putative different copies of the *rap-1a* gene. *Escherichia coli* strain BL21 was transformed with the plasmid constructions and colonies with the expected inserts were selected by direct colony PCR using vector primers: T7 and SP6. Recombinant plasmids were then isolated using the Nucleospin Plasmid kit (Macherey-Nagel, Düren, Germany) and both strands of the inserts were sequenced using vector primers (Eurofins, Genomics, Ebersberg, Germany). Then primers were designed to selectively amplify the different *rap-1a* gene copies of *B. capreoli* isolates (Table 4). Primers rap1-a1-fw or rap1-a2-fw were associated with primer rap1-rev to amplify the 3′ part of respective *rap-1a* copies. Primers rap1-a1-rev or rap1-a2-rev were associated with primer rap1-fw to amplify the 5′ part of *rap-1a* copies (same reaction and cycling conditions as above). PCR products were purified and sequenced as already mentioned.

4.4. Comparison of Ama-1 and Rap-1a DNA Sequences for B. divergens-Like Phylogenetic Group Members

The resulting *ama-1* and *rap-1a* DNA sequences of *B. capreoli*, *Babesia* sp. AR1 and *Babesia* sp. FR1 were aligned along with the published *ama-1* and *rap-1a* DNA sequences of *B. divergens* isolates using the ClustalW program as implemented in the Geneious R6 software.

4.5. Phylogenetic Analysis

Phylogenetic relationships within the *Babesia divergens*-like group were inferred using published sequences available in GenBank (Supplementary Table S1) and sequence data produced in the present study (18S rRNA, *ama-1* and *rap-1a* sequences). Sequences were aligned using Muscle as implemented in MEGA version X [65]. Phylogenetic analyses used a trimmed alignment of 1189 bp with complete deletion option for the 18S rRNA gene,

1728 bp and 1138 bp with complete deletion option for the *ama-1* and *rap-1a* coding sequences respectively. Maximum likelihood phylogenetic trees were produced using MEGA-X, with 1000 bootstrap replications based on the Tamura 3-parameter model [66] for the 18S rRNA gene and the *ama-1* gene, and based on the Kimura 2-parameter model [67] model for *rap-1a* gene. For the *ama-1* and *rap-1a* sequences, the three codon positions were included. The appropriate model of nucleotide substitution for ML analysis was selected based on the Bayesian Information Criterion (BIC) computed by MEGA-X.

4.6. Genbank Deposition

Nucleotidic sequences obtained in this study were submitted to GenBank with accession numbers MZ825347 and OK086051 for the 18S rRNA sequence of *Babesia* sp. FR1 and *Babesia* sp. AR1 respectively, MZ836259 and MZ836261 for the *ama-1* sequences of *Babesia* sp. AR1 and *Babesia* sp. FR1 respectively, MZ836258 and MZ836260 for the *rap-1a* sequences of *Babesia* sp. AR1 and *Babesia* sp. FR1 respectively. Accession numbers for *rap-1a* and *ama-1* sequences of *B. capreoli* are presented in Supplementary Table S1.

Supplementary Materials: The following are available online at https://www.mdpi.com/article/10.3390/pathogens10111433/s1, Table S1: Description of *B. divergens* (A) and *B. capreoli* (B) clonal lines used in the study and Genbank accession numbers. Figure S1: (A) Major differences in *ama-1* gene and AMA-1 protein sequences. (B) Major differences in *rap-1a* gene and RAP-1A protein sequences.

Author Contributions: Conceptualization, L.M. and M.-C.d.C.; methodology, C.B. and F.M.; validation, C.B., N.d.l.C. and L.M.; formal analysis, C.B.; investigation, C.B., V.P. and M.-C.d.C.; resources, V.P., F.M., M.-C.d.C. and L.M.; data curation, C.B.; writing—original draft preparation, C.B., M.-C.d.C. and L.M.; writing—review and editing, C.B., M.-C.d.C., N.d.l.C., F.M. and V.P..; visualization, F.M., C.B. and L.M.; supervision, L.M.; project administration, L.M.; funding acquisition, C.B., N.d.l.C. and L.M. All authors have read and agreed to the published version of the manuscript.

Funding: This research received no external funding.

Institutional Review Board Statement: Ethical review and approval were waived for this study, because this case report did not involve human subject research.

Informed Consent Statement: Written informed consent has been obtained from the patient to publish this paper.

Acknowledgments: The authors wish to thank M. Jouglin for technical support.

Conflicts of Interest: The authors declare no conflict of interest.

References

1. Schnittger, L.; Rodriguez, A.E.; Florin-Christensen, M.; Morrison, D.A. *Babesia*: A world emerging. *Infect. Genet. Evol.* **2012**, *12*, 1788–1809. [CrossRef] [PubMed]
2. Herwaldt, B.L.; de Bruyn, G.; Pieniazek, N.J.; Homer, M.; Lofy, K.H.; Slemenda, S.B.; Fritsche, T.R.; Persing, D.H.; Limaye, A.P. *Babesia divergens*-like infection, Washington State. *Emerg. Infect. Dis.* **2004**, *10*, 622–629. [CrossRef]
3. Herwaldt, B.; Persing, D.H.; Précigout, E.A.; Goff, W.L.; Mathiesen, D.A.; Taylor, P.W.; Eberhard, M.L.; Gorenflot, A.F. A fatal case of babesiosis in Missouri: Identification of another piroplasm that infects humans. *Ann. Intern. Med.* **1996**, *124*, 643–650. [CrossRef] [PubMed]
4. Vannier, E.G.; Diuk-Wasser, M.A.; Ben Mamoun, C.; Krause, P.J. Babesiosis. *Infect. Dis. Clin. N. Am.* **2015**, *29*, 357–370. [CrossRef]
5. Jiang, J.F.; Zheng, Y.C.; Jiang, R.R.; Li, H.; Huo, Q.B.; Jiang, B.G.; Sun, Y.; Jia, N.; Wang, Y.W.; Ma, L.; et al. Epidemiological, clinical, and laboratory characteristics of 48 cases of "*Babesia venatorum*" infection in China: A descriptive study. *Lancet Infect. Dis.* **2015**, *15*, 196–203. [CrossRef]
6. Wang, J.; Zhang, S.; Yang, J.; Liu, J.; Zhang, D.; Li, Y.; Luo, J.; Guan, G.; Yin, H. *Babesia divergens* in human in Gansu province, China. *Emerg. Microbes Infect.* **2019**, *8*, 959–961. [CrossRef] [PubMed]
7. Jia, N.; Zheng, Y.C.; Jiang, J.F.; Jiang, R.R.; Jiang, B.G.; Wei, R.; Liu, H.B.; Huo, Q.B.; Sun, Y.; Chu, Y.L.; et al. Human babesiosis caused by a *Babesia crassa*-like pathogen: A case series. *Clin. Infect. Dis.* **2018**, *67*, 1110–1119. [CrossRef]
8. Skrabalo, Z.; Deanovic, Z. Piroplasmosis in man; report of a case. *Doc. Med. Geogr. Trop.* **1957**, *9*, 11–16. [PubMed]
9. Gray, J.S. Identity of the causal agents of human babesiosis in Europe. *Int. J. Med. Microbiol.* **2006**, *296*, 131–136. [CrossRef]
10. Uguen, C.; Girard, L.; Brasseur, P.; Leblay, R. Human babesiosis in 1997. *Rev. Med. Interne* **1997**, *18*, 945–951. [CrossRef]

11. Herwaldt, B.L.; Cacciò, S.; Gherlinzoni, F.; Aspöck, H.; Slemenda, S.B.; Piccaluga, P.; Martinelli, G.; Edelhofer, R.; Hollenstein, U.; Poletti, G.; et al. Molecular characterization of a non-*Babesia divergens* organism causing zoonotic babesiosis in Europe. *Emerg. Infect. Dis.* **2003**, *9*, 942–948. [CrossRef]
12. Häselbarth, K.; Tenter, A.M.; Brade, V.; Krieger, G.; Hunfeld, K.P. First case of human babesiosis in Germany—Clinical presentation and molecular characterisation of the pathogen. *Int. J. Med. Microbiol.* **2007**, *297*, 197–204. [CrossRef] [PubMed]
13. Bläckberg, J.; Lazarevic, V.L.; Hunfeld, K.P.; Persson, K.E.M. Low-virulent *Babesia venatorum* infection masquerading as hemophagocytic syndrome. *Ann. Hematol.* **2018**, *97*, 731–733. [CrossRef] [PubMed]
14. Stahl, P.; Poinsignon, Y.; Pouedras, P.; Ciubotaru, V.; Berry, L.; Emu, B.; Krause, P.J.; Ben Mamoun, C.; Cornillot, E. Case report of the patient source of the *Babesia microti* R1 reference strain and implications for travelers. *J. Travel. Med.* **2018**, *25*, tax073. [CrossRef] [PubMed]
15. Hildebrandt, A.; Hunfeld, K.P.; Baier, M.; Krumbholz, A.; Sachse, S.; Lorenzen, T.; Kiehntopf, M.; Fricke, H.J.; Straube, E. First confirmed autochthonous case of human *Babesia microti* infection in Europe. *Eur. J. Clin. Microbiol. Infect. Dis.* **2007**, *26*, 595–601. [CrossRef]
16. Centeno-Lima, S.; do Rosário, V.; Parreira, R.; Maia, A.J.; Freudenthal, A.M.; Nijhof, A.M.; Jongejan, F. A fatal case of human babesiosis in Portugal: Molecular and phylogenetic analysis. *Trop. Med. Int. Health.* **2003**, *8*, 760–764. [CrossRef] [PubMed]
17. Corpelet, C.; Vacher, P.; Coudore, F.; Laurichesse, H.; Conort, N.; Souweine, B. Role of quinine in life-threatening *Babesia divergens* infection successfully treated with clindamycin. *Eur. J. Clin. Microbiol. Infect. Dis.* **2005**, *24*, 74–75. [CrossRef]
18. Haapasalo, K.; Suomalainen, P.; Sukura, A.; Siikamaki, H.; Jokiranta, T.S. Fatal babesiosis in man, Finland, 2004. *Emerg. Infect. Dis.* **2010**, *16*, 1116–1118. [CrossRef]
19. Gonzalez, L.M.; Rojo, S.; Gonzalez-Camacho, F.; Luque, D.; Lobo, C.A.; Montero, E. Severe babesiosis in immunocompetent man, Spain, 2011. *Emerg. Infect. Dis.* **2014**, *20*, 724–726. [CrossRef]
20. González, L.M.; Castro, E.; Lobo, C.A.; Richart, A.; Ramiro, R.; González-Camacho, F.; Luque, D.; Velasco, A.C.; Montero, E. First report of *Babesia divergens* infection in an HIV patient. *Int. J. Infect. Dis.* **2015**, *33*, 202–204. [CrossRef] [PubMed]
21. Tanyel, E.; Guler, N.; Hokelek, M.; Ulger, F.; Sunbul, M. A case of severe babesiosis treated successfully with exchange transfusion. *Int. J. Infect. Dis.* **2015**, *38*, 83–85. [CrossRef] [PubMed]
22. O'Connell, S.; Lyons, C.; Abdou, M.; Patowary, R.; Aslam, S.; Kinsella, N.; Zintl, A.; Hunfeld, K.P.; Wormser, G.P.; Gray, J.; et al. Splenic dysfunction from celiac disease resulting in severe babesiosis. *Ticks Tick Borne Dis.* **2017**, *8*, 537–539. [CrossRef]
23. Asensi, V.; González, L.M.; Fernández-Suárez, J.; Sevilla, E.; Navascués, R.Á.; Suárez, M.L.; Lauret, M.E.; Bernardo, A.; Carton, J.A.; Montero, E. A fatal case of *Babesia divergens* infection in Northwestern Spain. *Ticks Tick Borne Dis.* **2018**, *9*, 730–734. [CrossRef]
24. Kukina, I.V.; Zelya, O.P.; Guzeeva, T.M.; Karan, L.S.; Perkovskaya, I.A.; Tymoshenko, N.I.; Guzeeva, M.V. Severe babesiosis caused by *Babesia divergens* in a host with intact spleen, Russia, 2018. *Ticks Tick Borne Dis.* **2019**, *10*, 101262. [CrossRef]
25. Mørch, K.; Holmaas, G.; Frolander, P.S.; Kristoffersen, E.K. Severe human *Babesia divergens* infection in Norway. *Int. J. Infect. Dis.* **2015**, *33*, 37–38. [CrossRef] [PubMed]
26. Kukina, I.V.; Guzeeva, T.M.; Zelya, O.P.; Ganushkina, L.A. Fatal human babesiosis caused by *Babesia divergens* in an asplenic host. *IDCases* **2018**, *13*, e00414. [CrossRef]
27. Strizova, Z.; Havlova, K.; Patek, O.; Smrz, D.; Bartunkova, J. The first human case of babesiosis mimicking Reiter's syndrome. *Folia Parasitol.* **2020**, *67*, 1–5. [CrossRef]
28. Loutan, L.; Rossier, J.; Zufferey, G.; Cuénod, D.; Hatz, C.; Marti, H.P.; Gern, L. Human babesiosis: First case report in Switzerland. *Rev. Med. Suisse Romande* **1994**, *114*, 111–116. (In French)
29. Martinot, M.; Zadeh, M.M.; Hansmann, Y.; Grawey, I.; Christmann, D.; Aguillon, S.; Jouglin, M.; Chauvin, A.; De Briel, D. Babesiosis in immunocompetent patients, Europe. *Emerg. Infect. Dis.* **2011**, *17*, 114–116. [CrossRef]
30. Paleau, A.; Candolfi, E.; Souply, L.; De Briel, D.; Delarbre, J.M.; Lipsker, D.; Jouglin, M.; Malandrin, L.; Hansmann, Y.; Martinot, M. Human babesiosis in Alsace. *Med. Mal. Infect.* **2020**, *50*, 486–491. [CrossRef] [PubMed]
31. Lempereur, L.; Shiels, B.; Heyman, P.; Moreau, E.; Saegerman, C.; Losson, B.; Malandrin, L. A retrospective serological survey on human babesiosis in Belgium. *Clin. Microbiol. Infect.* **2015**, *21*, 96.e1–96.e7. [CrossRef]
32. Duh, D.; Petrovec, M.; Bidovec, A.; Avsic-Zupanc, T. Cervids as Babesiae hosts, Slovenia. *Emerg. Infect. Dis.* **2005**, *11*, 1121–1123. [CrossRef]
33. Malandrin, L.; Jouglin, M.; Sun, Y.; Brisseau, N.; Chauvin, A. Redescription of *Babesia capreoli* (Enigk and Friedhoff, 1962) from roe deer (*Capreolus capreolus*): Isolation, cultivation, host specificity, molecular characterisation and differentiation from *Babesia divergens*. *Int. J. Parasitol.* **2010**, *40*, 277–284. [CrossRef]
34. Beattie, J.F.; Michelson, M.L.; Holman, P.J. Acute babesiosis caused by *Babesia divergens* in a resident of Kentucky. *N. Engl. J. Med.* **2002**, *347*, 697–698. [CrossRef]
35. Burgess, M.J.; Rosenbaum, E.R.; Pritt, B.S.; Haselow, D.T.; Ferren, K.M.; Alzghoul, B.N.; Rico, J.C.; Sloan, L.M.; Ramanan, P.; Purushothaman, R.; et al. Possible transfusion-transmitted *Babesia divergens*-like/MO1 infection in an Arkansas patient. *Clin. Infect. Dis.* **2017**, *64*, 1622–1625. [CrossRef]
36. Herc, E.; Pritt, B.; Huizenga, T.; Douce, R.; Hysell, M.; Newton, D.; Sidge, J.; Losman, E.; Sherbeck, J.; Kaul, D.R. Probable locally acquired *Babesia divergens*-like infection in woman, Michigan, USA. *Emerg. Infect. Dis.* **2018**, *24*, 1558–1560. [CrossRef] [PubMed]
37. Goethert, H.K.; Telford, S.R., 3rd. Enzootic transmission of *Babesia divergens* among cottontail rabbits on Nantucket Island, Massachusetts. *Am. J. Trop. Med. Hyg.* **2003**, *69*, 455–460. [CrossRef] [PubMed]

38. Holman, P.J.; Spencer, A.M.; Droleskey, R.E.; Goethert, H.K.; Telford, S.R., 3rd. In vitro cultivation of a zoonotic *Babesia* sp. isolated from eastern cottontail rabbits (*Sylvilagus floridanus*) on Nantucket Island, Massachusetts. *J. Clin. Microbiol.* **2005**, *43*, 3995–4001. [CrossRef]
39. Holman, P.J.; Spencer, A.M.; Telford, S.R., 3rd; Goethert, H.K.; Allen, A.J.; Knowles, D.P.; Goff, W.L. Comparative infectivity of *Babesia divergens* and a zoonotic *Babesia divergens*-like parasite in cattle. *Am. J. Trop. Med. Hyg.* **2005**, *73*, 865–870. [CrossRef] [PubMed]
40. Spencer, A.M.; Goethert, H.K.; Telford, S.R., 3rd; Holman, P.J. In vitro host erythrocyte specificity and differential morphology of *Babesia divergens* and a zoonotic *Babesia* sp. from eastern cottontail rabbits (*Sylvilagus floridanus*). *J. Parasitol.* **2006**, *92*, 333–340. [CrossRef]
41. Holman, P.J. Phylogenetic and biologic evidence that *Babesia divergens* is not endemic in the United States. *Ann. N. Y. Acad. Sci.* **2006**, *1081*, 518–525. [CrossRef]
42. Hildebrandt, A.; Gray, J.S.; Hunfeld, K.P. Human babesiosis in Europe: What clinicians need to know. *Infection* **2013**, *41*, 1057–1072. [CrossRef]
43. Hildebrandt, A.; Zintl, A.; Montero, E.; Hunfeld, K.P.; Gray, J. Human Babesiosis in Europe. *Pathogens* **2021**, *10*, 1165. [CrossRef]
44. Jahfari, S.; Hofhuis, A.; Fonville, M.; van der Giessen, J.; van Pelt, W.; Sprong, H. Molecular Detection of tick-borne pathogens in humans with tick bites and erythema migrans, in the Netherlands. *PLoS Negl. Trop. Dis.* **2016**, *10*, e0005042. [CrossRef]
45. Moreau, E.; Bonsergent, C.; Al Dybiat, I.; Gonzalez, L.M.; Lobo, C.A.; Montero, E.; Malandrin, L. *Babesia divergens* apical membrane antigen-1 (BdAMA-1): A poorly polymorphic protein that induces a weak and late immune response. *Exp. Parasitol.* **2015**, *155*, 40–45. [CrossRef]
46. Sun, Y. Caractérisation moléculaire, localisation cellulaire et conservation des protéines impliquées dans le processus d'invasion des érythrocytes par *Babesia divergens*. Ph.D. Thesis, Nantes University, Nantes, France, 2010; 202p.
47. Bastian, S.; Jouglin, M.; Brisseau, N.; Malandrin, L.; Klegou, G.; L'Hostis, M.; Chauvin, A. Antibody prevalence and molecular identification of *Babesia* spp. in roe deer in France. *J. Wildl. Dis.* **2012**, *48*, 416–424. [CrossRef] [PubMed]
48. Krause, P.J. Human babesiosis. *Int. J. Parasitol.* **2019**, *49*, 165–174. [CrossRef]
49. Gorenflot, A.; Moubri, K.; Precigout, E.; Carcy, B.; Schetters, T.P. Human babesiosis. *Ann. Trop. Med. Parasitol.* **1998**, *92*, 489–501. [CrossRef] [PubMed]
50. L'Hostis, M.; Chauvin, A.; Valentin, A.; Marchand, A.; Gorenflot, A. Large scale survey of bovine babesiosis due to *Babesia divergens* in France. *Vet. Rec.* **1995**, *136*, 36–38. [CrossRef]
51. Agoulon, A.; Malandrin, L.; Lepigeon, F.; Vénisse, M.; Bonnet, S.; Becker, C.A.; Hoch, T.; Bastian, S.; Plantard, O.; Beaudeau, F. A Vegetation Index qualifying pasture edges is related to *Ixodes ricinus* density and to *Babesia divergens* seroprevalence in dairy cattle herds. *Vet. Parasitol.* **2012**, *185*, 101–109. [CrossRef] [PubMed]
52. González, L.M.; Estrada, K.; Grande, R.; Jiménez-Jacinto, V.; Vega-Alvarado, L.; Sevilla, E.; Barrera, J.; Cuesta, I.; Zaballos, Á.; Bautista, J.M.; et al. Comparative and functional genomics of the protozoan parasite *Babesia divergens* highlighting the invasion and egress processes. *PLoS Negl. Trop. Dis.* **2019**, *13*, e0007680. [CrossRef]
53. Zamoto-Niikura, A.; Tsuji, M.; Imaoka, K.; Kimura, M.; Morikawa, S.; Holman, P.J.; Hirata, H.; Ishihara, C. Sika deer carrying *Babesia* parasites closely related to *B. divergens*, Japan. *Emerg. Infect. Dis.* **2014**, *20*, 1398–1400. [CrossRef]
54. Zamoto-Niikura, A.; Tsuji, M.; Qiang, W.; Morikawa, S.; Hanaki, K.I.; Holman, P.J.; Ishihara, C. The *Babesia divergens* Asia lineage is maintained through enzootic cycles between *Ixodes persulcatus* and sika deer in Hokkaido, Japan. *Appl. Environ. Microbiol.* **2018**, *84*, e02491-17. [CrossRef] [PubMed]
55. Malandrin, L.; L'Hostis, M.; Chauvin, A. Isolation of *Babesia divergens* from carrier cattle blood using in vitro culture. *Vet. Res.* **2004**, *35*, 131–139. [CrossRef]
56. Dalrymple, B.P.; Casu, R.E.; Peters, J.M.; Dimmock, C.M.; Gale, K.R.; Böse, R.; Wright, I.G. Characterisation of a family of multi-copy genes encoding rhoptry protein homologues in *Babesia bovis*, *Babesia ovis* and *Babesia canis*. *Mol. Biochem. Parasitol.* **1993**, *57*, 181–192. [CrossRef]
57. Suarez, C.E.; Palmer, G.H.; Hötzel, I.; McElwain, T.F. Structure, sequence, and transcriptional analysis of the *Babesia bovis rap-1* multigene locus. *Mol. Biochem. Parasitol.* **1998**, *93*, 215–224. [CrossRef] [PubMed]
58. Suarez, C.E.; Palmer, G.H.; Florin-Christensen, M.; Hines, S.A.; Hötzel, I.; McElwain, T.F. Organization transcription, and expression of rhoptry associated protein genes in the *Babesia bigemina rap-1* locus. *Mol. Biochem. Parasitol.* **2003**, *127*, 101–112. [CrossRef]
59. Niu, Q.; Bonsergent, C.; Guan, G.; Yin, H.; Malandrin, L. Sequence and organization of the rhoptry-associated-protein-1 (*rap-1*) locus for the sheep hemoprotozoan *Babesia* sp. BQ1 Lintan (*B. motasi* phylogenetic group). *Vet. Parasitol.* **2013**, *198*, 24–38. [CrossRef]
60. Niu, Q.; Valentin, C.; Bonsergent, C.; Malandrin, L. Strong conservation of rhoptry-associated-protein-1 (RAP-1) locus organization and sequence among *Babesia* isolates infecting sheep from China (*Babesia motasi*-like phylogenetic group). *Infect. Genet. Evol.* **2014**, *28*, 21–32. [CrossRef]
61. Niu, Q.; Marchand, J.; Yang, C.; Bonsergent, C.; Guan, G.; Yin, H.; Malandrin, L. Rhoptry-associated protein (*rap-1*) genes in the sheep pathogen *Babesia* sp. Xinjiang: Multiple transcribed copies differing by 3′ end repeated sequences. *Vet. Parasitol.* **2015**, *211*, 158–169. [CrossRef]

62. Skuce, P.J.; Mallon, T.R.; Taylor, S.M. Molecular cloning of a putative rhoptry associated protein homologue from *Babesia divergens*. *Mol. Biochem. Parasitol.* **1996**, *77*, 99–102. [CrossRef]
63. Rodriguez, M.; Alhassan, A.; Ord, R.L.; Cursino-Santos, J.R.; Singh, M.; Gray, J.; Lobo, C.A. Identification and characterization of the RouenBd1987 *Babesia divergens* Rhopty-Associated Protein 1. *PLoS ONE* **2014**, *9*, e107727. [CrossRef]
64. Sun, Y.; Jouglin, M.; Bastian, S.; Chauvin, A.; Malandrin, L. Molecular cloning and genetic polymorphism of *Babesia capreoli* gene Bcp37/41, an ortholog of *Babesia divergens* merozoite surface antigen Bd37. *Vet. Parasitol.* **2011**, *178*, 184–191. [CrossRef] [PubMed]
65. Kumar, S.; Stecher, G.; Li, M.; Knyaz, C.; Tamura, K. MEGA X: Molecular evolutionary genetics analysis across computing platforms. *Mol. Biol. Evol.* **2018**, *35*, 1547–1549. [CrossRef] [PubMed]
66. Tamura, K. Estimation of the number of nucleotide substitutions when there are strong transition-transversion and G + C-content biases. *Mol. Biol. Evol.* **1992**, *9*, 678–687. [CrossRef]
67. Kimura, M. A simple method for estimating evolutionary rate of base substitutions through comparative studies of nucleotide sequences. *J. Mol. Evol.* **1980**, *16*, 111–120. [CrossRef] [PubMed]

pathogens

MDPI

Review

Experimental Infection of Ticks: An Essential Tool for the Analysis of *Babesia* Species Biology and Transmission

Sarah I. Bonnet [1,2,*] and Clémence Nadal [3,4]

1 Animal Health Department, INRAE, 37380 Nouzilly, France
2 Functional Genetics of Infectious Diseases Unit, Institut Pasteur, CNRS UMR 2000, Université de Paris, 75015 Paris, France
3 Epidemiology Unit, Laboratory for Animal Health, University Paris Est, 94700 Maisons-Alfort, France; clemence.nadal@anses.fr
4 Anses, INRAE, Ecole Nationale Vétérinaire d'Alfort, UMR BIPAR, Laboratoire de Santé Animale, 94700 Maisons-Alfort, France
* Correspondence: sarah.bonnet@inrae.fr

Abstract: Babesiosis is one of the most important tick-borne diseases in veterinary health, impacting mainly cattle, equidae, and canidae, and limiting the development of livestock industries worldwide. In humans, babesiosis is considered to be an emerging disease mostly due to *Babesia divergens* in Europe and *Babesia microti* in America. Despite this importance, our knowledge of *Babesia* sp. transmission by ticks is incomplete. The complexity of vectorial systems involving the vector, vertebrate host, and pathogen, as well as the complex feeding biology of ticks, may be part of the reason for the existing gaps in our knowledge. Indeed, this complexity renders the implementation of experimental systems that are as close as possible to natural conditions and allowing the study of tick-host-parasite interactions, quite difficult. However, it is unlikely that the development of more effective and sustainable control measures against babesiosis will emerge unless significant progress can be made in understanding this tripartite relationship. The various methods used to date to achieve tick transmission of *Babesia* spp. of medical and veterinary importance under experimental conditions are reviewed and discussed here.

Keywords: ticks; *Babesia* sp.; biological cycle; experimental transmission; experimental models

Citation: Bonnet, S.I.; Nadal, C. Experimental Infection of Ticks: An Essential Tool for the Analysis of Babesia Species Biology and Transmission. *Pathogens* **2021**, *10*, 1403. https://doi.org/10.3390/pathogens10111403

Academic Editors: Estrella Montero, Jeremy Gray, Cheryl Ann Lobo and Luis Miguel González

Received: 9 August 2021
Accepted: 26 October 2021
Published: 29 October 2021

1. Introduction

Babesiosis remains prevalent worldwide and represents an important threat for both humans and animals [1,2]. The disease, impacting mainly cattle, sheep, goat, equidae, canidaecanidae, and accidentally humans, is caused by apicomplexan parasites belonging to the *Babesia* genus that exclusively infect erythrocytes of their vertebrate hosts [3]. To date, more than 100 *Babesia* species have been identified [1]. *Babesia* spp. are transmitted by hard ticks—occasionally by blood transfusion—and require both a competent vertebrate and invertebrate host to maintain the transmission cycle [3].

Human babesiosis is caused by *Babesia microti*, a *Babesia crassa*-like pathogen, *Babesia divergens*, *Babesia duncani*, and *Babesia venatorum*, as well as other parasites closely genetically related to these pathogens, such as *B. divergens*-like, *B. duncani*-like, and *B. microti*-like [4]. Infections in otherwise healthy individuals is usually mild to moderate and most cases of severe disease occur in immunocompromised individuals. *B. microti* is endemic in the northeastern and upper midwestern regions of the United States, while *B. duncani* is present on the west coast of the country [4]. In Europe, most of the human cases are due to *B. divergens*, whereas in Asia they are due to *B. venatorum*, *B. crassa*-like, and *B. microti* [4]. In cattle, *Babesia* spp. have a significant worldwide economic, social, and epidemiological impact and include, among the most important species, *B. bovis*, *B. bigemina*, *Babesia major*, and *B. divergens* [5]. *B. bovis* and *B. bigemina* are present in many countries in Africa, Asia,

Australia, Central and South America, and Southern Europe between 40° N and 32° S. *B. major* is present in Europe, Northwest Africa and Asia, and *B. divergens* is present in northern Europe [5]. Ovine babesiosis due to *Babesia ovis* and *Babesia motasi* is considered as the most critical blood-borne parasitic disease of small ruminants in tropical and non-tropical regions (occurring in South-eastern Europe, North Africa, and Asia) [6]. In equids, *Babesia caballi* is (with *Theileria equi* and *Theileria haneyi*) the agent of equine piroplasmosis known to be endemic in several countries of Africa, Asia, the Americas, and mainly in the Mediterranean basin for Europe [7–9]. The disease represents a significant animal health issue and causes notable economic losses for the equine industry. Finally, babesiosis is one of the most important globally extended and quickly spreading tick-borne diseases in dogs worldwide. *Babesia canis* is the main cause of canine babesiosis in Europe and is only sporadically found around the world, whereas *Babesia gibsoni*, the most prevalent species, and *Babesia vogeli* have a global distribution. *Babesia rossi*, one of the most pathogenic species, is endemic in southern Africa [10].

The current approaches available for babesiosis control have many important limitations, including increased resistance to acaricides by ticks, as well as the numerous drawbacks of these acaricides and of the current vaccines and babesicidal drugs (e.g., efficacy, toxicity, environmental effects) [11]. The development of improved control measures against babesiosis is limited by the numerous and significant gaps in our understanding of the biology of *Babesia* spp., especially regarding molecular interaction between parasites, vectors, and vertebrate hosts, as well as the factors that may influence both the development and the transmission of the parasite [12]. To fill these gaps, it is essential to be able to reproduce the life cycle of *Babesia* species in controlled experimental conditions, including transmission by ticks [13,14]. In addition, the validation of new methods of interruption of the cycle requires that it can be first carried out entirely under such conditions. Finally, it is important to mention that despite the promise of in vitro culture systems [15], maintenance by in vitro culture [16] or needle-passage in the vertebrate host [17] in the absence of tick passage may generate significant changes in the parasite population, potentially creating a bias in research results.

Several laboratory studies that aimed to understand babesiosis pathogenesis have focused their interest on infecting laboratory animals through artificial parasite injection [18,19]. Regarding tick-parasite interaction, the great majority of studies carried out concern mainly epidemiological studies focusing on the detection of parasites in ticks collected into the field [20]. Some in vitro studies have also been performed in order to understand the interactions between parasites and the cells of their vertebrate [21–23] or invertebrate hosts [24–27]. However, and certainly because of the difficulties inherent to the studied model—including *Babesia* spp. culture, tick colony maintenance, and animal models—relatively few studies have been based on the establishment, under experimental conditions, of complete parasite transmission cycles from one vertebrate host to another via the tick bite. Thanks to the experimental models developed for that purpose, these few studies have nevertheless made significant advances in (1) the definition/confirmation of the vector competence of various tick species; (2) the understanding of the modalities of parasite acquisition and transmission by ticks; (3) the discovery of the molecular interactions between the parasite and its invertebrate hosts; (4) the evaluation of some control methods. The aim of this review is to summarize studies that include both tick infection on *Babesia*-infected animals and *Babesia* infection of ticks through artificial systems, and to comment on the major results they achieved.

2. General Description of the *Babesia* Life Cycle

Babesia spp. are transmitted by hard tick (ixodid) vectors. The tick vectors and reservoir hosts differ depending on *Babesia* sp. and geographical location considered [1]. Several tick species have been mentioned in the literature as vectors of *Babesia* sp., but, as shown in Table 1, vector competence through experimental transmission has not been validated for all of them. For those mentioned here as "suspected vectors" without realization of the complete transmission cycle under experimental conditions, their involvement is mostly based on epidemiological evidence (e.g., correlation of tick species presence with disease occurrence). Each of the three active stages of hard ticks (larva, nymph, and adult) takes a single blood meal from a vertebrate host in order to mature to the next stage or lay eggs for the female. Most of the tick species listed as confirmed or suspected vectors of some *Babesia* species are three-hosts ticks—meaning that they take their three blood meals on three different hosts. Some of them, however, have a two-host cycle such as some *Hyalomma* spp., *Rhipicephalus evertsi*, and *Rhipicephalus bursa*, whereas *Dermacentor nitens*, *Rhipicephalus* annulatus, *Rhipicephalus microplus*, and *Rhipicephalus decoloratus* are one-host ticks that use the same individual host animal for all active tick stages.

Table 1. Major *Babesia* species infecting humans, dogs, cattle, sheep, goat, and equids; their suspected or confirmed main vector and vertebrate hosts in the field; and the realization of the whole transmission cycle under experimental conditions.

Babesia spp.	Suspected or Confirmed Main Vectors	Main Vertebrate Hosts	Realization of the Complete Transmission Cycle Under Experimental Conditions
Babesia microti	*Ixodes persulcatus*	Human, rodent	ND
	Ixodes ovatus		ND
	Ixodes scapularis		[28]
	Ixodes trianguliceps		[29]
	Ixodes dammini		[30]
	Ixodes ricinus		[31,32]
	Rhipicephalus haemaphysaloides		[33]
	Haemaphysalis longicornis		[34]
Babesia divergens	*Ixodes ricinus*	Human, cattle	[35–39]
Babesia venatorum	*Ixodes ricinus*	Human, roe deer	[40]
Babesia duncani	*Dermacentor albipictus*	Human, mule deer	ND
Babesia bovis	*Rhipicephalus microplus*	Cattle, buffalo	[41]
	Rhipicephalus annulatus		ND
	Rhipicephalus geigyi		ND
Babesia bigemina	*Rhipicephalus annulatus*	Cattle, buffalo	[42]
	Rhipicephalus microplus		[43,44]
	Rhipicephalus decoloratus		[45–47]
	Rhipicephalus geigyi		ND
	Rhipicephalus evertsi		ND
Babesia major	*Haemaphysalis punctata*	Cattle	[48,49]
Babesia ovata	*Haemaphysalis longicornis*	Cattle	[50]
Babesia orientalis	*Rhipicephalus haemaphysaloides*	Water buffalo	ND
Babesia caballi	*Dermacentor nitens*	Horse, Donkey, Mule	[51,52]
	Dermacentor sp.		ND
	Hyalomma sp.		ND
	Rhipicephalus evertsi		[53]
Babesia ovis	*Rhipicephalus bursa*	Sheep and Goat	[54]
Babesia motasi	*Rhipicephalus bursa*	Sheep and Goat	ND
	Haemaphysalis punctata		ND
Babesia canis	*Dermacentor reticulatus*	Dog	[55–59]
	Haemaphysalis spp.		ND
	Hyalomma spp.		ND
Babesia gibsoni	*Haemaphysalis sp.*	Dog	ND
	Rhipicephalus sanguineus		ND
Babesia vogeli	*Rhipicephalus sanguineus*	Dog	ND
Babesia rossi	*Haemaphysalis elliptica*	Dog	[60]
	Rhipicephalus sanguineus		ND

ND: no identified data.

The *Babesia* life cycle includes both asexual multiplication in the erythrocytes of the vertebrate host and sexual reproduction in the tick vector [3,61]. The general life cycle of the *Babesia* species is summarized in Figure 1 for *Babesia* sensu stricto (s.s.) species.

Indeed, it is necessary to specify here that, quite recently, molecular phylogeny studies using the 18S rRNA gene have led to the division of *Babesia* species into two large groups: *Babesia* s.s. and *Babesia* sensu lato (s.l.). Species belonging to the latter group, such as *B. microti*, are not capable of transovarial transmission within the tick but only a transstadial mode of transmission [62,63]. Vertebrate hosts are infected by the injection of sporozoites present in tick saliva during the tick bite. Each sporozoite penetrates the cell membrane of an erythrocyte with the aid of a specialized apical complex. Once inside, the parasite produces two merozoites by a process of merogony. Merozoites are then intermittently released following erythrocyte lysis to infect new erythrocytes. The parasite may then persist asymptomatically within its host for several years or lead to acute disease. When they are ingested by the tick during the blood meal, some parasites present in infected erythrocytes (pre-gametocytes) undergo further development in the passage from host blood to the midgut of the tick vector to evolve into gametocytes. The sexual reproduction between gametocytes takes place in the tick gut and leads to a zygote that penetrates the gut epithelium, where further multiplication occurs, with development to motile and haploid kinetes that escape into the tick hemolymph. The kinetes then infect a variety of tick cell types and tissues, including the ovary in the female tick—for *Babesia* s.s. species—and the tick salivary glands, where successive cycles of asexual multiplication take place. In this last organ, sporozoite development usually only begins when the infected tick attaches to the vertebrate host. The ticks thus transmit the sporozoites to a new host during a new blood meal of the next life-stage for the ticks with several hosts or of the next generation after transovarian transmission for the one-host ticks.

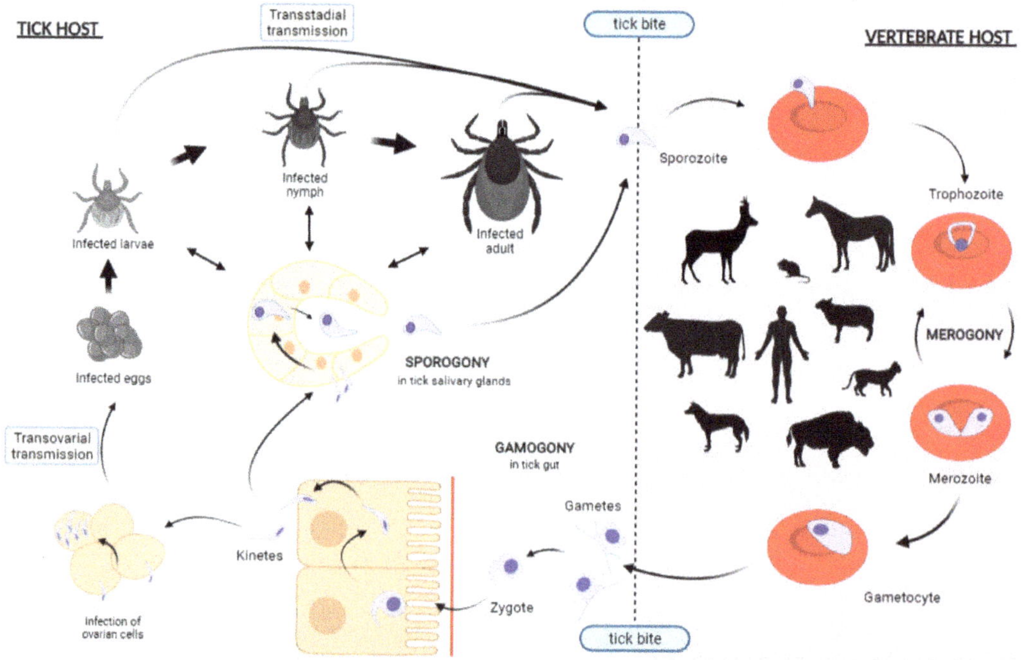

Figure 1. Life cycle of *Babesia* spp. sensu stricto. Vertebrate hosts are infected following the bite of an infected hard tick, through the invasion of the host erythrocytes by sporozoites excreted in the tick saliva. Inside the erythrocyte, sporozoites develop into trophozoites that undergo an asexual multiplication called merogony, ending in the formation of either merozoites that can infect other erythrocytes, or of gametocytes, which eventually develop into gametes. Infected erythrocytes are taken up by the tick during its blood meal, but only the gametocytes survive, and they then undergo further development, changing into gametes in the tick midgut. Then, sexual multiplication—gamogony—takes place with the fusion

of two gametes to form a motile zygote that enters the midgut epithelial cells to develop into motile kinetes through meiotic division. Kinetes disseminate to tick tissues, including ovarian and salivary gland cells. The invasion of tick ovaries results in transovarial transmission while those of salivary glands leads to transmission to the vertebrate host through injection of sporozoites with the saliva. *Babesia* microti-like species, which belong to *Babesia* spp. s.l. species, only invade the salivary glands, not the ovary. The schematic representation was made using the software biorender.com.

3. Experimental Models of *Babesia* Species—Transmission by Ticks

3.1. Tick Infestations on Babesia spp. Infected Animals

The first experiments to transmit *Babesia* spp. naturally were carried out by applying ticks suspected of being vectors on infected animals. Due to the huge economic importance of bovine babesiosis, these studies on vector competence for *Babesia* sp. were first conducted on species that infect cattle. Indeed, in 1893, two American researchers, Smith and Kilborne—the first authors to demonstrate the transmission of a disease organism from an arthropod to a mammalian host—showed the vector competence of *R.* annulatus for *B. bigemina* by placing ticks infected on animal onto naïve cattle that developed the associated disease [42]. Thereafter, different species of animals were used depending on the species of *Babesia* studied. Over time, the animal models and methodology used were refined to optimize the infection of both animals and ticks, and to comply with health and safety rules, and animal accommodation and tick containment methods during the tick feeding process have been the subject of several tests and evolutions (see examples in Figure 2A–F). In most cases, for cattle, animals were housed in individual, tick-proof pens surrounded by moats with or without detergent or insecticide [43,45]. Concerning the tick containment methods, in 1961, Callow and Hoyte used a hessian rug to protect the larvae until adult repletion to demonstrate the transmission of *B. bigemina* to cattle by *R. microplus* [43]. Ticks were either allowed to spread at will over the animal, or were confined to one site by releasing them under a fabric patch (nylon or organdie), which was glued along its edges to the flank of the bovine. A few years later, for the demonstration of the vector competence of *R. decoloratus* for *B. bigemina* in Kenya, ticks were fed on cattle until adult repletion by sprinkling larvae on the backs of the animals [45]. For the first experimental transmission of *B. divergens* by *Ixodes ricinus* achieved by Joyner et al in 1963, the ticks were contained in ear bags [36], a method also used later for sheep [64]. Regarding rodents, several laboratory studies involving complete transmission cycles of *B. microti* to the vertebrate host through the tick bite were performed [28–33]. In most instances, rodents were maintained over trays of water from which detached engorged ticks—applied by brush to animals—were harvested, whereas in some cases, ticks were contained in plastic capsules attached with different adhesives. For horses, the first studies aimed to validate the vector competence of *D. nitens* for *B. caballi* used larvae applied by brush on the animal [51], whereas in subsequent studies, tick feedings were accomplished by placing the larvae under a cloth patch glued to the back of the host [52].

The identification of a pathogen or pathogen DNA alone—which is even less convinc ing—in an arthropod cannot be sufficient to prove its ability to transmit this pathogen. Indeed, demonstrations of parasite presence in unfed field ticks, in tick salivary glands, eggs, or unfed larvae, while more convincing than detection in ticks collected from animals, also require confirmation only provided by the validation of vector competence in a controlled experimental model. The best illustration of this corresponds to the following studies performed in Iran in order to identify the vector of *B. ovis* to sheep. The kinetes of *B. ovis* were observed in hemolymph and egg smears of *Rhipicephalus sanguineus* and *Hyalomma marginatum* field ticks collected from sheep infected with *B. ovis* [69], so the vector competence of both tick species was further evaluated by placing pairs of adult ticks on sheep inoculated with *B. ovis,* but no transmission by any of the succeeding tick stages could be demonstrated, thus showing that these tick species are not vectors [64].

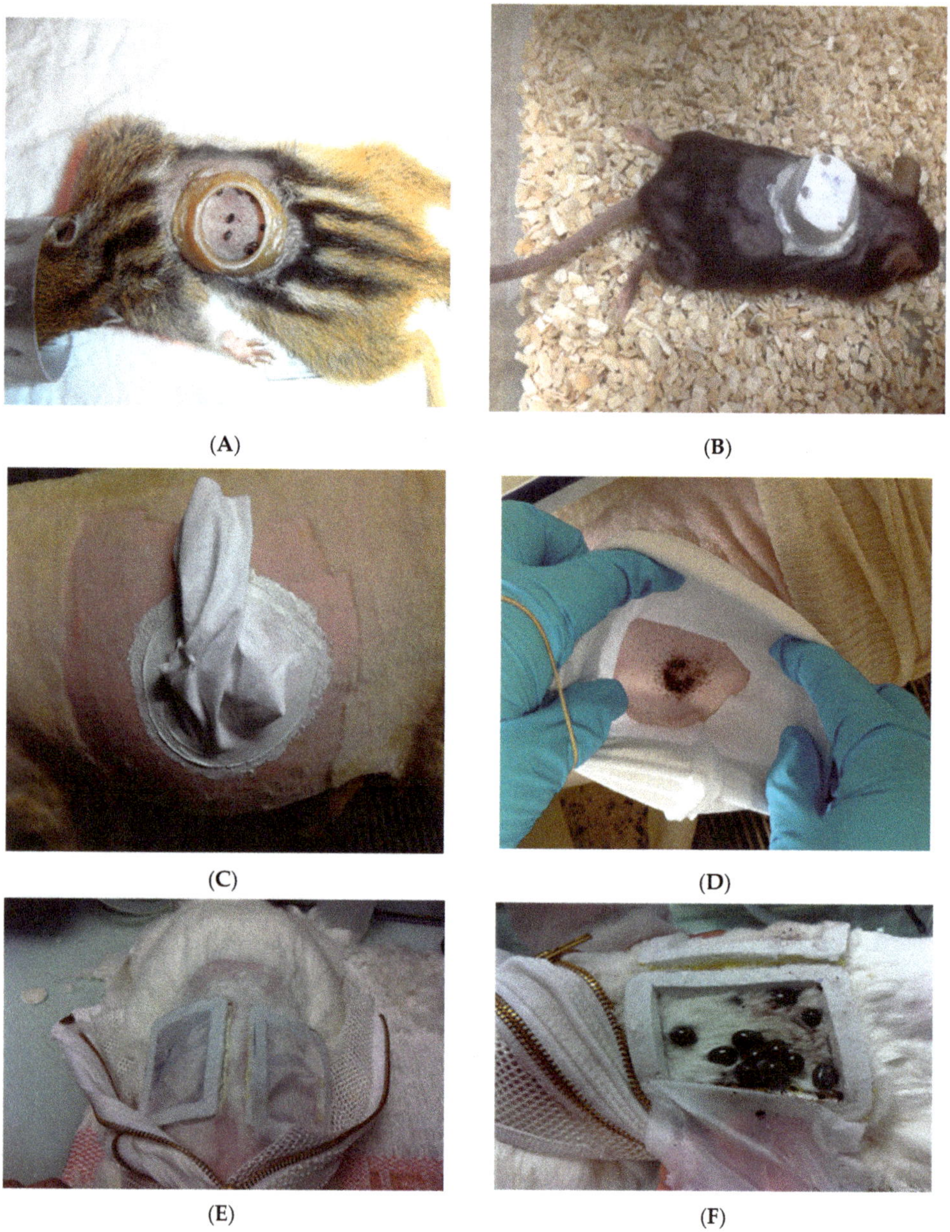

Figure 2. *Cont.*

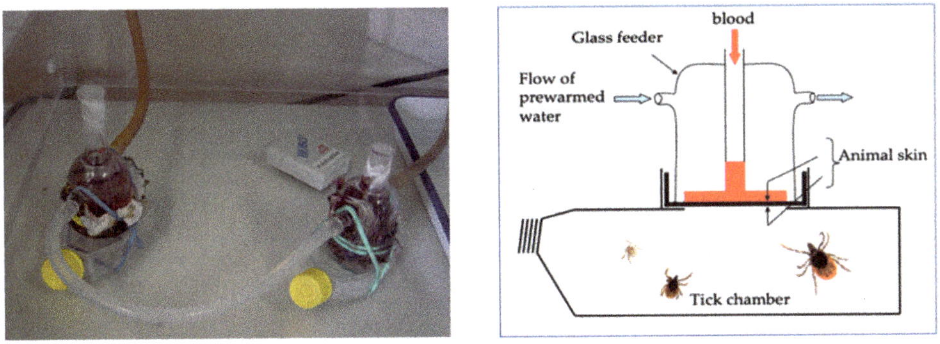

(G) (H)

Figure 2. Experimental feeding of *Ixodes ricinus* ticks on (**A**) Siberian chipmunks (*Tamias sibiricus barberi*) [65], (**B**) mouse [66], (**C,D**) sheep [67], (**E,F**) rabbit [68], and (**G,H**) a membrane artificial feeding system [35].

As recently reviewed by Gray and co-workers, the establishment of experimental models of pathogens transmission by ticks using live animals has led to significant advances in the understanding of transmission modalities and tick-parasite interactions [70]. For example, it allowed the demonstration that transovarial transmission does not occur in *B. microti*, leading to no longer classifying this parasite in *Babesia* spp. s.s. [31–33], and that, in *I. ricinus*, the infection only survives one molt [31]. Laboratory models have also demonstrated that *B. microti* may promote its transmission in rodents by enhancing the feeding success and survival of its tick vector, *Ixodes trianguliceps* [29]. Likewise, the establishment of the transmission of *B. divergens* by *I. ricinus* in a gerbil experimental model [35] provided proof of sexual development of *Babesia* through DNA measurements on the developmental stages of *B. divergens* in the blood of the vertebrate host and in the gut, hemolymph, and salivary glands of the tick vector [38,39]. In addition, several studies have been performed in order to establish which tick life stages are able to acquire and/or to transmit the parasite. Most of them have concluded that only adult stages were able to acquire *Babesia* sp. s.s. from infected animals, while all succeeding stages (larvae, nymphs, and adults) were able to re-transmit the parasites to susceptible animals [36,37,43,44,48]. However, Schwint and co-workers demonstrated that only the first of three subsequent generations from *D. nitens* females was able to transmit *B. caballi* to naïve horses, showing that the parasite is unable to persist in ticks without continuing alimentary infection of adult females [52], whereas other studies have also shown the acquisition of this parasite by nymphs of *R. evertsi* [53].

Models of transmission of *B. microti* to rodents via ticks in the laboratory have also made it possible to carry out studies on the phenomena of co-infections. In fact, a lower transmission efficiency of *B. microti* than *Borrelia burgdorferi* to *Ixodes dammini* from both hamsters [71] and white-footed mice [72] has been demonstrated. In the meantime, it was shown that ticks that fed on mice with these concurrent pathogen infections exhibited twice the incidence of *B. burgdorferi* infection compared with *B. microti* [72]. Twenty-five years later, however, this laboratory model also showed an increase of the frequency of *B. microti*-infected *Ixodes scapularis* (formerly *I. dammini*) nymphs when they fed as larvae on white-footed mice coinfected with *B. burgdorferi*, as well as an increase of *B. microti* parasitemia in co-infected mice [28]. This enhancement of *B. microti* establishment by *B. burgdorferi* has been attributed to an immunological conflict in the adaptive immune response of the vertebrate host against the two tick-borne pathogens [73].

The development of experimental models using animals also provided knowledge on the infection acquisition by the vertebrate host following a *Babesia*-infected tick bite. For example, by developing a laboratory model of *B. bovis* infection of calves through the bite of *R. microplus*-infected ticks, Smith and co-workers demonstrated, in 1978, that tick-induced infection was more severe than in calves infected with carrier blood, even when very low numbers of infected larvae were applied [41]. They attributed this difference in virulence to the large number of infective doses injected by each infected tick but Salivary-Assisted Transmission of tick-borne pathogens (see review in [74]) probably also contributed to this observation.

Although, compared to other pathogens, few molecular studies have involved *Babesia* parasites [70,75], experimental tick-transmission models of *Babesia* spp. using animals have also made it possible to identify molecules potentially involved in this transmission. Such studies are helping us to better understand the interactions involved and to identify potential targets for blocking parasite transmission. Thus, infection of *H. longicornis* on dogs infected with *B. gibsoni* has allowed to implicate a tick protein, longipain, in the transmission of the parasite by its vector [76], and to demonstrate that the vitellogenin receptor on the surface of tick oocytes is essential for its transovarial transmission [77]. Experimental models of *B. bovis* infection of cattle by *R. microplus* has also been used to study the function of the tick protein Bm86 during *B. bovis* infection [78]. In the same way, experimental tick infection models of both *B. bigemina* and *B. bovis*-infected cattle were used to perform functional genomics studies on *R. annulatus* and *R. microplus* genes that are differentially expressed in response to parasite infection [79,80].

Both the discovery and validation of methods to control the transmission of tick-borne pathogens require experimental designs that include complete transmission cycles. Regarding the *Babesia* spp. that infect cattle, experimental tick infection models for *B. bigemina*-infected cattle were used to evaluate the efficiency of some vaccine candidates and drugs against parasite transmission by *R. microplus* [81,82]. *Rhipicephalus microplus* experimentally infected with *B. bovis* were also used to demonstrate the inefficiency of the injectable and pour-on forms of both ivermectin and moxidectin to prevent parasite transmission by ticks [82]. In Argentina, Mangold and co-workers developed a laboratory model of *B. bovis* transmission to cattle by *R. microplus* in order to demonstrate the non-transmissibility to ticks of an attenuated vaccine strain of the parasite [83]. Several studies also involved experimental transmission of *B. canis* to dogs through the bite of infected *D. reticulatus* ticks in order to evaluate the usefulness of different acaricides to prevent parasite transmission [55–57,84], whereas similar experiments were performed regarding *B. canis* transmission by *R. sanguineus* [85,86], and *B. rossi* transmission by *Haemaphysalis elliptica* [60].

3.2. *Tick Infection through Artificial Feeding Systems*

The use of natural hosts for direct infection of ticks on infectious animals remains the best method to obtain conditions that are closest to the physiological reality of tick-borne pathogen transmission. However, firstly, ethical considerations lead us to limit the use of animals as much as possible. Secondly, in addition to the constraints associated with licensing the experiments and host specificity, obtaining the animals, keeping them in the laboratory, and handling them can be expensive and difficult or even impossible in the case of most species of wildlife. Finally, the difficulty of controlling parasitaemias of infected animals for the whole feeding period of the ticks is an important consideration. All these reasons have led to the development of artificial methods of tick infection in order to complete the lifecycle of tick-borne pathogens under laboratory conditions. Artificial feeding of ticks, mimicking the natural process, has been used for different purposes including tick rearing, the study of tick physiology and the effects of antibodies or drugs on tick physiology, functional genomic studies, and vaccine candidate discovery, as well as the analysis of tick-borne pathogen transmission (see review by Bonnet and Liu [13]). Nevertheless, relatively few studies have involved *Babesia* parasites. One of the factors limiting these studies is undoubtedly the need for successful in vitro cultivation of the *Babesia* species of interest [15].

The use of blood-filled capillary tubes placed over the mouthparts of ticks was first reported in 1938 by Gregson, who used this technique to collect saliva from *D. andersoni* [87].

Since then, this technique has been used to infect ticks with several tick-borne pathogens, mainly bacteria (see review in [13]). Although this infection process has the advantage of using the natural route of infection, i.e., the digestive tract of the tick, and allows control of the quantity of pathogen ingested, it is quite far from natural conditions because the tick absorbs a large amount of pathogen at once and this, regardless of the "true" full blood meal. The other drawback is that it requires the use of animals before or after infection to feed ticks to repletion. However, its use has led to some significant advances in the study of *Babesia* spp. transmission. In 1998, Inokuma and Kemp used the capillary feeding technique in order to infect *R. microplus* with *B. bigemina* [88]. Adult ticks were pre-fed on cattle and then *B. bigemina*-infected red blood cells were offered to the ticks using glass capillaries on a warm plate at 35 °C for 18 h in the dark. The authors subsequently demonstrated that ticks were able to acquire the parasite and to transmit it to their progeny. The capillary feeding technique has also been used by Antunes and co-workers in order to evaluate the impact of purified rabbit polyclonal antibodies on some *R. microplus* proteins associated with both tick physiology and tick infection by *B. bigemina* [89]. While an effect on tick weight and oviposition was observed, no effect was observed on pathogen DNA levels. However, this work has made it possible to set up an alternative system to the use of animals both to test vaccine candidates and to obtain essential data on tick-pathogen interaction, as this could also be done later with another protein, the calreticulin, identified as being involved in *B. bigemina* infection in *R. annulatus* ticks [90].

The membrane feeding technique—consisting of feeding ticks on blood or culture media through a membrane—was first developed by Pierce and Pierce in 1956 in order to feed *R. microplus* using embryonated hen eggs [91]. Since then, several membranes of animal or artificial origin have been used both to feed and to infect ticks with different pathogens (see review in [13]). In this case, as the pathogen is mixed in blood and absorbed throughout the blood meal via the digestive tract, the method mimics the natural conditions of tick infection more closely than other methods. Its main disadvantages, however, are the need to regularly change the blood used, and the need to use antibiotics and antifungals to avoid contamination. It is also necessary to test pathogen viability under these feeding conditions at regular intervals. In the case of artificial membranes such as silicone ones, feeding systems also need olfactory stimuli for attachment and feeding. Regarding their use to infect ticks with *Babesia* spp., and due to red blood cell sedimentation, it is important to note that this requires the placing of blood above the membrane to produce a continuous gravitational pressure, ensuring tick absorption of the intraerythrocytic parasites. In 2007, Bonnet and co-workers developed a skin-feeding technique using the skins of both gerbils (for larvae and nymphs) and rabbits (for nymphs and adults) to infect *I. ricinus* with *B. divergens* without the need for additional stimuli (Figure 2G,H) [35]. To our knowledge, this is the only membrane-feeding technique that has been used to date to infect ticks with *Babesia* spp. All tick instars were allowed to acquire the parasite from infected red blood cells maintained at 37 °C in a glass feeder through the animal skin until repletion. Contrary to what was previously observed [36,37], this system showed that in addition to adult females, *I. ricinus* larvae and nymphs can also acquire *B. divergens* infections, which persists transtadially in the subsequent nymphal and adult stages (as determined by the detection of DNA in their salivary glands). *Babesia divergens* DNA was also detected in eggs and larvae produced by females that had fed on parasitized blood, demonstrating the transovarial transmission of the parasite. Later, the use of this artificial tick infection system also allowed the discovery of molecular markers for *B. divergens* sexual stages [92,93]. Lastly, the same membrane feeding technique allowed the validation of the vector competence of *I. ricinus* for *Babesia* (EU1) *venatorum* [40].

Finally, in order to understand tick-*Babesia* interactions and to follow parasite development in the vector, Maeda and co-workers used a "semi-artificial" mouse skin membrane feeding technique to infect *H. longicornis* with *B. ovata* [94]. In this case, female adult ticks were first allowed to feed on the shaved back of mice, and after 4 to 5 days, a section of the mouse skin with the ticks attached was removed immediately after euthanasia, and set up in artificial feeding units. The ticks were then fed on a mix of media and *B. ovata*-infected red blood cells through the piece of mouse skin. This technique was then used to demonstrate the transovarial persistence of *B. ovata* DNA in *H. longicornis* [50]. Thus, the mixing of animal use and membrane feeding makes it possible to control the parasitemia of the meal offered to ticks, but does not prevent the use of live animals.

3.3. Tick Infection through Injection

Although this method is more distant from physiological reality than the ones previously detailed, some studies have also performed tick infections by injecting the pathogen through the cuticle of the tick. In addition to requiring live animals to feed ticks after the infection, this invasive method also has the disadvantage of a low survival rate of ticks after injection [95]. Nevertheless, its use by some authors has led to important results concerning *Babesia* spp. In 2018, Antunes and co-workers used a *R. bursa*-*B. ovis*-sheep infection model to characterize tick salivary gland genes that were differentially expressed in response to blood feeding and *B. ovis* infection [96]. In that experiment, female ticks were inoculated with *B. ovis* in the trochanter-coxae articulation and allowed to feed on rabbits. Vector competence was then confirmed by feeding *B. ovis*-infected ticks on a naïve lamb. This study allowed both increased understanding of the role of tick salivary gland genes in *Babesia* infections and identification of potential candidate vaccine antigens for innovative control strategies.

4. Conclusions

It is likely that vector competence for *Babesia* spp. has yet to be determined in some tick species. Furthermore, our understanding of the life cycles of *Babesia* spp. is still incomplete, especially regarding the intimate mechanisms of molecular dialogue between the parasite and its vertebrate and invertebrate hosts. Field experiments are less easy to control than those under laboratory conditions, and the gaps in our knowledge can probably only be filled by experimentally reproducing the transmission cycle as closely as possible to reality and by involving all three actors of the vectorial system. Indeed, this review has shown that the use of experimental systems for tick-borne pathogen infections that permit the complete transmission cycles of *Babesia* parasites has led to major scientific advances in the study of these pathogens. Despite these successes, efforts are still needed to standardize and simplify laboratory protocols to improve our ability to exploit tick artificial infection systems. It is hoped that, in the future, such models of artificial infection will be further developed in order to acquire new knowledge and develop new control strategies while avoiding the use of animals.

Author Contributions: Conceptualization, S.I.B.; formal analysis, S.I.B. and C.N.; writing—original draft preparation, S.I.B. and C.N.; writing—review and editing, S.I.B. and C.N.; supervision, S.I.B. All authors have read and agreed to the published version of the manuscript.

Funding: The PhD of CN is funded by the Institut Français du Cheval et de l'Equitation (IFCE) and by the Fonds Eperon.

Conflicts of Interest: The authors declare no conflict of interest. The funders had no role in the design of the study; in the collection, analyses, or interpretation of data; in the writing of the manuscript, or in the decision to publish the results.

References

1. Homer, M.J.; Aguilar-Delfin, I.; Telford, S.R., 3rd; Krause, P.J.; Persing, D.H. Babesiosis. *Clin. Microbiol. Rev.* **2000**, *13*, 451–469. [CrossRef]
2. Lobo, C.A.; Singh, M.; Rodriguez, M. Human babesiosis: Recent advances and future challenges. *Curr. Opin. Hematol.* **2020**, *27*, 399–405. [CrossRef]
3. Chauvin, A.; Moreau, E.; Bonnet, S.; Plantard, O.; Malandrin, L. *Babesia* and its hosts: Adaptation to long-lasting interactions as a way to achieve efficient transmission. *Vet. Res.* **2009**, *40*, 37. [CrossRef]
4. Krause, P.J. Human babesiosis. *Int. J. Parasitol.* **2019**, *49*, 165–174. [CrossRef] [PubMed]
5. Bock, R.; Jackson, L.; de Vos, A.; Jorgensen, W. Babesiosis of cattle. *Parasitology* **2004**, *129*, S247–S269. [CrossRef] [PubMed]

6. Yeruham, I.; Hadani, A.; Galker, F. Some epizootiological and clinical aspects of ovine babesiosis caused by *Babesia ovis*—A review. *Vet. Parasitol.* **1998**, *74*, 153–163. [CrossRef]
7. Tirosh-Levy, S.; Gottlieb, Y.; Fry, L.M.; Knowles, D.P.; Steinman, A. Twenty Years of Equine Piroplasmosis Research: Global Distribution, Molecular Diagnosis, and Phylogeny. *Pathogens* **2020**, *9*, 926. [CrossRef] [PubMed]
8. Nadal, C.; Bonnet, S.I.; Marsot, M. Eco-epidemiology of equine piroplasmosis and its associated tick vectors in Europe: A systematic literature review and a meta-analysis of prevalence. *Transbound. Emerg. Dis.* **2021**. [CrossRef]
9. Knowles, D.P.; Kappmeyer, L.S.; Haney, D.; Herndon, D.R.; Fry, L.M.; Munro, J.B.; Sears, K.; Ueti, M.W.; Wise, L.N.; Silva, M.; et al. Discovery of a novel species, *Theileria haneyi* n. sp., infective to equids, highlights exceptional genomic diversity within the genus *Theileria*: Implications for apicomplexan parasite surveillance. *Int. J. Parasitol.* **2018**, *48*, 679–690. [CrossRef]
10. Bilić, P.; Kuleš, J.; Barić, R.; Mrljak, V. Canine Babesiosis: Where Do We Stand? *Acta Vet.* **2018**, *68*, 127–160. [CrossRef]
11. Suarez, C.E.; Noh, S. Emerging perspectives in the research of bovine babesiosis and anaplasmosis. *Vet. Parasitol.* **2011**, *180*, 109–125. [CrossRef] [PubMed]
12. Rodriguez-Morales, A.J.; Bonilla-Aldana, D.K.; Escalera-Antezana, J.P.; Alvarado-Arnez, L.E. Research on Babesia: A bibliometric assessment of a neglected tick-borne parasite. *F1000Res* **2018**, *7*, 1987. [CrossRef]
13. Bonnet, S.I.; Liu, X.Y. Laboratory artificial infection of hard ticks: A tool for the analysis of tick-borne pathogen transmission. *Acarologia* **2012**, *52*, 453–464. [CrossRef]
14. de la Fuente, J.; Antunes, S.; Bonnet, S.; Cabezas-Cruz, A.; Domingos, A.G.; Estrada-Pena, A.; Johnson, N.; Kocan, K.M.; Mansfield, K.L.; Nijhof, A.M.; et al. Tick-Pathogen Interactions and Vector Competence: Identification of Molecular Drivers for Tick-Borne Diseases. *Front. Cell Infect. Microbiol.* **2017**, *7*, 114. [CrossRef]
15. Muller, J.; Hemphill, A. In vitro culture systems for the study of apicomplexan parasites in farm animals. *Int. J. Parasitol.* **2013**, *43*, 115–124. [CrossRef] [PubMed]
16. Sondgeroth, K.S.; McElwain, T.F.; Ueti, M.W.; Scoles, G.A.; Reif, K.E.; Lau, A.O. Tick passage results in enhanced attenuation of *Babesia bovis*. *Infect. Immun.* **2014**, *82*, 4426–4434. [CrossRef] [PubMed]
17. Stewart, N.P. Differences in the life cycles between a vaccine strain and an unmodified strain of *Babesia bovis* (Babes, 1889) in the tick *Boophilus microplus* (Canestrini). *J. Protozool.* **1978**, *25*, 497–501. [CrossRef]
18. Zaugg, J.L.; Kuttler, K.L. Experimental infections of *Babesia bigemina* in American bison. *J. Wildl. Dis.* **1987**, *23*, 99–102. [CrossRef]
19. Chauvin, A.; Valentin, A.; Malandrin, L.; L'Hostis, M. Sheep as a new experimental host for *Babesia divergens*. *Vet. Res.* **2002**, *33*, 429–433. [CrossRef]
20. Martinez-Garcia, G.; Santamaria-Espinosa, R.M.; Lira-Amaya, J.J.; Figueroa, J.V. Challenges in Tick-Borne Pathogen Detection: The Case for *Babesia* spp. Identification in the Tick Vector. *Pathogens* **2021**, *10*, 92. [CrossRef]
21. Sun, Y.; Moreau, E.; Chauvin, A.; Malandrin, L. The invasion process of bovine erythrocyte by *Babesia divergens*: Knowledge from an in vitro assay. *Vet. Res.* **2011**, *42*, 62. [CrossRef]
22. Spencer, A.M.; Goethert, H.K.; Telford, S.R., 3rd; Holman, P.J. In vitro host erythrocyte specificity and differential morphology of *Babesia divergens* and a zoonotic *Babesia* sp. from eastern cottontail rabbits (*Sylvilagus floridanus*). *J. Parasitol.* **2006**, *92*, 333–340. [CrossRef] [PubMed]
23. O'Connor, R.M.; Long, J.A.; Allred, D.R. Cytoadherence of *Babesia bovis*-infected erythrocytes to bovine brain capillary endothelial cells provides an in vitro model for sequestration. *Infect. Immun.* **1999**, *67*, 3921–3928. [CrossRef]
24. Maeda, H.; Hatta, T.; Alim, M.A.; Tsubokawa, D.; Mikami, F.; Kusakisako, K.; Matsubayashi, M.; Umemiya-Shirafuji, R.; Tsuji, N.; Tanaka, T. Initial development of *Babesia ovata* in the tick midgut. *Vet. Parasitol.* **2017**, *233*, 39–42. [CrossRef] [PubMed]
25. Bhat, U.K.; Mahoney, D.F.; Wright, I.G. The invasion and growth of *Babesia bovis* in tick tissue culture. *Experientia* **1979**, *35*, 752–753. [CrossRef] [PubMed]
26. Ribeiro, M.F.; Bastos, C.V.; Vasconcelos, M.M.; Passos, L.M. *Babesia bigemina*: In vitro multiplication of sporokinetes in *Ixodes scapularis* (IDE8) cells. *Exp. Parasitol.* **2009**, *122*, 192–195. [CrossRef] [PubMed]
27. de Rezende, J.; Rangel, C.P.; McIntosh, D.; Silveira, J.A.; Cunha, N.C.; Ramos, C.A.; Fonseca, A.H. In vitro cultivation and cryopreservation of *Babesia bigemina* sporokinetes in hemocytes of *Rhipicephalus microplus*. *Vet. Parasitol.* **2015**, *212*, 400–403. [CrossRef]
28. Dunn, J.M.; Krause, P.J.; Davis, S.; Vannier, E.G.; Fitzpatrick, M.C.; Rollend, L.; Belperron, A.A.; States, S.L.; Stacey, A.; Bockenstedt, L.K.; et al. *Borrelia burgdorferi* promotes the establishment of *Babesia microti* in the northeastern United States. *PLoS ONE* **2014**, *9*, e115494. [CrossRef]
29. Randolph, S.E. The effect of *Babesia microti* on feeding and survival in its tick vector, *Ixodes trianguliceps*. *Parasitology* **1991**, *102 Pt 1*, 9–16. [CrossRef]
30. Ruebush, T.K., 2nd; Piesman, J.; Collins, W.E.; Spielman, A.; Warren, M. Tick transmission of *Babesia microti* to rhesus monkeys (*Macaca mulatta*). *Am. J. Trop. Med. Hyg.* **1981**, *30*, 555–559. [CrossRef]
31. Gray, J.; von Stedingk, L.V.; Gurtelschmid, M.; Granstrom, M. Transmission studies of *Babesia microti* in *Ixodes ricinus* ticks and gerbils. *J. Clin. Microbiol.* **2002**, *40*, 1259–1263. [CrossRef]
32. Walter, G.; Weber, G. A study on the transmission (transstadial, transovarial) of *Babesia microti*, strain "Hannover i", in its tick vector, *Ixodes ricinus* (author's transl). *Tropenmed. Parasitol.* **1981**, *32*, 228–230. [PubMed]
33. Li, L.H.; Zhu, D.; Zhang, C.C.; Zhang, Y.; Zhou, X.N. Experimental transmission of *Babesia microti* by *Rhipicephalus haemaphysaloides*. *Parasites Vectors* **2016**, *9*, 231. [CrossRef]

34. Wu, J.; Cao, J.; Zhou, Y.; Zhang, H.; Gong, H.; Zhou, J. Evaluation on Infectivity of *Babesia microti* to Domestic Animals and Ticks Outside the *Ixodes* Genus. *Front. Microbiol.* **2017**, *8*, 1915. [CrossRef] [PubMed]
35. Bonnet, S.; Jouglin, M.; Malandrin, L.; Becker, C.; Agoulon, A.; L'Hostis, M.; Chauvin, A. Transstadial and transovarial persistence of *Babesia divergens* DNA in *Ixodes ricinus* ticks fed on infected blood in a new skin-feeding technique. *Parasitology* **2007**, *134*, 197–207. [CrossRef]
36. Joyner, L.P.; Davies, S.F.; Kendall, S.B. The Experimental Transmission of *Babesia divergens* by *Ixodes ricinus*. *Exp. Parasitol.* **1963**, *14*, 367–373. [CrossRef]
37. Donnelly, J.; Peirce, M.A. Experiments on the transmission of *Babesia divergens* to cattle by the tick *Ixodes ricinus*. *Int. J. Parasitol.* **1975**, *5*, 363–367. [CrossRef]
38. Lewis, D.; Young, E.R. The transmission of a human strain of *Babesia divergens* by *Ixodes ricinus* ticks. *J. Parasitol.* **1980**, *66*, 359–360. [CrossRef]
39. Mackenstedt, U.; Gauer, M.; Mehlhorn, H.; Schein, E.; Hauschild, S. Sexual cycle of *Babesia divergens* confirmed by DNA measurements. *Parasitol. Res.* **1990**, *76*, 199–206. [CrossRef]
40. Bonnet, S.; Brisseau, N.; Hermouet, A.; Jouglin, M.; Chauvin, A. Experimental in vitro transmission of *Babesia* sp. (EU1) by *Ixodes ricinus*. *Vet. Res.* **2009**, *40*, 21. [CrossRef] [PubMed]
41. Smith, R.D.; Osorno, B.M.; Brener, J.; De La Rosa, R.; Ristic, M. Bovine babesiosis: Severity and reproducibility of *Babesia bovis* infections induced by *Boophilus microplus* under laboratory conditions. *Res. Vet. Sci.* **1978**, *24*, 287–292. [CrossRef]
42. Smith, T.; Kilborne, F.L. Investigations into the nature, causation and prevention of Southern cattle fever. In *Ninth Annual Report of the Bureau of Animal Industry for the Year 1892*; Government Printing Office: Washington, DC, USA, 1893; pp. 177–304.
43. Callow, L.; Hoyte, H. Transmission experiments using *Babesia bigemina, Theileria mutans, Borrelia* sp. and the cattle tick, *Boophilus microplus*. *Aust. Vet. J.* **1961**, *37*, 381–390. [CrossRef]
44. Callow, L.L. *Babesia Bigemina* in Ticks Grown on Non-Bovine Hosts and Its Transmission to These Hosts. *Parasitology* **1965**, *55*, 375–381. [CrossRef]
45. Morzaria, S.P.; Young, A.S.; Hudson, E.B. *Babesia bigemina* in Kenya: Experimental transmission by *Boophilus decoloratus* and the production of tick-derived stabilates. *Parasitology* **1977**, *74*, 291–298. [CrossRef]
46. Akinboade, O.A.; Dipeolu, O.O.; Adetunji, A. Experimental transmission of *Babesia bigemina* and *Anaplasma marginale* to calves with the larvae of *Boophilus decoloratus*. *Zentralbl. Veterinarmed. B* **1981**, *28*, 329–332. [CrossRef]
47. Akinboade, O.A. Experimental transmission of *Babesia bigemina* in sheep using infective larval tick of *Boophilus decoloratus*. *Rev. Elev. Med. Vet. Pays. Trop.* **1981**, *34*, 271–273.
48. Morzaria, S.P.; Brocklesby, D.W.; Harradine, D.L. Experimental transmission of *Babesia major* by *Haemaphysalis punctata*. *Res. Vet. Sci.* **1977**, *23*, 261–262. [CrossRef]
49. Yin, H.; Lu, W.; Luo, J.; Zhang, Q.; Lu, W.; Dou, H. Experiments on the transmission of *Babesia major* and *Babesia bigemina* by *Haemaphysalis punctata*. *Vet. Parasitol.* **1996**, *67*, 89–98. [CrossRef]
50. Umemiya-Shirafuji, R.; Hatta, T.; Okubo, K.; Sato, M.; Maeda, H.; Kume, A.; Yokoyama, N.; Igarashi, I.; Tsuji, N.; Fujisaki, K.; et al. Transovarial persistence of *Babesia ovata* DNA in a hard tick, *Haemaphysalis longicornis*, in a semi-artificial mouse skin membrane feeding system. *Acta Parasitol.* **2018**, *63*, 433. [CrossRef]
51. Roby, T.O.; Anthony, D.W.; Thornton, C.W., Jr.; Holbrook, A.A. The Hereditary Transmission of *Babesia Caballi* in the Tropical Horse Tick, *Dermacentor Nitens* Neumann. *Am. J. Vet. Res.* **1964**, *25*, 494–499.
52. Schwint, O.N.; Knowles, D.P.; Ueti, M.W.; Kappmeyer, L.S.; Scoles, G.A. Transmission of *Babesia caballi* by *Dermacentor nitens* (Acari: Ixodidae) is restricted to one generation in the absence of alimentary reinfection on a susceptible equine host. *J. Med. Entomol.* **2008**, *45*, 1152–1155. [CrossRef]
53. de Waal, D.T.; Potgieter, F.T. The transstadial transmission of *Babesia caballi* by *Rhipicephalus evertsi evertsi*. *Onderstepoort. J. Vet. Res.* **1987**, *54*, 655–656.
54. Erster, O.; Roth, A.; Wolkomirsky, R.; Leibovich, B.; Savitzky, I.; Shkap, V. Transmission of *Babesia ovis* by different *Rhipicephalus bursa* developmental stages and infected blood injection. *Ticks Tick Borne Dis.* **2016**, *7*, 13–19. [CrossRef]
55. Jongejan, F.; Fourie, J.J.; Chester, S.T.; Manavella, C.; Mallouk, Y.; Pollmeier, M.G.; Baggott, D. The prevention of transmission of *Babesia canis canis* by *Dermacentor reticulatus* ticks to dogs using a novel combination of fipronil, amitraz and (S)-methoprene. *Vet. Parasitol.* **2011**, *179*, 343–350. [CrossRef] [PubMed]
56. Beugnet, F.; Halos, L.; Larsen, D.; Labuschagne, M.; Erasmus, H.; Fourie, J. The ability of an oral formulation of afoxolaner to block the transmission of *Babesia canis* by *Dermacentor reticulatus* ticks to dogs. *Parasites Vectors* **2014**, *7*, 283. [CrossRef]
57. Taenzler, J.; Liebenberg, J.; Roepke, R.K.; Heckeroth, A.R. Prevention of transmission of *Babesia canis* by *Dermacentor reticulatus* ticks to dogs after topical administration of fluralaner spot-on solution. *Parasites Vectors* **2016**, *9*, 234. [CrossRef]
58. Fourie, J.J.; de Vos, C.; Crafford, D.; Pollmeier, M.; Schunack, B. A study on the long-term efficacy of Seresto(R) collars in preventing *Babesia canis* (Piana & Galli-Valerio, 1895) transmission to dogs by infected *Dermacentor reticulatus* (Fabricius, 1794) ticks. *Parasites Vectors* **2019**, *12*, 139. [CrossRef]
59. Varloud, M.; Liebenberg, J.; Fourie, J. Early *Babesia canis* transmission in dogs within 24 h and 8 h of infestation with infected pre-activated male *Dermacentor reticulatus* ticks. *Parasites Vectors* **2018**, *11*, 41. [CrossRef] [PubMed]
60. Beugnet, F.; Lebon, W.; de Vos, C. Prevention of the transmission of *Babesia rossi* by *Haemaphysalis elliptica* in dogs treated with Nexgard((R)). *Parasite* **2019**, *26*, 49. [CrossRef]

61. Mehlhorn, H.; Shein, E. The piroplasms: Life cycle and sexual stages. *Adv. Parasitol.* **1984**, *23*, 37–103. [CrossRef]
62. Gray, J.; Weiss, M.L. *Babesia microti*. In *Emerging Protozoan Pathogens*; Naveed Ahmed, K., Ed.; Taylor & Francis: New York, NY, USA, 2007; pp. 303–349.
63. Jalovecka, M.; Sojka, D.; Ascencio, M.; Schnittger, L. *Babesia* Life Cycle—When Phylogeny Meets Biology. *Trends Parasitol.* **2019**, *35*, 356–368. [CrossRef]
64. Razmi, G.; Nouroozi, E. Transovarial Transmission of *Babesia ovis* by *Rhipicephalus sanguineus* and *Hyalomma marginatum*. *Iran J. Parasitol.* **2010**, *5*, 35–39.
65. Bonnet, S.; Choumet, V.; Masseglia, S.; Cote, M.; Ferquel, E.; Lilin, T.; Marsot, M.; Chapuis, J.L.; Vourc'h, G. Infection of Siberian chipmunks (*Tamias sibiricus barberi*) with *Borrelia* sp. reveals a low reservoir competence under experimental conditions. *Ticks Tick Borne Dis.* **2015**, *6*, 393–400. [CrossRef]
66. Almazan, C.; Simo, L.; Fourniol, L.; Rakotobe, S.; Borneres, J.; Cote, M.; Peltier, S.; Maye, J.; Versille, N.; Richardson, J.; et al. Multiple Antigenic Peptide-Based Vaccines Targeting *Ixodes ricinus* Neuropeptides Induce a Specific Antibody Response but Do Not Impact Tick Infestation. *Pathogens* **2020**, *9*, 900. [CrossRef] [PubMed]
67. Almazan, C.; Fourniol, L.; Rouxel, C.; Alberdi, P.; Gandoin, C.; Lagree, A.C.; Boulouis, H.J.; de la Fuente, J.; Bonnet, S.I. Experimental *Ixodes ricinus*-Sheep Cycle of *Anaplasma phagocytophilum* NV2Os Propagated in Tick Cell Cultures. *Front. Vet. Sci.* **2020**, *7*, 40. [CrossRef] [PubMed]
68. Almazan, C.; Bonnet, S.; Cote, M.; Slovak, M.; Park, Y.; Simo, L. A Versatile Model of Hard Tick Infestation on Laboratory Rabbits. *J. Vis. Exp.* **2018**. [CrossRef]
69. Razmi, G.R.; Naghibi, A.; Aslani, M.R.; Fathivand, M.; Dastjerdi, K. An epidemiological study on ovine babesiosis in the Mashhad suburb area, province of Khorasan, Iran. *Vet. Parasitol.* **2002**, *108*, 109–115. [CrossRef]
70. Gray, J.S.; Estrada-Pena, A.; Zintl, A. Vectors of Babesiosis. *Annu. Rev. Entomol.* **2019**, *64*, 149–165. [CrossRef]
71. Piesman, J. Intensity and duration of *Borrelia burgdorferi* and *Babesia microti* infectivity in rodent hosts. *Int. J. Parasitol.* **1988**, *18*, 687–689. [CrossRef]
72. Mather, T.N.; Telford, S.R., 3rd; Moore, S.I.; Spielman, A. *Borrelia burgdorferi* and *Babesia microti*: Efficiency of transmission from reservoirs to vector ticks (*Ixodes dammini*). *Exp. Parasitol.* **1990**, *70*, 55–61. [CrossRef]
73. Diuk-Wasser, M.A.; Vannier, E.; Krause, P.J. Coinfection by *Ixodes* Tick-Borne Pathogens: Ecological, Epidemiological, and Clinical Consequences. *Trends Parasitol.* **2016**, *32*, 30–42. [CrossRef]
74. Bonnet, S.; Kazimirova, M.; Richardson, R.; Simo, L. Tick saliva and its role in pathogen transmission. In *Skin and Arthropod Vectors*; Boulanger, N., Ed.; Elsevier: London, UK, 2018.
75. Liu, X.Y.; Bonnet, S.I. Hard tick factors implicated in pathogen transmission. *PLoS Negl. Trop. Dis.* **2014**, *8*, e2566. [CrossRef]
76. Tsuji, N.; Miyoshi, T.; Battsetseg, B.; Matsuo, T.; Xuan, X.; Fujisaki, K. A cysteine protease is critical for *Babesia* spp. transmission in *Haemaphysalis* ticks. *PLoS Pathog.* **2008**, *4*, e1000062. [CrossRef]
77. Boldbaatar, D.; Battsetseg, B.; Matsuo, T.; Hatta, T.; Umemiya-Shirafuji, R.; Xuan, X.; Fujisaki, K. Tick vitellogenin receptor reveals critical role in oocyte development and transovarial transmission of *Babesia* parasite. *Biochem. Cell Biol.* **2008**, *86*, 331–344. [CrossRef]
78. Bastos, R.G.; Ueti, M.W.; Knowles, D.P.; Scoles, G.A. The *Rhipicephalus (Boophilus) microplus* Bm86 gene plays a critical role in the fitness of ticks fed on cattle during acute *Babesia bovis* infection. *Parasites Vectors* **2010**, *3*, 111. [CrossRef]
79. Antunes, S.; Galindo, R.C.; Almazan, C.; Rudenko, N.; Golovchenko, M.; Grubhoffer, L.; Shkap, V.; do Rosario, V.; de la Fuente, J.; Domingos, A. Functional genomics studies of *Rhipicephalus (Boophilus) annulatus* ticks in response to infection with the cattle protozoan parasite, *Babesia bigemina*. *Int. J. Parasitol.* **2012**, *42*, 187–195. [CrossRef]
80. Heekin, A.M.; Guerrero, F.D.; Bendele, K.G.; Saldivar, L.; Scoles, G.A.; Dowd, S.E.; Gondro, C.; Nene, V.; Djikeng, A.; Brayton, K.A. The ovarian transcriptome of the cattle tick, *Rhipicephalus (Boophilus) microplus*, feeding upon a bovine host infected with *Babesia bovis*. *Parasites Vectors* **2013**, *6*, 276. [CrossRef]
81. Merino, O.; Almazan, C.; Canales, M.; Villar, M.; Moreno-Cid, J.A.; Galindo, R.C.; de la Fuente, J. Targeting the tick protective antigen subolesin reduces vector infestations and pathogen infection by *Anaplasma marginale* and *Babesia bigemina*. *Vaccine* **2011**, *29*, 8575–8579. [CrossRef]
82. Waldron, S.J.; Jorgensen, W.K. Transmission of *Babesia* spp. by the cattle tick (*Boophilus microplus*) to cattle treated with injectable or pour-on formulations of ivermectin and moxidectin. *Aust. Vet. J.* **1999**, *77*, 657–659. [CrossRef]
83. Mangold, A.J.; Aguirre, D.H.; Cafrune, M.M.; de Echaide, S.T.; Guglielmone, A.A. Evaluation of the infectivity of a vaccinal and a pathogenic *Babesia bovis* strain from Argentina to *Boophilus microplus*. *Vet. Parasitol.* **1993**, *51*, 143–148. [CrossRef]
84. Jongejan, F.; de Vos, C.; Fourie, J.J.; Beugnet, F. A novel combination of fipronil and permethrin (Frontline Tri-Act(R)/Frontect(R)) reduces risk of transmission of Babesia canis by Dermacentor reticulatus and of Ehrlichia canis by Rhipicephalus sanguineus ticks to dogs. *Parasites Vectors* **2015**, *8*, 602. [CrossRef]
85. Fourie, L.J.; Stanneck, D.; Horak, I.G. The efficacy of collars impregnated with flumethrin and propoxur against experimental infestations of adult *Rhipicephalus sanguineus* on dogs. *J. S. Afr. Vet. Assoc.* **2003**, *74*, 123–126. [CrossRef]
86. Estrada-Pena, A.; Reme, C. Efficacy of a collar impregnated with amitraz and pyriproxyfen for prevention of experimental tick infestations by *Rhipicephalus sanguineus*, *Ixodes ricinus*, and Ixodes *scapularis* in dogs. *J. Am. Vet. Med. Assoc.* **2005**, *226*, 221–224. [CrossRef]
87. Gregson, J. Notes on some phenomenal feeding of ticks. *Proc. Ent. Soc. Br. Columb.* **1938**, *34*, 8.

88. Inokuma, H.; Kemp, D.H. Establishment of *Boophilus microplus* infected with *Babesia bigemina* by using in vitro tube feeding technique. *J. Vet. Med. Sci.* **1998**, *60*, 509–512. [CrossRef]
89. Antunes, S.; Merino, O.; Mosqueda, J.; Moreno-Cid, J.A.; Bell-Sakyi, L.; Fragkoudis, R.; Weisheit, S.; Perez de la Lastra, J.M.; Alberdi, P.; Domingos, A.; et al. Tick capillary feeding for the study of proteins involved in tick-pathogen interactions as potential antigens for the control of tick infestation and pathogen infection. *Parasites Vectors* **2014**, *7*, 42. [CrossRef]
90. Antunes, S.; Merino, O.; Lerias, J.; Domingues, N.; Mosqueda, J.; de la Fuente, J.; Domingos, A. Artificial feeding of *Rhipicephalus microplus* female ticks with anti calreticulin serum do not influence tick and *Babesia bigemina* acquisition. *Ticks Tick Borne Dis.* **2015**, *6*, 47–55. [CrossRef]
91. Pierce, A.; Pierce, M. A note on the cultivation of *Boophilus microplus* (Canestrini, 1887) (Ixodidae: *Acarina*) on the embryonated hen egg. *Aust. Vet. J.* **1956**, *32*, 144–146. [CrossRef]
92. Becker, C.A.; Malandrin, L.; Depoix, D.; Larcher, T.; David, P.H.; Chauvin, A.; Bischoff, E.; Bonnet, S. Identification of three CCp genes in *Babesia divergens*: Novel markers for sexual stages parasites. *Mol. Biochem. Parasitol.* **2010**, *174*, 36–43. [CrossRef]
93. Becker, C.A.; Malandrin, L.; Larcher, T.; Chauvin, A.; Bischoff, E.; Bonnet, S.I. Validation of BdCCp2 as a marker for *Babesia divergens* sexual stages in ticks. *Exp. Parasitol.* **2013**, *133*, 51–56. [CrossRef]
94. Maeda, H.; Hatta, T.; Alim, M.A.; Tsubokawa, D.; Mikami, F.; Matsubayashi, M.; Miyoshi, T.; Umemiya-Shirafuji, R.; Kawazu, S.I.; Igarashi, I.; et al. Establishment of a novel tick-*Babesia* experimental infection model. *Sci. Rep.* **2016**, *6*, 37039. [CrossRef]
95. Rechav, Y.; Zyzak, M.; Fielden, L.J.; Childs, J.E. Comparison of methods for introducing and producing artificial infection of ixodid ticks (Acari: Ixodidae) with *Ehrlichia chaffeensis*. *J. Med. Entomol.* **1999**, *36*, 414–419. [CrossRef]
96. Antunes, S.; Couto, J.; Ferrolho, J.; Rodrigues, F.; Nobre, J.; Santos, A.S.; Santos-Silva, M.M.; de la Fuente, J.; Domingos, A. *Rhipicephalus bursa* Sialotranscriptomic Response to Blood Feeding and *Babesia ovis* Infection: Identification of Candidate Protective Antigens. *Front. Cell Infect. Microbiol.* **2018**, *8*, 116. [CrossRef]

pathogens

MDPI

Review

Preventing Transfusion-Transmitted Babesiosis

Evan M. Bloch [1,*], Peter J. Krause [2] and Laura Tonnetti [3]

1 Division of Transfusion Medicine, Department of Pathology, Johns Hopkins University, Baltimore, MD 21287, USA
2 Department of Epidemiology of Microbial Diseases, Yale School of Public Health, New Haven, CT 06520, USA; peter.krause@yale.edu
3 Scientific Affairs, American Red Cross, Holland Laboratories, Rockville, MD 21287, USA; Laura.Tonnetti@redcross.org
* Correspondence: ebloch2@jhmi.edu; Tel.: +1-410-614-4246

Abstract: *Babesia* are tick-borne intra-erythrocytic parasites and the causative agents of babesiosis. *Babesia*, which are readily transfusion transmissible, gained recognition as a major risk to the blood supply, particularly in the United States (US), where *Babesia microti* is endemic. Many of those infected with *Babesia* remain asymptomatic and parasitemia may persist for months or even years following infection, such that seemingly healthy blood donors are unaware of their infection. By contrast, transfusion recipients are at high risk of severe babesiosis, accounting for the high morbidity and mortality (~19%) observed in transfusion-transmitted babesiosis (TTB). An increase in cases of tick-borne babesiosis and TTB prompted over a decade-long investment in blood donor surveillance, research, and assay development to quantify and contend with TTB. This culminated in the adoption of regional blood donor testing in the US. We describe the evolution of the response to TTB in the US and offer some insight into the risk of TTB in other countries. Not only has this response advanced blood safety, it has accelerated the development of novel serological and molecular assays that may be applied broadly, affording insight into the global epidemiology and immunopathogenesis of human babesiosis.

Keywords: *Babesia*; blood transfusion; prevention; screening; babesiosis

Citation: Bloch, E.M.; Krause, P.J.; Tonnetti, L. Preventing Transfusion-Transmitted Babesiosis. *Pathogens* **2021**, *10*, 1176. https://doi.org/10.3390/pathogens10091176

Academic Editors: Estrella Montero, Jeremy Gray, Cheryl Ann Lobo and Luis Miguel González

Received: 31 July 2021
Accepted: 8 September 2021
Published: 13 September 2021

1. Introduction

Babesia are tick-borne apicomplexan parasites and the causative pathogens of the clinical illness, babesiosis. Over 100 species of *Babesia* infect a wide array of vertebrates, yet only six species have been implicated in human infections, of which *Babesia microti* is overwhelmingly predominant [1]. While *B. microti* has been reported frequently from the northeastern and northern midwestern United States (US), cases of babesiosis have been described globally [2]. Findings from *Babesia* surveillance and clinical case reporting suggest a significant increase in *B. microti* incidence in the United States (US) over the past two decades [3]. Factors that have been postulated for the emergence of *Babesia* include an increase in the deer population that amplifies the number of ticks, an increase in the human population, and building homes in tick infested areas [3–5]. *Babesia* was historically under-investigated, whereby greater attention (i.e., awareness) following its becoming a notifiable disease in many US states in 2011 likely contributed to the observed increase in cases.

Babesia are transmissible through blood transfusion [6]. The increase in reported cases of naturally acquired and transfusion-transmitted babesiosis (TTB) in the US drew the attention of the blood banking community, thus prompting over a decade of donor surveillance studies, along with the development of laboratory-based diagnostic and donor screening strategies to contend with TTB [7,8]. This culminated in 2019 with the publication of nonbinding recommendations from the US Food and Drug Administration (FDA) in favor of regional blood donor screening for *Babesia* in the US using an approved molecular assay [9]. Prior to the adoption of laboratory-based screening, *B. microti* was a leading infectious risk to the US blood supply. The risk of TTB in the US is now low as a result of routine testing for *Babesia* [10]. We describe the evolution of the response to TTB in the US as a means to contextualize the risk of *Babesia* in general with a view to guide future research efforts.

2. Epidemiology: Geographic Distribution, Seasonality, and Transmissibility

Babesia species have different geographic distributions. Cases of *B. microti* have been reported widely, notably in the northeastern and upper midwestern US, but also in other countries [11–15]. *Babesia duncani* occurs in the far western US [16]. *Babesia venatorum* and *Babesia crassa*-like agent have been reported in Europe and northeastern China [17–19]. *Babesia divergens/Babesia divergens*-like agents has been reported in Europe [17] and the United States [20]. *Babesia motasi*-like agent has been implicated in human cases in Korea [21].

2.1. Blood Donor Surveillance in the US

Beginning in the late 1990's, a series of surveillance studies were conducted to determine the seroprevalence of *Babesia* (specifically *B. microti*), as well as rates of parasitemia (using molecular positivity as a surrogate of active infection) specific to the blood donor population (Table 1). In one of the earliest studies, blood donors (n = 3490) in endemic and nonendemic areas of Connecticut were evaluated for *B. microti* [22]. In this study, 30 (0.9%) donors were confirmed positive for antibodies against *B. microti*; over half (10/19) of seropositive donors who were subsequently tested by PCR were shown to be positive [22]. In another study, about a fifth (21%) of 84 seropositive blood donors (IFA titers $\geq$ 64), who were followed for up to three years in Connecticut and Massachusetts, were found to be parasitemic [23]. Over the course of follow-up, protracted low-level parasitemia was variably and intermittently detectable.

Table 1. Transfusion-transmitted babesiosis: blood donor surveillance and follow-up studies in the United States.

Overview	Study Design	Location (s)	Year (s)	Major Finding	Reference
Donor surveillance (research)	3490 donations (1745 each fromendemic and nonendemic areas) were tested for *B. microti* antibodies using research-based enzyme immunoassay (EIA); supplemental IFA was used to conform EIA+ samples. Selected seropositive samples were evaluated using nested PCR.	CT, USA (endemic and nonendemic areas)	1999	30/3490 (0.9%) confirmed as seropositive (n = 24 [1.4%] vs. 6 [0.3%] in endemic and nonendemic areas, respectively). 10/19 (53%) of 19 seropositive donors PCR+.	Leiby et al. Transfusion 2005 [22]
Donor surveillance (research)	23,304 donations from 17,465 donors were tested by IFA.	CT and MA, USA	2000–2007	267/23,304 (1.1%) seroprevalence.	Johnson et al. Transfusion 2009 [24]
Donor surveillance (research)	Cross-sectional IFA (*B. microti* IgG) testing of blood donors with PCR testing of seroreactive donors and lookback investigation.	CT, USA	1999–2005	208/17,422 (1.2%) IFA+ 26/139 (18.7%) PCR+ 8/63 recipients were IFA and/or PCR+.	Johnson et al. Transfusion 2011 [25]
Donor screening and follow-up (research)	*B. microti* IFA (titers $\geq$ 64) were monitored up to 3 years for parasitemia by 2 PCR methods and hamster inoculation.	CT and MA, USA	2000 to 2004	18/84 (21.4%) donors parasitemic at follow-up; 9 had >1 specimen with evidence of parasitemia. Observation of protracted, intermittent, low-level parasitemia.	Leiby et al. Transfusion 2014 [23]
Hemovigilance study	Description of donor and recipient characteristics of suspected cases of TTB reported to American Red Cross.	USA (national)	2005 to 2007	Eighteen definite or probable B. microtiinfections with 5 fatalities 4/18 (24%). Nonresident donors had a history of travel to endemic areas.	Tonnetti et al. Transfusion 2009 [26]

Table 1. *Cont.*

Overview	Study Design	Location (s)	Year (s)	Major Finding	Reference
Donor surveillance with prospective follow-up (research)	Cross-sectional surveillance of consenting blood donors using RT-PCR and IFA (*B. microti* IgG); blood donors in VT (non or low-endemic state) used to establish specificity.	Southeast CT, USA VT, USA	2009	25/1002 (2.5%) IFA+ 3/1002 (0.3%) PCR+ (1 was IFA-negative). 1/1015 (0.1%) Vermont donors was IFA+.	Johnson et al. Transfusion 2013 [27]
Donor screening (real-time/operational)	Selective real-time donor screening with IFA and PCR units directed to neonates and pediatric sickle cell and thalassemia patients.	RI, USA	2010–2011	26/2113 (1.23%) representing 1783 blood donors were IFA+. 1 indeterminate PCR result (0.05%). No cases of TTB (vs. 7 cases of TTB out of 6500 unscreened units in targeted population using historical controls (2005–2010).	Young et al. Transfusion 2012 [7]
Investigation screening using donor sample repository	Paired samples screened by AFIA and PCR.	Nonendemic (AZ and OK), moderately endemic (MN and WI), and highly endemic (CT and MA) areas of the USA	2010 to 2011	Positivity (Seroreactivity and/or PCR+): Nonendemic: 0.025% (95% CI, 0.00–0.14%); Midendemic: 0.12% (95% CI, 0.04–0.28%); High endemic: 0.75% (95% CI, 0.53–1.03%). AFIA specificity 99.95% and 99.98% at cutoff of 1-in-64 and 1-in-128, respectively.	Moritz et al. Transfusion 2014 [28]
Validation study of EIA for blood donor screening	Retrospective testing of donor samples collected in high-risk endemic, lower-risk endemic, and nonendemic; EIA+ samples further tested by *B. microti* IFA, PCR, and peripheral blood smear examination.	Nonendemic area: AZ Lower-risk area: Manhattan and Brooklyn, NY High-risk endemic: Suffolk County, NY	2012	EIA repeat-reactive rates: Nonendemic area: 8/5000 (0.16%); Lower-risk area 27/5000 (0.54%); High-risk endemic: 46/5000 (0.92%).	Levin et al. Transfusion 2014 [29]
Donor screening (real-time/operational)	Donor screening with PCR and arrayed fluorescence immunoassay (AFIA).	CT, MA, MN, and WI, USA	2012 to 2016	700/220,749 donations screened positive, of which 15 (1 per 14,699 donations) were deemed to be window period infections (PCR+/AFIA-). Median estimated parasite load in WP donations 350 parasites/mL 3/10 (30%) WP donations infected hamsters.	Moritz et al. Transfusion 2017 [30]
Donor screening (real-time/operational)	Prospective AFIA and quantitative PCR testing of blood donors for *B. microti* DNA; assessment of parasitemia and infectivity using xeno-inoculation of hamsters. Prospective follow-up of test-reactive donors.	CT, MA, MN, and WI, USA	2012 to 2014	89,153 blood donation samples tested: 335 (0.38%) confirmed positive and 67/335 (20%) PCR-positive; 9 samples PCR+ but AFIA- (1 in 9906 screened), 27/93 (29%) reactive samples were infectious when inoculated into hamsters. At 1-year follow-up, DNA clearance had occurred in 86% of test-reactive donors but antibody seroreversion observed in only 8%.	Moritz et al. Transfusion 2016 [8]
Real time screening and donor notification	Screening blood donors with an investigational *B. microti* EIA. Repeat-reactive samples were retested by PCR, blood smear, IFA, and immunoblot assay. Findings were correlated with samples that had been collected from patients with established diagnoses of babesiosis.	NY, MN, and NM, USA, representing high endemic, moderately endemic, and nonendemic areas, respectively	2013	Rates of repeat reactivity by EIA: 38/ 13,757 (0.28%) NY; 7/4583 (0.15%) MN; 11/8363 (0.13%) NM. 9/56 EIA repeat-reactive donors positive by PCR. Assay specificity 99.93%. Sensitivity 91.1%.	Levin et al. Transfusion 2016 [31]

Table 1. *Cont.*

Overview	Study Design	Location (s)	Year (s)	Major Finding	Reference
Donor follow-up study	Prospective evaluation of seroreactive blood donors identified during study by Levin et al. [31]. Repeat testing (PCR, IFA, EIA, and blood smear) and completion of clinical questionnaire over the course of ~12 months of follow-up after reactive donation.	NY, MN, and NM, USA representing high endemic, moderately endemic and nonendemic areas respectively	2013–2014	37/60 (61.67%) eligible seroreactive donors enrolled, of whom, 20 (54%) completed the 12-month follow-up: 15/20 (75%) were still seroreactive at follow-up. 5/9 PCR+ donors participated in follow-up study: two remained positive at final follow-up (378 and 404 days). • Most seroreactive donors exhibited low-level seroreactivity that was stable or waning. • Level and pattern of reactivity correlated poorly with PCR positivity.	Bloch et al. Transfusion 2016 [32]
Donor screening (real-time/operational)	Donor screening with transcription-mediated amplification (Procleix Babesia assay, Grifols Diagnostic Solutions) in in 11 endemic states; minipool and individual donor testing evaluated.	11 endemic states, Washington DC and Florida	2017–2018Extended to 2019	61/176,608 donations confirmed positive (1 in 2895 donations). Extended screening 211/496,270 (1 in 2351 donations) confirmed positive. Detection of positive donations not restricted by season. 6 positive donations identified in individual testing also detected through pooled testing. 100% specificity (no false positives).	Tonnetti et al. Transfusion 2020 [33]

AFIA—arrayed fluorescent immunoassay (AFIA); IFA—indirect fluorescent antibody; EIA—enzyme immunoassay; PCR—polymerase chain reaction; TTB—transfusion-transmitted babesiosis; NA—not applicable; CT—Connecticut; MA—Massachusetts; MN—Minnesota; WI—Wisconsin; VT—Vermont; AZ—Arizona; NY—New York; NM—New Mexico; OK—Oklahoma; FL—Florida; RI—Rhode Island.

2.2. TTB in the US

Babesia are intraerythrocytic parasites and are readily transmissible through transfusion of any product containing red blood cells. TTB has been reported following transfusion of whole blood, packed red blood cells (RBCs), and even frozen RBCs [6]. Confirmed cases of TTB have not been ascribed to transfusion of apheresis platelets and acellular blood products such as plasma and cryoprecipitate [6]. Rare cases of TTB have been reported after transfusion of whole blood-derived platelets [6]. This may have been due to contamination of red cells and/or the presence of extraerythrocytic parasites [34]. The minimum infectious dose of *B. microti* that can cause TTB is low (10–100 parasites), based on murine models [35] (Table 2). TTB following transfusion of pediatric red cell aliquots and whole blood-derived platelets suggests that infectivity is high.

Table 2. Quantification of risk of transfusion transmitted babesiosis and assay development.

	Overview	Study Design	Major Finding	Reference
Efficacy of detection methods	Development of prototype EIA	Development of protype EIA using recombinant, immunodominant peptides BMN1-17 and MN-10.	69/72 (95.9%) IFA samples detected by EIA. 98/107 (91.5%) positive IgG blot samples detected using EIA. 53/63 (84.1%) positive IgM blot samples detected by EIA. All 12 PCR positive samples detected.	Houghton et al. Transfusion 2002 [36]
	Development of a real time PCR assay for detection of *B. microti*	Investigational study combining spiking experiments, probit analysis, and performance assessment using clinical sample panels.	Spiking experiment positive rate of detection: 445 copies/mL: 100%; 44.5 copies/mL: 97.5%; 4.45 copies/mL: 81%. The blinded probit analysis: detection rate: 95%: 12.92 parasites/2 mL; 50%: 1.52 parasites/2 mL of whole blood; Clinical samples: 13 of 21 samples were positive. Healthy donors: 0 of 48 positives.	Bloch et al. Transfusion 2013 [37]

Table 2. *Cont.*

	Overview	Study Design	Major Finding	Reference
	Development and validation of cobas *Babesia* assay (Roche diagnostics)	Evaluation of analytical performance of molecular assay (cobas *Babesia* assay, Roche diagnostics) targeting 4 major species of *Babesia* using individual and pooled samples Spiking experiments, cross-reactivity, and donor samples assessed to determine performance characteristics of the assay.	Limit of detection: *B. microti* 6.1 infected red blood cells (iRBC)/mL; *B. duncani* 50.2 iRBC/mL; *B. divergens* 26.1 iRBC/mL; *B. venatorum* 40.0 iRBC/mL. Specificity: ID-NAT: 99.999% (95% CI:99.996, 100); MP-NAT (6 donations): 100% (95% CI: 99.987, 100).	Stanley et al. Transfusion 2021 [38]
Parasite persistence in blood products	*Babesia* tolerance of storage conditions	*B. divergens* inoculated into blood bags containing leukoreduced red blood cells (RBCs) and stored at 4 °C for 0 to 31 days. Parasite viability assessed through interval sampling.	Viability maintained through 31 days of refrigerated storage despite altered morphology, reduction in parasitemia and lag to exponential growth.	Cursino-Santos et al. Transfusion 2014 [39]
Animal models for determining the risk of TTB.	Immunopathogenesis	6 Rhesus macaque monkeys were transfused with either hamster or monkey-passaged *B. microti*–infected red blood cells to simulate TTB	First detectable parasitemia 4 days in monkey-passaged cells (vs. 35 days in hamster passaged cells). Window period (detectable parasitemia by qPCR to detected antibody response): 10 to 17 days. Multilineage immune activation albeit not NK or Treg cells.	Gumber et al. Transfusion 2016 [40]
	Minimum infectious dose and kinetics of parasitemia	Murine model infected with different dilutions of *B. microti* parasitemic blood. Responses compared between immunocompetent and immunodeficient mice.	Peak parasitemia: 2×10^7 pRBCs/mL at 2 to 3 weeks and 5×10^8 pRBCs/mL at 6 weeks immunocompetent and immunodeficient, respectively. Chronic infection: fluctuating parasitemia in immunocompetent mice; high plateau parasitemia in immunodeficient mice. Minimum infectious dose: 100 parasitized RBCs in immunocompetent mice and 63 parasitized RBCs in immunodeficient mice; able to establish infection in all mice in respective cohorts.	Bakkour et al. Transfusion 2018 [35]

Abbreviations: IFA—indirect fluorescent antibody; EIA—enzyme immunoassay; PCR—polymerase chain reaction; TTB—transfusion-transmitted babesiosis; IDT—individual donor testing; MP-NAT—minipool nucleic acid testing.

To date, over 250 cases of TTB have been reported in the US, almost all (98%) of which were caused by *B. microti*. There are three reports of TTB due to *B. duncani* and one due to *B. divergens*-like parasites [20,41]. The risk of TTB is more widespread in the US than that associated with tick-borne transmission of parasites. Blood is often transfused far from where it is collected. It is not uncommon for blood products to cross state lines, where distribution is driven by clinical need, disproportionately being drawn toward major urban centers. In addition, residents from nonendemic areas may become asymptomatically infected during travel to endemic areas, return home, and donate blood [42]. *B. microti* can persist for long periods of time, even after standard antimicrobial therapy, whereby asymptomatic individuals may donate long after becoming infected [42,43]. These factors have accounted for cases of TTB in nonendemic states [44,45].

Natural acquisition of *Babesia* is predominantly seasonal, with peak incidence spanning late spring to early fall, following the life cycle of the tick vector. By contrast, cases of TTB are not strictly confined to peak periods of vector-borne transmission, although they still have a similar time distribution pattern as tick-borne disease, having been reported throughout the year [6,46]. Prolonged storage of blood components enables transfusion of parasitemic blood long after donor acquisition of infection and expands transmission time to include the entire calendar year [8,43]. In addition, the incubation period for development of symptoms after transfusion is as long as six months [6]. Furthermore, donor surveillance studies and prospective screening have also identified parasitemic donations (i.e., positive nucleic acid test) throughout the year, although positive donations still tend to occur from June to October [33].

3. The Risk of Transfusion-Transmitted Babesiosis outside of the US

To date, cases of TTB have been almost exclusively described in the US, with rare exceptions of reports in Japan and Canada (Table 3) [47]. Although it is well established that *Babesia* is globally ubiquitous, few studies have been undertaken to quantify risk of TTB outside of the US.

Table 3. Transfusion-transmitted babesiosis: blood donor surveillance and quantification of transfusion-associated risk outside of the United States.

Study Design	Overview	Location (s)	Year (s)	Major Finding	Reference
Case report	53 y old female transfused for anemia secondary to gastrointestinal bleeding; found to be due to tumor of small intestine.	Ontario, Canada	1998	Parasites demonstrated on blood smear and diagnosis of *B. microti* infection confirmed by PCR. Donor implicated (smear-, PCR-, and IFA-positive). The donor had been camping in Cape Cod, Massachusetts (USA)	Kain, et al. Canadian Medical Association Journal 2001 [47]
Case report	40 y old male transfused for gastric bleeding; 1 month later the patient was investigated for fever and hemolysis.	Japan	1998–1999	Parasites demonstrated on blood smear and diagnosis of *B. microti* infection confirmed by PCR. Donor implicated.	Matsui et al. Rinsho Ketsueki 2000 [14]
Pilot serosurvey	Retrospective IFA screening for *B. divergens and B. microti* IgG antibodies.	North and East Tyrol, Austria	Not stated	Total of 988 blood donors screened (cut-off titer 128). 21/988 (2.1%) seroreactive for IgG antibodies against *B. divergens*. 5/988 (0.6%) reactive against *B. microti*.	Sonnleitner et al. Transfusion 2014 [48]
Tick surveillance to guide donor serosurvey	Passive surveillance of ticks used to identify regions for tick drag sampling. All ticks were tested for *B. microti* using PCR. Blood donations from selected sites (based on tick testing and near-endemic US regions) tested for antibody to *B. microti*; donors subjected to questionnaire about risk travel and possible tick exposure.	Southern Manitoba, Ontario, Quebec, New Brunswick, and Nova Scotia, Canada	2013	13,993/26,260 (53%) donors at the selected sites tested; none were positive for antibody to *B. microti*. 41% reported travel to the United States.	O'Brien et al. Transfusion 2016 [49]
Pilot serosurvey	Retrospective IFA screening of blood donor samples for *B. microti* antibodies.	Heilongjiang Province, China	2016	888 whole blood and 112 platelet donor samples (n = 1000); 13/1000 (1.3%) donors were seroreactive; 0.8% at a titer of 64 and 0.05% at titer of 128.	Bloch et al. Vox Sanguinis 2018 [50]
Surveillance study	NAT (TMA) screening of 50,752 blood samples and IFA screening of a subset of TMA-nonreactive samples (14,758).	Canadian regions close to US border, including British Columbia, Alberta, Saskatchewan, Manitoba, Ontario, Quebec, and Nova Scotia	2018	1/50,752 TMA-reactive; 4/14,758 antibody-positive.	Tonnetti et al. Transfusion 2018 [51]
Pilot serosurvey	Retrospective IFA screening of blood donor plasma samples for *B. microti* IgG antibodies; initially reactive samples were further tested for *B. microti* IgG and IgM by immunoblot and *B. microti* DNA by PCR.	New South Wales and Queensland, Australia	2012–2013	0 (0%) confirmed positive. 5 initial reactive donors failed to confirm on repeat/confirmatory testing.	Faddy et al. Transfusion 2019 [52]

Table 3. *Cont.*

Study Design	Overview	Location (s)	Year (s)	Major Finding	Reference
Risk modelling study	Monte Carlo simulation used to estimate the number and proportion of *B. microti* infectious red blood cell units in Canada for three scenarios: base, localized incidence, and prevalence from donor data.	Canada	N/A	Expected NAT-positive donations per year (and clinically significant TTB): • Base scenario: 0.5 (0.08) (1 every 12.5 years). • Localized incidence scenario: 0.21(0.04) (about 1 every 25 years). • Donor study informed scenario: 4.6 (0.81)	O'Brien et al. Transfusion 2021 [53]

A seroprevalence study was undertaken of Tyrolean blood donors ($n = 988$): 2.1% were IgG-positive against the *B. divergens* complex and 0.6% were seropositive for *B. microti* [48]. While both species are causes of human infections, *B. divergens* has not been found to be transmitted through blood transfusion.

Canada has plausible risk given its proximity to endemic US states, as well as previously described autochthonous cases. In one study, passive surveillance was utilized to guide follow-up active surveillance and intervention [49]. Specifically, ~12,000 ticks that had been submitted by the public were tested for evidence of *Babesia* infection. Fourteen were found to be *B. microti*-positive, 10 of which originated in Manitoba. This guided selection of regions for active surveillance (2009–2014) using tick drag sampling. The ticks were tested by PCR: 6/361 (1.7%) were positive in Manitoba and 3/641 (0.5%) were positive in Quebec. None were positive from other sites. Blood donations (July and December, 2013) at selected sites near endemic US regions were tested for antibodies to *B. microti*. A donor questionnaire was used to enquire about travel-related risk and possible tick exposure. A total of 13,993/ 26,260 (53%) donors were tested, none of whom were found to have antibodies to *B. microti*. Further, almost half (47%) reported having visited forested areas in Canada and 41% had traveled to the US. During a more extensive study performed in 2018, over 50,000 donations that had been collected near the US border were tested for *Babesia* nucleic acid by transcription-mediated amplification (TMA). In addition, a subset of 14,758 TMA-nonreactive samples was also screened for *B. microti* antibodies. The study identified one TMA-reactive donation that had been collected in Winnipeg, Manitoba, the only region in Canada where autochthonous infections have been reported, and four antibody-positive donations in the TMA-negative group [51]. Collectively, these findings suggest that the risk of TTB is low in Canada and that a risk-based deferral for *Babesia* is not needed at the moment.

A study was conducted in blood donors in China [50]. Again, there is a plausible regional risk given prior reports of human babesiosis in China, as well as in Mongolia, Korea, and Japan [14,54–58]. A total of 1000 donor samples representing 888 whole blood and 112 platelet donations that had been collected in Heilongjiang province were evaluated by IFA against *B. microti:* 13/1000 (1.3%) were seroreactive.

In Australia, a fatal case of autochthonous babesiosis due to *B. microti* raised concern pertaining to the national blood supply [11,59]. A total of 7000 donations were tested for anti-*B. microti* IgG by IFA [52]. Initial reactive samples were subjected to *B. microti* IgG and IgM (immunoblot), as well as PCR. Five donors were initially reactive by IFA, none of whom were confirmed during repeat testing. All were PCR-negative. In addition, clinically suspected cases of babesiosis ($n = 29$) were also evaluated; none were *B. microti* IgG, IgM, or DNA positive.

4. Clinical Presentation

Clinically, about a fifth of *Babesia* infections in adult immunocompetent hosts are subclinical or manifest as mild flu-like illnesses that are not diagnosed and often clear without treatment [60]. Most patients experience a mild to moderate febrile illness that typically consists of fatigue, headache, chills, and sweats. However, selected patient subsets are at high risk of severe disease with complications. The latter include hemolytic anemia; cardiorespiratory, renal, and/or liver failure; disseminated intravascular coagulopathy; and death [2]. Transfusion recipients harbor many of the risk factors for severe or even fatal babesiosis, such as advanced age, comorbid cardiac or pulmonary disease, immunodeficiency due to asplenia, cancer, HIV/AIDS, or sickle cell disease [2]. This helps to explain the severity of illness and high fatality rate (~19%) associated with transfusion-transmitted babesiosis (TTB) [1,6,60]. Indeed, variability in reported fatality rates from babesiosis, in general, largely reflects a difference in clinical penetrance that is governed by the immune status of the host [61–63]. Importantly, transfusion of red blood cells and whole blood is indicated for the treatment of severe, decompensated anemia. Therefore, parasite-induced hemolysis that might otherwise be tolerated in the immunocompetent individual can have dire consequences in the transfusion recipient.

5. Prevention Strategies

5.1. Risk-Based Deferral

Historically, prevention of TTB has relied on donor selection (Table 4). Individuals who reported a history of babesiosis were permanently deferred from blood donation. This proved suboptimal, as evidenced by the number of cases of TTB that escaped detection using this approach. There are a number of reasons why this approach was problematic. For one, *Babesia* are able to persist chronically in donors without apparent adverse effects [42]. Even when clinically overt, the symptoms of babesiosis in immunocompetent adults are nonspecific. Risk factors for tick exposure are also nonspecific (e.g., outdoor activities, residence in highly endemic states), offering little diagnostic utility [32]. Vector (i.e., tick)-borne transmission is seasonal, largely aligning with the tick life cycle, whereby most infections occur late spring to early fall [2]. By contrast, cases of TTB are less prone to seasonality, given that blood can be stored for prolonged periods. Further, persistent, asymptomatic infection is well described, in some cases being detectable for more than two years following infection [42,43].

Table 4. Approaches to address the risk of TTB.

Approach	Strengths	Limitations
Risk-based deferral	Low cost Logistically simple	• Lack of specificity • High proportion of individuals are asymptomatic and parasitemia may be protracted • Most are unaware of past or active infection • Large number of reported cases of TTB in endemic areas
Peripheral blood smear	• Direct observation of parasites	• Not amenable to high-throughput donor screening • Low sensitivity • May lend itself to misdiagnosis, e.g., with *Plasmodium*
Serology	• Relatively low cost	• Poor correlation with active parasitemia risks intolerable rates of deferral in highly endemic areas • Limited cross-reactivity between *Babesia* species, such that other species may go undetected e.g., *B. duncani* • Variable performance of automated antibody tests in use that have largely been confined to the detection of *B. microti* antibodies • Rarity of selected species complicates validation of serological assays
Molecular methods	• Detectable RNA or DNA is a reasonable correlate of active parasitemia • Lower rates of reactivity than would be expected with serological testing, thus preventing high rates of donor deferral that would otherwise be encountered with serological testing • Central to blood donor screening policy in the US • Highly sensitive and specific, high-throughput licensed assays are available for donor screening; selected assays are also able to detect the major *Babesia* species using a single assay format • Enables donor reinstatement following deferral, i.e., after 2 years, if repeat testing is negative, individuals may be permitted to donate • Able to detect individuals in a pre-seroconversion window period	• Higher cost than serology • Imperfect correlate with active parasitemia, i.e., DNA/RNA may remain detectable following treatment or spontaneous resolution

Table 4. *Cont.*

Approach	Strengths	Limitations
Pathogen reduction	• FDA- and EU-approved photochemical inactivation technology is available for use in platelets and plasma; allowable as an alternative to molecular testing • Collateral benefits of pathogen reduction include efficacy against different classes of pathogens, including bacteria, thus addressing another major infectious risk to blood supply; also effective for prevention of transfusion-associated graft vs. host disease	• Absence of a licensed pathogen reduction technology for red blood cells and whole blood; TTB has not been ascribed to apheresis-collected platelets and plasma • High cost • Lower platelet yields as compared to standard platelet products

A history of tick bites is also a poor predictor of infection. Recall of tick bite is unreliable. One study observed no significant difference in *Babesia* seroprevalence between those who reported tick bites as compared to those who did not [64]. The investigators postulated that those who report tick exposure are the same group who take precautions against tick bites. Importantly, a high proportion of infections are ascribed to the bites from nymphs rather than adult ticks. Nymphal ticks are the size of poppy seeds, rendering them highly inconspicuous.

5.2. Laboratory-Based Methods for Donor Screening

Laboratory testing is necessary for any meaningful donor screening intervention. Laboratory approaches in routine use for clinical diagnosis of babesiosis (e.g., microscopy of peripheral blood smears and manual indirect fluorescent antibody [IFA] testing) are not suitable for donor screening. Microscopy is neither scalable nor sufficiently sensitive or specific to detect the low level of parasitemia that is often encountered in blood donors. Manual IFA testing is not amenable to high-throughput screening. Molecular testing for *Babesia* is a more suitable approach for blood donor screening but poses novel challenges. *Babesia*—unlike the major transfusion-transmitted viruses— is primarily red-cell-based, thereby requiring additional processing steps for optimal sensitivity of detection. Given the large numbers of donors, automation is critical. Therefore, a process needed to be devised to better access the target parasites in the infected red blood cells.

5.3. Serological Testing

The initial approach for evaluating *Babesia* in the blood donor population was focused on serology (i.e., antibody capture)—specifically of anti-*B. microti* antibodies— in endemic areas. Experimental research assays were developed for the detection of *B. microti*. One approach used an enzyme immunoassay (EIA) (i.e., targeting the recombinant protein BMN-17 and MN-10) [36]; the other employed a semi-automated IFA test [22]. Although less labor-intensive, the EIA assay showed poor specificity as compared to the semi-automated IFA test. By contrast, IFA testing is sensitive and specific and is still used today to supplement positive nucleic acid test results. The semi-automated version of the IFA test, the arrayed fluorescent immunoassay (AFIA), was applied successfully in a series of donor surveillance studies [8,10]. The combination of AFIA and real-time PCR were the first tests to receive FDA licensure for screening of blood donations, but have since been discontinued for blood screening by the manufacturer [65].

Another antibody test, an enzyme-linked immunoassay (ELISA), was developed to detect antibodies against *B. microti*. The assay employed four immunodominant peptides from the BMN1 family that had been shown to be immunodominant and highly specific to *B. microti* [36]. The assay was capable of detecting both IgM and IgG against *B. microti* [29]. In a pilot study, 15,000 blood donor samples from high-risk, low-risk, and nonendemic areas of New York State (5,000 each) were tested. Rates of reactivity following application of a revised cutoff were 0.92%, (46/5000), 0.54% (27/5000), and 0.16% (8/5000), respectively [29]. ELISA repeat-reactive samples were also tested by IFA with a concordance rate of 99.34%. Although the ELISA was evaluated in a formal IND (investigational new drug) trial, which was a preliminary step along the regulatory pathway to licensure, the assay was never licensed and is no longer in use.

5.4. Molecular Testing

Molecular testing better detects active infection/parasitemia than antibody testing. This is important because active infection rather than *Babesia* exposure alone (i.e., antibodies), is required for transmission by blood transfusion. Nevertheless, mitigation strategies for blood donors focused initially on serological methods. Molecular assays (i.e., nucleic acid testing or NAT) have been used since ~1999 to detect the major transfusion-transmissible viruses (e.g., HIV, hepatitis B, and hepatitis C viruses) [66]. Those agents are detectable in plasma. By contrast, *Babesia* are primarily intraerythrocytic, requiring additional processing of whole blood to ensure adequate target capture.

A variety of PCR research assays, from nested to real-time, have been developed using the 18S ribosomal RNA gene of *B. microti* as a target and used to determine parasitemia in antibody-positive blood donations during surveillance studies [27,67]. In most cases, these assays have been shown to be sensitive and specific; however, the methodologies used to access the red cell compartment represented a limiting factor for the sensitivity of these assays for blood donor screening. In addition, hemoglobin is also a known inhibitor of PCR [68]. The first real-time PCR assays for donor screening utilized an automated membrane-based isolation system (Taigen Bioscience) and had a limit of detection of 66 piroplasms per mL [8]. Later, larger manufacturers such as Grifols Diagnostics and Roche developed assays, and ultimately obtained FDA licensure [69,70]. These assays are exquisitely sensitive and specific, attaining limits of detection for *Babesia* as low as 2–3 parasites/mL [66]. Both assays can detect ribosomal DNA or RNA of four major species of *Babesia* that infect humans (*B. microti*, *B. divergens*, *B. duncani*, and *B. venatorum*) [38]. The assays can be performed on an automated platform and in pools of 6 (Cobas Babesia, Roche Diagnostics) to 16 samples (Procleix Babesia assay, Grifols diagnostic solutions), allowing for the screening of large numbers of donations. One of the two assays in current use (Cobas Babesia, Roche Diagnostics) employs proprietary whole blood collection tubes containing lysing agents [38].

6. Economic Impact

The cost implications of donor screening have been assessed in three studies undertaken by different groups. The first study examined four different testing strategies as applied to endemic areas: universal antibody screening, universal molecular screening, universal combined testing (antibody/molecular), and recipient-risk-targeted combined (antibody/molecular) testing [71]. The strategies were compared to the then-current standard practice of using a questionnaire. The authors concluded that use of a questionnaire was most wasteful, followed by a risk-targeted combined approach. Universal molecular screening would incur an incremental cost-effectiveness ratio (ICER) of $26,000 to $44,000/quality adjusted life year (QALY) and would serve to prevent 24 to 31 TTB cases/100,000 units transfused, incurring no wastage. The combined approach would be more effective, albeit at a higher cost. By contrast, antibody-based screening was lower in cost, yet was less effective and incurred higher wastage than the molecular options.

The second analysis evaluated the cost utility of a similar repertoire of screening approaches in endemic areas [72]. The results were substantially different. For one, the ICER for combined testing as compared to antibody screening was in excess of $8.7 million, preventing 3.6 cases of TTB per 100,000 units transfused. Universal endemic antibody screening was projected to prevent 3.39 cases of TTB at an ICER of $760,000/QALY when compared to the recipient-risk-targeted strategy. The authors concluded that antibody was the most cost-effective strategy when applying the threshold of cost effectiveness specific to transfusion safety initiatives in the US, i.e., $1 million/QALY.

The third study examined the cost-utility of different screening strategies, both by mode of testing (IFA, ELISA, PCR), as well as extent of geographic inclusion [73]. The authors concluded that even a strategy that was to be confined to highly endemic states would likely exceed the implicit threshold for cost-effectiveness of $1 million per QALY.

7. US Policy

Babesiosis has long been recognized as posing a risk to the US blood supply [9,74]. However, availability of validated tests that were of sufficient level of performance for donor screening, impeded rapid adoption of preventive strategies [75]. In 2019, the US FDA published their recommendations, thus supporting regional molecular screening of blood donors in 14 states and Washington DC using any of the approved assays [9]. Over 95% of all cases of TTB and 99% of clinical cases of babesiosis have occurred in the selected locations. The recommendations also allowed for pathogen reduction (PR) as an alternative to laboratory testing. At the time of this writing, at least one PR technology had been FDA approved for use in plasma and platelets. Of note, neither plasma nor apheresis platelets pose significant—if any—risk of transfusion transmission. A history or babesiosis or a positive test for *Babesia* previously led to permanent deferral from blood donation. Under the new guidance, donor re-entry is allowable after 2 years in the event that the donor has not had a positive test result for *Babesia* during the interval, remains negative by requalification using one of the licensed *Babesia* NAT assays, and meets all other eligibility criteria for blood donation [9].

8. Discussion

Successful strategies to reduce the risk of the major transfusion-transmitted viruses (e.g., HIV, hepatitis B, and C viruses) have rendered blood transfusion remarkably safe, at least in the US and other high-income countries [66,76]. These successful strategies have contributed to the investigation of risk posed by other pathogens (e.g., *Babesia*) and classes of pathogens (e.g., bacteria) to the blood supply. Implementation of donor screening for *Babesia* in the US has been a success, having —arguably— removed one of the last major transfusion-transmissible infections, thus serving to advance blood transfusion safety nationally.

Nonetheless, the donor screening policy was long overdue. A potential contributing factor for the delayed development of *Babesia* blood screening assays was the evolution of *T. cruzi* screening in the US. *T. cruzi*, the causative parasite for Chagas disease, is transfusion-transmissible. The agent is endemic to Central and South America, where longstanding public health efforts coupled with serological testing of blood donors have contributed to a decline in cases [77]. Universal donor screening for Chagas disease began in the US in 2006. Following implementation, studies determined the risk in the US to be low. This prompted a revision of the policy at that time to restrict screening to first-time donor testing only. While rational in outlook, that shift in policy impaired commercial investment in testing. The downstream effect may have been the later, tepid support from the major test manufacturers—at least initially—for *Babesia* testing. Instead, the larger blood collection agencies, such as American Red Cross, Vitalant (then Blood Systems), and New York Blood Center, partnered with small businesses to develop assays.

The path to regulatory approval and development of a screening policy for *Babesia* took almost a decade. By way of comparison, implementation of routine testing for West Nile Virus in 2003 (lauded as a major success) took less than a year from recognition of transfusion-transmitted disease [78], a timeline bettered by the later adoption of screening for Zika in 2016 within weeks [79–81]. Of note, Zika has yet to show any evidence of clinical effect following the rare accounts of possible transfusion transmission. Collectively, this underscores the myriad of factors and competing priorities that guide blood transfusion policy, not all of which are scientific in nature [82].

While there may be an element of closure on TTB in the US, *Babesia* remain global pathogens. *Babesia* species have been described in both ticks and animal populations over a wide geographic distribution spanning the Americas, Europe, Asia, Africa, and Australia [2,11–13,17,55,58,83]. Outside of the US, perception of risk is low and the US remains the only country to have implemented blood donor screenings [77]. Over the last two decades, only six studies (and two case reports) pertaining to TTB have originated outside of the US (Table 3). Those studies did not find comparable risk to that encountered in the US [49,52,53]. Nonetheless, surveillance is lacking, with a grossly skewed geographic sampling that remains focused on the US. One of the challenges that previously impeded surveillance was the lack of diagnostic tools that could be applied to high-throughput testing. The advent of licensed, high-performance commercial *Babesia* PCR and TMA assays should enable testing across a more diverse geography, with the caveat that implementation of molecular testing, even for research use, is challenging for low- and middle-income countries [84]. While robust molecular assays may be available, the lack of local expertise and infrastructure may still necessitate the transfer of samples to settings where equipment is available.

9. Conclusions

Babesia are major transfusion-transmissible parasites. A concerted effort by the blood banking community has yielded effective policy and testing strategies that have been integrated into routine donation practices in the US. Nonetheless, these efforts have not been matched elsewhere and deserve greater attention from the international blood banking community. Further, the lessons learned from *Babesia* (e.g., related to sample preparation, thus enabling automated testing of an intraerythrocytic pathogen) can be applied to *Plasmodium* (malaria), a related parasite that remains a leading cause of transfusion-associated morbidity in much of the World.

Author Contributions: Conceptualization, E.M.B.; data curation, E.M.B.; writing—original draft preparation, E.M.B.; writing—review and editing, E.M.B.; P.J.K. and L.T. All authors have read and agreed to the published version of the manuscript.

Funding: EMB is supported by National Heart Lung and Blood Institute 1K23HL151826 (EMB). PJK is supported in part by the Gordon and Llura Gund Foundation.

Conflicts of Interest: EMB reports personal fees and nonfinancial support from Terumo BCT, Grifols Diagnostics Solutions, and Abbott Laboratories outside of the submitted work; EMB is a member of the United States Food and Drug Administration (FDA) Blood Products Advisory Committee. Any views or opinions that are expressed in this manuscript are that of the author's, based on his own scientific expertise and professional judgment; they do not necessarily represent the views of either the Blood Products Advisory Committee or the formal position of FDA, and also do not bind or otherwise obligate or commit either the Advisory Committee or the Agency to the views expressed. PJK reports research collaboration with Gold Standard Diagnostics. LT has no relevant conflicts of interest to disclose.

References

1. Homer, M.J.; Aguilar-Delfin, I.; Telford, S.R., 3rd; Krause, P.J.; Persing, D.H. Babesiosis. *Clin. Microbiol. Rev.* **2000**, *13*, 451–469. [CrossRef]
2. Vannier, E.; Krause, P.J. Human babesiosis. *N. Engl. J. Med.* **2012**, *366*, 2397–2407. [CrossRef] [PubMed]
3. Krause, P.J.; Auwaerter, P.G.; Bannuru, R.R.; Branda, J.A.; Falck-Ytter, Y.T.; Lantos, P.M.; Lavergne, V.; Meissner, H.C.; Osani, M.C.; Rips, J.G.; et al. Clinical Practice Guidelines by the Infectious Diseases Society of America (IDSA): 2020 Guideline on Diagnosis and Management of Babesiosis. *Clin. Infect. Dis.* **2020**, *72*, e49–e64. [CrossRef]
4. Menis, M.; Whitaker, B.I.; Wernecke, M.; Jiao, Y.; Eder, A.; Kumar, S.; Xu, W.; Liao, J.; Wei, Y.; MaCurdy, T.E.; et al. Babesiosis Occurrence Among United States Medicare Beneficiaries, Ages 65 and Older, During 2006–2017: Overall and by State and County of Residence. *Open Forum Infect. Dis.* **2020**, *8*, ofaa608. [CrossRef] [PubMed]
5. Ingram, D.; Crook, T. Rise in Babesiosis Cases, Pennsylvania, USA, 2005–2018. *Emerg. Infect. Dis. J.* **2020**, *26*, 1703. [CrossRef]
6. Herwaldt, B.L.; Linden, J.V.; Bosserman, E.; Young, C.; Olkowska, D.; Wilson, M. Transfusion-associated babesiosis in the United States: A description of cases. *Ann. Intern. Med.* **2011**, *155*, 509–519. [CrossRef]
7. Young, C.; Chawla, A.; Berardi, V.; Padbury, J.; Skowron, G.; Krause, P.J. Preventing transfusion-transmitted babesiosis: Preliminary experience of the first laboratory-based blood donor screening program. *Transfusion* **2012**, *52*, 1523–1529. [CrossRef] [PubMed]
8. Moritz, E.D.; Winton, C.S.; Tonnetti, L.; Townsend, R.L.; Berardi, V.P.; Hewins, M.E.; Weeks, K.E.; Dodd, R.Y.; Stramer, S.L. Screening for *Babesia* microti in the U.S. Blood Supply. *N. Engl. J. Med.* **2016**, *375*, 2236–2245. [CrossRef] [PubMed]
9. FDA. Recommendations for Reducing the Risk of Transfusion-Transmitted Babesiosis. 2019. Available online: https://www.fda.gov/regulatory-information/search-fda-guidance-documents/recommendations-reducing-risk-transfusion-transmitted-babesiosis (accessed on 5 September 2021).

10. Tonnetti, L.; Townsend, R.L.; Deisting, B.M.; Haynes, J.M.; Dodd, R.Y.; Stramer, S.L. The impact of *Babesia* microti blood donation screening. *Transfusion* **2019**, *59*, 593–600. [CrossRef] [PubMed]
11. Senanayake, S.N.; Paparini, A.; Latimer, M.; Andriolo, K.; Dasilva, A.J.; Wilson, H.; Xayavong, M.V.; Collignon, P.J.; Jeans, P.; Irwin, P.J. First report of human babesiosis in Australia. *Med. J. Aust.* **2012**, *196*, 350–352. [CrossRef] [PubMed]
12. Peniche-Lara, G.; Balmaceda, L.; Perez-Osorio, C.; Munoz-Zanzi, C. Human Babesiosis, Yucatan State, Mexico, 2015. *Emerg. Infect. Dis.* **2018**, *24*, 2061–2062. [CrossRef]
13. Gabrielli, S.; Totino, V.; Macchioni, F.; Zuniga, F.; Rojas, P.; Lara, Y.; Roselli, M.; Bartoloni, A.; Cancrini, G. Human Babesiosis, Bolivia, 2013. *Emerg. Infect. Dis.* **2016**, *22*, 1445–1447. [CrossRef]
14. Matsui, T.; Inoue, R.; Kajimoto, K.; Tamekane, A.; Okamura, A.; Katayama, Y.; Shimoyama, M.; Chihara, K.; Saito-Ito, A.; Tsuji, M. First documentation of transfusion-associated babesiosis in Japan. *Rinsho Ketsueki* **2000**, *41*, 628–634.
15. Hildebrandt, A.; Hunfeld, K.P.; Baier, M.; Krumbholz, A.; Sachse, S.; Lorenzen, T.; Kiehntopf, M.; Fricke, H.J.; Straube, E. First confirmed autochthonous case of human *Babesia* microti infection in Europe. *Eur. J. Clin. Microbiol. Infect. Dis.* **2007**, *26*, 595–601. [CrossRef]
16. Swei, A.; O'Connor, K.E.; Couper, L.I.; Thekkiniath, J.; Conrad, P.A.; Padgett, K.A.; Burns, J.; Yoshimizu, M.H.; Gonzales, B.; Munk, B.; et al. Evidence for transmission of the zoonotic apicomplexan parasite *Babesia* duncani by the tick Dermacentor albipictus. *Int. J. Parasitol.* **2019**, *49*, 95–103. [CrossRef]
17. Hildebrandt, A.; Gray, J.S.; Hunfeld, K.P. Human babesiosis in Europe: What clinicians need to know. *Infection* **2013**, *41*, 1057–1072. [CrossRef]
18. Strasek-Smrdel, K.; Korva, M.; Pal, E.; Rajter, M.; Skvarc, M.; Avsic-Zupanc, T. Case of *Babesia* crassa-Like Infection, Slovenia, 2014. *Emerg. Infect. Dis.* **2020**, *26*, 1038–1040. [CrossRef] [PubMed]
19. Jiang, J.F.; Zheng, Y.C.; Jiang, R.R.; Li, H.; Huo, Q.B.; Jiang, B.G.; Sun, Y.; Jia, N.; Wang, Y.W.; Ma, L.; et al. Epidemiological, clinical, and laboratory characteristics of 48 cases of "*Babesia* venatorum" infection in China: A descriptive study. *Lancet Infect. Dis.* **2015**, *15*, 196–203. [CrossRef]
20. Burgess, M.J.; Rosenbaum, E.R.; Pritt, B.S.; Haselow, D.T.; Ferren, K.M.; Alzghoul, B.N.; Rico, J.C.; Sloan, L.M.; Ramanan, P.; Purushothaman, R.; et al. Possible Transfusion-Transmitted *Babesia* divergens-like/MO-1 Infection in an Arkansas Patient. *Clin. Infect. Dis.* **2017**, *64*, 1622–1625. [CrossRef] [PubMed]
21. Hong, S.H.; Kim, S.Y.; Song, B.G.; Rho, J.R.; Cho, C.R.; Kim, C.N.; Um, T.H.; Kwak, Y.G.; Cho, S.H.; Lee, S.E. Detection and characterization of an emerging type of *Babesia* sp. similar to *Babesia* motasi for the first case of human babesiosis and ticks in Korea. *Emerg. Microbes Infect.* **2019**, *8*, 869–878. [CrossRef] [PubMed]
22. Leiby, D.A.; Chung, A.P.; Gill, J.E.; Houghton, R.L.; Persing, D.H.; Badon, S.; Cable, R.G. Demonstrable parasitemia among Connecticut blood donors with antibodies to *Babesia* microti. *Transfusion* **2005**, *45*, 1804–1810. [CrossRef]
23. Leiby, D.A.; Johnson, S.T.; Won, K.Y.; Nace, E.K.; Slemenda, S.B.; Pieniazek, N.J.; Cable, R.G.; Herwaldt, B.L. A longitudinal study of *Babesia* microti infection in seropositive blood donors. *Transfusion* **2014**, *54*, 2217–2225. [CrossRef]
24. Johnson, S.T.; Cable, R.G.; Tonnetti, L.; Spencer, B.; Rios, J.; Leiby, D.A. Seroprevalence of *Babesia* microti in blood donors from *Babesia*-endemic areas of the northeastern United States: 2000 through 2007. *Transfusion* **2009**. [CrossRef]
25. Johnson, S.T.; Cable, R.G.; Leiby, D.A. Lookback investigations of *Babesia* microti-seropositive blood donors: Seven-year experience in a *Babesia*-endemic area. *Transfusion* **2012**, *52*, 1509–1516. [CrossRef]
26. Tonnetti, L.; Eder, A.F.; Dy, B.; Kennedy, J.; Pisciotto, P.; Benjamin, R.J.; Leiby, D.A. Transfusion-transmitted *Babesia* microti identified through hemovigilance. *Transfusion* **2009**, *49*, 2557–2563. [CrossRef]
27. Johnson, S.T.; Van Tassell, E.R.; Tonnetti, L.; Cable, R.G.; Berardi, V.P.; Leiby, D.A. *Babesia* microti real-time polymerase chain reaction testing of Connecticut blood donors: Potential implications for screening algorithms. *Transfusion* **2013**, *53*, 2644–2649. [CrossRef]
28. Moritz, E.D.; Winton, C.S.; Johnson, S.T.; Krysztof, D.E.; Townsend, R.L.; Foster, G.A.; Devine, P.; Molloy, P.; Brissette, E.; Berardi, V.P.; et al. Investigational screening for *Babesia* microti in a large repository of blood donor samples from nonendemic and endemic areas of the United States. *Transfusion* **2014**, *54*, 2226–2236. [CrossRef] [PubMed]
29. Levin, A.E.; Williamson, P.C.; Erwin, J.L.; Cyrus, S.; Bloch, E.M.; Shaz, B.H.; Kessler, D.; Telford, S.R., 3rd; Krause, P.J.; Wormser, G.P.; et al. Determination of *Babesia* microti seroprevalence in blood donor populations using an investigational enzyme immunoassay. *Transfusion* **2014**, *54*, 2237–2244. [CrossRef] [PubMed]
30. Moritz, E.D.; Tonnetti, L.; Hewins, M.E.; Berardi, V.P.; Dodd, R.Y.; Stramer, S.L. Description of 15 DNA-positive and antibody-negative "window-period" blood donations identified during prospective screening for *Babesia* microti. *Transfusion* **2017**, *57*, 1781–1786. [CrossRef]
31. Levin, A.E.; Williamson, P.C.; Bloch, E.M.; Clifford, J.; Cyrus, S.; Shaz, B.H.; Kessler, D.; Gorlin, J.; Erwin, J.L.; Krueger, N.X.; et al. Serologic screening of United States blood donors for *Babesia* microti using an investigational enzyme immunoassay. *Transfusion* **2016**, *56*, 1866–1874. [CrossRef]
32. Bloch, E.M.; Levin, A.E.; Williamson, P.C.; Cyrus, S.; Shaz, B.H.; Kessler, D.; Gorlin, J.; Bruhn, R.; Lee, T.H.; Montalvo, L.; et al. A prospective evaluation of chronic *Babesia* microti infection in seroreactive blood donors. *Transfusion* **2016**, *56*, 1875–1882. [CrossRef]
33. Tonnetti, L.; Young, C.; Kessler, D.A.; Williamson, P.C.; Reik, R.; Proctor, M.C.; Bres, V.; Deisting, B.; Bakkour, S.; Schneider, W.; et al. Transcription-mediated amplification blood donation screening for *Babesia*. *Transfusion* **2020**, *60*, 317–325. [CrossRef]

34. Pantanowitz, L.; Cannon, M.E. Extracellular *Babesia* microti parasites. *Transfusion* **2001**, *41*, 440. [CrossRef]
35. Bakkour, S.; Chafets, D.M.; Wen, L.; Muench, M.O.; Telford, S.R., 3rd; Erwin, J.L.; Levin, A.E.; Self, D.; Bres, V.; Linnen, J.M.; et al. Minimal infectious dose and dynamics of *Babesia* microti parasitemia in a murine model. *Transfusion* **2018**, *58*, 2903–2910. [CrossRef]
36. Houghton, R.L.; Homer, M.J.; Reynolds, L.D.; Sleath, P.R.; Lodes, M.J.; Berardi, V.; Leiby, D.A.; Persing, D.H. Identification of *Babesia* microti-specific immunodominant epitopes and development of a peptide EIA for detection of antibodies in serum. *Transfusion* **2002**, *42*, 1488–1496. [CrossRef]
37. Bloch, E.M.; Lee, T.H.; Krause, P.J.; Telford, S.R., 3rd; Montalvo, L.; Chafets, D.; Usmani-Brown, S.; Lepore, T.J.; Busch, M.P. Development of a real-time polymerase chain reaction assay for sensitive detection and quantitation of *Babesia* microti infection. *Transfusion* **2013**, *53*, 2299–2306. [CrossRef]
38. Stanley, J.; Stramer, S.L.; Erickson, Y.; Cruz, J.; Gorlin, J.; Janzen, M.; Rossmann, S.N.; Straus, T.; Albrecht, P.; Pate, L.L.; et al. Detection of *Babesia* RNA and DNA in whole blood samples from US blood donations. *Transfusion* **2021**. [CrossRef]
39. Cursino-Santos, J.R.; Alhassan, A.; Singh, M.; Lobo, C.A. *Babesia*: Impact of cold storage on the survival and the viability of parasites in blood bags. *Transfusion* **2014**, *54*, 585–591. [CrossRef]
40. Gumber, S.; Nascimento, F.S.; Rogers, K.A.; Bishop, H.S.; Rivera, H.N.; Xayavong, M.V.; Devare, S.G.; Schochetman, G.; Amancha, P.K.; Qvarnstrom, Y.; et al. Experimental transfusion-induced *Babesia* microti infection: Dynamics of parasitemia and immune responses in a rhesus macaque model. *Transfusion* **2016**, *56*, 1508–1519. [CrossRef]
41. Bloch, E.M.; Herwaldt, B.L.; Leiby, D.A.; Shaieb, A.; Herron, R.M.; Chervenak, M.; Reed, W.; Hunter, R.; Ryals, R.; Hagar, W.; et al. The third described case of transfusion-transmitted *Babesia* duncani. *Transfusion* **2012**, *52*, 1517–1522. [CrossRef]
42. Bloch, E.M.; Kumar, S.; Krause, P.J. Persistence of *Babesia* microti Infection in Humans. *Pathogens* **2019**, *8*, 102. [CrossRef] [PubMed]
43. Krause, P.J.; Spielman, A.; Telford, S.R., 3rd; Sikand, V.K.; McKay, K.; Christianson, D.; Pollack, R.J.; Brassard, P.; Magera, J.; Ryan, R.; et al. Persistent parasitemia after acute babesiosis. *N. Engl. J. Med.* **1998**, *339*, 160–165. [CrossRef]
44. Ngo, V.; Civen, R. Babesiosis acquired through blood transfusion, California, USA. *Emerg. Infect. Dis.* **2009**, *15*, 785–787. [CrossRef] [PubMed]
45. Cangelosi, J.J.; Sarvat, B.; Sarria, J.C.; Herwaldt, B.L.; Indrikovs, A.J. Transmission of *Babesia* microti by blood transfusion in Texas. *Vox Sang.* **2008**, *95*, 331–334. [CrossRef] [PubMed]
46. Tonnetti, L.; Townsend, R.L.; Dodd, R.Y.; Stramer, S.L. Characteristics of transfusion-transmitted *Babesia* microti, American Red Cross 2010–2017. *Transfusion* **2019**, *59*, 2908–2912. [CrossRef]
47. Kain, K.C.; Jassoum, S.B.; Fong, I.W.; Hannach, B. Transfusion-transmitted babesiosis in Ontario: First reported case in Canada. *Can. Med. Assoc. J.* **2001**, *164*, 1721–1723.
48. Sonnleitner, S.T.; Fritz, J.; Bednarska, M.; Baumgartner, R.; Simeoni, J.; Zelger, R.; Schennach, H.; Lass-Florl, C.; Edelhofer, R.; Pfister, K.; et al. Risk assessment of transfusion-associated babesiosis in Tyrol: Appraisal by seroepidemiology and polymerase chain reaction. *Transfusion* **2014**, *54*, 1725–1732. [CrossRef]
49. O'Brien, S.F.; Delage, G.; Scalia, V.; Lindsay, R.; Bernier, F.; Dubuc, S.; Germain, M.; Pilot, G.; Yi, Q.L.; Fearon, M.A. Seroprevalence of *Babesia* microti infection in Canadian blood donors. *Transfusion* **2016**, *56*, 237–243. [CrossRef]
50. Bloch, E.M.; Yang, Y.; He, M.; Tonnetti, L.; Liu, Y.; Wang, J.; Guo, Y.; Li, H.; Leiby, D.A.; Shan, H.; et al. A pilot serosurvey of *Babesia* microti in Chinese blood donors. *Vox Sang.* **2018**, *113*, 345–349. [CrossRef]
51. Tonnetti, L.; O'Brien, S.F.; Grégoire, Y.; Proctor, M.C.; Drews, S.J.; Delage, G.; Fearon, M.A.; Brès, V.; Linnen, J.M.; Stramer, S.L. Prevalence of *Babesia* in Canadian blood donors: June–October 2018. *Transfusion* **2019**, *59*, 3171–3176. [CrossRef]
52. Faddy, H.M.; Rooks, K.M.; Irwin, P.J.; Viennet, E.; Paparini, A.; Seed, C.R.; Stramer, S.L.; Harley, R.J.; Chan, H.T.; Dennington, P.M.; et al. No evidence for widespread *Babesia* microti transmission in Australia. *Transfusion* **2019**, *59*, 2368–2374. [CrossRef]
53. O'Brien, S.F.; Drews, S.J.; Yi, Q.L.; Bloch, E.M.; Ogden, N.H.; Koffi, J.K.; Lindsay, L.R.; Gregoire, Y.; Delage, G. Risk of transfusion-transmitted *Babesia* microti in Canada. *Transfusion* **2021**. [CrossRef] [PubMed]
54. Zhou, X.; Li, S.G.; Wang, J.Z.; Huang, J.L.; Zhou, H.J.; Chen, J.H.; Zhou, X.N. Emergence of human babesiosis along the border of China with Myanmar: Detection by PCR and confirmation by sequencing. *Emerg. Microbes Infect.* **2014**, *3*, e55. [CrossRef]
55. Zhou, X.; Xia, S.; Huang, J.L.; Tambo, E.; Zhuge, H.X.; Zhou, X.N. Human babesiosis, an emerging tick-borne disease in the People's Republic of China. *Parasites Vectors* **2014**, *7*, 509. [CrossRef] [PubMed]
56. Wei, Q.; Tsuji, M.; Zamoto, A.; Kohsaki, M.; Matsui, T.; Shiota, T.; Telford, S.R., 3rd; Ishihara, C. Human babesiosis in Japan: Isolation of *Babesia* microti-like parasites from an asymptomatic transfusion donor and from a rodent from an area where babesiosis is endemic. *J. Clin. Microbiol.* **2001**, *39*, 2178–2183. [CrossRef]
57. Hong, S.H.; Anu, D.; Jeong, Y.I.; Abmed, D.; Cho, S.H.; Lee, W.J.; Lee, S.E. Molecular detection and seroprevalence of *Babesia* microti among stock farmers in Khutul City, Selenge Province, Mongolia. *Korean J. Parasitol.* **2014**, *52*, 443–447. [CrossRef] [PubMed]
58. Kim, J.Y.; Cho, S.H.; Joo, H.N.; Tsuji, M.; Cho, S.R.; Park, I.J.; Chung, G.T.; Ju, J.W.; Cheun, H.I.; Lee, H.W.; et al. First case of human babesiosis in Korea: Detection and characterization of a novel type of *Babesia* sp. (KO1) similar to ovine babesia. *J. Clin. Microbiol.* **2007**, *45*, 2084–2087. [CrossRef]
59. Paparini, A.; Senanayake, S.N.; Ryan, U.M.; Irwin, P.J. Molecular confirmation of the first autochthonous case of human babesiosis in Australia using a novel primer set for the beta-tubulin gene. *Exp. Parasitol.* **2014**, *141*, 93–97. [CrossRef]

60. Krause, P.J.; McKay, K.; Gadbaw, J.; Christianson, D.; Closter, L.; Lepore, T.; Telford, S.R., 3rd; Sikand, V.; Ryan, R.; Persing, D.; et al. Increasing health burden of human babesiosis in endemic sites. *Am. J. Trop. Med. Hyg.* **2003**, *68*, 431–436. [CrossRef]
61. Mareedu, N.; Schotthoefer, A.M.; Tompkins, J.; Hall, M.C.; Fritsche, T.R.; Frost, H.M. Risk Factors for Severe Infection, Hospitalization, and Prolonged Antimicrobial Therapy in Patients with Babesiosis. *Am. J. Trop. Med. Hyg.* **2017**, *97*, 1218–1225. [CrossRef]
62. Rosner, F.; Zarrabi, M.H.; Benach, J.L.; Habicht, G.S. Babesiosis in splenectomized adults. Review of 22 reported cases. *Am. J. Med.* **1984**, *76*, 696–701. [CrossRef]
63. Krause, P.J.; Gewurz, B.E.; Hill, D.; Marty, F.M.; Vannier, E.; Foppa, I.M.; Furman, R.R.; Neuhaus, E.; Skowron, G.; Gupta, S.; et al. Persistent and relapsing babesiosis in immunocompromised patients. *Clin. Infect. Dis.* **2008**, *46*, 370–376. [CrossRef] [PubMed]
64. Leiby, D.A.; Chung, A.P.; Cable, R.G.; Trouern-Trend, J.; McCullough, J.; Homer, M.J.; Reynolds, L.D.; Houghton, R.L.; Lodes, M.J.; Persing, D.H. Relationship between tick bites and the seroprevalence of *Babesia* microti and Anaplasma phagocytophila (previously Ehrlichia sp.) in blood donors. *Transfusion* **2002**, *42*, 1585–1591. [CrossRef] [PubMed]
65. FDA. March 6, 2018 Approval Letter—*Babesia* microti AFIA/*Babesia*. 2018. Available online: https://www.fda.gov/files/vaccines%2C%20blood%20%26%20biologics/published/March-6--2018-Approval-Letter---Babesia-microti-AFIA-Babesia-microti-AFIA-for-Blood-Donor-Screening.pdf (accessed on 5 September 2021).
66. Busch, M.P.; Bloch, E.M.; Kleinman, S. Prevention of transfusion-transmitted infections. *Blood* **2019**, *133*, 1854–1864. [CrossRef]
67. Tonnetti, L.; Thorp, A.M.; Deisting, B.; Bachowski, G.; Johnson, S.T.; Wey, A.R.; Hodges, J.S.; Leiby, D.A.; Mair, D. *Babesia* microti seroprevalence in Minnesota blood donors. *Transfusion* **2013**, *53*, 1698–1705. [CrossRef] [PubMed]
68. Al-Soud, W.A.; Rådström, P. Purification and characterization of PCR-inhibitory components in blood cells. *J. Clin. Microbiol.* **2001**, *39*, 485–493. [CrossRef]
69. FDA. BLA APPROVAL January 24, 2019. 2019. Available online: https://www.accessdata.fda.gov/scripts/cder/daf/index.cfm?event=overview.process&ApplNo=021083 (accessed on 5 September 2021).
70. FDA. Cobas *Babesia*. Available online: https://www.fda.gov/vaccines-blood-biologics/cobas-babesia (accessed on 5 September 2021).
71. Bish, E.K.; Moritz, E.D.; El-Amine, H.; Bish, D.R.; Stramer, S.L. Cost-effectiveness of *Babesia* microti antibody and nucleic acid blood donation screening using results from prospective investigational studies. *Transfusion* **2015**, *55*, 2256–2271. [CrossRef]
72. Simon, M.S.; Leff, J.A.; Pandya, A.; Cushing, M.; Shaz, B.H.; Calfee, D.P.; Schackman, B.R.; Mushlin, A.I. Cost-effectiveness of blood donor screening for *Babesia* microti in endemic regions of the United States. *Transfusion* **2014**, *54*, 889–899. [CrossRef]
73. Goodell, A.J.; Bloch, E.M.; Krause, P.J.; Custer, B. Costs, consequences, and cost-effectiveness of strategies for *Babesia* microti donor screening of the US blood supply. *Transfusion* **2014**, *54*, 2245–2257. [CrossRef]
74. Gubernot, D.M.; Nakhasi, H.L.; Mied, P.A.; Asher, D.M.; Epstein, J.S.; Kumar, S. Transfusion-transmitted babesiosis in the United States: Summary of a workshop. *Transfusion* **2009**, *49*, 2759–2771. [CrossRef]
75. FDA. Report of Blood Product Advisory Committee Meeting July 26, 2010. 2010. Available online: https://www.aabb.org/regulatory-and-advocacy/regulatory-affairs/government-advisory-regulatory-meetings/blood-products-advisory-committee/bpac-meeting-100726 (accessed on 5 September 2021).
76. Dodd, R.Y.; Crowder, L.A.; Haynes, J.M.; Notari, E.P.; Stramer, S.L.; Steele, W.R. Screening Blood Donors for HIV, HCV, and HBV at the American Red Cross: 10-Year Trends in Prevalence, Incidence, and Residual Risk, 2007 to 2016. *Transfus. Med. Rev.* **2020**, *34*, 81–93. [CrossRef]
77. Leiby, D.A.; O'Brien, S.F.; Wendel, S.; Nguyen, M.L.; Delage, G.; Devare, S.G.; Hardiman, A.; Nakhasi, H.L.; Sauleda, S.; Bloch, E.M. International survey on the impact of parasitic infections: Frequency of transmission and current mitigation strategies. *Vox Sang.* **2019**, *114*, 17–27. [CrossRef] [PubMed]
78. Pealer, L.N.; Marfin, A.A.; Petersen, L.R.; Lanciotti, R.S.; Page, P.L.; Stramer, S.L.; Stobierski, M.G.; Signs, K.; Newman, B.; Kapoor, H.; et al. Transmission of West Nile virus through blood transfusion in the United States in 2002. *N. Engl. J. Med.* **2003**, *349*, 1236–1245. [CrossRef]
79. Kuehnert, M.J.; Basavaraju, S.V.; Moseley, R.R.; Pate, L.L.; Galel, S.A.; Williamson, P.C.; Busch, M.P.; Alsina, J.O.; Climent-Peris, C.; Marks, P.W.; et al. Screening of Blood Donations for Zika Virus Infection—Puerto Rico, April 3–June 11, 2016. *MMWR Morb. Mortal Wkly. Rep.* **2016**, *65*, 627–628. [CrossRef]
80. Galel, S.A.; Williamson, P.C.; Busch, M.P.; Stanek, D.; Bakkour, S.; Stone, M.; Lu, K.; Jones, S.; Rossmann, S.N.; Pate, L.L.; et al. First Zika-positive donations in the continental United States. *Transfusion* **2017**, *57*, 762–769. [CrossRef]
81. Saa, P.; Proctor, M.; Foster, G.; Krysztof, D.; Winton, C.; Linnen, J.M.; Gao, K.; Brodsky, J.P.; Limberger, R.J.; Dodd, R.Y.; et al. Investigational Testing for Zika Virus among U.S. Blood Donors. *N. Engl. J. Med.* **2018**, *378*, 1778–1788. [CrossRef]
82. Bloch, E.M.; Ness, P.M.; Tobian, A.A.R.; Sugarman, J. Revisiting Blood Safety Practices Given Emerging Data about Zika Virus. *N. Engl. J. Med.* **2018**, *378*, 1837–1841. [CrossRef]
83. Bloch, E.M.; Kasubi, M.; Levin, A.; Mrango, Z.; Weaver, J.; Munoz, B.; West, S.K. *Babesia* microti and Malaria Infection in Africa: A Pilot Serosurvey in Kilosa District, Tanzania. *Am. J. Trop. Med. Hyg.* **2018**, *99*, 51–56. [CrossRef] [PubMed]
84. Weimer, A.; Tagny, C.T.; Tapko, J.B.; Gouws, C.; Tobian, A.A.R.; Ness, P.M.; Bloch, E.M. Blood transfusion safety in sub-Saharan Africa: A literature review of changes and challenges in the 21st century. *Transfusion* **2019**, *59*, 412–427. [CrossRef] [PubMed]

pathogens

MDPI

Review

Sickle Cell Anemia and *Babesia* Infection

Divya Beri [1], Manpreet Singh [1], Marilis Rodriguez [1], Karina Yazdanbakhsh [2] and Cheryl Ann Lobo [1,*]

1 Department of Blood Borne Parasites, Lindsley F. Kimball Research Institute, New York Blood Center, New York, NY 100065, USA; dberi@nybc.org (D.B.); msingh@nybc.org (M.S.); mrodriguez@nybc.org (M.R.)
2 Department of Complement Biology, Lindsley F. Kimball Research Institute, New York Blood Center, New York, NY 100065, USA; kyazdanbakhsh@nybc.org
* Correspondence: clobo@nybc.org

Abstract: *Babesia* is an intraerythrocytic, obligate Apicomplexan parasite that has, in the last century, been implicated in human infections via zoonosis and is now widespread, especially in parts of the USA and Europe. It is naturally transmitted by the bite of a tick, but transfused blood from infected donors has also proven to be a major source of transmission. When infected, most humans are clinically asymptomatic, but the parasite can prove to be lethal when it infects immunocompromised individuals. Hemolysis and anemia are two common symptoms that accompany many infectious diseases, and this is particularly true of parasitic diseases that target red cells. Clinically, this becomes an acute problem for subjects who are prone to hemolysis and depend on frequent transfusions, like patients with sickle cell anemia or thalassemia. Little is known about *Babesia*'s pathogenesis in these hemoglobinopathies, and most parallels are drawn from its evolutionarily related *Plasmodium* parasite which shares the same environmental niche, the RBCs, in the human host. In vitro as well as in vivo *Babesia*-infected mouse sickle cell disease (SCD) models support the inhibition of intra-erythrocytic parasite proliferation, but mechanisms driving the protection of such hemoglobinopathies against infection are not fully studied. This review provides an overview of our current knowledge of *Babesia* infection and hemoglobinopathies, focusing on possible mechanisms behind this parasite resistance and the clinical repercussions faced by *Babesia*-infected human hosts harboring mutations in their globin gene.

Keywords: *Babesia*; sickle-cell anemia; hemolysis; haemoglobinopathies

Citation: Beri, D.; Singh, M.; Rodriguez, M.; Yazdanbakhsh, K.; Lobo, C.A. Sickle Cell Anemia and *Babesia* Infection. *Pathogens* **2021**, *10*, 1435. https://doi.org/10.3390/pathogens10111435

Academic Editors: Estrella Montero, Jeremy Gray, Luis Miguel González and Lawrence S. Young

Received: 5 October 2021
Accepted: 1 November 2021
Published: 4 November 2021

1. Introduction

Human babesiosis is a zoonotic disease in which the natural acquisition of human cases is most often the result of an interaction with established zoonotic cycles [1,2]. A number of factors have contributed to the emergence of human babesiosis, including increased awareness among physicians, changing ecology, and an increased population of immuno-compromised individuals who exhibit severe disease. *Babesia* belongs to the Phylum Alveolata, Class Apicomplexa Family Piroplasmida and Genus *Babesia* which comprises more than 100 classified species. The four identified *Babesia* species that can infect humans are: *B. microti*, *B. divergens*, *B. duncani* and *B. venatorum*. As molecular techniques are becoming more available and accessible, new species described as "*microti*-like" or "*divergens*-like" are being described [3].

Babesia is an intra-erythrocytic parasite that causes malaria-like symptoms in infected people. *Plasmodium*, the causative agent of malaria, is the most studied Apicomplexan parasite and, like *Babesia*, resides within red blood cells. *Plasmodium* has a long association with its human host dating back to the first report in 1857 [4]. As the erythrocyte provides the parasite with the infra-structure to grow and multiply, it is expected that any perturbation to the cell should impact parasite homeostasis and viability. Clinical, epidemiological, and genome-wide association studies have identified multiple polymorphisms in the globin protein of hemoglobin within the red blood cell (RBC), commonly referred to as hemoglobinopathies, that attenuate or completely abrogate malaria pathogenesis.

Malaria has thus imposed extreme selective pressure on the human genome, far more than any other infectious disease, and the RBC has been the prime target for evolutionary adaptation. The evolutionary proximity of *Plasmodium* and *Babesia* [5], and the fact that they both infect RBCs, raises important clinical questions of *Babesia* infections in patients harboring hemoglobinopathies.

In this paper, we review the literature documenting the effects of hemoglobinopathies on the life cycle of the *Babesia* parasite, using both in vitro and in vivo models of *Babesia* infection. We provide an overview of available clinical cases of the severity of *Babesia* infection in patients harboring these mutations and emphasize why it is essential to focus research in this area. We also describe plausible mechanisms that could exert this protective effect and discuss ways we can use this double-edged sword to develop better therapeutics against blood-borne parasites.

2. Pathogenesis and Anemia in Babesiosis

Hemolytic anemia is the central feature of sickle cell anemia (SCA) that contributes to its severe clinical outcomes. Epidemiological studies and basic research point to the pathogenic role of intravascular hemolysis as the primary cause of clinical complications in SCA. Interestingly, the primary pathological event in babesiosis is also hemolysis, resulting in hemolytic anemia and jaundice. In the absence of aggressive intervention, the anoxia and toxic effects that follow often lead to organ failure and death. Parasitemias do not always relate directly to the degree of anemia, suggesting that erythrocyte destruction is not only due to lysis of infected cells or their removal by splenic and liver macrophages, but also due to lysis of bystander cells which might be a significant contributing factor to the process. Some symptoms, such as fever, myalgia, renal insufficiency, coagulopathy, and hypotension, that occur in *B. microti* infections with parasitemias of less than 1%, may be caused by excessive production of pro-inflammatory cytokines, as also seen in malaria [6,7].

Clinical features in heavy infections, particularly those caused by another major human species, *B. divergens*-like parasites occurring in immuno-compromised patients, exhibit acute illness that appears suddenly with hemoglobinuria as a presenting symptom [8,9]. The clinical presentation also includes persistent non-periodic high fever (40–41 °C), shaking chills, intense sweats, headaches, myalgia, and lumbar and abdominal pain. Jaundice may develop as a result of the high level of hemolysis; vomiting and diarrhea may be present, and the toxins and anoxia, resulting from the hemolysis and the host immunological response, may cause respiratory, cardiac, renal, or hepatic failure [10–12]. The few known infections with *B. venatorum* have shown similar though generally milder manifestations [12].

In our previous report of *B. microti* infections in mice, we reported the increase in hemolysis in *Babesia*-infected mice, which was highly accentuated in mice harboring the SCA genotype, as observed by significantly reduced hematocrit and enhanced hemoglobinuria in these mice [13]. Therefore, these studies indicate that hemolysis is a central mechanism of clinical manifestations of both babesiosis and SCA individually, which is further accentuated and becomes life-threatening in *Babesia* infections in SCA mice/humans.

We found in our infected SCA mouse model that they mount an equally robust adaptive immune response despite exhibiting low parasitemia. This underscores the importance of examining both the fate of *B microti* and the immunological consequences of parasite infection in individuals with SCA to establish whether a similar hyperimmune response against the parasite occurs in humans too. Patients with SCA require transfusions, with some undergoing chronic transfusion therapy, placing them at greater risk of acquiring transfusion-transmitted infections like babesiosis. Thus, these individuals, if transfused from an infected donor, would be exposed to a larger infectious dose compared with a tick bite. The outcome of these infections, whether one of immune protection mediated by the first infection or a more deleterious pathological sequel, is required to be studied to establish effective treatments for these patients [13].

Laboratory findings that are consistent with mild-to-moderate hemolytic anemia include a low hematocrit, low hemoglobin level, low haptoglobin level, elevated reticulocyte count, and elevated lactate dehydrogenase level [14]. Thrombocytopenia is commonly observed. The illness usually lasts for 1 or 2 weeks, but fatigue may persist for months. Asymptomatic parasitemia may persist for several months after standard therapy is initiated or for more than a year if the patient does not receive treatment. Illness may relapse in severely immuno-compromised patients despite 7 to 10 days of antimicrobial therapy and may persist for more than a year if not adequately treated [15].

Patients infected by *B. microti* show a wider range of signs and symptoms. A study on Block Island, Rhode Island, USA, concluded that about 25% of adults and 50% of children are asymptomatic or only show very mild 'flu-like' symptoms in cases that may not result in medical consultation and are therefore rarely diagnosed [16]. At the other end of the spectrum, very severe manifestations, similar to those seen in *B. divergens* infections, may occur in patients who have been splenectomized, are receiving immune-suppressive therapy, or are elderly. These cases typically show high fever, chills, night sweats, myalgia, hemolytic anemia, and hemoglobinuria [17]. Life-threatening complications include acute respiratory failure, disseminated intra-vascular coagulation, congestive heart failure, coma, and renal failure [18]. Immuno-compromised individuals are also likely to develop persistent relapsing disease despite treatment [15]. The symptoms caused by *B. duncani* and related parasites (CA1–4) closely resemble those of *B. microti* infections [19].

3. *Babesia* and the Red Blood Cell

When *Babesia* sporozoites are first injected into the human host, they target the host RBCs immediately, unlike *Plasmodium* spp. which are required to undergo an exo-erythrocytic phase in hepatic cells. Furthermore, *Babesia*-infected RBCs remain circulating in the peripheral blood stream, including regularly passing through the hosts' spleen, and do not sequester to the fine capillaries of the bone marrow or organs. It is the parasite's ability to first recognize and then invade host RBCs that is central to human babesiosis, and the parasites invade RBCs using multiple complex interactions between parasite proteins and the host cell surface, which are not fully elucidated yet [20]. Once inside the RBC, the parasite begins a cycle of maturation and growth exhibited by intense intra-cellular proliferation leading to populations described as 1N, 2N, 4N and >4N [21]. The parasite population can expand inside the RBCs or egress at multiple points in the life cycle [21]. Previous work from our lab has led to the development of synchronized parasite populations and showed the sequential progression of the seven morphological forms of *B. divergens* in culture along with the dynamics of parasite proliferation and differentiation. These processes are maintained through controls that secure the constituent infected-RBC populations in strict ratios to enable rapid movement between new invasion events or further intra-RBC development and replication cycles, as dictated by the environment of the parasite. The early stages of the cycle are morphologically indistinguishable from *Plasmodium* spp., with both appearing as ring-like parasites. However, unlike *Plasmodium*, *Babesia* exhibits plasticity in its life cycle and is thus able to swiftly respond to environmental conditions like host RBCs and nutritional availabilities [22].

4. Hemoglobinopathies

For intracellular parasites, the environment of host red cells plays a key role in the development and success of the pathogen; therefore, perturbations in the RBCs are most likely to modify parasite survival and viability. For blood-borne parasites like *Plasmodium* and *Babesia*, the environments of the RBC, membrane proteins, and hemoglobin, the primary oxygen carrier, are important determinants of parasite success. Human hemoglobin is comprised of alpha and beta globin chains encoded from multiple globin genes. The α-globin gene cluster is at the end of chromosome 16 and contains three genes. The human β-globin gene cluster consists of five genes arranged in chromosome 11 in the same order in which they are expressed during human development: ϵ, Gγ-, Aγ-, δ-, and β-globin gene. The Hb switching event which occurs after birth in the β-globin cluster leads to the suppression of the γ-globin gene accompanied by the complementary increase of the previously silent β-globin gene. Understanding the regulation of Hb switching can have direct therapeutic applications for sickle cell disease in which the γ-globin gene can functionally substitute for mutations in the β-globin gene of these diseases [23]. Hemoglobinopathies are genetic disorders of the globin protein and are classified as structural hemoglobin variants including HbS, HbC and HbE, as described ahead, or thalassemia syndromes [24]. The term 'thalassaemias' collectively refers to several different genetic mutations that result in either reduced or absent expression of one or more of these globin alleles. Specifically, individuals described as having 'α-thalassaemia' have a loss of one or more α-globin allele(s). Additionally, there is also HbH disease (loss of 3 α-globin alleles) and, finally, hydrops fetalis (loss of all 4 α-globin alleles), which leads to the death of the fetus in the uterus. Individuals with mutations in HBB can also have a range of genetic defects referred to as 'β-thalassaemia', including β-thalassaemia minor (reduced expression of one β-globin allele), and β-thalassaemia major (reduced expression of both β-globin alleles) [25].

Sickle cell disease (SCD) is the most common monogenic blood disorder of hemoglobin synthesis, encompassing the single replacement mutation of glutamic acid at position 6 of the β-globin chain by valine (HbSS genotype) [26–28]. The hallmark of SCD is "the sickle-shaped" red blood cells due to the polymerization of mutated sickle hemoglobin (HbS) under low oxygen tension. Chronic blood transfusion is one of the most effective treatments in SCD and results in the reduction of the frequency of acute pain episodes and acute chest syndrome but causes a dramatic increase in the risk of transfusion-transmitted infection [29]. The HbSS and HbAS (heterozygous) genotypes are commonly found in populations from sub-Saharan Africa. The Hemoglobin C (HbC) mutation (HbAC–heterozygotes; HbCC–homozygotes) also involves a point mutation at the 6th codon in the HBB gene, resulting in a glutamic acid to lysine substitution and is most common in West Africa, with prevalence reported as high as 15% in parts of Burkina Faso [30]. The Hemoglobin E (HbE) mutation is a point mutation that results in a glutamic acid to lysine switch at position 26 of the HBB gene and is most commonly found in parts of Southeast Asia and India and reaches a prevalence of up to 60% in some areas [31,32]. HbS, HbC, and HbE are characterized as structural hemoglobin variants. The major human hemoglobinopathies and related genetic mutations are summarized in Table 1. According to CDC Reports in 2010, the total incidence estimate for sickle cell trait was 15.5 cases per 1000 births in USA, ranging from 0.8 cases per 1000 births in Montana to 34.1 cases per 1000 births in Mississippi. The U.S. incidence estimate for sickle cell trait (based on information provided by 13 states) was 73.1 cases per 1000 black newborns, 3.0 cases per 1000 white newborns, and 2.2 cases per 1000 Asian or Pacific Islander newborns. The incidence estimate for Hispanic ethnicity was 6.9 cases per 1000 Hispanic newborns. The total number of babies born with sickle cell trait in 2010 was estimated to be greater than 60,000. The study showed that as many as 1.5% of babies born in the United States have the sickle cell trait [33]. With approximately 7% of the worldwide population being carriers, hemoglobinopathies are the most common monogenic diseases and one of the world's major health problems. This makes it very essential to understand the pathogenesis of blood-borne parasites in human hosts harboring these mutations in their RBCs.

Table 1. Major hemoglobinopathies and related genetic mutations.

Hemoglobinopathy	**Mutation**	**Position**
HbS	Glutamic Acid to Valine	β-6
HbC	Glutamic Acid to Lysine	β-6
HbE	Glutamic Acid to Lysine	β-26
Thalassemia	**Gene Modifications**	**Disease Name**
α-Thalassemia	- - / - α	HbH disease
	- - / - -	α-Thalassemia major
β-Thalassemia	β°/β	β-Thalassemia minor
	β°/β°	β-Thalassemia major

Denotes: (-) loss of α-globin gene. (β°) loss of β-globin [34,35].

5. Natural Resistance against Blood-Borne Parasites

The long association and co-evolution of the malaria parasite with humans is reflected in the fact that almost all examples of molecular evolution in humans, like sickle cell anemia, G6PD-deficiency, and thalassemia, are attributed to a selection of mutations that attenuate malaria pathogenesis. Though these mutations lead to unpleasant consequences, as of 2015 it was estimated that about 4.4 million people have sickle cell disease, while an additional 43 million have sickle cell traits [36]. Zones that are endemic for malaria have a high proportion of humans carrying these mutations either in the homozygous form (the subject suffers from the disease caused due to the mutation) or heterozygous form (one copy of normal gene and one copy of mutated gene). These genes have all arisen in areas in which falciparum malaria is endemic, and their rise to high levels of prevalence is thought to result from their conferring significant degrees of protection against this dreaded pathogen. It is well-established that the homozygotes suffer from sickling of RBCs but do not support the rapid growth of the parasite; however, in rare cases, subjects with SCD and malaria can suffer from hyper-hemolytic crisis [37]. Heterozygotes do not suffer from sickling and have lesser severity of malaria. AS subjects can get malaria, but the number of parasitized cells is low, and they rarely suffer from cerebral malaria or severe anemia [37]. The enhanced resistance of persons with sickle traits to falciparum malaria is substantial. Infected AS children have lower parasite densities than AA children and are 50–90% less likely to progress to a severe form of malaria or to die from the disease [38]. *Babesia*'s association with hemoglobinopathies is not completely understood but is an important field of research as hemolytic anemia is common in hemoglobinopathies and can be life-threatening when coupled with *Babesia* infection.

There have been several explanations as to why β-globin might confer resistance to malaria. Researchers have reported that parasitized AS cells sickle more readily and show enhanced HbS polymerization under hypoxic conditions and are therefore removed from circulation. Further, it has been shown that parasites are fragile and killed by these HbS polymers. A compelling cause of reduced parasite load in AS and SS RBCs is the extent of oxidative damage which is inherent in these host cells added to the oxidative stress due to parasite growth; the cumulative oxidant damage can cause considerable damage to the host RBC and impairment of parasite development [39]. Interestingly, accumulated reactive oxygen species (ROS)-mediated damage is a common mechanism shared by AS, SS, G6PD-deficient, β- and α-thalassemia RBCs in mediating resistance to malaria [40,41]. However, the mechanism for ROS-mediated protection in malaria remains elusive. It was also observed that AS RBCs parasitized with *P. falciparum* late stages bound to human microvascular endothelial cells and blood monocytes half as effectively as did comparably infected AA RBCs. Moreover, infected AS RBCs displayed slightly reduced and highly uneven distribution of expression of PfEMP-1 on their surface. There is also evidence based on host microRNAs playing a role in protection in AS and SS RBCs [38,42–50]. There have been several plausible mechanisms proposed for resistance of hemoglobinopathic RBCs to malaria, but little is known about *Babesia* in this regard. Given the parallels between the two parasites, it is tempting to speculate that they might share mechanisms of resistance to growth in hemoglobinopathic RBCs.

6. *Babesia* and the Sickle Red Cell

The RBC serves as the home for this intra-erythrocytic parasite for its entire life cycle in the human host. The interactions between the parasite and the RBC can be classified into three broad areas: invasion, growth and maturation within the RBC, and egress. Previous studies from our group have examined these phases of the intra-erythrocytic lifecycle of *Babesia divergens* in homozygous SS and heterozygous AS human blood [51]. While the invasion was similar across all RBCs, there was atypical population progression, a potential loss of merozoite infectivity, and defective egress of the parasite in SS cells (as explained in Figure 1). Unlike previous reports in *Plasmodium*, AS cells supported invasion, growth, and egress of *Babesia* much like AA cells. While parasites grew from their characteristic 1N to

2N, 4N and >4N populations in AA and AS cells, in SS host cells beyond 24 h, the majority of the parasites were stuck in the 1N phase as demonstrated in Figure 1. Interestingly, even when parasites growing in SS RBCs were supplemented with fresh AA RBCs, they did not grow [51]. This indicates that the initial invasion and growth in SS host cells programs the parasite irreversibly to poor growth and/or defects in egress. Our work on the mouse model using *B. microti* also showed poor growth of the parasite in mice harboring the SS gene (HbSS-Townes mice), and normal growth in AS mice when compared to the wildtype AA mice [13]. For AA and AS mice, parasitemias peaked on day 7 of infection, while the SS mice exhibited a sluggish increase in parasitemias. In all three genotypes, parasites were cleared by day 21 and all mice survived. Interestingly, while the parasitemia was 4–5-fold lower in SS mice, the extent of immune response mounted was the same in AA, AS and SS mice. The adaptive immune response was measured by a robust GC reaction and significant expansion of TFH cells. Currently, it is not known how these SS mice respond to subsequent *Babesia* infection. This becomes especially critical to understand as babesiosis is primarily a transfusion-transmitted infection and since several sickle cell patients undergo repeated blood transfusions, they may be exposed to a parasite load that could be more than the parasites in one tick bite.

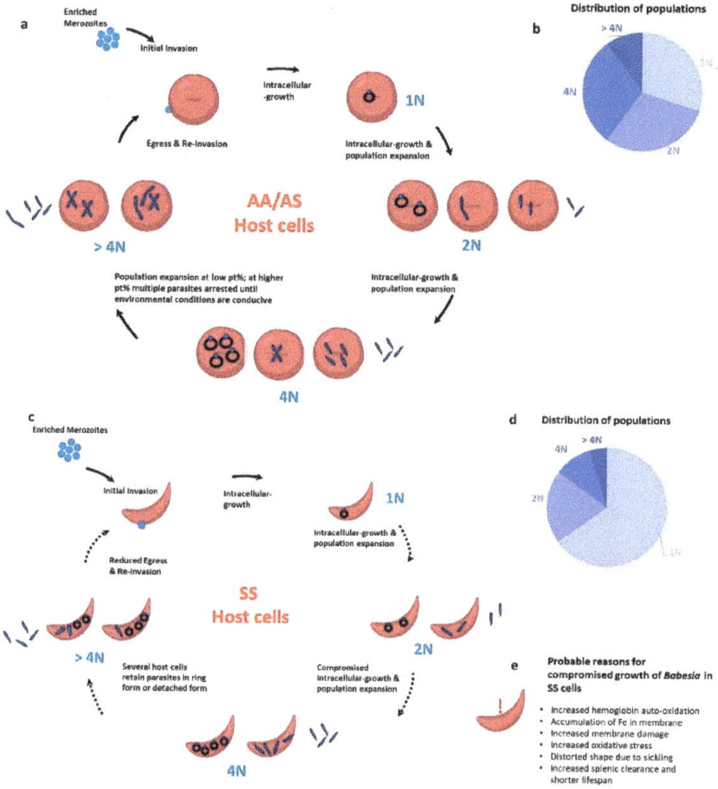

Figure 1. *Babesia* infection progression in wild type (AA) RBCs, heterozygous for sickle cell anemia (AS) RBCs, and homozygous for sickle cell anemia (SS) RBCs. (**a**) In AA and AS host cells, the merozoite invades and the parasite develops inside the RBCs to 1N, 2N, 4N and >4N populations. Egress can take place at 2N, 4N or >4N stage. (**b**) The distribution percentage of 1N, 2N and 4N parasites is similar. (**c**) In SS host RBCs, parasites mostly retain their "ring form" and very few "Maltese cross" forms are seen. (**d**) As shown in the pie chart, a high population of parasites get stuck in the 1N form. (**e**) List of probable reasons for compromised growth of *Babesia* parasites in SS cells.

CDC reported that from 1979 to 2009, 159 transfusion-related *Babesia microti* cases were identified, most (77%) of which were from 2000 to 2009 [52]. A recent review in 2016 has summarized the state-wise seropositivity of *B. microti* in the blood used for transfusion in the USA [53]. However, no data are available on the number of sickle patients transfused with *Babesia*-contaminated blood.

7. Clinical SCA and Babesiosis

There have been scattered case reports of babesiosis in sickle cell patients transmitted via blood transfusions. Transfusion-acquired babesiosis can result in severe hemolytic anemia in patients with sickle cell disease. The infection can be difficult to treat and may require a prolonged treatment duration [54]. A recent study presented a case of two sickle cell patients who had delayed diagnosis post transfusion due to confusing symptoms: as patients who receive chronic transfusions are also at risk for the development of allo- and autoantibodies, the hemolytic anemia caused by the former can often obscure a different pathophysiology, such as babesiosis, which occurred with these patients. In another case, diagnosis took 4 months for a patient with HbSS and babesiosis, after repeated visits to the hospital [54,55]. Another study reported a young female with HbSC who presented in the emergency department multiple times with pain and shortness of breath, eventually developing unresponsiveness and a brief episode of pulseless electrical activity. She was admitted to the intensive care unit with multisystem organ failure and found to have diffuse ischemic strokes. Infectious workup revealed disseminated anaplasmosis and babesiosis, which had likely caused sickle cell crisis. The patient continued to show a significant neurologic burden, despite months of treatment [56]. Evidently, with increased awareness about babesiosis among physicians and more sensitive diagnostic tests available, the number of case reports on babesiosis have increased. Given that there is a significant incidence of SCA carriers/other hemoglobinopathies in *Babesia*-endemic zones (like north-eastern USA) who require frequent transfusions, it becomes increasingly necessary to understand *Babesia* pathogenesis in such subjects.

8. Plausible Mechanisms for Resistance of *Babesia* in Sickle Cells

From previous work of our group, the outstanding question is why the parasite exhibits developmental/egress abnormalities when growing in a sickle cell as opposed to a wild type AA RBC host. There are multiple possible causes for this: It is well known that sickle cells have a high burden of oxidative stress due to repeated polymerization and depolymerization of hemoglobin. It is also well known that a wide variety of intracellular pathogens like *Plasmodium*, *Mycobacterium*, and several viruses impose redox stress on their host cells. Therefore, unfavorable host cell conditions, like increased hemoglobin autoxidation, accumulation of iron in membranes, increased membrane damage, and a shorter red cell life span, could justify the reason why SS cells do not promote growth of the *Babesia* species. Further, the bystander effect, whereby uninfected RBCs are also affected leading to increased hemolysis, has been widely described in malaria. It is possible that in SS subjects there is an accentuated bystander effect leading to massive hemolysis and therefore unfavorable conditions for the parasite to grow and proliferate. It is also possible that invasion/growth of the parasite modifies the shape of the sickling RBCs, making them more prone to splenic removal. Our study in the mouse model has clearly shown that even though parasitemias are much lower in SS mice as compared to AA mice, the adaptive immune response is almost as severe; therefore, the heightened immune response against the parasite might be another SS-specific strategy to abrogate the growth of *Babesia*. In future studies, it would be interesting to monitor the growth of *Babesia* in other hemoglobinopathic disorders like thalassemia and RBC enzymopathy like G6PD-deficiency, both of which are known to afford resistance to malaria. However, unlike *Plasmodium*, AS mice showed no protection against babesiosis and followed the same parasite growth curve both in vitro and in vivo. Thus, from the current experiments, heterozygotes for the mutated beta globin gene do not seem to be protected against babesiosis.

9. Concluding Remarks and Future Directions

Hemoglobin-associated genetic disorders affect millions throughout the world and are concentrated in humans living in malaria-endemic countries. However, as borders of countries are becoming more porous, these genetic traits are now seen throughout the world. For several years, researchers have observed that hemoglobinopathies afford protection from malaria and the studies from our group in *Babesia* also point in that direction. Given the evolutionary proximity between these two parasites, it is possible that resistance to their growth in SS cells has a common mechanism. Further studies are needed to understand if the growth of *Babesia* parasites in thalassemic RBCs and those with an inherent deficiency in the G6PD enzyme is similarly impaired and to determine how these mutations hinder intra-erythrocytic parasite growth. These results will provide researchers with an opportunity to discover the Achilles' heel of two deadly parasites and learn how nature has evolved a way to protect against these diseases. Uncovering the mechanism behind this protection will lead us to a better understanding of their pathogenesis as well as in designing better drugs against these parasites. As described above, multiple mechanisms of resistance against parasite proliferation in sickle cells may operate to confer protection. A detailed study of these pathways is needed to identify the main pathways in *Babesia*-infected red cells and this, in turn, will shed light on the intricate interplay between polymorphisms of the human host red cells and intruding parasites.

Funding: This research was funded by National Institutes of Health P01 HL149626 (K.Y. and C.A.L.) and R01HL140625 (C.A.L.) and a grant from BNY Mellon (K.Y. and C.A.L.).

Institutional Review Board Statement: Not applicable.

Informed Consent Statement: Not applicable.

Data Availability Statement: Not applicable.

Conflicts of Interest: The authors declare no conflict of interest.

References

1. Lobo, C.A.; Cursino-Santos, J.R.; Alhassan, A.; Rodrigues, M. *Babesia*: An Emerging Infectious Threat in Transfusion Medicine. *PLoS Pathog.* **2013**, *9*, e1003387. [CrossRef]
2. Ord, R.L.; Lobo, C.A. Human Babesiosis: Pathogens, Prevalence, Diagnosis, and Treatment. *Curr. Clin. Microbiol. Rep.* **2015**, *2*, 173–181. [CrossRef]
3. Yabsley, M.J.; Shock, B.C. Natural history of Zoonotic *Babesia*: Role of wildlife reservoirs. *Int. J. Parasitol. Parasites Wildl.* **2013**, *2*, 18–31. [CrossRef]
4. Arrow, K.J.; Panosian, C.; Gelband, H. (Eds.) *Saving Lives, Buying Time: Economics of Malaria Drugs in an Age of Resistance*; National Academies Press: Washington, DC, USA, 2004.
5. Lau, A.O. An overview of the *Babesia*, *Plasmodium* and *Theileria* genomes: A comparative perspective. *Mol. Biochem. Parasitol.* **2009**, *164*, 1–8. [CrossRef]
6. Clark, I.A.; Jacobson, L.S. Do babesiosis and malaria share a common disease process? *Ann. Trop. Med. Parasitol.* **1998**, *92*, 483–488. [CrossRef]
7. Raju, M.; Salazar, J.C.; Leopold, H.; Krause, P.J. Atovaquone and Azithromycin Treatment for Babesiosis in an Infant. *Pediatr. Infect. Dis. J.* **2007**, *26*, 181–183. [CrossRef]
8. Slovut, D.P.; Benedetti, E.; Matas, A.J. Babesiosis and Hemophagocytic Syndrome in an Asplenic Renal Transplant Recipient. *Transplantation* **1996**, *62*, 537–539. [CrossRef]
9. Brasseur, P.; Gorenflot, A. Human babesiosis in Europe. *Memórias Inst. Oswaldo Cruz* **1992**, *87*, 131–132. [CrossRef]
10. Zintl, A.; Mulcahy, G.; Skerrett, H.E.; Taylor, S.M.; Gray, J.S. *Babesia divergens*, a Bovine Blood Parasite of Veterinary and Zoonotic Importance. *Clin. Microbiol. Rev.* **2003**, *16*, 622–636. [CrossRef]
11. Borggraefe, I.; Yuan, J.; Telford, S.R., 3rd; Menon, S.; Hunter, R.; Shah, S.; Spielman, A.; Gelfand, J.A.; Wortis, H.H.; Vannier, E. *Babesia microti* Primarily Invades Mature Erythrocytes in Mice. *Infect. Immun.* **2006**, *74*, 3204–3212. [CrossRef]
12. Hunfeld, K.-P.; Hildebrandt, A.; Gray, J.S. Babesiosis: Recent insights into an ancient disease. *Int. J. Parasitol.* **2008**, *38*, 1219–1237. [CrossRef]
13. Yi, W.; Bao, W.; Rodriguez, M.; Liu, Y.; Singh, M.; Ramlall, V.; Cursino-Santos, J.R.; Zhong, H.; Elton, C.M.; Wright, G.J.; et al. Robust adaptive immune response against *Babesia microti* infection marked by low parasitemia in a murine model of sickle cell disease. *Blood Adv.* **2018**, *2*, 3462–3478. [CrossRef]
14. Akel, T.; Mobarakai, N. Hematologic manifestations of babesiosis. *Ann. Clin. Microbiol. Antimicrob.* **2017**, *16*, 6. [CrossRef]

15. Krause, P.J.; Gewurz, B.E.; Hill, D.; Marty, F.M.; Vannier, E.; Foppa, I.M.; Furman, R.R.; Neuhaus, E.; Skowron, G.; Gupta, S.; et al. Persistent and Relapsing Babesiosis in Immunocompromised Patients. *Clin. Infect. Dis.* **2008**, *46*, 370–376. [CrossRef]
16. Lantos, P.M.; Krause, P.J. Babesiosis: Similar to Malaria but Different. *Pediatr. Ann.* **2002**, *31*, 192–197. [CrossRef]
17. White, D.J.; Talarico, J.; Chang, H.G.; Birkhead, G.S.; Heimberger, T.; Morse, D.L. Human babesiosis in New York State: Review of 139 hospitalized cases and analysis of prognostic factors. *Arch. Intern. Med.* **1998**, *158*, 2149–2154. [CrossRef]
18. Hatcher, J.C.; Greenberg, P.D.; Antique, J.; Jimenez-Lucho, V.E. Severe Babesiosis in Long Island: Review of 34 Cases and Their Complications. *Clin. Infect. Dis.* **2001**, *32*, 1117–1125. [CrossRef]
19. Kjemtrup, A.M.; Conrad, P.A. Human babesiosis: An emerging tick-borne disease. *Int. J. Parasitol.* **2000**, *30*, 1323–1337. [CrossRef]
20. Lobo, C.A.; Cursino-Santos, J.R.; Singh, M.; Rodriguez, M. *Babesia divergens*: A Drive to Survive. *Pathogens* **2019**, *8*, 95. [CrossRef]
21. Cursino-Santos, J.R.; Singh, M.; Pham, P.; Rodriguez, M.; Lobo, C.A. *Babesia divergens* builds a complex population structure composed of specific ratios of infected cells to ensure a prompt response to changing environmental conditions. *Cell. Microbiol.* **2015**, *18*, 859–874. [CrossRef]
22. Cursino-Santos, J.R.; Singh, M.; Pham, P.; Lobo, C.A. A novel flow cytometric application discriminates among the effects of chemical inhibitors on various phases of *Babesia divergens* intraerythrocytic cycle. *Cytom. Part A* **2017**, *91*, 216–231. [CrossRef]
23. Cao, A.; Moi, P. Regulation of the Globin Genes. *Pediatr. Res.* **2002**, *51*, 415–421. [CrossRef]
24. Kohne, E. Hemoglobinopathies. *Dtsch. Aerzteblatt Int.* **2011**, *108*, 532–540. [CrossRef]
25. Taylor, S.M.; Cerami, C.; Fairhurst, R.M. Hemoglobinopathies: Slicing the Gordian Knot of *Plasmodium falciparum* Malaria Pathogenesis. *PLoS Pathog.* **2013**, *9*, e1003327. [CrossRef]
26. Booth, C.; Inusa, B.; Obaro, S.K. Infection in sickle cell disease: A review. *Int. J. Infect. Dis.* **2010**, *14*, e2–e12. [CrossRef]
27. Kato, G.J.; Piel, F.B.; Reid, C.D.; Gaston, M.H.; Ohene-Frempong, K.; Krishnamurti, L.; Smith, W.R.; Panepinto, J.A.; Weatherall, D.J.; Costa, F.F.; et al. Sickle cell disease. *Nat. Rev. Dis. Prim.* **2018**, *4*, 18010. [CrossRef]
28. Rees, D.C.; Williams, T.N.; Gladwin, M.T. Sickle-cell disease. *Lancet* **2010**, *376*, 2018–2031. [CrossRef]
29. Noubouossie, D.; Key, N.S.; Ataga, K.I. Coagulation abnormalities of sickle cell disease: Relationship with clinical outcomes and the effect of disease modifying therapies. *Blood Rev.* **2016**, *30*, 245–256. [CrossRef]
30. Piel, F.B.; Patil, A.P.; Howes, R.E.; Nyangiri, O.A.; Gething, P.W.; Dewi, M.; Temperley, W.H.; Williams, T.N.; Weatherall, D.J.; Hay, S. Global epidemiology of sickle haemoglobin in neonates: A contemporary geostatistical model-based map and population estimates. *Lancet* **2013**, *381*, 142–151. [CrossRef]
31. Williams, T.N.; Weatherall, D.J. World Distribution, Population Genetics, and Health Burden of the Hemoglobinopathies. *Cold Spring Harb. Perspect. Med.* **2012**, *2*, a011692. [CrossRef]
32. Goheen, M.M.; Campino, S.; Cerami, C. The role of the red blood cell in host defence against falciparum malaria: An expanding repertoire of evolutionary alterations. *Br. J. Haematol.* **2017**, *179*, 543–556. [CrossRef]
33. Ojodu, J.; Hulihan, M.M.; Pope, S.N.; Grant, A.M.; Centers for Disease Control and Prevention. Incidence of sickle cell trait—United States, 2010. *MMWR Morb. Mortal. Wkly. Rep.* **2014**, *63*, 1155–1158.
34. Chonat, S.; Quinn, C.T. Current Standards of Care and Long Term Outcomes for Thalassemia and Sickle Cell Disease. *Neurobiol. Essent. Fat. Acids* **2017**, *1013*, 59–87. [CrossRef]
35. Wiwanitkit, V. Single amino acid substitution in important hemoglobinopathies does not disturb molecular function and biological process. *Int. J. Nanomed.* **2008**, *3*, 225–227. [CrossRef]
36. Sundd, P.; Gladwin, M.T.; Novelli, E.M. Pathophysiology of Sickle Cell Disease. *Annu. Rev. Pathol. Mech. Dis.* **2019**, *14*, 263–292. [CrossRef]
37. Luzzatto, L. Sickle Cell Anaemia and Malaria. *Mediterr. J. Hematol. Infect. Dis.* **2012**, *4*, e2012065. [CrossRef]
38. Bunn, H.F. The triumph of good over evil: Protection by the sickle gene against malaria. *Blood* **2013**, *121*, 20–25. [CrossRef]
39. Díaz-Castillo, A.; Contreras-Puentes, N.; Alvear-Sedán, C.; Moneriz-Pretell, C.; Rodríguez-Cavallo, E.; Mendez-Cuadro, D. Sickle Cell Trait Induces Oxidative Damage on *Plasmodium falciparum* Proteome at Erythrocyte Stages. *Int. J. Mol. Sci.* **2019**, *20*, 5769. [CrossRef] [PubMed]
40. Senok, A.; Nelson, E.; Li, K.; Oppenheimer, S. Thalassaemia trait, red blood cell age and oxidant stress: Effects on *Plasmodium falciparum* growth and sensitivity to artemisinin. *Trans. R. Soc. Trop. Med. Hyg.* **1997**, *91*, 585–589. [CrossRef]
41. Cyrklaff, M.; Srismith, S.; Nyboer, B.; Burda, K.; Hoffmann, A.; Lasitschka, F.; Adjalley, S.; Bisseye, C.; Simpore, J.; Mueller, A.-K.; et al. Oxidative insult can induce malaria-protective trait of sickle and fetal erythrocytes. *Nat. Commun.* **2016**, *7*, 13401. [CrossRef] [PubMed]
42. Luzzatto, L.; Nwachuku-Jarrett, E.; Reddy, S. Increased Sickling of Parasitised Erythrocytes as Mechanism of Resistance against Malaria in the Sickle-Cell Trait. *Lancet* **1970**, *295*, 319–322. [CrossRef]
43. Roth, E.F., Jr.; Friedman, M.; Ueda, Y.; Tellez, I.; Trager, W.; Nagel, R.L. Sickling Rates of Human as Red Cells Infected in Vitro with *Plasmodium falciparum* Malaria. *Science* **1978**, *202*, 650–652. [CrossRef] [PubMed]
44. Friedman, M.J. Erythrocytic mechanism of sickle cell resistance to malaria. *Proc. Natl. Acad. Sci. USA* **1978**, *75*, 1994–1997. [CrossRef]
45. Pasvol, G.; Weatherall, D.J.; Wilson, R.J.M. Cellular mechanism for the protective effect of haemoglobin S against *P. falciparum* malaria. *Nat. Cell Biol.* **1978**, *274*, 701–703. [CrossRef]
46. Friedman, M.J. Ultrastructural Damage to the Malaria Parasite in the Sickled Cell. *J. Protozool.* **1979**, *26*, 195–199. [CrossRef] [PubMed]
47. Griffiths, M.J.; Ndungu, F.; Baird, K.L.; Muller, D.P.R.; Marsh, K.; Newton, C. Oxidative stress and erythrocyte damage in Kenyan children with severe *Plasmodium falciparum* malaria. *Br. J. Haematol.* **2001**, *113*, 486–491. [CrossRef]

48. Hebbel, R.P. Beyond hemoglobin polymerization: The red blood cell membrane and sickle disease pathophysiology. *Blood* **1991**, *77*, 214–237. [CrossRef]
49. Fairhurst, R.M.; Baruch, D.I.; Brittain, N.J.; Ostera, G.R.; Wallach, J.S.; Hoang, H.L.; Hayton, K.; Guindo, A.; Makobongo, M.O.; Schwartz, O.M.; et al. Abnormal display of PfEMP-1 on erythrocytes carrying haemoglobin C may protect against malaria. *Nat. Cell Biol.* **2005**, *435*, 1117–1121. [CrossRef] [PubMed]
50. Cholera, R.; Brittain, N.J.; Gillrie, M.R.; Lopera-Mesa, T.M.; Diakité, S.A.S.; Arie, T.; Krause, M.A.; Guindo, A.; Tubman, A.; Fujioka, H.; et al. Impaired cytoadherence of *Plasmodium falciparum*-infected erythrocytes containing sickle hemoglobin. *Proc. Natl. Acad. Sci. USA* **2008**, *105*, 991–996. [CrossRef]
51. Santos, J.R.C.; Singh, M.; Senaldi, E.; Manwani, D.; Yazdanbakhsh, K.; Lobo, C.A. Altered parasite life-cycle processes characterize *Babesia divergens* infection in human sickle cell anemia. *Haematologica* **2019**, *104*, 2189–2199. [CrossRef]
52. Herwaldt, B.L.; Linden, J.V.; Bosserman, E.; Young, C.; Olkowska, D.; Wilson, M. Transfusion-Associated Babesiosis in the United States: A Description of Cases. *Ann. Intern. Med.* **2011**, *155*, 509–519. [CrossRef] [PubMed]
53. Levin, A.E.; Krause, P.J. Transfusion-transmitted babesiosis: Is it time to screen the blood supply? *Curr. Opin. Hematol.* **2016**, *23*, 573–580. [CrossRef] [PubMed]
54. Karkoska, K.; Louie, J.; Appiah-Kubi, A.O.; Wolfe, L.; Rubin, L.; Rajan, S.; Aygun, B. Transfusion-transmitted babesiosis leading to severe hemolysis in two patients with sickle cell anemia. *Pediatr. Blood Cancer* **2018**, *65*, e26734. [CrossRef]
55. Bloch, E.M.; Herwaldt, B.L.; Leiby, D.A.; Shaieb, A.; Herron, R.M.; Chervenak, M.; Reed, W.; Hunter, R.; Ryals, R.; Hagar, W.; et al. The third described case of transfusion-transmitted *Babesia duncani*. *Transfusion* **2012**, *52*, 1517–1522. [CrossRef]
56. Herbst, J.; Crissinger, T.; Baldwin, K. Diffuse Ischemic Strokes and Sickle Cell Crisis Induced by Disseminated Anaplasmosis: A Case Report. *Case Rep. Neurol.* **2019**, *11*, 271–276. [CrossRef] [PubMed]

pathogens

Review

Technologies for Detection of *Babesia microti*: Advances and Challenges

Scott Meredith, Miranda Oakley and Sanjai Kumar *

Laboratory of Emerging Pathogens, Division of Emerging and Transfusion-Transmitted Diseases, Office of Blood Research and Review, Food and Drug Administration, Silver Spring, MD 20993, USA; Scott.Meredith@fda.hhs.gov (S.M.); Miranda.Oakley@fda.hhs.gov (M.O.)
* Correspondence: Sanjai.Kumar@fda.hhs.gov

Abstract: The biology of intraerythrocytic *Babesia* parasites presents unique challenges for the diagnosis of human babesiosis. Antibody-based assays are highly sensitive but fail to detect early stage *Babesia* infections prior to seroconversion (window period) and cannot distinguish between an active infection and a previously resolved infection. On the other hand, nucleic acid-based tests (NAT) may lack the sensitivity to detect window cases when parasite burden is below detection limits and asymptomatic low-grade infections. Recent technological advances have improved the sensitivity, specificity and high throughput of NAT and the antibody-based detection of *Babesia*. Some of these advances include genomics approaches for the identification of novel high-copy-number targets for NAT and immunodominant antigens for superior antigen and antibody-based assays for *Babesia*. Future advances would also rely on next generation sequencing and CRISPR technology to improve *Babesia* detection. This review article will discuss the historical perspective and current status of technologies for the detection of *Babesia microti*, the most common *Babesia* species causing human babesiosis in the United States, and their implications for early diagnosis of acute babesiosis, blood safety and surveillance studies to monitor areas of expansion and emergence and spread of *Babesia* species and their genetic variants in the United States and globally.

Keywords: *Babesia microti*; antibody-based assays; nucleic acid tests; multiplex detection; next generation sequencing

Citation: Meredith, S.; Oakley, M.; Kumar, S. Technologies for Detection of *Babesia microti*: Advances and Challenges. *Pathogens* **2021**, *10*, 1563. https://doi.org/10.3390/pathogens10121563

Academic Editors: Estrella Montero, Jeremy Gray and Cheryl Ann Lobo

Received: 5 October 2021
Accepted: 29 November 2021
Published: 30 November 2021

1. Introduction

Babesia microti is an intraerythrocytic, apicomplexan parasite that is the primary agent responsible for human babesiosis in the United States. *B. microti* is transmitted sporadically in many temperate regions of the world, but its prevalence is highest in New England and the northern Midwest region of the United States [1–4]. In spite of its global transmission and public health impact, *B. microti* infections often remain undetected, resulting in undiagnosed or delayed diagnosis of acute babesiosis cases, which could be fatal in vulnerable individuals, and asymptomatic chronic infections, which present a risk to blood safety. At the time of the discovery of the parasites responsible for babesiosis in livestock in 1888, diagnosis relied on the then-new technology of microscopic examination of stained blood films [5]. The first case of human babesiosis was identified in 1957, and an outbreak on Nantucket Island established the disease in the United States [6–11]. Since this time, disease prevalence has increased sharply from only a few cases a year to as many as 2418 in the United States in 2019 [12]. Detection technologies have improved accordingly, but the biology of *B. microti*. and its infection kinetics in humans present unique challenges that have not been fully met by any one detection technology.

Advancements in the technologies for *B. microti* detection have improved diagnostic capability, primarily by making the reliable identification of low-grade early infections for clinical diagnosis possible and the monitoring of treatment. In addition, superior assay sensitivity provides a valuable tool to identify blood donors with chronic, low-grade infections, as the *B. microti* parasite is one of the most commonly transfusion-transmitted pathogens in United States. In this review article, we discuss the advances in detection methods for *B. microti*, in the context of clinical diagnosis, epidemiology and molecular surveillance, and blood safety since the discovery of the parasite over 130 years ago. The field of *Plasmodium* parasite detection and epidemiology is more advanced compared to *Babesia*. Given the biological similarities and detection challenges, we have drawn parallels and applied lessons from this pathogen throughout the article.

2. *Babesia microti* Biology and Detection Challenges

The dynamics of the natural course of human babesial infection has still yet to be fully defined in absence of a human challenge model. Our knowledge of the kinetics of infection and parasite burden mostly comes from observations in clinical and epidemiological studies and data from asymptomatic blood donors in endemic areas. From a clinical standpoint, it is assumed that most symptomatic babesiosis cases develop within 1 to 4 weeks following exposure, but clinicians are recommended to consider babesial infection in patients with tick bites within the previous six months [13]. Furthermore, tick bites are often unnoticed, which, in addition to complicating diagnosis, makes extrapolation of the incubation period difficult [13]. Transfusion-transmitted babesiosis (TTB) cases provide a more definitive timepoint for acquisition of the infection, though patients are not monitored for infection early after transfusion before the onset of symptoms. Nevertheless, in these cases, evidence suggests that the incubation period of *B. microti* prior to the appearance of illness ranges from one to nine weeks in most cases, though one patient did not develop symptoms until six months after transfusion of infected blood product [14].

The intraerythrocytic nature of *B. microti* infection presents several challenges to effective detection of the parasite. Blood film microscopy and xenodiagnosis are the most direct methods for *Babesia* diagnosis. Parasite nucleic acid and antigen detection are considered the reliable biomarkers of active infection, whereas antibodies can be indicative of active infection or a previously resolved infection. After a tick bite or transfusion of infected blood product, parasitemia remains below detectable limit during the early phase of infection (window period), followed by a relatively higher parasitemia (acute) phase and finally a persistent (chronic) infection in some individuals (Figure 1).

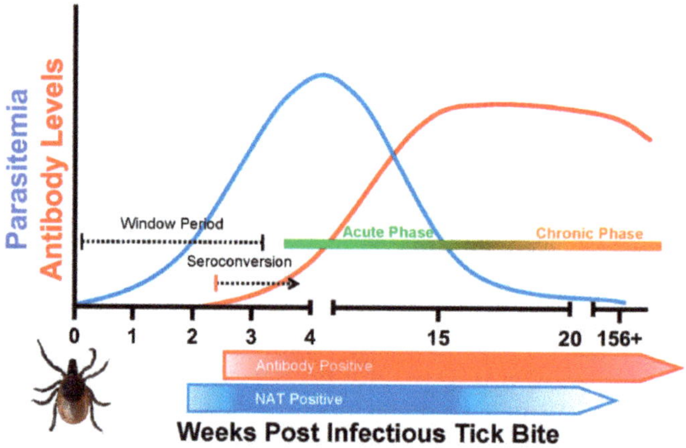

Figure 1. A schematic of course of *Babesia microti* infection and induction and duration of antibody response after an infectious tick bite in a healthy human host. The time frame for the window period (time to infectious bite to first detection of parasitemia), acute phase and chronic phase of infection are based on the observations from clinical cases, epidemiological studies and follow up studies in transfusion-transmitted infections.

Experimental infection of rhesus monkeys is the only available data describing early *B. microti* infection kinetics in primates. Intravenous inoculation resulted in parasitemia detectable by microscopy in seven of eight monkeys after prepatent periods ranging from 15 to 46 days [15]. On the other hand, infection transmitted via tick bite was established in four of five monkeys after a prepatent period of 13 to 28 days [16]. In these studies, blood film microscopy was the only tool employed to determine the early infection, and it is not known when molecular assays would have become effective.

In humans, parasite burdens higher than 1% are commonly observed in acute severe babesiosis patients. A review of 139 human babesiosis cases requiring hospitalization found a significant correlation between disease severity and parasitemia $\geq$ 4% [17]. While high parasitemias are a useful marker in identifying risk of severe outcomes, severe cases can develop in individuals with lower parasitemias. Another case series of 34 patients with babesiosis requiring hospitalization found the median parasitemia in these severe cases to be 7.6%, though individuals ranged from 0.1% to 30%; anemia was more strongly correlated with severe outcomes than parasitemia [18]. Parasitemia has been observed as high as 85% in an asplenic individual [19].

The proportion of *Babesia* infections that persist as asymptomatic, chronic infections is not clearly known. In one study on Block Island (Rhode Island), one-third of *Babesia* infections were asymptomatic [20], although the sample size was too small to draw firm conclusions. In addition, in endemic areas, the contribution of reinfection to chronic parasitemia has not been investigated. Nonetheless, results from limited clinical observations and donor screening for *Babesia* by nucleic acid-based test (NAT) assays are beginning to shed some light on the duration of the persistence of *B. microti* infections in asymptomatic individuals living in endemic areas. In one case report, *B. microti* infection, based on polymerase chain reaction (PCR) results, may persist for up to 27 months without overt clinical illness [21]. However, in an investigational study on blood donors in endemic areas, in the majority of NAT-positive donors the parasitemic period was reported to last from 2–7 months by a PCR-based test [22]. In contrast to the acute parasitemic phase, parasite burden during persistent chronic infection phase is significantly lower, but wide ranging and generally not detectable by microscopy. Results from one study (based on extrapolations from a laboratory-based PCR assay) showed the presence of 5 parasites to 3 million parasites per mL in asymptomatic blood donors in endemic areas [22].

The detection of early infection prior to seroconversion (window period cases) is even more challenging and important for early diagnosis and treatment, particularly in vulnerable population groups. Thus, a combination of detection biomarkers and further technological advances would be required for early diagnosis, epidemiology and to monitor the genetic diversity and geographical spread of human babesiosis in the United States and globally.

3. Detection Techniques

In the near century and a half since the identification of the parasites that would come to populate the *Babesia* genus, the methods used for detection of the parasites in blood samples have, obviously, become much more sensitive. This became especially true in the latter half of the 20th century as human babesiosis emerged from a medical curiosity to a true public health threat. Modern molecular techniques are at least 10- to 20-fold more sensitive compared to those used at the time of the identification of the parasites, and new technologies on the horizon promise to increase sensitivity while optimizing time and resource economy, providing adaptable platforms with the possibility of multiplexing and possibly elucidating correlations between biomarkers and clinical status or outcomes (Figure 2).

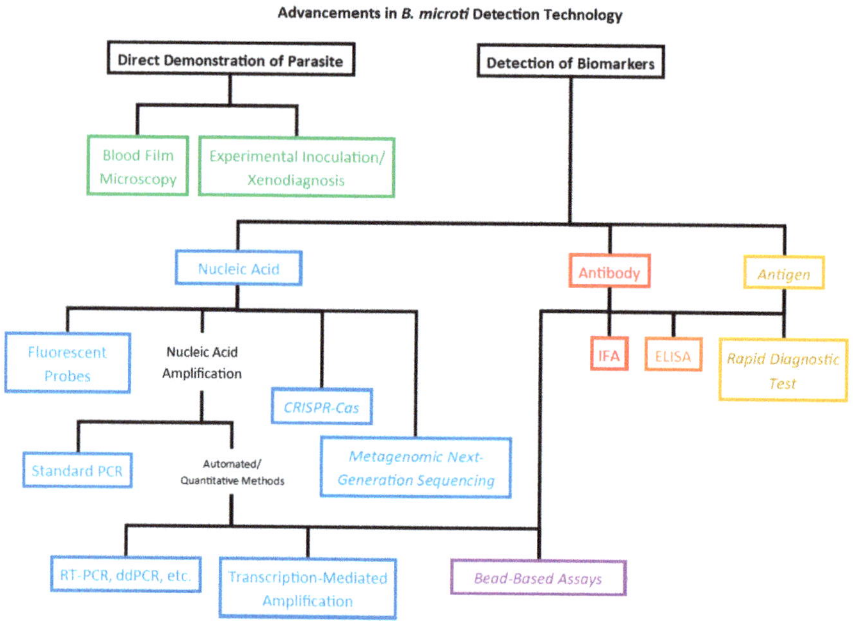

Figure 2. Diagram depicting developments in *B. microti* detection technology. Detection of biomarkers of infection are classified according to the type of biomarker: nucleic acid (blue), antibody (red), or antigen (yellow). Bead-based methods (purple) can be adapted for detection of either nucleic acid or antibody, while ELISA (orange) can be used to detect antibody or antigen. Technologies in italics have been developed for other pathogens and are proposed for detection of *B. microti* but have not yet been effectively adapted.

3.1. Direct Demonstration of B. microti Parasites

3.1.1. Experimental Inoculation

Xenodiagnosis and experimental inoculation have long been tools for the diagnosis of babesial infection. Babes employed Robert Koch's third postulate, requiring reproduction of the disease upon inoculation into a healthy, susceptible host in his initial identification of *Babesia* parasites. He did not observe clinical signs in inoculated cattle or other large livestock, though he did see significant disease in inoculated rabbits [5]. Hamsters have been used for the experimental inoculation of *B. microti*, while gerbils, splenectomized calves, and SCID mice are used when appropriate for other *Babesia* species [23,24]. Direct observation of parasites on a blood film is generally easier and much less time consuming for all but the lowest parasitemia cases, as the inoculation of susceptible animal models will take 7–10 days before appreciable amplification of the parasites can be detected. In addition, procuring animals for each diagnosis is significantly more expensive and resource-intensive. Nevertheless, experimental inoculation was a common alternate diagnostic technique for low-parasitemia cases for nearly 100 years until the advent of highly sensitive serological and molecular procedures for *Babesia* detection [24,25].

3.1.2. Blood Film Microscopy

The discovery of the *Babesia* parasite in 1888 by Babes was slightly preceded by the identification of many other blood-borne pathogens, most notably the human malaria parasite in 1880 by Alphonse Levaran [26]. On a Giemsa-stained blood film, the abundant *B. microti* ring-like trophozoites resemble those of *P. falciparum*, though *Babesia* spp. rings tend to be larger with more variation in size and shape. Additionally, *Babesia* spp. rings do not contain pigment and may be vacuolated. Trophozoites divide by binary fission, usually twice, producing a cruciform merozoite structure known as a tetrad or "Maltese Cross" (Figure 3). This form is rare but is pathognomic of *Babesia* infection [27].

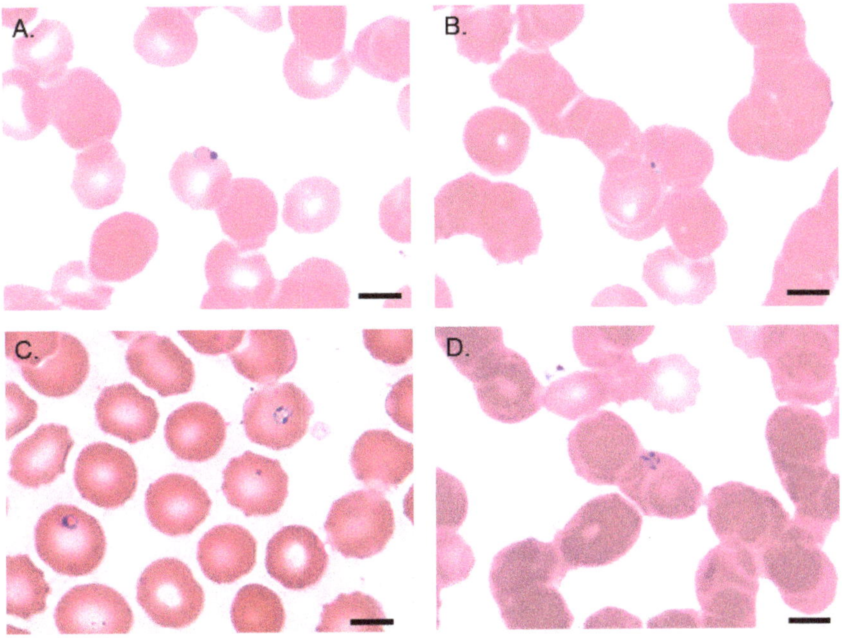

Figure 3. Images from a Giemsa-stained blood film from a human infected with *B. microti*. Trophozoites appear in (**A**) ring forms or in (**B**) mature, amoeboid forms. Merozoites can be seen as (**C**) a multinucleated body during division or as (**D**) tetrads, called the "Maltese Cross" form, following two rounds of division. Scale bar represents 5 μm.

In the case of malaria, the limit of detection of a thick blood smear is approximately 10–50 parasites/μL (at least 0.0002% parasitemia), while a thin blood smear alone is roughly 20–40 times less sensitive even under ideal conditions [28]. Furthermore, it has been estimated that the practical limit of detection in a routine diagnostic screen is closer to 100 parasites/μL (0.002% parasitemia) [29,30]. The limit of detection by microscopy has not been determined for *Babesia*. However, similarities in parasite morphology and the blood film preparation method indicate a limit of detection comparable to *Plasmodium* detection by microscopy. Therefore, even if a potential *B. microti*-infected sample is screened with a thick smear and confirmed by thin smear, the risk of failing to identify parasites in prepatent or convalescent stages or among asymptomatic carriers is large. Parasitemia is frequently less than 1%, especially early in infection when treatment is often sought [31], so while blood films can be valuable for confirmation of diagnoses in a low-volume setting, higher-throughput and more sensitive techniques are needed to meet the need presented by the emergence of *B. microti* as a public health threat.

3.2. Detection of Biomarkers of B. microti Infection

3.2.1. Nucleic Acid-Based Assays

Since the early 1990s, methods for molecular detection based on the PCR amplification of *B. microti* genes have been tested and validated [24,32–34]. The results have shown that molecular methods provide a superior option for the detection of *B. microti* than blood film microscopy. Notably, the increased sensitivity of molecular detection methods has improved the detection of low-grade early infections (window period cases) and chronic infections [22,35]. While complete data are not available for *Babesia* spp. detection, the

World Health Organization Methods Manual for the evaluation of *P. falciparum* blood smears indicates that approximately 0.333 μL of blood is screened in a standard thick smear, yielding a limit of detection of roughly 20 parasites per μL [36]. By comparison, even early PCR protocols for *P. falciparum* detection could reliably detect 20 times fewer parasites from a 10-fold smaller sample volume [37]. In addition, molecular methods are better suited for the species differentiation of different *Babesia* strains, as differentiation by microscopy can be difficult or impossible [38].

Recent advances in *B. microti* genomics and detection technologies have led to the development of assays of higher sensitivity and high-throughput platforms for diagnosis, molecular surveillance and blood safety. The adaptation of real-time PCR technology to *B. microti* detection increased the sensitivity dramatically over standard PCR techniques [33]; an early diagnostic RT-PCR protocol exhibited a limit of detection that was roughly ten-fold lower than standard PCR [39,40].

The sample volume used in the assay is another major consideration that determines the sensitivity and limit of detection of an assay. While Persing et al. detected roughly 3 parasites in a 50 μL standard PCR reaction, Bloch et al. calculated a limit of detection of 12.92 parasites per 2 mL of blood by their RT-PCR protocol [33,40]. This equates to roughly 0.39 parasites per 50 μL, which emphasizes the potential impact of sampling error on the sensitivity of molecular detection methods; the procedure may be extraordinarily sensitive, but the sample size may be too small to contain target nucleic acid.

The droplet digital PCR platform has been adapted to *B. microti* detection and achieves sensitivity and limits of detection comparable to RT-PCR [40,41]. In addition, transcription-mediated amplification has been employed in an FDA-licensed detection assay for *B. microti* and has a 95% detection limit of approximately 3 parasites per mL [35].

The *B. microti* genome sequence was first published in 2012 [42]. Analyses revealed a genome of approximately 6.5 Mbp encoding around 500 polypeptides, which is the smallest of all Apicomplexan nuclear genomes [42]. A combination of genomics-based antigen discovery and computational sequence analyses have allowed for the identification of novel high-copy-number conserved detection targets, which was previously not available [42–44]. For example, the 18S ribosomal RNA gene is the most commonly used amplification target for *Babesia* spp. detection [33,35,41]. Recently, high-copy-number BMN family genes were evaluated for analytical sensitivity by RT-PCR. In this study, the 18S rRNA gene produced a limit of detection of 30.9 parasites per mL, while the BMN primer set detected as few as 10.0 parasites per mL [45]. Table 1 summarizes the sensitivity of blood film microscopy, experimental inoculation and nucleic acid-based detection of *Babesia* parasites in blood.

Table 1. Limit of detection for direct observation and molecular methods of detection of *Babesia microti*.

Method	Target	Limit of Detection	Reference
Blood Film		20–100 pRBCs */μL	[28–30]
Experimental Inoculation		63 pRBCs/inoculation [into mice]	[46]
Fluorescent Nucleic Acid Probes		100 pg DNA (~30 parasites)[*B. bovis* **]	[47]
PCR	18S rRNA	3 parasites/50 μL	[33]
RT-PCR	18S rRNA	12.92 parasites/2 mL	[40]
	BMN genes	10 pRBCs/mL	[45]
ddPCR	18S rRNA	10 copies	[41]
TMA	18S rRNA	3 pRBCs/mL	[35]

* Parasitized red blood cells. ** No data are available for *B. microti*; this technique was applied for animal *Babesia* species.

To better understand genetic diversity and evolutionary relationships, investigators have begun to sequence the *B. microti* genome from parasite isolates collected from around the world. In one comprehensive study, the complete genome sequencing of 42 *B. microti* samples from different parts of the world showed extensive genetic diversity [48]. As anticipated, *B. microti* samples from the continental US are genetically distant from samples from Alaska, Russia and Japan. In the U.S., deep genetic divergence was noted between samples from the Northeast and the Midwest. Minimal genetic diversity was noted among the New England samples, though three sub-populations exist: Nantucket, mainland New England and the R1 reference group [48]. A study based on a 32 single nucleotide polymorphism (SNP) barcode assay supported previous findings and identified two distinct lineages among the New England and Midwestern *B. microti* parasites [49]. SNP-based barcode assays developed from genome-wide sequencing of recently circulating *B. microti* isolates could be an important surveillance tool to monitor genetic diversity in clinical cases and in the expanding areas of transmission.

It is anticipated that novel high-copy-number conserved gene targets identified by genome analyses, multiplexing for simultaneous detection of *Babesia* species and sub-populations circulating in an area and technological advances including detection target enrichment in a sample would further improve the sensitivity, specificity and applicability of *B. microti* NAT assays for diagnosis, surveillance and blood safety purposes.

3.2.2. Antigen Detection Assays

Antigens expressed by an invading pathogen serve as a reliable biomarker to detect an active infection for many pathogens. Antigen-based rapid detection tests (RDT) are a mainstay of malaria diagnosis in endemic areas. No laboratory-based or commercial RDT for the diagnosis of *B. microti* is available, though potential biomarkers of infection have been identified. In 2000, Lodes et al. screened *B. microti* antigens for immunoreactivity in serological tests [50]; Homer et al. later verified the antigenicity of several novel antigens with the aim of supporting the development of a diagnostic assay [51]. *B. microti* alpha-helical cell surface protein 1 (BmBAHCS1, also known as BmGPI12 [52], BMN1-9 [50] and BmSA1 [53]), a secreted *B. microti* antigen, was identified by Cornillot et al. as the most sensitive antigen for the detection of active infections [52]. Anti-BmBAHCS1 antibodies can be detected in serum as early as 4 (IgM) to 8 (IgG) days following infection in mice, indicating that the detection of the antigen could reduce the window period before the development of a detectable antibody titer [43,52].

Thekkiniath et al. developed an antigen capture assay for the detection of BmBAHCS1 that had a limit of detection of 20 pg/μL in in vitro samples [54]. However, it only identified six of seven clinical samples, failing to detect a sample with a parasitemia of 0.3% [54]. Therefore, further improvements to the assay are required before its widespread adoption. Applications of a combination of genome-wide screening, transcriptional profiling and antigenic characterization in functional assays has led to identification of a large number of immunodominant excreted and secreted and surface-anchored *B. microti* antigens that deserve evaluation as biomarker(s) of active infection [43,44,50,55,56].

Antigen-detection technology is highly advanced for malaria diagnosis. According to the World Health Organization, in 2019, 348 million malaria RDTs were sold globally [57]. The majority of malaria RDTs are based on the plasmodium falciparum histidine-rich protein-2 (PfHRP-2), which is the most reliable marker available for the diagnosis of acute and asymptomatic P. falciparum infections in endemic settings. However, recently, an alarming number of reports indicate deletions of the PfHRP2/PfHRP3 gene and a reduced sensitivity of the HRP-2 based RDTs, thus threatening the effectiveness of HRP-2 based RDTs as a public health tool against malaria [58,59]. These results strongly indicate that *B. microti* antigen-based detection assays should also rely on multiple antigens to offset potential sensitivity loss due emerging polymorphism in target antigens.

In summary, there has been no systematic approach to explore the potential of antigens as biomarkers for diagnosis of human babesiosis. If adequately sensitive and specific, antigen detection-based assays could be an attractive option for the rapid clinical diagnosis and detection of asymptomatic chronic infections in endemic areas.

3.2.3. Antibody-Based Assays

Antibodies are the most sensitive and reliable markers for detection of *Babesia* exposure, albeit with potential limitations in detection in the early phase of infection prior to seroconversion and inability to distinguish between active infection and previously resolved infections. In the early 1970s, several groups began developing indirect immunofluorescence assay (IFA) for the detection of the antibodies indicative of *Babesia* infection in animals, as human babesiosis was rare and considered a curious, if relatively insignificant zoonosis [60–62]. By the end of the decade, enough human cases had been identified in residents of Nantucket Island to make the establishment of a standardized protocol for indirect immunofluorescent detection of antibodies directed at *B. microti* antigens necessary and feasible [25,63]. Among antibody-based tests, IFA has been demonstrated to be the most sensitive and detect 100% of blood film-positive acute babesiosis cases and is expected to be highly sensitive in detecting donors with asymptomatic *Babesia* infections, whereas antibody titers are maintained by a low-grade infection [22,25].

However, there has been debate in the literature surrounding the threshold distinguishing active from cleared infections. Chisolm et al. developed the first sensitive and specific technique for the immunofluorescent detection of antibody specific for antigens on the surface of infected erythrocytes and determined that active cases in the acute phase of infection can be loosely defined by a detectable IgG antibody titer of $\geq$1:1024 [63]. Boustani and Gelfand recommend a titer of $\geq$1:256 as suggestive of acute infection, while the Centers for Disease Control and Prevention adds that samples from individuals epidemiologically linked to *B. microti* exposure need only exhibit reactivity at a titer of $\geq$1:64 to be considered a babesiosis case [64,65].

Inter-genus cross-reactivity in indirect immunofluorescence assays is usually low when detecting anti-*B. microti* antibodies, and cross-reactivity with other *Babesia* species is often observed only at lower dilutions [63].

B. microti-specific IgG may persist for months or years following infection, which, while valuable for serosurveys that are largely agnostic to the time of infection, could complicate the use of serological tests for diagnostic or donor screening purposes [66]. Ruebush et al. characterized the development of an antibody response to *B. microti* with respect to the onset of symptoms and found that the peak antibody titer was reached around three to four weeks following the onset of symptoms, after which titers decreased over the next several months [67]. The rate of antibody titer decrease was different for each patient and was not correlated with initial antibody titer or severity of illness. One patient was followed for six years after illness and still had an appreciable antibody titer [67]. In a more recent large investigational study, the median time of seroreversion (IFA titer of less than 1:64) in blood donors was 17.1 months [22].

Enzyme-linked immunosorbent assay (ELISA) protocols have been developed for the detection of *B. microti*-specific antibodies using antigens harvested from infected hamsters [68] or mice [69] or using recombinant proteins [44,50,53,70]. The most common antigens exploited by serological assays have been those of the BMN family [50,53]. Historically, compared to IFA, ELISA has been considered less sensitive and specific in detecting acute babesiosis and asymptomatic infections, indicating the need to identify additional immunodominant *B. microti* antigens for use as synthetic peptides or recombinant protein(s) as coating antigens. Recently, a combination of three novel immunodominant *B. microti* antigens (*Babesia microti* Maltese Cross form related protein 1 [BmMCFRP1], *Babesia microti* serine reactive antigen 1 [BmSERA1], and *Babesia microti* piroplasm β-Strand domain 1 [BmPiβS]), when used in combination with the previously described immunodominant antigen BmBAHCS1, yielded 100% sensitivity in the detection of *B. microti*-positive serum samples by ELISA [44].

Thus, it appears that multiple antigens may be needed to achieve the desired sensitivity for an automated alternative to IFA for human babesiosis. Another consideration is the identification of *B. microti* antigens that associated with antibody responses induced during the early phase of infection and could also distinguish between active and resolved infections. To date, no studies have investigated a temporal correlation of parasitemia or clinical condition with titer of antibodies to specific *B. microti* antigens throughout the course of infection. Assays based on such antigens would have a high prognostic value and applications in identifying asymptomatically infected individuals in endemic areas.

4. Multiplex Assays

Multiplex assays for *B. microti* have become quite common, as the ability to distinguish between it and other tick-borne diseases in a given area has become more vital. Multiplex PCR assays using standard PCR protocols and fragment size differentiation have been employed for decades [71], but now the RT-PCR platform can easily be adapted to distinguish separate species with the use of fluorescent probes specific for distinct target genes. Historically, these assays have been of particular use in veterinary fields, as livestock and domesticated animals tend to be exposed to a far greater breadth of tick-borne pathogens that need to be distinguished [71,72]. Another application of multiplex PCR assays is for the surveillance of the tick population in a given region to establish the probable rate of exposure to given pathogens [73,74]. RT-PCR techniques routinely detect as few as 10 copies per sample in multiplex assays [74].

Multiplex PCR assays for the detection of tick-borne pathogens in humans are being developed. Buchan et al. evaluated a high definition PCR (HDPCR) panel which contained primers for amplification of target genes of nine species and species groups of tick-borne pathogens [75]. The panel is intended to be an adjunct diagnostic resource for the differentiation of clinical cases suspected to be caused by tick-borne pathogens. The researchers validating the panel observed 100% specificity relative to gold-standard PCR assays for several of the pathogens but did not observe any samples positive for *B. microti* in 530 whole blood specimens, despite high sensitivity among simulated single- and co-infected blood samples. Sensitivity for *Borrelia burgdorferi* was lacking at only 44% relative to standard PCR [75]. It remains to be established whether the lack of detection to *B. microti* is due to performance of the assay or is indicative of the low prevalence of infection among the sample population.

The Luminex bead platform provides an attractive alternative to RT-PCR for multiplex detection assays, as conjugation to xMAP beads allows for the concentration and enhanced differentiation of PCR products. A commercial multiplex bead assay was validated by Livengood et al. for the surveillance of genus- and species-level infection rates of *I. scapularis* ticks [76]. The assay has not been applied to human samples to date. Limits of detection in ticks varied widely across species, but as few as four copies of the *B. microti* target gene (18S rRNA) could be detected [76].

Another application of the multiplex bead assay is the conjugation of recombinantly expressed antigens to spectrally distinct luminescent beads for the detection of antibody specific for each pathogen in a sample. This technique has been applied to differentiation of *B. microti, B. duncani,* and *B. divergens* exposure in human samples [77]. Similar to bead-based PCR techniques, bead-based antibody assays capitalize on the large surface area of the beads for capturing and concentrating the antigen-specific antibody, while relying on species specificity that appears to be characteristic of most human *Babesia* species [76–81].

5. Novel and Future Technologies

5.1. Next Generation Sequencing

Next generation sequencing (NGS) has revolutionized all aspects of medicine. NGS is also being extensively evaluated for the diagnosis and tracking of infectious diseases. The metagenomics NGS (mNGS) is an unbiased approach for the detection of bacteria, fungi, viruses and parasites in clinical samples [82–84]. This approach combines the genome sequencing of genetic materials in a biological sample, bioinformatics analysis for exclusion of human reads and pathogen identification based on sequence alignment to a curated database [85]. While mNGS has been successfully applied for pathogen detection including discovery of novel pathogens in clinical samples, sensitivity, specificity and high-cost considerations must be addressed for the routine application of this approach for the routine diagnosis of infection diseases including human babesiosis.

5.2. CRISPR Technology

The CRISPR-Cas system is a component of prokaryotic adaptive immunity that protects microbes from invading bacteriophage or plasmid DNA by specifically cleaving foreign genetic elements [86]. In this system, RNA encoding a memorized sequence of foreign DNA "guides" a caspase to a matching target sequence from an invading phage or plasmid that is then destroyed by degradation. Due to its ability to edit genomes, the CRISPR-Cas system has been applied to develop therapeutics to treat genetic diseases. In recent years, the CRISPR-Cas system has also been utilized to develop a new class of rapid, inexpensive, easy-to-use detection systems with high sensitivity and specificity.

The CRISPR-Cas systems of some bacteria contain caspases that collaterally cleave single-stranded nucleic acid in addition to targeting foreign genetic elements. Cas12a and Cas13a (formally C2c2) indiscriminately cleave single-stranded DNA [87] and single-stranded RNA [88], respectively. These systems have been used to develop CRISPR collateral cleavage-based molecular detection platforms where the cleavage of an amplified target pathogen sequence activates collateral cleavage of single-stranded fluorescent or colorimetric reporter molecules. DNA endonuclease-targeted CRISPR trans reporter (DETECTR) [87] and Specific High-Sensitivity Enzymatic Reporter unLOCKing (SHERLOCK) [89] are two diagnostic platforms that use Cas12a and Cas13a to detect DNA and RNA, respectively.

To date, CRISPR-based diagnostics have not been applied to the detection of *Babesia*. However, Cunningham et al. used SHERLOCK CRISPR collateral cleavage-based diagnostics to develop a fast, low-cost deployable assay capable of *Plasmodium* detection, species differentiation and drug-resistance genotyping [90]. This CRISPR-based SHERLOCK assay uses an isothermal RPA reaction to generate double-stranded DNA amplicons of the target sequence, in vitro transcription of RPA product to produce single-stranded RNA (ssRNA) targets and the collateral cleavage of fluorescent or colorimetric RNA reporter molecules to produce a detection signal. When compared to real-time PCR, the *P. falciparum* SHERLOCK assay achieved 94% sensitivity and 94% specificity.

The CRISPR technology warrants the evaluation of species-differentiating detection of human *Babesia* spp. in a high-throughput platform for diagnostic and donor screening purposes.

6. Blood Donor Screening

Transfusion-transmitted babesiosis (TTB) is caused by the transfusion of blood and blood products collected from an asymptomatically infected donor. The first case of TTB was reported in 1979 [91]. Since then, more than 250 reported cases of TTB have been reported in the U.S. [10,92–94]. Data collected from the national babesiosis surveillance program and other published reports indicate that the clinical burden, areas of transmission and risk to the U.S. blood supply are increasing [10,35,93–95]. The intraerythrocytic nature of the parasite and lack of knowledge on minimum parasite burden in the asymptomatic chronic phase of infection present unique challenges in detecting *Babesia* infection in blood donors.

In the past 15 years, laboratory-based NAT and antibody tests have been applied to assess *B. microti* risk in random blood donors in endemic areas. These studies have been useful to gain information on the relative value of NAT and antibodies in identifying asymptomatically infected donors and have shed light on the relationship between seropositivity and parasitemia and the seasonality of transmission in endemic areas [96–98]. More recently, two large prospective studies conducted under Investigational New Drug protocols have further enhanced our understanding of the prevalence of *B. microti* infections in asymptomatic healthy blood donors and the rate of window period cases in endemic areas and nonendemic states [22,35,99]. In one investigational study, a total of 89,153 blood donations were screened in four *Babesia* endemic states. Of these, 335 (0.38%) were positive by IFA, and 67 were also PCR positive (20% of IFA+; 0.075% total). A total of nine blood donations were IFA negative but PCR positive (window period cases; 0.01%). Interestingly, 86% of all PCR-positive donors became DNA negative in a one year follow up, while only 8% had seroreversion during the same period, confirming that antibodies continues to persist long after parasitemia clearance [22]. The second investigational study was conducted in 11 endemic states plus Washington D.C. and Florida (nonendemic). Of the 176,926 blood donations initially screened, 61 were confirmed to be positive. Among these samples, 35 (57%; 0.020% of total) were PCR positive and 59 (97%; 0.033% of total) were antibody positive, and 2 (3%; 0.001% of total) were PCR positive but antibody negative (window period cases) [35]. These prospective investigational studies have clearly shown that donor screening for *Babesia* infection allowed for the identification of potentially infectious blood units and thus a valuable tool to minimize the TTB risk to blood supply. Additionally, results complied from the surveillance programs [10,92,93] and investigational studies [22,96] have shown that while tick-borne transmission is seasonal, parasitemic donors can be found year-round. The other finding from these studies indicates that due to travels to endemic areas from nonendemic areas and interstate transport of blood, TTB risk exits outside the outside the bounds of recognized endemic states [100,101].

In May 2019, the FDA issued a guidance document recommending screening blood donors for evidence of *Babesia* infection in 14 high-risk states plus Washington, D.C. through the use of a licensed *Babesia* NAT assay. The effectiveness of regional donor screening for *Babesia* by a licensed NAT assay will be determined based on a significant reduction in the TTB cases in United States.

7. Assay Validation

Generally, freshly collected *B. microti* patient samples of known parasite count (by microscopy) are not available for assay validation for diagnosis or blood donor screening. Therefore, the validation of detection assays typically relies on *B. microti* parasites propagated in mice or hamsters and spiked into whole human blood. A reference panel consisting of whole blood spiked with *B. microti* parasites harvested from mice was used to support the licensure of two NAT assays intended for screening blood donations *for B. microti*. By comparison, nucleic acid standards for assay validation of other pathogens, such as Hepatitis C virus (HVC) [102] and human immunodeficiency virus 1 (HIV-1) [103], rely on high-titer isolates from clinical cases or blood product donations. These isolates may be expanded in vitro prior to dilution in human plasma. Efforts should be made to develop validated reference panels based on *B. microti*-infected red blood cells and/or nucleic acid (DNA and RNA) prepared from blood samples from babesiosis patients. Such reference panels should be validated in collaborative studies and made available to assay developers in academia and industry.

8. Conclusions

Genomics-based antigen discovery and the incorporation of technological advancements have led to the development of superior NAT and antibody-based assays for human diagnosis. Likewise, the availability of highly sensitive and specific, high-throughput *Babesia* NAT assays have, for the first time, allowed regional donor screening for *Babesia* in endemic states.

Antibody assays based on novel *Babesia* antigens may shorten the window period and allow us to distinguish between acute, persistent chronic and a previously resolved infections.

Antigen-detection based assays in multiplex ELISA format and as RDTs for diagnostics and blood donor screening are awaiting development. It is anticipated that the next generation of assays would also incorporate technological advances offered by mNGS and CRISPR technology.

Author Contributions: Each author made substantial contributions to the conceptualization and writing of the manuscript. All authors have read and agreed to the published version of the manuscript.

Funding: This research was funded by the Food and Drug Administration Intramural Research Program (#6001).

Institutional Review Board Statement: Not applicable.

Informed Consent Statement: Not applicable.

Data Availability Statement: Not applicable.

Acknowledgments: The authors would like to acknowledge Kazuyo Takeda for providing the microscopy images. The views expressed here are those of the authors and do not represent those of the Food and Drug Administration.

Conflicts of Interest: The authors declare no conflict of interest.

References

1. Homer, M.J.; Aguilar-Delfin, I.; Telford, S.R., 3rd; Krause, P.J.; Persing, D.H. Babesiosis. *Clin. Microbiol. Rev.* **2000**, *13*, 451–469. [CrossRef]
2. Hunfeld, K.-P.; Hildebrandt, A.; Gray, J.S. Babesiosis: Recent insights into an ancient disease. *Int. J. Parasitol.* **2008**, *38*, 1219–1237. [CrossRef]
3. Vannier, E.; Krause, P.J. Human babesiosis. *N. Engl. J. Med.* **2012**, *366*, 2397–2407. [CrossRef]
4. Zhou, X.; Hong-Xiang, Z.; Huang, J.-L.; Tambo, E.; Zhuge, H.-X.; Zhou, X.-N. Human babesiosis, an emerging tick-borne disease in the People's Republic of China. *Parasites Vectors* **2014**, *7*, 1–10. [CrossRef]
5. Babes, V. Sur l'hemoglobinuria bacterienne des boeufs. *Comptes Rendus De L'académie Des Sci.* **1888**, *107*, 693–694.
6. Skrabalo, Z.; Deanovic, Z. Piroplasmosis in man; report of a case. *Doc. Med. Geogr. Trop.* **1957**, *9*, 11–16. [PubMed]
7. Telford, S.R.; Gorenflot, A.; Brasseur, P.; Spielman, A. Babesial infections in humans and wildlife. In *Parasitic Protozoa*, 2nd ed.; Kreier, J.P., Ed.; Academic Press: San Diego, CA, USA, 1993; pp. 1–47.
8. Scholtens, R.G.; Gleason, N.; Braff, E.H.; Healy, G.R. A case of babesiosis in man in the United States. *Am. J. Trop. Med. Hyg.* **1968**, *17*, 810–813. [CrossRef]
9. Piesman, J.; Spielman, A. Human babesiosis on Nantucket Island: Prevalence of *Babesia microti* in ticks. *Am. J. Trop. Med. Hyg.* **1980**, *29*, 742–746. [CrossRef] [PubMed]
10. Gray, E.B.; Herwaldt, B.L. Babesiosis surveillance—United States, 2011–2015. *MMWR Surveill. Summ.* **2019**, *68*, 1–11. [CrossRef] [PubMed]
11. Western, K.A.; Benson, G.D.; Gleason, N.N.; Healy, G.R.; Schultz, M.G. Babesiosis in a Massachusetts Resident. *N. Engl. J. Med.* **1970**, *283*, 854–856. [CrossRef]
12. Centers for Disease Control and Prevention (CDC). Surveillance for Babesiosis—United States, 2019 Annual Summary. 2021. Available online: https://www.cdc.gov/parasites/babesiosis/resources/Surveillance_Babesiosis_US_2019.pdf. (accessed on 23 November 2021).
13. Vannier, E.G.; Diuk-Wasser, M.A.; Ben Mamoun, C.; Krause, P.J. Babesiosis. *Infect. Dis. Clin. North Am.* **2015**, *29*, 357–370. [CrossRef]
14. Vannier, E.; Krause, P.J. 100—Babesiosis. In *Hunter's Tropical Medicine and Emerging Infectious Disease (Ninth Edition)*; Magill, A.J., Hill, D.R., Solomon, T., Ryan, E.T., Eds.; W.B. Saunders: London, UK, 2013; pp. 761–763.
15. Ruebush, T.K., 2nd; Collins, W.E.; Healy, G.R.; Warren, M. Experimental *Babesia microti* infections in non-splenectomized *Macaca mulatta*. *J. Parasitol.* **1979**, *65*, 144–146. [PubMed]
16. Ii, T.K.R.; Warren, M.; Spielman, A.; Collins, W.E.; Piesman, J. Tick Transmission of *Babesia microti* to Rhesus Monkeys (*Macaca mulatta*). *Am. J. Trop. Med. Hyg.* **1981**, *30*, 555–559. [CrossRef]
17. White, D.J.; Talarico, J.; Chang, H.-G.; Birkhead, G.S.; Heimberger, T.; Morse, D.L. Human babesiosis in New York State: Review of 139 hospitalized cases and analysis of prognostic factors. *Arch. Intern. Med.* **1998**, *158*, 2149–2154. [CrossRef]
18. Hatcher, J.C.; Greenberg, P.D.; Antique, J.; Jimenez-Lucho, V.E. Severe babesiosis in Long Island: Review of 34 cases and their complications. *Clin. Infect. Dis.* **2001**, *32*, 1117–1125. [CrossRef]
19. Sun, T.; Tenenbaum, M.J.; Greenspan, J.; Teichberg, S.; Wang, R.T.; Degnan, T.; Kaplan, M.H. Morphologic and clinical observations in human infection with *Babesia microti*. *J. Infect. Dis.* **1983**, *148*, 239–248. [CrossRef]
20. Krause, P.J.; McKay, K.; Gadbaw, J.; Christianson, D.; Closter, L.; Lepore, T.; Telford, S.R., 3rd; Sikand, V.; Ryan, R.; Persing, D.; et al. Increasing health burden of human babesiosis in endemic sites. *Am. J. Trop. Med. Hyg.* **2003**, *68*, 431–436. [CrossRef]
21. Krause, P.J.; Spielman, A.; Telford, S.R., 3rd; Sikand, V.K.; McKay, K.; Christianson, D.; Pollack, R.J.; Brassard, P.; Magera, J.; Ryan, R.; et al. Persistent parasitemia after acute babesiosis. *N. Engl. J. Med.* **1998**, *339*, 160–165. [CrossRef] [PubMed]

22. Moritz, E.D.; Winton, C.S.; Tonnetti, L.; Townsend, R.L.; Berardi, V.P.; Hewins, M.-E.; Weeks, K.E.; Dodd, R.Y.; Stramer, S.L. Screening for *Babesia microti in* the U.S. blood supply. *N. Engl. J. Med.* **2016**, *375*, 2236–2245. [CrossRef]
23. Gorenflot, A.; Moubri, K.; Precigout, E.; Carcy, B.; Schetters, T.P. Human babesiosis. *Ann. Trop. Med. Parasitol.* **1998**, *92*, 489–501. [CrossRef]
24. Krause, P.J.; Telford, S., 3rd; Spielman, A.; Ryan, R.; Magera, J.; Rajan, T.V.; Christianson, D.; Alberghini, T.V.; Bow, L.; Persing, D. Comparison of PCR with blood smear and inoculation of small animals for diagnosis of *Babesia microti* parasitemia. *J. Clin. Microbiol.* **1996**, *34*, 2791–2794. [CrossRef]
25. Krause, P.J.; Telford, S.R., 3rd; Ryan, R.; Conrad, P.A.; Wilson, M.; Thomford, J.W.; Spielman, A. Diagnosis of babesiosis: Evaluation of a serologic test for the detection of *Babesia microti* antibody. *J. Infect. Dis.* **1994**, *169*, 923. [CrossRef]
26. Laveran, A. *Un nouveau parasite trouvé dans le sang des malades atteints de fièvre palustre: Origine parasitaire des accidents de l'impaludisme*; J.-B. Baillière: Paris, France, 1881.
27. Healy, G.R.; Ruebush, T.K., 2nd. Morphology of *Babesia microti* in human blood smears. *Am. J. Clin. Pathol.* **1980**, *73*, 107–109. [CrossRef]
28. Trampuz, A.; Jereb, M.; Muzlovic, I.; Prabhu, R.M. Clinical review: Severe malaria. *Crit. Care* **2003**, *7*, 315–323. [CrossRef]
29. Wongsrichanalai, C.; Barcus, M.J.; Muth, S.; Sutamihardja, A.; Wernsdorfer, W.H. A review of malaria diagnostic tools: Microscopy and rapid diagnostic test (RDT). *Am. J. Trop. Med. Hyg.* **2007**, *77*, 119–127. [CrossRef] [PubMed]
30. Bell, D.; Wongsrichanalai, C.; Barnwell, J.W. Ensuring quality and access for malaria diagnosis: How can it be achieved? *Nat. Rev. Microbiol.* **2006**, *4*, S7–S20. [CrossRef] [PubMed]
31. Vannier, E.; Gewurz, B.E.; Krause, P.J. Human babesiosis. *Infect. Dis. Clin. North Am.* **2008**, *22*, 469–488. [CrossRef]
32. Persing, D.H. PCR detection of *Babesia microti*. In *Diagnostic Molecular Microbiology: Principles and Applications*; Persing, D.H., Tenover, F.C., White, T.J., Eds.; American Society for Microbiology: Washington, DC, USA, 1993; pp. 475–479.
33. Persing, D.H.; Mathiesen, D.; Marshall, W.F.; Telford, S.R.; Spielman, A.; Thomford, J.W.; Conrad, P.A. Detection of *Babesia microti* by polymerase chain reaction. *J. Clin. Microbiol.* **1992**, *30*, 2097–2103. [CrossRef]
34. Wang, G.; Villafuerte, P.; Zhuge, J.; Visintainer, P.; Wormser, G.P. Comparison of a quantitative PCR assay with peripheral blood smear examination for detection and quantitation of *Babesia microti* infection in humans. *Diagn. Microbiol. Infect. Dis.* **2015**, *82*, 109–113. [CrossRef]
35. Tonnetti, L.; Young, C.; Kessler, D.A.; Williamson, P.C.; Reik, R.; Proctor, M.C.; Brès, V.; Deisting, B.; Bakkour, S.; Schneider, W.; et al. Transcription-mediated amplification blood donation screening for *Babesia*. *Transfusion* **2020**, *60*, 317–325. [CrossRef] [PubMed]
36. World Health Organization & UNICEF/UNDP/World Bank/WHO Special Programme for Research and Training in Tropical Diseases. Microscopy for the Detection, Identification and Quantification of Malaria Parasites on Stained Thick and Thin Blood Films in Research Settings (Version 1.0): Procedure: Methods Manual. World Health Organization. 2015. Available online: https://apps.who.int/iris/handle/10665/163782 (accessed on 14 November 2021).
37. Sethabutr, O.; Brown, A.E.; Panyim, S.; Kain, K.C.; Webster, H.K.; Echeverria, P. Detection of plasmodium falciparum by polymerase chain reaction in a field study. *J. Infect. Dis.* **1992**, *166*, 145–148. [CrossRef]
38. Hoare, C.A. Comparative aspects of human babesiosis. *Trans. R. Soc. Trop. Med. Hyg.* **1980**, *74*, 143–148. [CrossRef]
39. Wang, G.; Wormser, G.P.; Zhuge, J.; Villafuerte, P.; Ip, D.; Zeren, C.; Fallon, J.T. Utilization of a real-time PCR assay for diagnosis of *Babesia microti* infection in clinical practice. *Ticks Tick Borne Dis.* **2015**, *6*, 376–382. [CrossRef]
40. Bloch, E.M.; Lee, T.-H.; Krause, P.J.; Telford, S.R., 3rd; Montalvo, L.; Chafets, D.; Usmani-Brown, S.; Lepore, T.J.; Busch, M.P. Development of a real-time polymerase chain reaction assay for sensitive detection and quantitation of *Babesia microti* infection. *Transfusion* **2013**, *53*, 2299–2306. [CrossRef] [PubMed]
41. Wilson, M.; Glaser, K.C.; Adams-Fish, D.; Boley, M.; Mayda, M.; Molestina, R.E. Development of droplet digital PCR for the detection of *Babesia microti* and *Babesia duncani*. *Exp. Parasitol.* **2015**, *149*, 24–31. [CrossRef]
42. Cornillot, E.; Hadj-Kaddour, K.; Dassouli, A.; Noel, B.; Ranwez, V.; Vacherie, B.; Augagneur, Y.; Bres, V.; Duclos, A.; Randazzo, S.; et al. Sequencing of the smallest apicomplexan genome from the human pathogen *Babesia microti*. *Nucleic Acids Res.* **2012**, *40*, 9102–9114. [CrossRef] [PubMed]
43. Silva, J.C.; Cornillot, E.; McCracken, C.; Usmani-Brown, S.; Dwivedi, A.; Ifeonu, O.O.; Crabtree, J.; Gotia, H.T.; Virji, A.Z.; Reynes, C.; et al. Genome-wide diversity and gene expression profiling of *Babesia microti* isolates identify polymorphic genes that mediate host-pathogen interactions. *Sci. Rep.* **2016**, *6*, 35284. [CrossRef]
44. Verma, N.; Puri, A.; Essuman, E.; Skelton, R.; Anantharaman, V.; Zheng, H.; White, S.; Gunalan, K.; Takeda, K.; Bajpai, S.; et al. Antigen discovery, bioinformatics and biological characterization of novel immunodominant *Babesia microti* antigens. *Sci. Rep.* **2020**, *10*, 9598. [CrossRef] [PubMed]
45. Grabias, B.; Clement, J.; Krause, P.J.; Lepore, T.; Kumar, S. Superior real-time polymerase chain reaction detection of *Babesia microti* parasites in whole blood utilizing high-copy BMN antigens as amplification targets. *Transfusion* **2018**, *58*, 1924–1932. [CrossRef]
46. Bakkour, S.; Chafets, D.M.; Wen, L.; Muench, M.; Telford, S.R., 3rd; Erwin, J.L.; Levin, A.E.; Self, D.; Brès, V.; Linnen, J.M.; et al. Minimal infectious dose and dynamics of *Babesia microti* parasitemia in a murine model. *Transfusion* **2018**, *58*, 2903–2910. [CrossRef] [PubMed]
47. McLaughlin, G.L.; Edlind, T.D.; Ihler, G.M. Detection of *Babesia bovis* using DNA hybridization1. *J. Protozool.* **1986**, *33*, 125–128. [CrossRef]

48. Lemieux, J.E.; Tran, A.D.; Freimark, L.; Schaffner, S.F.; Goethert, H.; Andersen, K.G.; Bazner, S.; Lisa, F.; McGrath, G.; Sloan, L.; et al. A global map of genetic diversity in *Babesia microti* reveals strong population structure and identifies variants associated with clinical relapse. *Nat. Microbiol.* **2016**, *1*, 1–7. [CrossRef]
49. Baniecki, M.L.; Moon, J.; Sani, K.; Lemieux, J.E.; Schaffner, S.F.; Sabeti, P.C. Development of a SNP barcode to genotype *Babesia microti* infections. *PLOS Negl. Trop. Dis.* **2019**, *13*, e0007194. [CrossRef]
50. Lodes, M.J.; Houghton, R.L.; Bruinsma, E.S.; Mohamath, R.; Reynolds, L.D.; Benson, D.R.; Krause, P.J.; Reed, S.G.; Persing, D.H. Serological expression cloning of novel immunoreactive antigens of *Babesia microti*. *Infect. Immun.* **2000**, *68*, 2783–2790. [CrossRef]
51. Homer, M.J.; Lodes, M.J.; Reynolds, L.D.; Zhang, Y.; Douglass, J.F.; McNeill, P.D.; Houghton, R.L.; Persing, D.H. Identification and characterization of putative secreted antigens from *Babesia microti*. *J. Clin. Microbiol.* **2003**, *41*, 723–729. [CrossRef] [PubMed]
52. Cornillot, E.; Dassouli, A.; Pachikara, N.; Lawres, L.; Renard, I.; Francois, C.; Randazzo, S.; Brès, V.; Garg, A.; Brancato, J.; et al. A targeted immunomic approach identifies diagnostic antigens in the human pathogen *Babesia microti*. *Transfusion* **2016**, *56*, 2085–2099. [CrossRef] [PubMed]
53. Luo, Y.; Jia, H.; Terkawi, M.A.; Goo, Y.-K.; Kawano, S.; Ooka, H.; Li, Y.; Yu, L.; Cao, S.; Yamagishi, J.; et al. Identification and characterization of a novel secreted antigen 1 of *Babesia microti* and evaluation of its potential use in enzyme-linked immunosorbent assay and immunochromatographic test. *Parasitol. Int.* **2011**, *60*, 119–125. [CrossRef] [PubMed]
54. Thekkiniath, J.; Mootien, S.; Lawres, L.; Perrin, B.A.; Gewirtz, M.; Krause, P.J.; Williams, S.; Doggett, J.S.; Ledizet, M.; Ben Mamoun, C. BmGPAC, an antigen capture assay for detection of active *Babesia microti* infection. *J. Clin. Microbiol.* **2018**, *56*, e00067-18. [CrossRef]
55. Homer, M.J.; Bruinsma, E.S.; Lodes, M.J.; Moro, M.H.; Telford, S., 3rd; Krause, P.J.; Reynolds, L.D.; Mohamath, R.; Benson, D.R.; Houghton, R.L.; et al. A polymorphic multigene family encoding an immunodominant protein from *Babesia microti*. *J. Clin. Microbiol.* **2000**, *38*, 362–368. [CrossRef]
56. Puri, A.; Bajpai, S.; Meredith, S.; Aravind, L.; Krause, P.J.; Kumar, S. *Babesia microti*: Pathogen genomics, genetic variability, immunodominant antigens, and pathogenesis. *Front. Microbiol.* **2021**, *12*, 697669. [CrossRef]
57. *World Malaria Report 2020: 20 Years of Global Progress and Challenges*; World Health Organization: Geneva, Switzerland, 2020.
58. Berhane, A.; Anderson, K.; Mihreteab, S.; Gresty, K.; Rogier, E.; Mohamed, S.; Hagos, F.; Embaye, G.; Chinorumba, A.; Zehaie, A.; et al. Major threat to malaria control programs by *Plasmodium falciparum* lacking histidine-rich protein 2, eritrea. *Emerg. Infect. Dis.* **2018**, *24*, 462–470. [CrossRef] [PubMed]
59. Pati, P.; Dhangadamajhi, G.; Bal, M.; Ranjit, M. High proportions of pfhrp2 gene deletion and performance of HRP2-based rapid diagnostic test in Plasmodium falciparum field isolates of Odisha. *Malar. J.* **2018**, *17*, 394. [CrossRef] [PubMed]
60. Leeflang, P.; Perié, N.M. Comparative immunofluorescent studies on 4 *Babesia* species of cattle. *Res. Vet. Sci.* **1972**, *13*, 342–346. [CrossRef]
61. Goldman, M.; Pipano, E.; Rosenberg, A.S. Fluorescent antibody tests for *Babesia bigemina* and *B. berbera*. *Res. Vet. Sci.* **1972**, *13*, 77–81. [CrossRef]
62. Cox, F.E.; Turner, S.A. Antigenic relationships between the malaria parasites and piroplasms of mice as determined by the fluorescent-antibody technique. *Bull. World Health Organ.* **1970**, *43*, 337–340.
63. Chisholm, E.S.; RuebushIi, T.K., 2nd; Sulzer, A.J.; Healy, G.R. *Babesia microti* infection in man: Evaluation of an indirect immunofluorescent antibody test. *Am. J. Trop. Med. Hyg.* **1978**, *27*, 14–19. [CrossRef]
64. Boustani, M.R.; Gelfand, J.A. Babesiosis. *Clin. Infect. Dis.* **1996**, *22*, 611–615. [CrossRef]
65. Centers for Disease Control and Prevention. Babesiosis (Babesia spp.) 2011 CASE definition. Available online: https://ndc.services.cdc.gov/case-definitions/babesiosis-2011/ (accessed on 30 September 2021).
66. Tonnetti, L.; Johnson, S.; Cable, R.; Rios, J.; Spencer, B.; Leiby, D. Natural history study (NHS) of *Babesia microti* in *Connecticut blood donors*. *Transfusion* **2009**, *49*, 35A–36A.
67. Ruebush, T.K., 2nd; Chisholm, E.S.; Sulzer, A.J.; Healy, G.R.; Ii, T.K.R. Development and persistence of antibody in persons infected with *Babesia microti*. *Am. J. Trop. Med. Hyg.* **1981**, *30*, 291–292. [CrossRef]
68. Loa, C.C.; Adelson, M.E.; Mordechai, E.; Raphaelli, I.; Tilton, R.C. Serological diagnosis of human babesiosis by IgG enzyme-linked immunosorbent assay. *Curr. Microbiol.* **2004**, *49*, 385–389. [CrossRef]
69. Meeusen, E.; Lloyd, S.; Soulsby, E. Antibody levels in adoptively immunized mice after infection with *Babesia microti* or injection with antigen fractions. *Aust. J. Exp. Biol. Med. Sci.* **1985**, *63 Pt 3*, 261–272. [CrossRef]
70. Houghton, R.L.; Homer, M.J.; Reynolds, L.D.; Sleath, P.R.; Lodes, M.J.; Berardi, V.; Leiby, D.A.; Persing, D.H. Identification of *Babesia microti*-specific immunodominant epitopes and development of a peptide EIA for detection of antibodies in serum. *Transfusion* **2002**, *42*, 1488–1496. [CrossRef] [PubMed]
71. Figueroa, J.; Chieves, L.; Johnson, G.; Buening, G. Multiplex polymerase chain reaction based assay for the detection of *Babesia bigemina, Babesia bovis* and *Anaplasma marginale* DNA in bovine blood. *Vet. Parasitol.* **1993**, *50*, 69–81. [CrossRef]
72. Parodi, P.; Corbellini, L.G.; Leotti, V.B.; Rivero, R.; Miraballes, C.; Riet-Correa, F.; Venzal, J.M.; Armúa-Fernández, M.T. Validation of a multiplex PCR assay to detect *Babesia* spp. and *Anaplasma marginale* in cattle in Uruguay in the absence of a gold standard test. *J. Vet. Diagn. Investig.* **2020**, *33*, 73–79. [CrossRef] [PubMed]
73. Rodríguez, I.; Burri, C.; Noda, A.; Douet, V.; Gern, L. Multiplex PCR for molecular screening of *Borrelia burgdorferi* sensu lato, *Anaplasma* spp. and *Babesia* spp. *Ann. Agric. Environ. Med.* **2015**, *22*, 642–646. [CrossRef]

74. Tokarz, R.; Tagliafierro, T.; Cucura, D.M.; Rochlin, I.; Sameroff, S.; Lipkin, W.I. Detection of *Anaplasma phagocytophilum*, *Babesia microti*, *Borrelia burgdorferi*, *Borrelia miyamotoi*, and Powassan Virus in ticks by a multiplex real-time reverse transcription-PCR assay. *mSphere* **2017**, *2*, e00151-17. [CrossRef]
75. Buchan, B.W.; Jobe, D.A.; Mashock, M.; Gerstbrein, D.; Faron, M.L.; Ledeboer, N.A.; Callister, S.M. Evaluation of a novel multiplex high-definition PCR assay for detection of tick-borne pathogens in whole-blood specimens. *J. Clin. Microbiol.* **2019**, *57*, e00513-19. [CrossRef]
76. Livengood, J.; Hutchinson, M.L.; Thirumalapura, N.; Tewari, D. Detection of *Babesia*, *Borrelia*, *Anaplasma*, and *Rickettsia* spp. in adult black-legged ticks (*Ixodes scapularis*) from Pennsylvania, United States, with a luminex multiplex bead assay. *Vector Borne Zoonotic Dis.* **2020**, *20*, 406–411. [CrossRef]
77. Priest, J.W.; Moss, D.M.; Won, K.; Todd, C.W.; Henderson, L.; Jones, C.C.; Wilson, M. Multiplex assay detection of immunoglobulin G antibodies that recognize *Babesia microti* antigens. *Clin. Vaccine Immunol.* **2012**, *19*, 1539–1548. [CrossRef]
78. Duh, D.; Jelovšek, M.; Županc, T.A. Evaluation of an indirect fluorescence immunoassay for the detection of serum antibodies against *Babesia divergens* in humans. *Parasitology* **2006**, *134*, 179–185. [CrossRef] [PubMed]
79. Persing, D.H.; Herwaldt, B.L.; Glaser, C.; Lane, R.S.; Thomford, J.W.; Mathiesen, D.; Krause, P.J.; Phillip, D.F.; Conrad, P.A. Infection with a babesia-like organism in Northern California. *N. Engl. J. Med.* **1995**, *332*, 298–303. [CrossRef]
80. Herwaldt, B.L.; Persing, D.H.; Precigout, E.A.; Goff, W.L.; Mathiesen, D.A.; Taylor, P.W.; Eberhard, M.L.; Gorenflot, A.F. A fatal case of babesiosis in Missouri: Identification of another piroplasm that infects humans. *Ann. Intern. Med.* **1996**, *124*, 643–650. [CrossRef]
81. Herwaldt, B.L.; de Bruyn, G.; Pieniazek, N.J.; Homer, M.; Lofy, K.H.; Slemenda, S.B.; Fritsche, T.R.; Persing, D.H.; Limaye, A.P. *Babesia divergens*–like Infection, Washington State. *Emerg. Infect. Dis.* **2004**, *10*, 622–629. [CrossRef]
82. Wilson, M.; Naccache, S.N.; Samayoa, E.; Biagtan, M.; Bashir, H.; Yu, G.; Salamat, S.M.; Somasekar, S.; Federman, S.; Miller, S.; et al. Actionable diagnosis of neuroleptospirosis by next-generation sequencing. *N. Engl. J. Med.* **2014**, *370*, 2408–2417. [CrossRef]
83. Doan, T.; Wilson, M.R.; Crawford, E.D.; Chow, E.D.; Khan, L.M.; Knopp, K.A.; O'Donovan, B.D.; Xia, D.; Hacker, J.K.; Stewart, J.M.; et al. Illuminating uveitis: Metagenomic deep sequencing identifies common and rare pathogens. *Genome Med.* **2016**, *8*, 1–9. [CrossRef]
84. Greninger, A.L.; Naccache, S.N.; Federman, S.; Yu, G.; Mbala, P.; Bres, V.; Stryke, D.; Bouquet, J.; Somasekar, S.; Linnen, J.M.; et al. Rapid metagenomic identification of viral pathogens in clinical samples by real-time nanopore sequencing analysis. *Genome Med.* **2015**, *7*, 1–13. [CrossRef] [PubMed]
85. Gu, W.; Miller, S.; Chiu, C.Y. Clinical metagenomic next-generation sequencing for pathogen detection. *Annu. Rev. Pathol. Mech. Dis.* **2019**, *14*, 319–338. [CrossRef] [PubMed]
86. Mojica, F.J.M.; Díez-Villaseñor, C.; García-Martínez, J.; Soria, E. Intervening sequences of regularly spaced prokaryotic repeats derive from foreign genetic elements. *J. Mol. Evol.* **2005**, *60*, 174–182. [CrossRef] [PubMed]
87. Chen, J.S.; Ma, E.; Harrington, L.B.; Da Costa, M.; Tian, X.; Palefsky, J.M.; Doudna, J.A. CRISPR-Cas12a target binding unleashes indiscriminate single-stranded DNase activity. *Science* **2018**, *360*, 436–439. [CrossRef]
88. Abudayyeh, O.O.; Gootenberg, J.S.; Konermann, S.; Joung, J.; Slaymaker, I.M.; Cox, D.B.T.; Shmakov, S.; Makarova, K.S.; Semenova, E.; Minakhin, L.; et al. C2c2 is a single-component programmable RNA-guided RNA-targeting CRISPR effector. *Science* **2016**, *353*, aaf5573. [CrossRef]
89. Gootenberg, J.S.; Abudayyeh, O.O.; Lee, J.W.; Essletzbichler, P.; Dy, A.J.; Joung, J.; Verdine, V.; Donghia, N.; Daringer, N.M.; Freije, C.A.; et al. Nucleic acid detection with CRISPR-Cas13a/C2c2. *Science* **2017**, *356*, 438–442. [CrossRef]
90. Cunningham, C.H.; Hennelly, C.M.; Lin, J.T.; Ubalee, R.; Boyce, R.M.; Mulogo, E.M.; Hathaway, N.; Thwai, K.L.; Phanzu, F.; Kalonji, A.; et al. A novel CRISPR-based malaria diagnostic capable of Plasmodium detection, species differentiation, and drug-resistance genotyping. *EBioMedicine* **2021**, *68*, 103415. [CrossRef]
91. Jacoby, G.A.; Hunt, J.V.; Kosinski, K.S.; Demirjian, Z.N.; Huggins, C.; Etkind, P.; Marcus, L.C.; Spielman, A. Treatment of transfusion-transmitted babesiosis by exchange transfusion. *N. Engl. J. Med.* **1980**, *303*, 1098–1100. [CrossRef] [PubMed]
92. Herwaldt, B.L.; Linden, J.V.; Bosserman, E.; Young, C.; Olkowska, D.; Wilson, M. Transfusion-associated babesiosis in the United States: A description of cases. *Ann. Intern. Med.* **2011**, *155*, 509–519. [CrossRef] [PubMed]
93. Linden, J.V.; Prusinski, M.; Crowder, L.; Tonnetti, L.; Stramer, S.L.; Kessler, D.A.; White, J.; Shaz, B.; Olkowska, D. Transfusion-transmitted and community-acquired babesiosis in New York, 2004 to 2015. *Transfusion* **2018**, *58*, 660–668. [CrossRef]
94. Mintz, E.D.; Anderson, J.F.; Cable, R.G.; Hadler, J.L. Transfusion-transmitted babesiosis: A case report from a new endemic area. *Transfusion* **1991**, *31*, 365–368. [CrossRef]
95. Menis, M.; Forshee, R.A.; Kumar, S.; Mckean, S.; Warnock, R.; Izurieta, H.S.; Gondalia, R.; Johnson, C.; Mintz, P.D.; Walderhaug, M.O.; et al. Babesiosis occurrence among the elderly in the United States, as recorded in large medicare databases during 2006–2013. *PLoS ONE* **2015**, *10*, e0140332. [CrossRef]
96. Johnson, S.T.; Cable, R.G.; Tonnetti, L.; Spencer, B.; Rios, J.; Leiby, D.A. Transfusion complications: Seroprevalence of *Babesia microti* in blood donors from *Babesia*-endemic areas of the northeastern United States: 2000 through 2007. *Transfusion* **2009**, *49*, 2574–2582. [CrossRef]
97. Leiby, D.A.; Chung, A.P.; Gill, J.E.; Houghton, R.L.; Persing, D.H.; Badon, S.; Cable, R.G. Demonstrable parasitemia among Connecticut blood donors with antibodies to *Babesia microti*. *Transfusion* **2005**, *45*, 1804–1810. [CrossRef] [PubMed]

98. Leiby, D.A.; Johnson, S.T.; Won, K.Y.; Nace, E.K.; Slemenda, S.B.; Pieniazek, N.J.; Cable, R.G.; Herwaldt, B.L. A longitudinal study of *Babesia microti* infection in seropositive blood donors. *Transfusion* **2014**, *54*, 2217–2225. [CrossRef]
99. Levin, A.E.; Williamson, P.C.; Bloch, E.M.; Clifford, J.; Cyrus, S.; Shaz, B.; Kessler, D.; Gorlin, J.; Erwin, J.L.; Krueger, N.X.; et al. Serologic screening of United States blood donors for *Babesia microti* using an investigational enzyme immunoassay. *Transfusion* **2016**, *56*, 1866–1874. [CrossRef] [PubMed]
100. Cangelosi, J.J.; Sarvat, B.; Sarria, J.C.; Herwaldt, B.L.; Indrikovs, A.J. Transmission of *Babesia microti* by blood transfusion in Texas. *Vox Sang.* **2008**, *95*, 331–334. [CrossRef] [PubMed]
101. Ngo, V.; Civen, R. Babesiosis acquired through blood transfusion, California, USA. *Emerg. Infect. Dis.* **2009**, *15*, 785–787. [CrossRef] [PubMed]
102. Expert Committee on Biological Standardization. A collaborative study to evaluate the proposed 6th WHO International Standard for Hepatitis C Virus (HCV) RNA for nucleic acid amplification techniques (NAT). *World Health Organization.* 2019. Available online: https://www.who.int/biologicals/expert_committee/BS.2019.2358_6thHCVIS_WHOECBS_July2019.pdf (accessed on 21 November 2021).
103. Expert Committee on Biological Standardization. International collaborative study to establish the 4th WHO International Standard for HIV-1 NAT assays. *World Health Organization.* 2017. Available online: https://apps.who.int/iris/handle/10665/260256 (accessed on 21 November 2021).

pathogens

MDPI

Review

Major Surface Antigens in Zoonotic *Babesia*

Stephane Delbecq

Centre de Biologie Structurale, Faculté de Pharmacie, University of Montpellier, UMR CNRS 5048, 34090 Montpellier, France; stephane.delbecq@umontpellier.fr

Abstract: Human babesiosis results from a combination of tick tropism for humans, susceptibility of a host to sustain *Babesia* development, and contact with infected ticks. Climate modifications and increasing diagnostics have led to an expanded number of *Babesia* species responsible for human babesiosis, although, to date, most cases have been attributed to *B. microti* and *B. divergens*. These two species have been extensively studied, and in this review, we mostly focus on the antigens involved in host–parasite interactions. We present features of the major antigens, so-called Bd37 in *B. divergens* and BmSA1/GPI12 in *B. microti*, and highlight the roles of these antigens in both host cell invasion and immune response. A comparison of these antigens with the major antigens found in some other Apicomplexa species emphasizes the importance of glycosylphosphatidylinositol-anchored proteins in host–parasite relationships. GPI-anchor cleavage, which is a property of such antigens, leads to soluble and membrane-bound forms of these proteins, with potentially differential recognition by the host immune system. This mechanism is discussed as the structural basis for the protein-embedded immune escape mechanism. In conclusion, the potential consequences of such a mechanism on the management of both human and animal babesiosis is examined.

Keywords: glycosylphosphatidylinositol; protein structure; antigen

Citation: Delbecq, S. Major Surface Antigens in Zoonotic *Babesia*. *Pathogens* **2022**, *11*, 99. https://doi.org/10.3390/pathogens11010099

Academic Editors: Estrella Montero, Jeremy Gray, Cheryl Ann Lobo and Luis Miguel González

Received: 8 October 2021
Accepted: 11 January 2022
Published: 15 January 2022

1. Introduction

Human babesiosis has been mainly reported in North America and Europe and has been increasingly identified in Asia [1]. On other continents, either the underestimation of diagnosis or a low risk level could explain the low rate of detected human babesiosis. As a zoonotic disease transmitted by ticks, human babesiosis results from the encounter of a parasitized vector with a susceptible host [2]. The current epidemiology of human diseases is driven by tick tropism for humans, parasites circulating in the tick population, and frequency of tick bites in shared areas (for leisure, work, or home locations). Such a situation is well illustrated by *B. divergens* human babesiosis in Europe, where a tick bite by infected *Ixodes ricinus* leads to transmission, but severe disease mainly develops in spleen-deficient patients. The *B. divergens* parasite will not pursue its development in immunocompetent humans, so human-to-human or human-to-animal transmission is considered very unlikely. In North America, severe human babesiosis caused by *B. microti* is also a great concern for immunocompromised humans, ranging from neonates to the elderly. But in the case of *B. microti*, which is able to infect immunocompetent patients, asymptomatic human carriers lead to transfusional babesiosis risk.

Some *Babesia* species have been proven to develop in human blood, but for a vast number of species, the ability to invade human red blood cells remains unknown. In addition to the well-known *B. microti* and *B. divergens*, the parasites *B. duncani* and *B. venatorum* are recognized as occasional human pathogens [3]. The latter parasites have both been recognized as relatively new *Babesia* species that can invade a human host and cause clinical diseases, but many human cases are diagnosed as babesiosis without clear identification of the parasite. A recent example described patient cases of babesiosis associated with *B. odocoilei*, a parasite closely related to *B. divergens* [4]. This report highlighted the need for an accurate diagnosis assay, efficient care of babesiosis cases, evaluation of the risk level, and adaptation of prophylaxis. Babesiosis treatment will not be the same in the case of a splenectomized patient infected by *B. divergens* compared with an immunocompetent human infected with *B. microti*, at least in terms of emergency measures. Additionally, emergence of new *Babesia* species infecting humans have to be monitored to avoid potential transfusional risk.

Babesia have biological features that make them unique among Apicomplexa, but they also have the same requirements as other intracellular parasites, i.e., to invade a host cell and escape the immune system. A critical step for the blood stages of *Babesia* parasites is the interval between the release of merozoites from red blood cells and successful invasion of new erythrocytes [5]. During this short period of time, merozoites are flowing in the blood stream and their surfaces are coated with erythrocyte-binding proteins exposed to immune effectors, such as antibodies. Thus, the surfaces of merozoites represent an interface between the parasite and the host cells, to which the parasite has to bind while avoiding the antibodies. Among the molecules exposed at the surfaces of merozoites, at least some glycosylphosphatidylinositol-anchored proteins (GPI-AP) can meet these contradictory requirements. These proteins are anchored at the surfaces of the merozoites, providing erythrocyte-binding sites potentially used for host cell invasion. Via mechanisms not fully determined yet, the GPI anchor allows GPI-AP to be released from the plasma membrane of the parasite. As a soluble form, the shed protein could be bound to an antibody which, then, would not interfere with the parasite. These features of GPI-AP produced by parasites highlight their critical role in successful parasite development inside the host, but also their high potential as a target for vaccine or diagnostic tools.

Human babesiosis represents only a part of all the Apicomplexa-borne disease cases, compared with animal babesiosis (cattle, dog, etc.), malaria (humans), and many other animal or human infections. Therefore, knowledge of human babesiosis could benefit from a comparative analysis with other parasites using similar mechanisms. In this paper, we review some information about *Babesia* parasites from various hosts, focusing on GPI-AP and their dual role in invasion and immune escape. Two major antigens from the species most frequently found in humans (*B. microti* and *B. divergens*) are then presented and their features compared. These two antigens, Bd37 and BmSA1, highlight the crucial role of GPI-AP in host relationships and their high potential as a target for medical intervention. From the comparative analysis of these two proteins, critical points could be determined in order to decipher the multiple functions of such antigens. This will open discussion about the possibility of standardizing current serological assays for known human babesiosis and also speed up the process of identifying antigens of high potential for diagnosis and/or vaccination.

2. Glycosylphosphatidylinositol-Anchored Proteins Are Important Antigens for Invasion and Immune Escape

In recent years, there has been significant progress in genomics and phylogeny of *Babesia*, leading to improved parasite classification [6]. Comparisons of clinical observations and biological mechanisms to study the evolutional history of each parasite will certainly help to join disparate elements into a more comprehensive picture. In particular, comparative analyses of the proteins involved in host–parasite interactions, structure determinations, and functional analyses need to be extended [7].

Briefly, focusing on GPI-anchored proteins expressed by Apicomplexa, the importance of their role in host–parasite relationships is quite well known. *Plasmodium* is outside the scope of this paper, but the example of the RTS,S vaccine highlights the role of these antigens. The RTS,S vaccine is based on the GPI-anchored circumsporozoite protein (CSP) and is currently one of the most advanced recombinant vaccines in clinical trials [8]. The GPI-anchor by itself also induces an immune response in the host, in the absence of antigenic proteins [9]. Indeed, the non-protein part of the GPI anchor remains understudied in *Babesia* despite a significant role in host–parasite interactions, as evidenced in other Apicomplexa [10–12]. The structure of the GPI anchor has been determined in some *Babesia* species, either experimentally or by analysis of the GPI metabolic pathway [13–15]. The organization of GPI-AP at the cell surface in raft or other patterns remains to be determined, as well as potential heterogeneity in the anchor bound to proteins (either glycosidic or lipidic). The fate of these proteins during parasite invasion of erythrocytes and the antigen protein shedding mechanisms also need further studies.

Some studies on *Babesia* have been driven by the need to prevent babesiosis in animals, mostly cattle or dogs [16]. The classic vaccine research scheme starts from live, attenuated, or killed parasites as antigens and progresses towards the use of recombinant molecules, either protein or nucleic acids. This process leads to the identification of various antigens that can induce protective immune responses, ranging from an avirulent parasite strain to a recombinant protein. For example, soluble parasite antigens (SPAs) have often been used as a source for crude vaccine preparations containing shed GPI-anchored proteins. In most of these efficient vaccines, the role of highly immunogenic proteins has been highlighted, and in most of the cases, the relevant proteins are GPI-anchored (Table 1).

The results obtained from various *Babesia* species have helped to define major antigens as GPI-anchored proteins with high-level expression, high abundance in the extracellular space (culture supernatants or plasma of infected host), and high immunogenicity. Another critical feature is the function of these proteins in the host cell invasion process [17]. Interestingly, in two of the main parasites responsible for human babesiosis, such major antigens have been identified. A comparative analysis of these major antigens in the two human parasites *Babesia microti* and *Babesia divergens* (Table 2) could be an opportunity to establish a common reference and classification of antigens.

Table 1. Some examples of major antigens found in *Babesia* sp. These proteins are all GPI-anchored at the surface of merozoites and are released into host blood or in vitro culture supernatants (++: evidence of high potential, +/−: no clear evidence or no data supporting high potential).

Babesia **Species**	**Protein**	**Expression Level**	**Diagnostic Potential**	**Vaccine Potential**	**Ref.**
B. divergens	Bd37	++	++	++	[18]
B. microti	BmSA1/GPI12	++	++	++	[19]
B. bovis	MSA1	++	++	++	[20]
B. bigemina	Gp45	++	++	++	[21]
B. canis	Bc28	++	++	+/−	[22]
B. canis	BcMSA/CBA	+/−	+/−	++	[23,24]

Table 2. Comparison between Bd37 and BmSA1 features (+: effective activity, −: no activity).

	Bd37	**BmGPI12/BmSA1**
Related genes in genome	2 to 6 genes (need further analysis)	BMN family (>15 members) Not all are GPI-anchored
Protein global structure	mainly α-helical protein (2jo7)	BAHCS domain (α-helical)
GPI anchor core structure	Man2-GlcN	Man2-GlcN
GPI lipid moiety	palmitate	not determined
Erythrocyte binding activity	+	+
Growth-inhibitory antibodies	−	+
Early detected by antibodies	+	+
In vivo protection	effective or not	Effective or not
Secreted form	soluble	vesicle-bound and soluble

3. The Major Antigen in *Babesia divergens*: Bd37 Protein

Babesia divergens, as the main cause of bovine babesiosis in Europe and potentially fatal human infections, has been extensively studied. Research efforts towards a bovine vaccine have led to the identification of the main antigen, named Bd37, according to the molecular weight of this protein (around 37 kDa) [18]. In the first attempts to obtain an efficient vaccine, in vitro culture supernatants were used as vaccine antigens. These experiments demonstrated the high protective potential of such crude antigenic preparations [25]. A critical parameter to obtain such efficient vaccines was the inclusion of the adjuvant saponin, which was found to induce a protective response. Such a crude antigenic preparation contains both secreted antigens and shed proteins and also proteins released from lysed or dying parasites. Despite the undefined composition of in vitro culture supernatants, sometimes referred to as soluble parasite antigens (SPAs) or excreted/secreted antigens (E/S antigens), they offer the possibility for successful development of a vaccine [26]. At the same time, a similar strategy for the *Leishmania* vaccine development in dogs was also successful, leading to a commercial product [27]. Another example is the vaccine developments against canine babesiosis that have also led to a commercial product [28].

A *Babesia* vaccine based on in vitro culture supernatants, or on live parasites, requires an established long-term culture system for consistent production of antigens [29,30]. A significant drawback of this production process is the availability of a critical cell substrate, i.e., the erythrocytes. Moreover, the potential presence of an infectious element in the production process, for example, a cattle vaccine used in human food-producing animals, could be an issue in terms of product safety. Therefore, a high priority is the identification of protective components in in vitro culture supernatants, which will later be produced by biotechnological methods and safer processes.

In the case of *B. divergens*, a traditional strategy was to purify relevant molecules from in vitro supernatants [25]. Using size-exclusion chromatography, separation of crude supernatants has led to several fractions that have been tested in vaccine experiments. A fraction (called F4) containing antigens with molecular weights ranging from 17 to 50 kDa has been shown to induce a protective response in gerbils [31].

Therefore, after successful purification of native Bd37 from in vitro culture supernatants, and the characterization of this protein, some immunological detection tools have been generated, including immune serum and the so-called F4.2F8 monoclonal antibody, which was raised against the protective F4 fraction from the supernatant, hence the name of the mAb [32]. Interestingly, mAb F4.2F8 greatly reduced clinical signs. To obtain the coding sequence of the Bd37 antigen, a cDNA library from *B. divergens* merozoite mRNA was screened with immune serum [33]. Although this type of library could introduce a large bias in the representation of cell transcripts, positive clones contain sequences directly expressible in bacteria.

When Bd37 was identified, no *B. divergens* genome data were available as they were released in 2014 [34,35]. In addition, the proteomic analyses of a complex mixture with low abundance of parasite molecules among large amounts of host proteins is still highly challenging. Therefore, the systematic identification of other GPI-AP of *B. divergens* has not been published yet, although some Bd37-related genes can be found in released genomes [36,37].

The production of a recombinant Bd37 protein without the use of a parasite in vitro culture was a milestone in the development of an industrial vaccine for cattle. Moreover, this recombinant vaccine induced an immune protection broader than that induced by the supernatant and was efficient against all the tested strains [38]. Nevertheless, a striking difference in recombinant vaccine antigen potency was observed, i.e., the protective immune response was only induced by a protein containing a hydrophobic peptide. Thus, such proteins associated with saponin are thought to mimic the merozoite surface and elicit an efficient immune response that is able to impair parasite development and onset of disease. In contrast, the Bd37 recombinant protein with similar immunogenicity but devoid of a hydrophobic tail induced an inefficient response, leaving parasites unaffected [39]. These results highlight a potential protein-embedded immune escape mechanism used by

B. divergens parasites, in which Bd37 released in a soluble form (Figure 1A) acts as a shield for the Bd37-coated merozoite surface (Figure 1C).

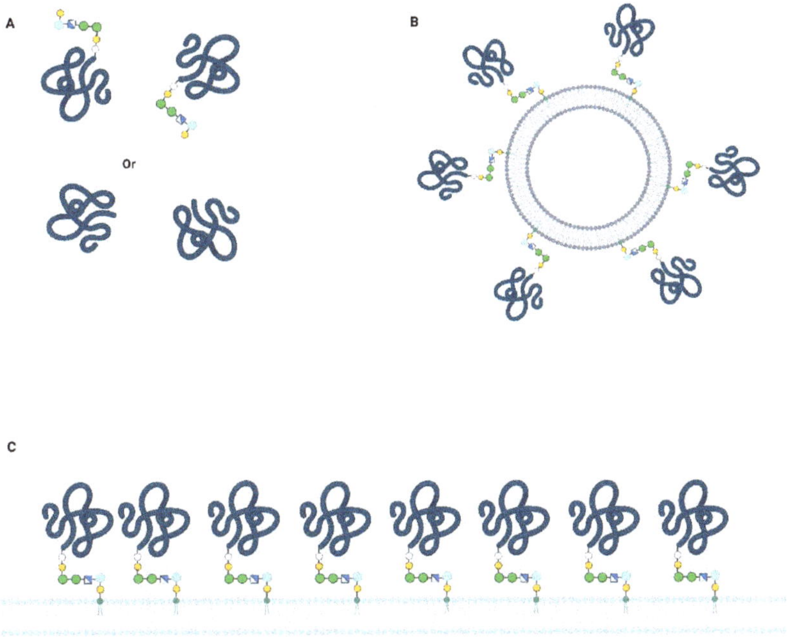

Figure 1. Different physical presentations of major GPI-anchored antigens in *Babesia*. Protein concentration, orientation, and degrees of freedom could influence interactions between antigens and antibodies or erythrocyte surface: (**A**) Soluble protein free in the blood and in vitro culture supernatants (e.g., Bd37 and BmSA1); shed by proteolytic or phospholipase cleavage (**B**) extracellular vesicle released by parasite, coated with GPI-anchored proteins (e.g.,: BmSA12); (**C**) GPI-anchored proteins at the plasma membrane of merozoite (either on the entire cell surface or on lipid rafts).

The erythrocyte-binding function of Bd37 and the high vaccine potency of the cognate recombinant protein prompted the elucidation of the three-dimensional (3D) structure of this antigen [40]. This protein bears a protruding unstructured region in the N-terminal part of the molecule, followed by an alpha-helical domain. The structured core of the protein is organized into three subdomains stuck together by salt bridges, suggesting the possibility of conformational changes. Considering the membrane-bound form of Bd37, packed at the merozoite surface, the binding of relevant antibodies could be impaired by steric hindrance, while free soluble proteins are dispersed and fully exposed (Figure 1A,C). At the molecular level, a conformational change of Bd37 could also occur when merozoite and erythrocyte surfaces are in close vicinity, potentially inducing electrostatic bond modifications. Such a potential conformational change would expose erythrocyte-binding sites that are otherwise hidden from antibodies. Another possibility is that a conformational change leads to the displacement of bound antibodies in favor of erythrocyte receptors, making a humoral response useless for the host. Although further studies are required to totally decipher these mechanisms, the intrinsic properties of Bd37 integrate requirements for both immune escape and erythrocyte-binding functions.

4. The Major Antigen in *Babesia microti*: BmSA1/GPI12 Protein

A vaccine against *B. microti* for human use is not considered the best tool for human babesiosis management, in contrast to *B. divergens* and cattle babesiosis, for which vaccine research has been extensive. Therefore, in *B. microti*, research on GPI anchored antigens has been more focused on their use for detection. Nevertheless, first attempts to identify relevant antigens have rapidly led to a much more complex panel of molecules than those found in *B. divergens* [41]. Since the first genome annotation, which was published in 2012, genomic data on this parasite have been generated, including the genome analysis of several isolates [42]. These data allow better characterization of the parasite proteome and metabolic pathways, including the protein post-translational modification machinery. The immune response against *B. microti* and the most relevant antigens have been reviewed previously [43]; therefore, in this paper, we focus on one of the most characterized antigens without ignoring the role of other proteins.

BmR1_03g00785, named BmGPI12, has been identified as a GPI-anchored antigen from the *Babesia microti* R1 strain using a bioinformatics strategy based on targeting signal recognition at the N and C terminal position in amino acid sequences [44]. This strategy has been used on *B. bovis* to predict around 20 GPI-AP, a number similar to the predicted GPI-anchored proteome in *B. microti* [17]. A sequence comparison analysis indicated almost complete identity with previously identified BmSA1 in other *B. microti* strains [45]. When the human antibody response against different predicted proteins was evaluated, the high immunogenicity of this protein relative to other antigens was demonstrated [44]. In addition, strong similarities with antigens from the BMN family, which are proteins identified in the *B. microti* MN1 strain after serological screening, were observed [46]. The history and features of the BMN antigens were recently reviewed, and the name of BmBAHCS1 (*Babesia* alpha-helical cell surface) was suggested for BmR1_03g00785 [47]. The 3D structure of this antigen has not yet been experimentally determined, but sequence analysis has indicated an unstructured part, followed by an alpha-helical domain. This organization is relatively similar to the Bd37 protein, in which a disordered region is N-terminally added to a structured core of an alpha-helical protein. Another common feature shared with Bd37 is its early recognition by antibodies during the rise of an immune response [44,48].

The analysis of BmHACS1/GPI12/SA1 (henceforth referred to as BmSA1 for readability) expression in *B. microti* has revealed an unusual mechanism for releasing proteins in culture supernatants as vesicle-anchored antigens [49]. Thus, this GPI-anchored antigen has a classic cellular distribution of merozoite surface protein released into soluble form, as well as membrane-bound protein on small vesicles (Figure 1B). These vesicles appear to be loaded with some other antigens, strongly suggesting a role in host immune system manipulation. Neither soluble nor vesicle-bound BmSA1 could be involved in erythrocyte invasion without physical connection to the merozoite. These forms of the protein are produced at a high rate and therefore could be exploited as a diagnostic marker of active infection [50].

There have been some attempts to evaluate the potential of BmSA1 as a vaccine antigen and to determine the inhibitory growth potency of antibodies [51]. Showing some similarities with Bd37 in *B. divergens* vaccine experiments, the immune response elicited by recombinant BmSA1 could either be protective or with negligible effect on the infection course [52]. In some cases, antibodies against this protein could inhibit in vitro culture, suggesting blocking of the essential interaction with the host erythrocyte. The direct interaction of the recombinant protein with erythrocytes has been demonstrated, definitively making BmSA1 a major antigen of *B. microti* [19].

5. Protein-Embedded Immune Escape Mechanism: Membrane-Bound Versus Soluble Antigen

Merozoite surface proteins function as an interface between host and parasite by interacting with the immune system through effectors (antibodies, cell receptors etc.). Among these proteins exposed to the immune system are erythrocyte-binding proteins, which, in order to maintain their cell interaction ability, have limited evolutionary opportunities. This functional restraint counteracts the trend to diversify antigen sequences in response to immune pressure. Recently, the initial interaction of merozoite proteins with erythrocytes, just prior to invasion, has been documented at the cell scale in *B. divergens* [53]. This initial step seems to allow transitory interactions (quite like "touch-and-go" binding to red blood cells) or induce the wrapping of the erythrocyte membrane around the parasite, possibly triggering the invasion sequence. Such wrapping could be the consequence of a coordinated multiple low-affinity interaction between GPI-anchored merozoite proteins and erythrocyte surfaces. It is possible that such low-affinity interaction occurring at one point on the merozoite surface, possibly involving only a few proteins, can spread to other close proteins, leading to a large contact zone with erythrocytes.

The functional constraint to bind to the surface of erythrocytes limits sequence variation (polymorphism or antigenic variation mechanism) in such a protein domain, whereas their exposure to antibodies applies a selective pressure to develop escape mechanisms [7]. A common feature of both major antigens, Bd37 and BmSA1, is their ability to induce strong immune responses, although their effects against parasite development and disease onset are highly variable. The *B. divergens* vaccine model, using recombinant Bd37 with or without a hydrophobic tail, shifts the immune response from totally inefficient to a full protective immunity [39]. There is a similar situation in *B. microti*, for which different experiments have evaluated the immune response induced by various types of recombinant BmSA1 proteins and adjuvants [51,52]. In both cases, the host immune system (mostly from gerbils and mice in experimental vaccine trials) was able to raise a protective response depending on the antigen vaccine used. On one hand, the protein-embedded immune mechanism acting in GPI-anchored proteins could drive the immune system response toward soluble or vesicle-anchored antigens, almost obliterating the protective response against merozoites. On the other hand, an efficient vaccine would drive the immune response toward merozoite surface-bound proteins, either impairing the infection or at least leading to parasitemia decay and disease recovery. The balance between protective and non-protective response could then rely on the dynamics of interactions with antibodies (conformational changes) or on the local concentration of membrane-bound proteins in contrast to dispersed soluble proteins.

In both *B. divergens* and *B. microti* species, a monoclonal antibody directed against Bd37 and BmSA1, respectively, can interfere in vivo with the target parasite. The protective effect of such monoclonal antibodies could result from the high concentration of antibody against a single epitope, or from better interaction with the membrane-bound antigen than with the soluble form. The binding of an antibody to its cognate antigen can be greatly affected by the physical state of the protein, either membrane-bound or soluble [54]. This is especially the case for GPI-anchored proteins, as these proteins could be packed in a membrane raft of potentially high density or homogeneously spread on the cell surface, which could have an impact on antibody binding (Figure 1C) [55]. For vesicle-bound antigens, it remains to be determined if the protein density and orientation are similar to the plasma membrane-bound proteins, and the interactions with antibodies would need to be characterized.

The conformational changes in Bd37 and the potential shift in functional properties of the protein, according to such a structural dynamics, are reminiscent of protein allostery, mainly described in enzymes but applicable to antigens [56]. The nature of the GPI anchor is probably the basis of the immune escape mechanism embedded in Bd37, inducing modifications in the conformational dynamics of the protein when bound to the membrane or released in soluble form. The influence of the GPI anchor on the conformational dynamics and functional properties has been shown in the prion protein, which could exist as both a membrane-bound and soluble protein [57,58]. Another level of complexity may be represented by the structural diversity of the GPI anchor. Thus, varying anchors may be attached to the protein according to the C-terminal signal processing sequence, with varying impact on protein properties [59].

In addition to protein structure, the type of GPI anchor could have an impact on the antigen presentation at the parasite surface and then affect the function of such antigen [60,61]. The genome of *B. divergens* has been released and analyzed, confirming that Bd37 is a member of a small group of related genes [36]. One of the questions is to determine the membrane pattern (localization, density, orientation, etc.) of these Bd37-related proteins and determine whether or not their GPI-anchors are identical. The diversity of the GPI-anchor structure in the different GPI-anchored proteins from parasites has not yet been extensively studied. GPI-anchor structure has an impact on protein shedding, which leads to the release of protein as soluble antigen, and potentially on the protein organization at the surface of the parasite [59–61]. Thus, determining, at a proteome scale, the specificity or the identity of the GPI-anchor type for each antigen will be a major milestone in the understanding of host–parasite molecular interactions.

Deciphering all the characteristics of a protective immune response is challenging, while predicting which antigen formulation will induce such protective response is even more complex. Nevertheless, there is growing evidence suggesting that mimicking the membrane-bound form of antigens instead of the soluble form is one of the keys to achieving protective immunity [62]. In the Bd37 (*B. divergens*) vaccine model, a single recombinant antigen can switch between an efficient or inefficient vaccine according to the formulation. In most of the other Apicomplexa vaccine experimental models, there is not such a great difference, in clinical signs or parasitemia, between protective and non-protective immune responses. A general trend of results in the literature indicates that a membrane-bound antigen is generally better than soluble molecules. This could be recombinant molecules, attenuated or killed whole parasites, or crude antigen preparations formulated with adjuvant. GPI-anchored Bd37 expressed on the surface of a live, heterologous recombinant vaccine (*Trypanosoma theileri*) was able to induce a protective immune response in cattle, illustrating the importance of a membrane-bound form in vaccine potency [63]. Another example is the Gp60 protein of *Cryptosporidium*, which has been expressed in *Tetrahymena* [64]. An increase in local antigen density could potentially also account for the high protection rate obtained with the R21 CSP-based vaccine [65]. These examples illustrate the importance of vaccine formulation and antigen expression to obtain efficient, protective immune responses.

6. Use of Major *Babesia* Antigens in the Management of Human Babesiosis: Polymorphism and Cross-Reactions

As previously mentioned, human babesiosis cases occur at the crossroad of vector, parasite, and host biology, which are evolving parameters due to climate change. Therefore, the distribution of endemic babesiosis areas will certainly change, together with the potential emergence of new zoonotic *Babesia* species. In contrast to animal babesiosis, for which a vaccine is the best control method, human babesiosis mainly needs detection tools and a risk mitigation system. Improved mapping of the high prevalence areas for parasites and vectors, together with public information, would certainly lower infection rates. In addition, rapid and reliable diagnostic assays are greatly needed both for the prevention of babesiosis (for example in blood screening for transfusion) and for patient healthcare. Acute human babesiosis requires quick parasite identification in patients before a humoral immune response can develop. A splenectomized patient with *B. divergens* babesiosis should need additional healthcare compared to an immunocompetent patient with *B. microti* babesiosis. However, there is significant interest in serological assays that could be used for epidemiological analyses.

It should be noted that the *B. microti* R1 strain was isolated in France from a patient coming from North America [41]. Therefore, people who travel and become infected with various species of *Babesia* may need an appropriate diagnostic test far from the source of the infection area [66]. This supports the development of a broad diagnostic system that is able to detect as many different species as possible [67]. Molecular tools could detect almost all *Babesia* species, depending on the oligonucleotides used in a PCR, but serological assays are much more challenging. In addition to the number of species to be included, the polymorphism of each antigen could impair the detection of antibodies raised against distantly related parasites [37]. Therefore, an ideal "universal" serological assay should probably use different recombinant proteins, covering most species and strains encountered in patients, and be delivered in a multiplexed format. A panel of recombinant proteins could advantageously be included in a *Babesia* antigen toolbox, which would be useful for the development of serodiagnostic assays, but also for basic research on protein structure determination and functional analysis.

According to the results obtained with Bd37 and BmSA1 in two *Babesia* species, achieving a broad, multiplexed, serological assay might not be as difficult as expected. In addition to classic immunofluorescence assays using native antigens from in vitro cultures or infected animals, recombinant proteins have been successfully used in serological assays [68,69]. Some initial studies on *B. divergens* antigens have compared the immune response raised in different hosts and demonstrated a similar profile of recognized proteins [48]. Thus, a standardized serological assay could be efficiently developed in parallel for both cattle and humans, using a common panel of recombinant proteins, therefore reducing costs. Moreover, despite the polymorphism found on Bd37, the recombinant protein based on the Rouen 1987 sequence is able to bind antibodies elicited against various strains, suggesting that a few antigens, or possibly only one, would allow the achievement of a broad-spectrum serological assay for *B. divergens*. In the case of *B. microti*, the BmSA1 antigen seems to detect antibodies against many different strains [45].

Other species can cause human babesiosis, for example *B. duncani* and *B. venatorum*, but also new emerging species, for which major antigens have not yet been characterized or even identified. Extrapolating results from other *Babesia* species (Table 1), there is a high probability of finding relevant diagnostic antigens for a serological assay among the GPI-anchored proteome of these parasites [15]. Achieving an efficient recombinant vaccine is not the main objective for managing human babesiosis; efforts should focus on the main antibody targets with high expression levels that are most favorable for diagnostic assays. In vitro cultivation of *B. duncani* will ensure enough biological material for genome, transcriptome, and proteome analyses, as well as in-cell experiments [70]. Concerning *B. microti*, a long-term in vitro cultivation system is not available yet, as for many other species. However, the identification of a major antigen and quickly including it in a serodiagnostic toolbox, in the case of a new emerging species, will remain highly challenging. Progress in genome sequencing methods and annotation pipelines would help researchers avoid the in vitro cultivation bottleneck and allow them to generate data from limited samples.

7. Conclusions

Major antigens in *Babesia*, such as erythrocyte-binding proteins with high immunogenicity, have mostly been found in the GPI-anchored proteome. The Bd37 protein was identified in *B. divergens* using a classic and time-consuming approach based on in vitro cultivation of the parasite, but genome analysis and recombinant protein expression have speeded up the process, as described for the BmSA1 protein from *B. microti*. These antigens, expressed as recombinant proteins, could form the basis of high-performance serodiagnostic assays.

These two antigens highlight the role of GPI-anchored proteins in *Babesia* biology and the complexity of their functional relationships with the host. Protein structure and dynamics, proteome organization, carbohydrate heterogeneity and GPI-anchor diversity, polymorphism, and antibody cross-reactivity need to be further explored to decipher such complex interactions. The first step of erythrocyte invasion relies on GPI-anchored parasite proteins, and in addition to major antigens, there are many other molecules with still unknown roles. Achieving a complete atlas of GPI-anchored proteins, including quantitative expression data, cellular and membrane organization, mechanisms and rates of soluble protein release, and protein and anchor structure, should be an important milestone. The knowledge about these proteins can then be applied to their usage in diagnostic or therapeutic applications as vaccines.

The immune response against these major antigens, at cell and antibody level, also deserves further studies. In particular, the definition of correlates of protection is needed to differentiate a protective from a non-protective response. The identification of biomarkers associated to immune protection is a prerequisite to the development of a predictive assay for the protection status of a subject, either human or animal. As an example, current IFAT or ELISA serological assays can detect antibodies against intraerythrocytic merozoites or recombinant proteins in sera from protected but also unprotected animals without evidencing differences between them. Considering that neutralization assays (growth-inhibitory assays) are not satisfying and need rather large amounts of the sample, the development of differentiating immune status assays for *Babesia* has high interest and could then be extrapolated to other Apicomplexa parasites.

There is a need to keep the basic science effort on *Babesia* at a high level, in particular, in a climate change context. The complete antigenic landscape, displayed by a GPI-anchored proteome in membrane-bound or soluble state, and the role of major antigens in this immune interface are still not fully understood. This knowledge is nevertheless critical to select and properly express recombinant antigens that could lead to efficient vaccines. Although well-established models have to be maintained to allow in-depth experiments, it should be anticipated that new parasite species could emerge, and then methods should be set up to ensure quick and efficient management of these human babesiosis cases. Currently, the generation of large data sets (annotated genome, transcriptome etc.) for a new species requires the propagation of the parasite to obtain sufficient amounts of biological material (DNA, RNA etc). Otherwise, GPI proteome prediction strategy based on hydrophobic signal recognition (which does not need sequence homologies) can be applied to many pathogens [71]. Until now, such data cannot easily be obtained from clinical human samples; therefore, animal inoculation continues to be used to isolate parasites. Although not needed for routine analysis, it should be performed in the case of an unknown parasite or atypical babesiosis, even if current animal models probably do not reflect the entire range of human susceptibility to *Babesia* species.

For serological analysis, whatever the commercial outcome, a panel of recombinant antigens should be the most efficient tools to cover the broad range of human *Babesia* parasites. Such an antigen toolbox will grow with each new protein or parasite described and should allow the definition of a common framework for serological assay development. The current markets of diagnostic assays for human and animal babesiosis are not the same, but it will be interesting to discuss a common toolbox extracted from scientific knowledge, based on a comparison between *Babesia* species. As discussed in this paper, major antigens and cognate antibodies could be used for vaccines, various types of serological assays, and antigen capture assays. This could be used to define biomarkers of protection, biomarkers of exposition, or biomarkers of active infection, which will be useful for human and animal babesiosis management.

Funding: This research received no external funding; all results were previously published.

Institutional Review Board Statement: Not applicable.

Informed Consent Statement: Not applicable.

Data Availability Statement: Not applicable.

Acknowledgments: The members of the Vaccine Against Parasite research team are acknowledged for their participation in this work.

Conflicts of Interest: The author declares no conflict of interest.

References

1. Lobo, C.A.; Singh, M.; Rodriguez, M. Human babesiosis: Recent advances and future challenges. *Curr. Opin. Hematol.* **2020**, *27*, 399–405. [CrossRef]
2. Homer, M.J.; Aguilar-Delfin, I.; Telford, S.R., 3rd; Krause, P.J.; Persing, D.H. Babesiosis. *Clin. Microbiol. Rev.* **2000**, *13*, 451–469. [CrossRef]
3. Young, K.M.; Corrin, T.; Wilhelm, B.; Uhland, C.; Greig, J.; Mascarenhas, M.; Waddell, L.A. Zoonotic *Babesia*: A scoping review of the global evidence. *PLoS ONE* **2019**, *14*, e0226781. [CrossRef]

4. Scott, J.D.; Sajid, M.S.; Pascoe, E.L.; Foley, J.E. Detection of *Babesia odocoilei* in humans with babesiosis symptoms. *Diagnostics* **2021**, *11*, 947. [CrossRef]
5. Conesa, J.J.; Sevilla, E.; Terrón, M.C.; González, L.M.; Gray, J.; Pérez-Berná, A.J.; Carrascosa, J.L.; Pereiro, E.; Chichón, F.J.; Luque, D.; et al. Four-dimensional characterization of the *Babesia divergens* asexual life cycle, from the trophozoite to the multiparasite stage. *mSphere* **2020**, *5*, e00928-20. [CrossRef]
6. Jalovecka, M.; Sojka, D.; Ascencio, M.; Schnittger, L. *Babesia* life cycle—When phylogeny meets biology. *Trends Parasitol.* **2019**, *35*, 356–368. [CrossRef]
7. Anantharaman, V.; Iyer, L.M.; Balaji, S.; Aravind, L. Adhesion molecules and other secreted host-interaction determinants in *Apicomplexa*: Insights from comparative genomics. *Int. Rev. Cytol.* **2007**, *262*, 1–74. [CrossRef]
8. Hoffman, S.L.; Vekemans, J.; Richie, T.L.; Duffy, P.E. The march toward malaria vaccines. *Am. J. Prev. Med.* **2015**, *49*, S319–S333. [CrossRef] [PubMed]
9. Schofield, L.; Hewitt, M.C.; Evans, K.; Siomos, M.-A.; Seeberger, P.H. Synthetic GPI as a candidate anti-toxic vaccine in a model of malaria. *Nature* **2002**, *418*, 785–789. [CrossRef] [PubMed]
10. Azzouz, N.; Gerold, P.; Schwarz, R.T. Metabolic labeling and structural analysis of glycosylphosphatidylinositols from parasitic protozoa. *Methods Mol. Biol.* **2019**, *1934*, 145–162. [CrossRef] [PubMed]
11. Debierre-Grockiego, F.; Schwarz, R.T. Immunological reactions in response to apicomplexan glycosylphosphatidylinositols. *Glycobiology* **2010**, *20*, 801–811. [CrossRef]
12. Gerold, P.; Schofield, L.; Blackman, M.J.; Holder, A.A.; Schwarz, R.T. Structural analysis of the glycosyl-phosphatidylinositol membrane anchor of the merozoite surface proteins-1 and -2 of *Plasmodium falciparum*. *Mol. Biochem. Parasitol.* **1996**, *75*, 131–143. [CrossRef]
13. Rodríguez, A.E.; Couto, A.; Echaide, I.; Schnittger, L.; Florin-Christensen, M. *Babesia bovis* contains an abundant parasite-specific protein-free glycerophosphatidylinositol and the genes predicted for its assembly. *Vet. Parasitol.* **2010**, *167*, 227–235. [CrossRef]
14. Debierre-Grockiego, F.; Smith, T.K.; Delbecq, S.; Ducournau, C.; Lantier, L.; Schmidt, J.; Brès, V.; Dimier-Poisson, I.; Schwarz, R.T.; Cornillot, E. *Babesia divergens* glycosylphosphatidylinositols modulate blood coagulation and induce Th2-biased cytokine profiles in antigen presenting cells. *Biochimie* **2019**, *167*, 135–144. [CrossRef]
15. Nathaly Wieser, S.; Schnittger, L.; Florin-Christensen, M.; Delbecq, S.; Schetters, T. Vaccination against babesiosis using recombinant GPI-Anchored proteins. *Int. J. Parasitol.* **2019**, *49*, 175–181. [CrossRef]
16. Florin-Christensen, M.; Suarez, C.E.; Rodriguez, A.E.; Flores, D.A.; Schnittger, L. Vaccines against bovine babesiosis: Where we are now and possible roads ahead. *Parasitology* **2014**, *141*, 1563–1592. [CrossRef]
17. Rodriguez, A.E.; Florin-Christensen, M.; Flores, D.A.; Echaide, I.; Suarez, C.E.; Schnittger, L. The glycosylphosphatidylinositol-anchored protein repertoire of *Babesia bovis* and its significance for erythrocyte invasion. *Ticks Tick Borne Dis.* **2014**, *5*, 343–348. [CrossRef] [PubMed]
18. Carcy, B.; Precigout, E.; Valentin, A.; Gorenflot, A.; Schrevel, J. A 37-Kilodalton Glycoprotein of *Babesia divergens* is a major component of a protective fraction containing low-molecular-mass culture-derived exoantigens. *Infect. Immun.* **1995**, *63*, 811–817. [CrossRef] [PubMed]
19. Li, M.; Ao, Y.; Guo, J.; Nie, Z.; Liu, Q.; Yu, L.; Luo, X.; Zhan, X.; Zhao, Y.; Wang, S.; et al. Surface Antigen 1 is a crucial secreted protein that mediates *Babesia microti* invasion into host cells. *Front. Microbiol.* **2019**, *10*, 3046. [CrossRef]
20. Hines, S.A.; Palmer, G.H.; Jasmer, D.P.; McGuire, T.C.; McElwain, T.F. Neutralization-sensitive merozoite surface antigens of *Babesia bovis* encoded by members of a polymorphic gene family. *Mol. Biochem. Parasitol.* **1992**, *55*, 85–94. [CrossRef]
21. McElwain, T.F.; Perryman, L.E.; Musoke, A.J.; McGuire, T.C. Molecular characterization and immunogenicity of neutralization-sensitive *Babesia bigemina* merozoite surface proteins. *Mol. Biochem. Parasitol.* **1991**, *47*, 213–222. [CrossRef]
22. Yang, Y.-S.; Murciano, B.; Moubri, K.; Cibrelus, P.; Schetters, T.; Gorenflot, A.; Delbecq, S.; Roumestand, C. Structural and functional characterization of bc28.1, major erythrocyte-binding protein from *Babesia canis* merozoite surface. *J. Biol. Chem.* **2012**, *287*, 9495–9508. [CrossRef]
23. Zhou, M.; Cao, S.; Luo, Y.; Liu, M.; Wang, G.; Moumouni, P.F.A.; Jirapattharasate, C.; Iguchi, A.; Vudriko, P.; Terkawi, M.A.; et al. Molecular identification and antigenic characterization of a merozoite surface antigen and a secreted antigen of *Babesia canis* (BcMSA1 and BcSA1). *Parasit. Vectors* **2016**, *9*, 257. [CrossRef]
24. Moubri, K.; Kleuskens, J.; Van de Crommert, J.; Scholtes, N.; Van Kasteren, T.; Delbecq, S.; Carcy, B.; Précigout, E.; Gorenflot, A.; Schetters, T. Discovery of a recombinant *Babesia canis* supernatant antigen that protects dogs against virulent challenge infection. *Vet. Parasitol.* **2018**, *249*, 21–29. [CrossRef]
25. Valentin, A.; Precigout, E.; L'Hostis, M.; Carcy, B.; Gorenflot, A.; Schrevel, J. Cellular and humoral immune responses induced in cattle by vaccination with *Babesia divergens* culture-derived exoantigens correlate with protection. *Infect. Immun.* **1993**, *61*, 734–741. [CrossRef]
26. James, M.A. Application of exoantigens of *Babesia* and *Plasmodium* in vaccine development. *Trans. R. Soc. Trop. Med. Hyg.* **1989**, *83*, 67–72. [CrossRef]
27. Lemesre, J.-L.; Holzmuller, P.; Cavaleyra, M.; Gonçalves, R.B.; Hottin, G.; Papierok, G. Protection against experimental visceral leishmaniasis infection in dogs immunized with purified excreted secreted antigens of *Leishmania infantum* promastigotes. *Vaccine* **2005**, *23*, 2825–2840. [CrossRef]
28. Schetters, T. Vaccination against canine babesiosis. *Trends Parasitol.* **2005**, *21*, 179–184. [CrossRef]

29. Alvarez, J.A.; Rojas, C.; Figueroa, J.V. An overview of current knowledge on in vitro *Babesia* cultivation for production of live attenuated vaccines for bovine babesiosis in Mexico. *Front. Vet. Sci.* **2020**, *7*, 364. [CrossRef] [PubMed]
30. Grande, N.; Precigout, E.; Ancelin, M.L.; Moubri, K.; Carcy, B.; Lemesre, J.L.; Vial, H.; Gorenflot, A. Continuous in vitro culture of *Babesia divergens* in a serum-free medium. *Parasitology* **1997**, *115*, 81–89. [CrossRef] [PubMed]
31. Gorenflot, A.; Precigout, E.; Bissuel, G.; Lecointre, O.; Brasseur, P.; Vidor, E.; L'Hostis, M.; Schrevel, J. Identification of major *Babesiadivergens* polypeptides that induce protection against homologous challenge in gerbils. *Infect. Immun.* **1990**, *58*, 4076–4082. [CrossRef] [PubMed]
32. Precigout, E.; Delbecq, S.; Vallet, A.; Carcy, B.; Camillieri, S.; Hadj-Kaddour, K.; Kleuskens, J.; Schetters, T.; Gorenflot, A. Association between sequence polymorphism in an epitope of *Babesia divergens* Bd37 exoantigen and protection induced by passive transfer. *Int. J. Parasitol.* **2004**, *34*, 585–593. [CrossRef] [PubMed]
33. Delbecq, S.; Precigout, E.; Vallet, A.; Carcy, B.; Schetters, T.P.M.; Gorenflot, A. *Babesia divergens*: Cloning and biochemical characterization of Bd37. *Parasitology* **2002**, *125*, 305–312. [CrossRef]
34. Cuesta, I.; González, L.M.; Estrada, K.; Grande, R.; Zaballos, Á.; Lobo, C.A.; Barrera, J.; Sanchez-Flores, A.; Montero, E. High-quality draft genome sequence of *Babesia divergens*, the etiological agent of cattle and human babesiosis. *Genome Announc.* **2014**, *2*, e01194-14. [CrossRef] [PubMed]
35. Jackson, A.P.; Otto, T.D.; Darby, A.; Ramaprasad, A.; Xia, D.; Echaide, I.E.; Farber, M.; Gahlot, S.; Gamble, J.; Gupta, D.; et al. The evolutionary dynamics of variant antigen genes in *Babesia* reveal a history of genomic innovation underlying host-parasite interaction. *Nucleic Acids Res.* **2014**, *42*, 7113–7131. [CrossRef] [PubMed]
36. González, L.M.; Estrada, K.; Grande, R.; Jiménez-Jacinto, V.; Vega-Alvarado, L.; Sevilla, E.; de la Barrera, J.; Cuesta, I.; Zaballos, Á.; Bautista, J.M.; et al. Comparative and functional genomics of the protozoan parasite *Babesia divergens* highlighting the invasion and egress processes. *PLoS Negl. Trop. Dis.* **2019**, *13*, e0007680. [CrossRef] [PubMed]
37. Carcy, B.; Précigout, E.; Schetters, T.; Gorenflot, A. Genetic basis for GPI-Anchor merozoite surface antigen polymorphism of *Babesia* and resulting antigenic diversity. *Vet. Parasitol.* **2006**, *138*, 33–49. [CrossRef] [PubMed]
38. Hadj-Kaddour, K.; Carcy, B.; Vallet, A.; Randazzo, S.; Delbecq, S.; Kleuskens, J.; Schetters, T.; Gorenflot, A.; Precigout, E. Recombinant protein Bd37 protected gerbils against heterologous challenges with isolates of *Babesia divergens* polymorphic for the Bd37 gene. *Parasitology* **2007**, *134*, 187–196. [CrossRef]
39. Delbecq, S.; Hadj-Kaddour, K.; Randazzo, S.; Kleuskens, J.; Schetters, T.; Gorenflot, A.; Précigout, E. Hydrophobic moeties in recombinant proteins are crucial to generate efficient saponin-based vaccine against apicomplexan *Babesiadivergens*. *Vaccine* **2006**, *24*, 613–621. [CrossRef]
40. Delbecq, S.; Auguin, D.; Yang, Y.-S.; Löhr, F.; Arold, S.; Schetters, T.; Précigout, E.; Gorenflot, A.; Roumestand, C. The solution structure of the adhesion protein Bd37 from *Babesia divergens* reveals structural homology with eukaryotic proteins involved in membrane trafficking. *J. Mol. Biol.* **2008**, *375*, 409–424. [CrossRef]
41. Cornillot, E.; Hadj-Kaddour, K.; Dassouli, A.; Noel, B.; Ranwez, V.; Vacherie, B.; Augagneur, Y.; Brès, V.; Duclos, A.; Randazzo, S.; et al. Sequencing of the smallest apicomplexan genome from the human pathogen *Babesia microti*. *Nucleic Acids Res.* **2012**, *40*, 9102–9114. [CrossRef]
42. Silva, J.C.; Cornillot, E.; McCracken, C.; Usmani-Brown, S.; Dwivedi, A.; Ifeonu, O.O.; Crabtree, J.; Gotia, H.T.; Virji, A.Z.; Reynes, C.; et al. Genome-wide diversity and gene expression profiling of *Babesia microti* isolates identify polymorphic genes that mediate host-pathogen interactions. *Sci. Rep.* **2016**, *6*, 35284. [CrossRef] [PubMed]
43. Puri, A.; Bajpai, S.; Meredith, S.; Aravind, L.; Krause, P.J.; Kumar, S. *Babesia microti: Pathogen* genomics, genetic variability, immunodominant antigens, and pathogenesis. *Front. Microbiol.* **2021**, *12*, 697669. [CrossRef] [PubMed]
44. Cornillot, E.; Dassouli, A.; Pachikara, N.; Lawres, L.; Renard, I.; Francois, C.; Randazzo, S.; Brès, V.; Garg, A.; Brancato, J.; et al. A targeted immunomic approach identifies diagnostic antigens in the human pathogen *Babesia Microti*. *Transfusion* **2016**, *56*, 2085–2099. [CrossRef] [PubMed]
45. Luo, Y.; Jia, H.; Terkawi, M.A.; Goo, Y.-K.; Kawano, S.; Ooka, H.; Li, Y.; Yu, L.; Cao, S.; Yamagishi, J.; et al. Identification and characterization of a novel secreted antigen 1 of *Babesia microti* and evaluation of its potential use in enzyme-linked immunosorbent assay and immunochromatographic test. *Parasitol. Int.* **2011**, *60*, 119–125. [CrossRef] [PubMed]
46. Lodes, M.J.; Houghton, R.L.; Bruinsma, E.S.; Mohamath, R.; Reynolds, L.D.; Benson, D.R.; Krause, P.J.; Reed, S.G.; Persing, D.H. Serological expression cloning of novel immunoreactive antigens of *Babesia microti*. *Infect. Immun.* **2000**, *68*, 2783–2790. [CrossRef] [PubMed]
47. Verma, N.; Puri, A.; Essuman, E.; Skelton, R.; Anantharaman, V.; Zheng, H.; White, S.; Gunalan, K.; Takeda, K.; Bajpai, S.; et al. Antigen discovery, bioinformatics and biological characterization of novel immunodominant *Babesia microti* antigens. *Sci. Rep.* **2020**, *10*, 9598. [CrossRef]
48. Gorenflot, A.; Brasseur, P.; Precigout, E.; L'Hostis, M.; Marchand, A.; Schrevel, J. Cytological and immunological responses to *Babesia divergens* in different hosts: Ox, gerbil, man. *Parasitol. Res.* **1991**, *77*, 3–12. [CrossRef]
49. Thekkiniath, J.; Kilian, N.; Lawres, L.; Gewirtz, M.A.; Graham, M.M.; Liu, X.; Ledizet, M.; Ben Mamoun, C. Evidence for vesicle-mediated antigen export by the human pathogen *Babesia microti*. *Life Sci. Alliance* **2019**, *2*, e201900382. [CrossRef]
50. Thekkiniath, J.; Mootien, S.; Lawres, L.; Perrin, B.A.; Gewirtz, M.; Krause, P.J.; Williams, S.; Doggett, J.S.; Ledizet, M.; Ben Mamoun, C. BmGPAC, an antigen capture assay for detection of active *Babesia microti* infection. *J. Clin. Microbiol.* **2018**, *56*, e00067-18. [CrossRef]

51. Elton, C.M.; Rodriguez, M.; Ben Mamoun, C.; Lobo, C.A.; Wright, G.J. A library of recombinant Babesia microti cell surface and secreted proteins for diagnostics discovery and reverse vaccinology. *Int. J. Parasitol.* **2019**, *49*, 115–125. [CrossRef]
52. Man, S.; Fu, Y.; Guan, Y.; Feng, M.; Qiao, K.; Li, X.; Gao, H.; Cheng, X. Evaluation of a major surface antigen of *Babesia microti* merozoites as a vaccine candidate against *Babesia* infection. *Front. Microbiol.* **2017**, *8*, 2545. [CrossRef]
53. Sevilla, E.; González, L.M.; Luque, D.; Gray, J.; Montero, E. Kinetics of the invasion and egress processes of *Babesia divergens*, observed by time-lapse video microscopy. *Sci. Rep.* **2018**, *8*, 14116. [CrossRef]
54. Bütikofer, P.; Malherbe, T.; Boschung, M.; Roditi, I. GPI-Anchored proteins: Now you see 'em, now you don't. *FASEB J.* **2001**, *15*, 545–548. [CrossRef]
55. Bar, L.; Dejeu, J.; Lartia, R.; Bano, F.; Richter, R.P.; Coche-Guérente, L.; Boturyn, D. Impact of antigen density on recognition by monoclonal antibodies. *Anal. Chem.* **2020**, *92*, 5396–5403. [CrossRef]
56. James, L.C.; Tawfik, D.S. Conformational diversity and protein evolution—A 60-year-old hypothesis revisited. *Trends Biochem. Sci.* **2003**, *28*, 361–368. [CrossRef]
57. Elfrink, K.; Ollesch, J.; Stöhr, J.; Willbold, D.; Riesner, D.; Gerwert, K. Structural changes of membrane-anchored native PrP(C). *Proc. Natl. Acad. Sci. USA* **2008**, *105*, 10815–10819. [CrossRef] [PubMed]
58. Puig, B.; Altmeppen, H.; Glatzel, M. The GPI-Anchoring of PrP: Implications in sorting and pathogenesis. *Prion* **2014**, *8*, 11–18. [CrossRef]
59. Puig, B.; Altmeppen, H.C.; Linsenmeier, L.; Chakroun, K.; Wegwitz, F.; Piontek, U.K.; Tatzelt, J.; Bate, C.; Magnus, T.; Glatzel, M. GPI-Anchor signal sequence influences PrPC sorting, shedding and signalling, and impacts on different pathomechanistic aspects of prion disease in mice. *PLoS Pathog.* **2019**, *15*, e1007520. [CrossRef] [PubMed]
60. Bradley, J.E.; Chan, J.M.; Hagood, J.S. Effect of the GPI anchor of human Thy-1 on antibody recognition and function. *Lab. Investig.* **2013**, *93*, 365–374. [CrossRef] [PubMed]
61. Miyagawa-Yamaguchi, A.; Kotani, N.; Honke, K. Each GPI-Anchored protein species forms a specific lipid raft depending on its GPI attachment signal. *Glycoconj. J.* **2015**, *32*, 531–540. [CrossRef]
62. Fotoran, W.L.; Kleiber, N.; Müntefering, T.; Liebau, E.; Wunderlich, G. Production of glycosylphosphatidylinositol-anchored proteins for vaccines and directed binding of immunoliposomes to specific cell types. *J. Venom. Anim. Toxins Incl. Trop. Dis.* **2020**, *26*, e20200032. [CrossRef] [PubMed]
63. Mott, G.A.; Wilson, R.; Fernando, A.; Robinson, A.; MacGregor, P.; Kennedy, D.; Schaap, D.; Matthews, J.B.; Matthews, K.R. Targeting cattle-borne zoonoses and cattle pathogens using a novel trypanosomatid-based delivery system. *PLoS Pathog.* **2011**, *7*, e1002340. [CrossRef]
64. Elguero, M.E.; Tomazic, M.L.; Montes, M.G.; Florin-Christensen, M.; Schnittger, L.; Nusblat, A.D. The *Cryptosporidium parvum* gp60 glycoprotein expressed in the ciliate *Tetrahymena thermophila* is immunoreactive with sera of calves infected with *Cryptosporidium* oocysts. *Vet. Parasitol.* **2019**, *271*, 45–50. [CrossRef] [PubMed]
65. Datoo, M.S.; Natama, M.H.; Somé, A.; Traoré, O.; Rouamba, T.; Bellamy, D.; Yameogo, P.; Valia, D.; Tegneri, M.; Ouedraogo, F.; et al. Efficacy of a low-dose candidate malaria vaccine, R21 in adjuvant Matrix-M, with seasonal administration to children in Burkina Faso: A Randomised Controlled Trial. *Lancet* **2021**, *397*, 1809–1818. [CrossRef]
66. Guirao-Arrabal, E.; González, L.M.; García-Fogeda, J.L.; Miralles-Adell, C.; Sánchez-Moreno, G.; Chueca, N.; Anguita-Santos, F.; Muñoz-Medina, L.; Vinuesa-García, D.; Hernández-Quero, J.; et al. Imported babesiosis caused by *Babesia microti*—A Case Report. *Ticks Tick Borne Dis.* **2020**, *11*, 101435. [CrossRef] [PubMed]
67. Tokarz, R.; Mishra, N.; Tagliafierro, T.; Sameroff, S.; Caciula, A.; Chauhan, L.; Patel, J.; Sullivan, E.; Gucwa, A.; Fallon, B.; et al. A multiplex serologic platform for diagnosis of tick-borne diseases. *Sci. Rep.* **2018**, *8*, 3158. [CrossRef] [PubMed]
68. González, L.M.; Castro, E.; Lobo, C.A.; Richart, A.; Ramiro, R.; González-Camacho, F.; Luque, D.; Velasco, A.C.; Montero, E. First report of *Babesia divergens* infection in an HIV patient. *Int. J. Infect. Dis.* **2015**, *33*, 202–204. [CrossRef] [PubMed]
69. Al-Nazal, H.A.; Cooper, E.; Ho, M.F.; Eskandari, S.; Majam, V.; Giddam, A.K.; Hussein, W.M.; Islam, M.T.; Skwarczynski, M.; Toth, I.; et al. Pre-clinical evaluation of a whole-parasite vaccine to control human babesiosis. *Cell Host Microbe* **2021**, *29*, 894–903.e5. [CrossRef] [PubMed]
70. Abraham, A.; Brasov, I.; Thekkiniath, J.; Kilian, N.; Lawres, L.; Gao, R.; DeBus, K.; He, L.; Yu, X.; Zhu, G.; et al. Establishment of a continuous in vitro culture of *Babesia duncani* in human erythrocytes reveals unusually high tolerance to recommended therapies. *J. Biol. Chem.* **2018**, *293*, 19974–19981. [CrossRef]
71. Tomazic, M.L.; Rodriguez, A.E.; Lombardelli, J.; Poklepovich, T.; Garro, C.; Galarza, R.; Tiranti, K.; Florin-Christensen, M.; Schnittger, L. Identification of novel vaccine candidates against *Cryptosporidiosis* of neonatal bovines by reverse vaccinology. *Vet. Parasitol.* **2018**, *264*, 74–78. [CrossRef] [PubMed]

pathogens

MDPI

Article

Babesia microti Immunoreactive Rhoptry-Associated Protein-1 Paralogs Are Ancestral Members of the Piroplasmid-Confined RAP-1 Family

Reginaldo G. Bastos [1,*], Jose Thekkiniath [2], Choukri Ben Mamoun [3], Lee Fuller [2], Robert E. Molestina [4], Monica Florin-Christensen [5,6], Leonhard Schnittger [5,6], Heba F. Alzan [1,7,8] and Carlos E. Suarez [1,9,*]

1 Department of Veterinary Microbiology and Pathology, College of Veterinary Medicine, Washington State University, Pullman, WA 99164, USA; heba.alzan@wsu.edu
2 Fuller Laboratories, 1312 East Valencia Drive, Fullerton, CA 92831, USA; jose.thekkiniath@fullerlabs.net (J.T.); Lee.Fuller@fullerlabs.net (L.F.)
3 Section of Infectious Diseases, Department of Internal Medicine, Yale School of Medicine, New Haven, CT 06520, USA; choukri.benmamoun@yale.edu
4 Protistology Laboratory, American Type Culture Collection, Manassas, VA 10801, USA; rmolestina@atcc.org
5 Consejo Nacional de Investigaciones Científicas y Técnicas (CONICET), Buenos Aires C1033AAJ, Argentina; jacobsen.monica@inta.gob.ar (M.F.-C.); schnittger.leonhard@inta.gob.ar (L.S.)
6 Instituto de Patobiología Veterinaria, CICVyA, INTA-Castelar, Hurlingham, Buenos Aires C1033AAE, Argentina
7 Parasitology and Animal Diseases Department, National Research Center, Dokki, Giza 12622, Egypt
8 Tick and Tick-Borne Disease Research Unit, National Research Center, Dokki, Giza 12622, Egypt
9 Animal Disease Research Unit, United States Department of Agricultural—Agricultural Research Service, Pullman, WA 99164, USA
* Correspondence: reginaldo_bastos@wsu.edu (R.G.B.); carlos.suarez@usda.gov (C.E.S.)

Citation: Bastos, R.G.; Thekkiniath, J.; Ben Mamoun, C.; Fuller, L.; Molestina, R.E.; Florin-Christensen, M.; Schnittger, L.; Alzan, H.F.; Suarez, C.E. *Babesia microti* Immunoreactive Rhoptry-Associated Protein-1 Paralogs Are Ancestral Members of the Piroplasmid-Confined RAP-1 Family. *Pathogens* **2021**, *10*, 1384. https://doi.org/10.3390/pathogens10111384

Academic Editors: Estrella Montero, Jeremy Gray, Cheryl Ann Lobo and Luis Miguel González

Received: 17 September 2021
Accepted: 23 October 2021
Published: 26 October 2021

Abstract: *Babesia*, *Cytauxzoon* and *Theileria* are tick-borne apicomplexan parasites of the order Piroplasmida, responsible for diseases in humans and animals. Members of the piroplasmid rhoptry-associated protein-1 (pRAP-1) family have a signature cysteine-rich domain and are important for parasite development. We propose that the closely linked *B. microti* genes annotated as BMR1_03g00947 and BMR1_03g00960 encode two paralogue pRAP-1-like proteins named BmIPA48 and Bm960. The two genes are tandemly arranged head to tail, highly expressed in blood stage parasites, syntenic to *rap-1* genes of other piroplasmids, and share large portions of an almost identical ~225 bp sequence located in their 5′ putative regulatory regions. BmIPA48 and Bm960 proteins contain a N-terminal signal peptide, share very low sequence identity (<13%) with pRAP-1 from other species, and harbor one or more transmembrane domains. Diversification of the piroplasmid-confined *prap-1* family is characterized by amplification of genes, protein domains, and a high sequence polymorphism. This suggests a functional involvement of pRAP-1 at the parasite-host interface, possibly in parasite adhesion, attachment, and/or evasion of the host immune defenses. Both BmIPA48 and Bm960 are recognized by antibodies in sera from humans infected with *B. microti* and might be promising candidates for developing novel serodiagnosis and vaccines.

Keywords: *Babesia microti*; BmIPA48; BMR1_03g00960; piroplasmid rhoptry-associated protein-1 (pRAP-1); human babesiosis

1. Introduction

Babesia, *Cytauxzoon* and *Theileria* are tick-borne apicomplexan piroplasmid parasites of vertebrates that invade and reproduce asexually in erythrocytes. These parasites are a major concern to human and animal health and cause an important economic burden worldwide. *Babesia* parasites are responsible for acute and persistent hemolytic disease in several wild and domestic vertebrate species, including human. While *Theileria* parasites are transmitted transstadially by ticks, *sensu stricto* (s.s.) *Babesia* spp. are transovarially and, in some species, also transstadially, transmitted. Other piroplasmids, such as *B. microti*, are defined as *sensu lato* (s.l.) *Babesia* parasites, based on their transstadial mode of transmission and the absence of schizont stages in their life cycles [1–3].

Human babesiosis is an emergent worldwide zoonosis caused by several *Babesia* spp., including the s.s. *B. divergens* and the s.l. *B. microti*, the latter of which is the predominant agent in the Northeastern and Midwest regions of the US [4,5]. As for other piroplasmids, the life cycle of *B. microti* is dixenic, involving an invertebrate definitive host and a vertebrate host. In the US, the primary vertebrate host is the white-footed mouse (*Peromyscus leucopus*) and the invertebrate host is a tick of the genus *Ixodes*, such as *I. scapularis*. However, humans are accidental and dead-end hosts when bitten by infected ticks. Importantly, human-to-human transmission of *B. microti* may occur via contaminated blood transfusions [6,7]. Due to climate change and human activity, the geographic distribution of *I. scapularis*, and hence of *B. microti*, is expanding rapidly in the US [8]. In addition, the finding of vertical transmission in the white-footed mouse indicates a potentially relevant way of parasite dissemination without the participation of the tick vector [9]. The disease caused by *B. microti* in humans may vary from asymptomatic or subclinical to acute and chronic manifestations, which can be lethal in immunocompromised patients. Clinical manifestations of acute human babesiosis include fever, hemolytic anemia, acute respiratory distress and multiorgan dysfunction [10]. Because of the expansion of the tick habitat and the constant increase in cases of human babesiosis in the US, there is a need to develop vaccines and improved diagnostics against *B. microti*, which requires identification of conserved immunogenic proteins in this apicomplexan parasite.

Apicomplexan parasites, including *B. microti*, are equipped with an apical complex with at least three distinct secretory organelles known as the rhoptries, micronemes, and spherical bodies or dense granules. These organelles play an essential role in host cell invasion by the parasite [11]. Once the parasite is committed to invasion, it is quickly and actively propelled inside the target cell by the activity of an actin motor, with intervention of the cytoskeletal structures of the parasite [12]. Rhoptry proteins are probably involved in the formation of the parasitophorous vacuole (PV), a membranous structure separating the parasite from the cytoplasm of the host cell, that disappears quickly upon invasion in *Babesia* parasites [13]. Remarkably, *B. microti* also developed a mechanism for vesicle-mediated antigen export generating an interlacement of vesicles which extends from the plasma membrane of the parasite into the cytoplasm of the host erythrocyte [14]. Few rhoptry proteins have been so far identified and characterized in *Babesia* parasites. Initial studies performed mainly in *B. bovis* and *B. bigemina* were focused on the functional role of rhoptry-associated protein-1s (RAP-1s), which were later identified in all piroplasmids, including other *Babesia* spp., *Theileria* spp. and *Cytauxzoon felis* [15–23]. We hereby refer to these proteins as piroplasmid RAP-1s (pRAP-1s). It is possible that the function of these piroplasmid-specific proteins is needed to support unique features of the parasite life cycle, such as parasite-attachment to the erythrocyte, dissolution of the PV in *Babesia*, the zipper-mediated invasion of *Theileria*, or other events that may be related to erythrocyte invasion and egress [24,25]. The *prap-1* gene superfamily encodes the paralogs *rap-1* and RAP-1-related antigens (*rra*) in *B. bovis* [26]. Plasmodial RAP-1 shares the same denomination with pRAP-1s, but they are unrelated non-homologous proteins [27]. Since pRAP-1 proteins are highly immunogenic and can be targeted for neutralization-sensitive antibodies, they may be attractive candidates for diagnostic assays or subunit vaccines against *Babesia* and *Theileria* parasites [16,28–34].

The piroplasmid-specific RAP-1 family domain (PF03085) contains a characteristic motif of four cysteine (Cys) residues and a single conserved tyrosine (Tyr) residue. Other definitions of the members of this protein family are based on localization or function, which are still waiting experimental confirmation. Although the pRAP-1 proteins have been identified and annotated in genomes of *Babesia* spp. s.s., *Cytauxzoon felis*, and *Theileria* spp. parasites, they remain not fully identified in the genome of the s.l. parasite *B. microti*. A RAP putative protein (XP_021337499) was annotated in the genome of *B. microti*, but this protein, which is homologous to *Plasmodium* and *Toxoplasma* RAPs, lacks the characteristic motifs of the members of the *Babesia/Theileria* pRAP-1 superfamily [35]. Thus, the presence of canonical *Babesia/Theileria* pRAP-1 genes has yet to be reported in *B. microti*. We hypothesized that, like *Babesia* and *Theileria* parasites, the genome of *B. microti* also includes genes encoding for pRAP-1 or pRAP-1-like proteins. Furthermore, because of the relatively distant phylogenetic relationship of *B. microti* with piroplasmid parasites such as *Babesia* s.s. and *Theileria* s.s. [1], we propose that the pRAP-1-like proteins encoded by *B. microti* may have diverged dramatically from the pRAP-1 molecules expressed in other piroplasmids, resulting in a low non-significant sequence identity, but conservation of important structural features. Indeed, neither a common BLASTp nor a Pfam search resulted in hit or domain report, respectively. Therefore, we carried out alternative search strategies on the *B. microti* genome based on the previously detected conserved synteny in the genome regions of piroplasmid parasites where the *prap-1* loci are encoded and found two head-to-tail oriented linked genes, BMR1_03g00947 and BMR1_03g00960, encoding for proteins with structural characteristics that are compatible with the pRAP-1 molecules. Although the database searches did not result in hits, synteny analysis and the presence of highly conserved amino acid residues of structural importance organized as the Cys-rich domains of the pRAP-1s proteins strongly suggest that the presented two genes encode for pRAP-1 homologs in *B. microti*. Since these putative *B. microti* pRAP-1 proteins lack significant sequence identity with pRAP-1 domains of other pRAP-1s, we designated them pRAP-1-like proteins. For the aforementioned reasons, *B. microti* pRAP-1-like proteins have previously remained unnoticed, though these proteins have been identified and shown to be expressed in *B. microti* merozoites [35,36].

2. Results

2.1. Two Tandemly Arranged RAP-1 Syntenic Genes of B. microti Encode Proteins Containing Non-Canonical Piroplasmid RAP-1 Cys-Rich Domains

The piroplasmid RAP-1 proteins contain a characteristic Cys-rich domain, signal peptide, and other short conserved sequence motifs. The salient features of some typical pRAP-1 and RRA representatives of this family are schematized in Figure S1. In this study, we first searched the predicted proteome of the *B. microti* R1 strain for the identification of proteins containing pRAP-1 Cys motifs using Delta-Blast analysis against a query of the *B. bigemina* RAP-1c Cys-rich domain (CLGSKDEHHCASQIAAYVARCKE), also typical for the pRAP-1s of *B. bovis* (Figure 1). This search revealed a hit with the hypothetical protein encoded by gene BMR1_03g00960, here referred to as Bm960 (Figure 1). This finding prompted us to investigate the corresponding gene locus for the presence of other *rap-1* related genes and for synteny with *B. bovis*, *B. bigemina* and *T. equi rap-1* loci. Sequence analysis revealed that the BMR1_03g00947 gene, reffered to as BmIPA48 (Figure S1), located immediately next to Bm960, and separated by an 800-bp intergenic region, encodes for a protein also containing a similar RAP-1-like Cys-rich region, including a key conserved Tyr residue in its amino terminal (Figure 1, Figure 2B,C and Figure S2).

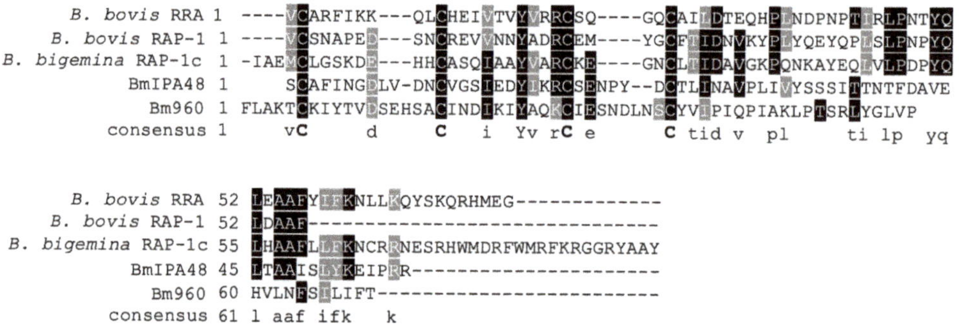

Figure 1. Representative figure of the comparisons performed with the pRAP-1 Cys-rich motif among babesial rRAP-1 proteins and the newly identified *B. microti* putative pRAP-1. The comparisons include the Cys-rich regions of *B. bovis* RRA, *B. bovis* RAP-1, *B. bigemina* RAP-1c, and the *B. microti* RAP-1- like proteins BmIPA48 and Bm960.

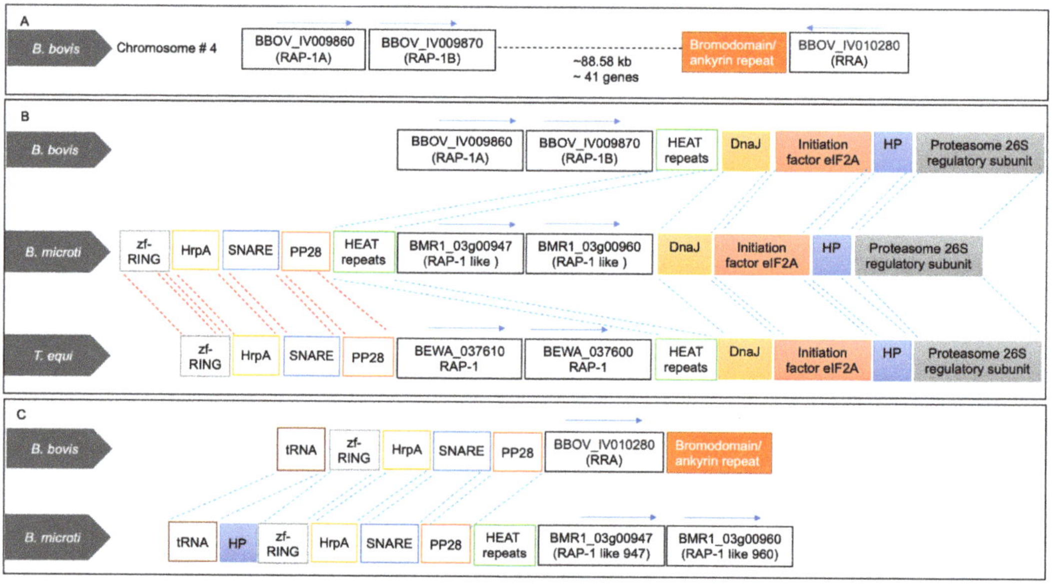

Figure 2. Synteny map of the *rap-1* locus of *T. equi*, putative *rap-1 B. microti*, and typical s.s. *B. bovis*. (**A**) Structure of the *prap-1* and *rra* genes localized in the chromosome 4 of *B. bovis*. (**B**) Conserved synteny among the *rap-1* loci of *B. bovis* and *T. equi* and the BMR1_03g00960 (BmIPA48) and BMR1_03g00947 (Bm960) genes of *B. microti*, that encode for proteins containing the typical Cys-rich region of the pRAP-1 proteins. (**C**) Conserved synteny among the *B. bovis rra* and the *B. microti* BMR1_03g00960 and BMR1_03g00947 genes.

As shown in Figure 2A, the chromosome 4 of *B. bovis* contains two identical head-to-tail arranged *prap-1* genes, and a single gene encoding for the RRA protein. These two loci are separated by a 88.5 kb intervening region containing ~41 genes. A comparison between the rap-1 loci of *B. bovis* and *T. equi* with the *B. microti* locus containing BmIPA48 and Bm960 genes is shown in Figure 2B. This illustration shows full synteny in the 5′ and 3′ ends of the *B. microti* BmIPA48 and Bm960 gene locus and the *prap-1* locus of *T. equi*. In Figure 2C we illustrate partial synteny of the 3′ end of the *B. microti* genes and the rra locus of *B. bovis*. Besides the presence of the unique Cys-rich regions, there was no significant sequence similarity among the putative pRAP-1 proteins encoded by the BmIPA48 and Bm960 genes (Figure S2). However, the alignment shows conserved Cys, Tyr, and other typical residues of the pRAP-1 proteins in the NT-region of the molecules, as well as other short amino acid motifs (Figure S2). The protein encoded by gene BMR1_ BmIPA48 also contains a series of tandem repeats in its C-terminal region, a feature that is shared with the *B. bovis* RAP-1 proteins (Figure 3 and Figure S3). Strikingly, sequence analysis of the non-coding regions immediately upstream of genes BmIPA48 and Bm960 revealed conservation of a 300-bp sequence (Figure 3 and Figure S4), suggesting that expression of these two proteins might be coordinated, despite their non-relatedness in sequence. In addtion, secondary structure sequence analysis performed in silico using TMpred suggests that BmIPA48 contains a signal peptide (aa 4–24) and a putative transmembrane (TM) region (aa 164–186) (Figure 4). Since no TM domains were previously reported in this protein, the prediction was confirmed using the alternative algorithm Phobius, which also showed the presence of a TM domain in the same region (Figure S6). Bm960 protein also contains a predicted signal peptide, two TM domains, and lack a predicted GPI anchor attachment site (Figure 4). Collectively, these features are fully consistent with expression on the surface of the parasite, as previously predicted [35].

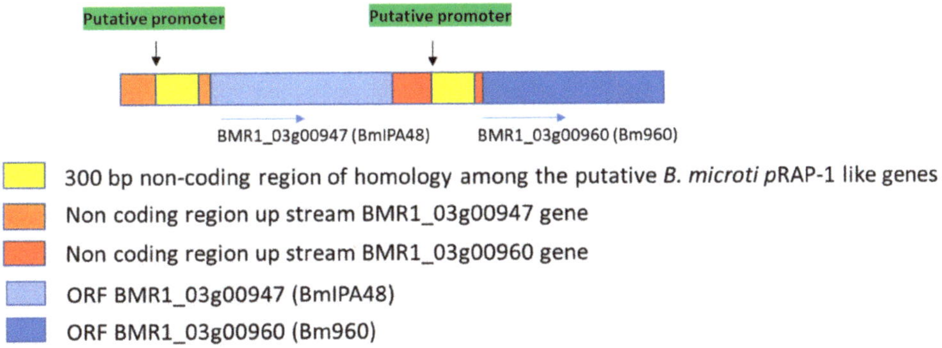

Figure 3. Schematic representation of the locus encoding for the *B. microti* RAP-1 putative proteins BmIPA48 and Bm960. A ~300 bp region upstream the two ORFs is repeated (yellow boxes).

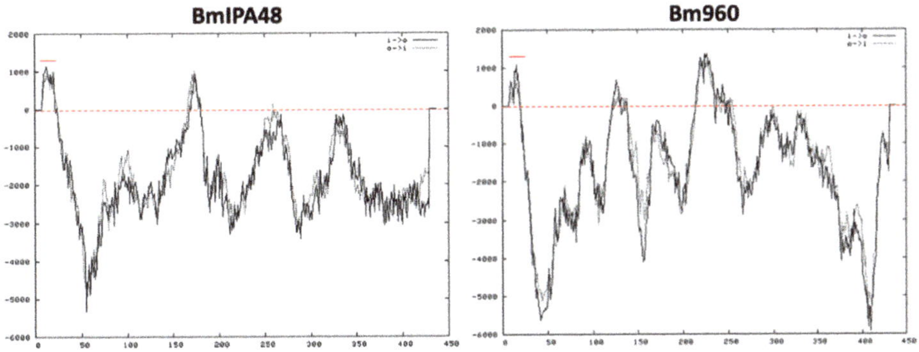

Figure 4. Predicted secondary structure of the pRAP-1-like proteins BmIPA48 and Bm960 using the Program TMpred. Predicted location of signal peptide (SP) is marked with a red bar. A dashed red line marks the boundary between predicted hydrophilic and hydrophobic transmembrane regions of the proteins.

2.2. *Significance of Synteny Relationships among rap-1 and rra Genes of Babesia and Theileria*

After identifying BmIPA48 and Bm960 as two *B. microti* encoded proteins containing non-canonical piroplasmid RAP-1 Cys-rich domains, we perfomed synteny analysis of these genes. Results showed a remarkable synteny conservation of the *rap-1* locus in piroplasmids (Figure 2). The BmIPA48 and Bm960 locus is in close vicinity with 3 genes that are also in the neighborhood of the *rap-1* genes in *B. bovis* and *Theileria* spp. (Figure 2). Moreover, one of these neighboring genes, encoding for the platelet-derived GF associated protein, is also associated with the locus of the *rra* gene of *B. bovis*. The schematic representation of the *rap-1* loci of *B. microti*, *Theileria* and *Babesia* s.s. in Figure 2 suggests the occurrence of a mechanism of genomic rearrangement in a chromosome of an ancestral *Babesia* organism that resulted in the insertion of an intervening region (~88 kb) encoding 41 genes in the case of *B. bovis* (Figure 2A).

2.3. Phylogeny of Piroplasmid RAP-1 Proteins Recapitulates Piroplasmid Phylogeny

Next, we inferred on the phylogenetic relationship between amino acid sequences of pRAP-1-like BmIPA48 and Bm960 (Clade I, *B. microti*-group: *B. microti* RI) with that of pRAP-1 proteins encoded in available reference genomes of piroplasmid species belonging to Clade II (Western clade: *B. duncani* WA), Clade III (Cytauxzoon: *C. felis* Winnie), Clade IV (Equus group: *T. equi* WA1), Clade V (*Theileria* s.s: *T. annulata* Ankara C9, *T. parva* Muguga, and *T. orientalis* Shintoku), and Clade VI (*Babesia* s.s.: *B. bovis* T2Bo, *B. ovata* Miyake, *B. bigemina* Bond, *Babesia* sp. Xinjiang) (Clades as defined by Schnittger et al. 2012 [1], Jalovecka et al. 2019 [3]) (Figure 5). Based on the assumption that *B. microti* is distantly related to other piroplasmid species, the tree was rooted using *B. microti* RI RAP-1-like BmIPA48 as an outgroup. As can be seen in Figure 5, the constructed pRAP-1 protein tree recapitulates phylogenetic lineages of piroplasmids as previously reported [1]. However, Bm960 places with a low bootstrap (bs: 34) as sister taxon to remaining *Babesia* s.s. pRAP-1 proteins due to its low sequence identity with other pRAP-1 proteins.

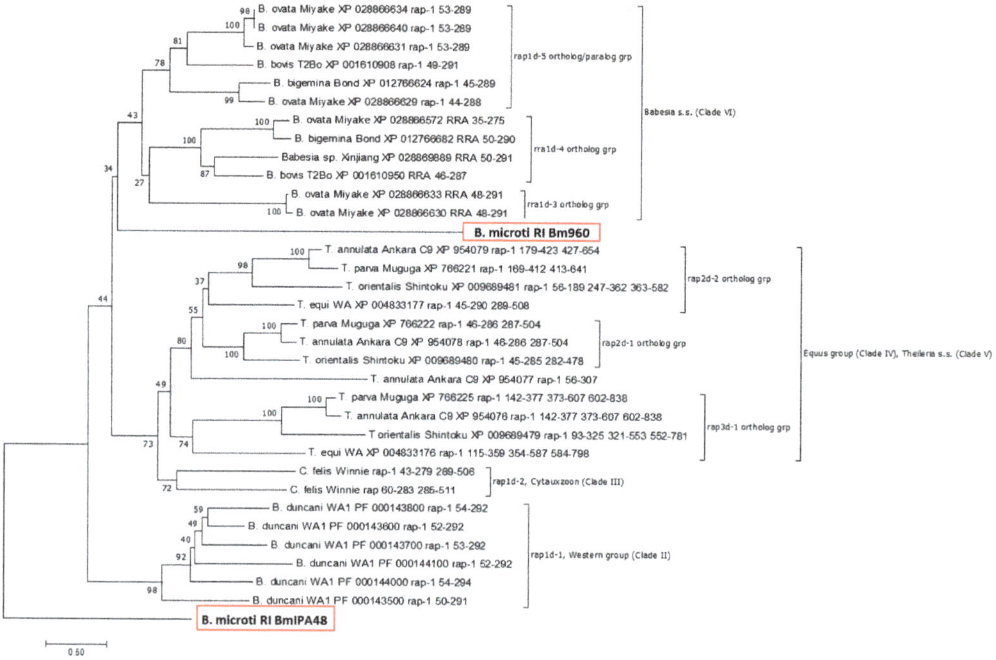

Figure 5. Phylogenetic neighbor joining tree inferred using amino acid sequences of pRAP-1 from the reference genomes of s.s. *Babesia* (Clade VI), s.s. *Theileria* (Clade V), *T. equi* (Clade IV), *C. felis* (Clade III), and *B. duncani* (Clade II) and the *B. microti* RAP-1 proteins BmIPA48 and Bm960 (bold fonts, red boxes). Bootstrap values of 1000 replicates are shown next to the branches. BmIPA48 is used as outgroup. The scale gives the evolutionary distance used to construct the tree.

Because of the expansion in the number of pRAP-1 domains in *Theileria* and *Cytauxzoon*, here we propose a new nomenclature for this gene family, which is based on the number of pRAP-1 domains in encoded proteins and shown in Figures 3 and 5. Thus, *rap1d*, *rap2d*, and *rap3d* genes encode for pRAP-1 proteins that comprise of a single (as seen in *B. microti*, Clade I; *B. duncani*, Clade V; and *Babesia* s.s., Clade VI), a tandemly repeated (as seen in *Cytauxzoon*, Clade III; *T. equi*, Clade IV, and *Theileria* s.s. Clade V), or tandemly triplicated pRAP-1 domains (*T. equi*, Clade IV, and *Theileria* s.s. Clade V), respectively (Table 1). Furthermore, an additional number refers to the placement into different orthologous groups within each piroplasmid phylogenetic lineage (Figure 5).

Table 1. Correlation of *rap* domain architecture and number of *rap-1* paralogs with phylogenetic classification of piroplasmids.

Species (Reference Genome)	Clade (Sensu Schnittger et al. 2012)	*rap-1* Domain Architectures	Number of *rap-1* Paralogs	Nomenclature (Proposed)
B. microti	I (*B. microti*-group)	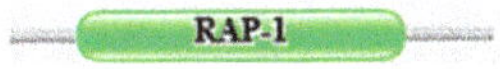	2×	*rap1d*-like
B. duncani	II (Western group	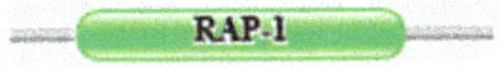	6×	*rap1d-1*
C. felis	III (*Cytauxzoon*)	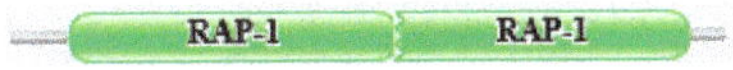	2×	*rap1d-2*
T. equi	IV (Equus group)	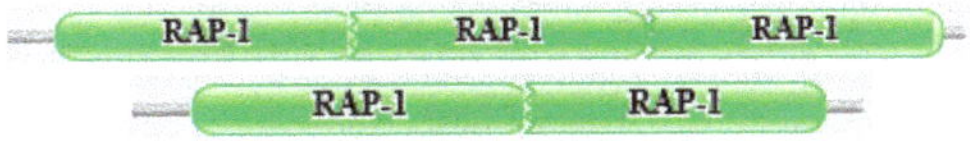	1× 1×	*rap2d-1* *rap3d-1*
T. annulata *T. parva* *T. orientalis*	V (*Theileria* s.s.)	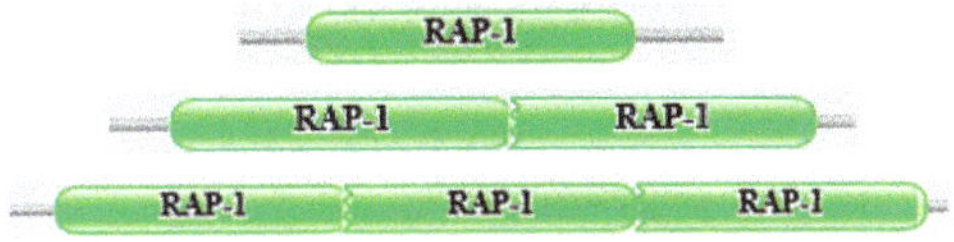	Ta:1×, Tp:1×,To:0 Ta:2×,Tp:2×,To:2× Ta:1×, Tp:1×,To:2×	*rap2d-2* *rap2d-1* *rap3d-1*
B. bovis *B. bigemina* *B. ovata* *Babesia* sp. Xinjiang	VI (*Babesia* s.s.)	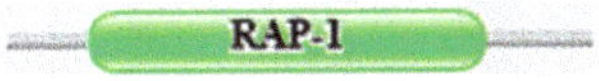	3× 2× 8× 1×	*rap1d-3* *rap1d-4* *rap1d-5*

Interestingly, two orthologous groups of *Babesia* s.s. (*rap1d-3* and *rap1d-4*) correspond with chromosomal rearrangements that have resulted in the generation of RRA proteins, which, although their pRAP-1 domain is complete, are shortened at their C-terminal end and are only found in *Babesia* s.s. (Figure 1). As shown in Figure 2, *Babesia* parasites contain two or more copies of pRAP-1 and a single additional RRA located ~40–80 kb from the pRAP-1 locus, separated by the insertion of an intervening sequence (Figure 2A). Results show that this is not the case for *Theileria* parasites, which did not undergo the splitting of the *rap-1* locus due to chromosome rearrangements and thus, lack *rra* genes (Figure 2A).

2.4. BmIPA48 and Bm960 Are Immunogenic during Infection in Humans

A previous study identified BmIPA48 and Bm960 proteins as possible biomarkers of acute infection by using a combination of nanoparticle harvesting technology and mass spectrometry on blood derived from *B. microti* infected hamsters [37]. Even though the antigenicity of Bm960 was not investigated in detail, the protein was not recognized by global antibody screening in rodent models. Bm960 was found to be highly polymorphic among strains [35], and to be present in the plasma of infected hamsters [36], confirming that it is a component of the secretome of the parasite. So far, the immunogenicity of BmIPA48 and Bm960 proteins has remained unknown in *B. microti*-infected humans. We then investigated whether sera from B. microti infected humans contain antibodies that recognize these two proteins. To this end, we expressed and purified recombinant HIS-tagged truncated forms of BmIPA48 and Bm960 proteins. The recombinant proteins were analyzed in ELISA and immunoblot using previously characterized sera from *B. microti*-infected humans (Figure 6). Antibodies from four *B. microti*-infected individuals recognized BmIPA48 and Bm960 in ELISA. Immunoblot analysis showed that antibodies from infected humans reacted with a product of expected size of BmIPA48 and Bm960 recombinant proteins, as recognized by control anti-HIS monoclonal antibody (Figure 6).

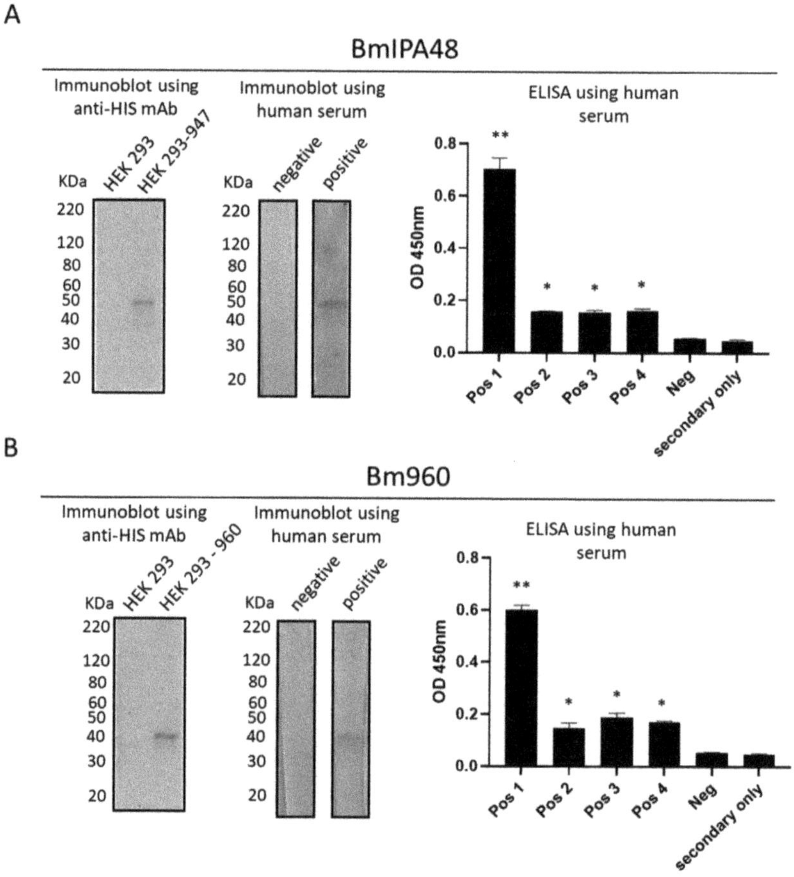

Figure 6. Immunogenicity of BmIPA48 and Bm960 in *B. microti*-infected humans. Expression of the recombinant BmIPA48 and Bm960 containing a HIS-tag in the immunoblots was demonstrated using an anti-HIS monoclonal antibody (panels (**A**,**B**), respectively). A control lysate of cells not expressing the recombinant protein was included as a negative control (HEK 293). Immunoblots were incubated with human *B. microti* positive and negative sera. ELISAs were performed with four positive (Pos 1, Pos 2, Pos 3, and Pos4) and one negative (Neg) human serum samples were tested. A control sample incubated only with secondary anti-human IgG serum (secondary only) was also included in the ELISA analysis. ** $p < 0.001$. * $p < 0.01$.

3. Discussion

In this study we identified two pRAP-1 in *B. microti*, named BmIPA48 and Bm960. Previous work indicated that BmIPA48 and Bm960 are highly expressed by *B. microti* merozoites and present in the parasite secretome [35]. The BMR1_03g00947 protein was previously identified erroneously as an orthologue of the *P. falciparum* gene PF3D7_1324300, and given the designation of BmIPA48, which is kept in the present study to avoid confusion [35,36]. However, alignment of PF3D7_1324300 and BmIPA48 reveals that their similarity is limited mainly to the glycine residues located in the tandem repeat regions of the two proteins (Figure S5). The tandem repeat region in PF3D7_1324300 is not pan-conserved among *Plasmodium* proteins, suggesting that it might lack functional or structural relevance, but instead, it may work as a decoy for the immune system of the host. This observation also suggests that the repeat segment may be a result of convergent evolution, and thus BmIPA48 might not be a true orthologue of PF3D7_1324300. Also, BmIPA48 contains non-synonymous polymorphisms, including a variable microsatellite region, that is highly antigenic and secreted, as part of tubes of vesicles during infection in mice [14,35]. In addition, electron microscopy analysis demonstrated that BmIPA48 is localized inside lipid-rich vesicles, which is consistent with their exclusive association with a membrane fraction. Also, IFA shows association of BmIPA48 with the cytoplasm of infected erythrocytes [37]. The presence of previously unnoticed TM domains in BmIPA48 is compatible with the association and export of this protein via lipid-rich vesicles to the cytoplasm of host erythrocytes and eventually to the outside of the host cell, as previously reported [14].

Considering that random gene location associations among four gene loci are highly unlikely in genomes larger than 8 Mb as those of *Babesia* and *Theileria* parasites, the data strongly suggest that the BmIPA48 and Bm960 genes are positional equivalents of the *Babesia-Theileria rap-1* genes. The biological significance of conserved gene synteny remains undefined. However, co-localization of genes may be important in epigenetic mechanisms and may influence the topology of the chromatin, which in turn can heavily influence coordinated gene expression and gene evolution. It is possible that the presence of syntenic genes results in the advantages of sharing regulatory mechanisms [38]. Sequence analysis of the non-coding regions immediately upstream of BmIPA48 and Bm960 showed conservation of a 300-bp sequence, suggesting a potential coordinated expression of these genes. Notably, a similar feature was found in other *Babesia* tandemly arranged and closely related or identical gene pairs or triplets, such as the *B. bovis rap-1s*, *msa-2s*, and *ef-1α*, that share common 5′ untranslated regions [15,39–41].

A remarkable synteny conservation of the *rap-1* locus in piroplasmids is shown by the data in our study (Figure 2). In addition, the insertion of an intervening region may have resulted in the splitting of the original *rap-1* locus, favoring independent gene evolution of the two identical copies of *rap-1* and *rra* genes [15,26,42]. A similar gene organization is found in *B. bigemina* with a *rra* gene separated by a similar large intervening region from a highly diversified and complex *rap-1* locus [17]. Interestingly, the intervening region between *rra* and *rap-1* in *Babesia* parasites is located ~100 kb upstream in the same chromosome in the *B. microti*, as well as in the *T. equi* genomes. However, all the *rap-1* genes are located together in a single cluster in this group of organisms, which also lack *rra* genes. Altogether, comparative analysis of the locus encoding *B. microti* BmIPA48 and Bm960 proteins with the loci of *Babesia* and *Theileria rap-1* genes provides interesting insights on the synteny and the evolution of the genome of these parasites.

Results from the phylogenetic analysis supports the notion that Bm960 cannot be defined as pRAP-1 based on sequence identity, but only due to structural conservations and synteny. Importantly, it can also be concluded from the phylogenetic tree that pRAP-1 is a relatively complex highly polymorphic protein family that underwent multiple duplications into large gene families of paralogs, tandem duplications and triplications of the pRAP-1 cys-rich domain, and a substantial nucleotide diversification, resulting in the existence of multiple highly polymorphic pRAP-1 domains. Thus, this protein family displays a considerable complexity, typically observed for molecules that play a pivotal functional role in the parasite-host interface, such as adhesion, attachment, and invasion, or the interaction with the host immune defense [43]. We hypothesize that the generation of diversification of pRAP-1 proteins is driven by a strong positive selection to optimize adhesion and attachment to their different hosts, as is required for the evolution of parasite host-specificity. The different copy number of pRAP-1 domains in a single protein may represent an adaptation strategy to different hosts and life cycles, enabling the parasites to invade different host species and cells. *C. felis* has two tandemly arranged pRAP-1 proteins containing canonical domains, while most *Theileria* has pRAP-1 proteins with tandemly duplicated or triplicated pRAP-1 domains. Both the *C. felis* and *Theileria* pRAP-1 domains contain 4 conserved Cys residues and a single conserved Tyr residue, as originally described in *Babesia* [15,17,26]. Considering that certain pRAP-1 features correspond with the phylogenetic classification of piroplasmid species, this finding may be exploited for the development of specific diagnostic tests. Furthermore, pRAP-1 proteins with a duplicated and/or triplicated domain architecture specify the piroplasmid lineages *Cytauxzoon*, *Theileria equi*, and *Theileria* s.s. and contrast with those that encode exclusively single-domain pRAP-1s, such as *Babesia* s.s. and *Babesia* s.l. [1].

B. microti contains two *prap-1*-like genes located as a single cluster in the region of the genome where s.s. *Babesia* and *Theileria* organisms contain their *prap-1* genes. These two genes have a fully conserved synteny and identical flanking genes as *Theileria* parasites, as shown in Figure 2A. This implies that the aforementioned genome rearrangements resulted in an independent evolution of RRA encoding genes, which likely occurred after *Babesia* organisms emerged as separate species from a common *Babesia* and *Theileria* ancestor. This notion is further supported by the observation that all proteins segregating into the *rap1d-3* and the *rap1d-4* orthologous groups represent RRA proteins since, although they contain a complete pRAP-1 domain, are shortened at the C-terminal end (Figure 1). This strongly suggests that the ancient RRA protein has lost its C-terminal partly due to chromosomal rearrangement and places this event before the diversification of the RRA proteins.

Considering that the antigenicity of BmIPA48 and Bm960 was not previously investigated [35–37,39], here we examined sera from *B. microti*-infected humans for the presence of antibodies against these proteins. Collectively, results of ELISA and immunoblot indicate that BmIPA48 and Bm960 are immunogenic during infection in humans, and thus should be considered for further testing as possible candidates for serological diagnosis of human babesiosis caused by *B. microti*. In addition, because of their previously established high degree of expression, surface localization, conservation, and immunogenicity, BmIPA48 and Bm960 proteins might also be promising candidates for the development of vaccines that may prevent human babesiosis.

4. Materials and Methods

4.1. Expression of Recombinant B. microti pRAP-1 like Proteins

The predicted proteins encoded by *B. microti* BMR1_03g00947 and BMR1_03g00960 (GenBank accession numbers: XP_021338473 and XP_021338474, respectively), here referred to as BmIPA48 and Bm960, respectively, were analyzed by the Kyte-Doolittle scale for the presence of hydrophobic regions as previously described [44]. As a result, 105 nt and 84 nt-long fragments located at the 5′ end of BMR1_03g00947 and BMR1_03g00960, correspondingly, encoding hydrophobic peptide segments, were excluded from the cloning and protein expression experiments described in this work. The resulting nucleotide sequences were codon-optimized for mammalian cell expression, synthesized by GenArt Gene Synthesis (Thermo Fisher Scientific, Waltham, MA, USA) and cloned into pcDNA3.4. Recombinant plasmids containing either truncated BMR1_03g00947 (pcDNA3.4/947) or truncated BMR1_03g00960 (pcDNA3.4/960) were fully sequenced to confirm the presence of the target genes in frame with the cytomegalovirus promoter (data not shown). Subsequently, HEK 293 cells were transiently transfected with either pcDNA3.4/947 or pcDNA3.4/960 using polyethylenimine, as described elsewhere [45]. Expression of the recombinant truncated proteins (BmIPA48tr and Bm960tr) was confirmed by immunoblot using the anti-6xHis monoclonal antibody (clone AD1.1.10) (Bio-Rad, Hercules, CA, USA). Recombinant BmIPA48tr and Bm960tr were purified using the HisPur™ Cobalt Purification Kit following the manufacturer's protocol (Thermo Fisher Scientific). After purification, the recombinant proteins were dialyzed using the Slide-A-Lyzer™ Dialysis cassettes (Thermo Fisher Scientific) and stored at −80 °C until use for ELISA and immunoblot.

4.2. Human Serum Samples

Unidentified human patient serum samples were submitted to Fuller Laboratories from Labcorp, NC for anti-*B. microti* IgG determination. No clinical data were provided for any of the specimens.

4.3. ELISA Procedure

Antigen dilution was performed by mixing 8 µL of recombinant BmIPA48 antigen (approx. 0.5 µg/µL) in 500 µL PBS buffer followed by two-fold dilutions 1:2, 1:4 and 1:8. For Bm960, 4 µL of the recombinant antigen (approx. 1 µg/µL) was mixed in 500 µL PBS buffer, and then diluted two-fold 1:2, 1:4 and 1:8. Two neighboring strips of the ELISA plate were coated with 100 µL/well of 1:4 and 1:8 antigen dilutions. The antigen-coated plates were incubated at room temperature (23–25 °C) overnight, then back coated by adding 100 µL/well WellChampion (Microwell Plate Blocker/Stabilizer, Kementec, Copenhagen, Denmark) to each well for 5–10 min. Plates were then decanted and allowed to dry overnight in a dark low-humidity room before use. Negative serum control was obtained from a non-reactive unidentified human patient, which tested negative in confirmatory IFA analysis. Positive controls ($n = 4$) corresponded to anti-*B. microti* IgG and IgM reactive unidentified human sera with IFA endpoint titers > 1:1024 (cat. BMG-120, Fuller Laboratories, Fullerton, CA, USA). IFA testing utilized both hamster in vivo and human type O in vitro antigen (US 10,087,412 B2 patent). All sera were diluted 1:100 in sample diluent (PBS/2 mg/mL bovine serum albumin/0.1% Tween-20). One hundred µL aliquots of diluted sera were added to ELISA plate microwells. Two rows of microwells were filled with sample diluent and were used for secondary antibody controls. Plates were covered to minimize evaporation and incubated for 60 min at room temperature. Then, plates were washed four times with wash buffer (PBS/0.1% Tween-20). One hundred µL of a working dilution of anti-human IgG (γ-chain-specific)-horseradish peroxidase (HRP) conjugate (SFG-1X, Fuller Labs) were added to each well, and the plate was covered and incubated for 30 min at RT in the dark. Microwells were washed as above and 100 µL TMB substrate was added to each well. Reactions were allowed to proceed for exactly 10 min in the dark and interrupted by adding 100 µL Stop solution (0.36 N sulfuric acid). Absorbance at 450 nm was read in a microplate reader (MultiSkan MCC/340, Titertek, Pforzheim, Germany). Absorbance values of *B. microti* positive and negative sera were compared by Student's *t*-test using Prism version 6 (GraphPad Software, San Diego, CA, USA).

4.4. Immunoblot Analysis

For human serum analysis, aliquots (45 µL) of recombinant BmIPA48 and Bm960 antigens were separated using 10% Mini-PROTEAN® TGX™ Precast Protein Gels (Bio-Rad, Cat #4561034) and transferred to PVDF membranes. Membranes were blocked with 5% milk, cut into strips, and individually incubated overnight at 4 °C with *B. microti*-positive or negative patient sera, in a 1:250 dilution. Membranes were then washed with PBS/0.1% Tween-20 and incubated for 1 h with HRP-conjugated secondary antibody (1:10,000 dilution). Following additional washings, membranes were incubated with Opti-4CN substrate diluted in 1-part Opti-4CN diluent and 9 parts distilled water (Bio-Rad, Cat# 1708235) for 5–30 min until the desired the signal was obtained.

4.5. Bioinformatic Analysis

Secondary sequence analysis was performed using TMpred Server (vital-it.ch, accessed on 1 August 2021) and Phobius (phobius.sbc.su.se, accessed on 1 August 2021). Prediction of GPI anchor signals was carried out using PredGPI (gpcr.biocomp.unibo.it/predgpi/, accessed on 1 August 2021). Synteny studies were carried out by exploring the Piroplasma DB database (piroplasmadb.org/piro/app, accessed on 1 August 2021).

4.6. Phylogenetic Analysis

The amino acid sequence of *B. bovis* T2Bo RAP-1 (XP_001610908) was used in a BLASTp search, adjusting parameter settings to piroplasmid sequences (taxid:5863) and reference proteins to identify homologs in completely sequenced genomes of piroplasmid species. The genomes analyzed included *B. bigemina* strain Bond [46], *B. bovis* strain T2Bo [47], *B. ovata* strain Miyake [48], *B. microti* strain RI [35], *C. felis* strain Winnie [49], *T. annulata* strain Ankara [50], *T. equi* strain WA [51], *T. orientalis* strain Shintoku [52], and *T. parva* strain Muguga [53]. In addition, RAP-1 sequences of *B. duncani* were retrieved by courtesy from yet public unavailable genomes (*B. duncani* strain WA1: Choukri Ben Mamoun, Yale School of Medicine, New Haven, CT, USA). Finally, BmIPA48 and Bm960 were identified by delta Blast using a RAP-1 region containing 4 conserved Cys, as described before.

Altogether 34 amino acid sequences were aligned by Muscle (www.ebi.ac.uk/Tools/msa/muscle/, accessed on 30 July 2021). In order to estimate evolutionary distances, the JTT+G (G = 5.93) was determined as best model by BIC criteria and applied [54]. After eliminating all positions with gaps and missing data, the remaining 212 positions were used for estimation of a neighbor joining tree [55]. The phylogenetic analysis was carried out using MEGA7 [56].

5. Conclusions

Findings in this study suggest that *rap-1* genes appeared early in the evolution of piroplasmid parasites, implying that expression of *prap-1* and *prap-1*-like genes is required for sustaining the life cycle of these organisms. Two tandemly arranged genes separated by an 800 bp intergenic region that includes a highly conserved putative promoter region are located in a region of the *B. microti* genome with strong synteny to the *prap-1* locus of *Babesia* and *Theileria* parasites. The organization of these two *prap-1*-like *B. microti* genes is reminiscent of the organization of the *prap-1* locus in *B. bovis* [15]. This feature, together with the presence of a single Cys-rich pRAP-1 motif in the encoded proteins resembles pRAP-1/RRA proteins of *Babesia*, rather than *Theileria*, parasites, but with identical synteny to *Theileria* parasites. The presence of a shared 300-bp region in the putative regulatory DNA regions suggests that the expression of these genes might be co-regulated. Both *B. microti* proteins contain TM domains and signal peptides, which is consistent with extracellular vesicle localization. Previous work showed that Bm960 is secreted into the sera of infected mice [35] and that BmIPA48 is strongly immunogenic in infected hamsters [14,36]. The gene structure comparison and phylogenetic analysis of the *prap-1* locus among distinct piroplasmid parasites allowed valuable insights on the genetic mechanisms involved in the evolution of the members of this piroplasmid-confined gene family. Importantly, this work also confirmed that antibodies in *B. microti*-infected humans recognized the recombinant forms of both proteins, so their potential as candidates for diagnostic assays and vaccines should be further explored.

Supplementary Materials: The following are available online at https://www.mdpi.com/article/10.3390/pathogens10111384/s1, Figure S1. Schematic representation of the structural features of RAP-1 and RRA proteins, Figure S2. Amino acid sequence alignment between the BmIPA48 and Bm960 RAP-1 like proteins, Figure S3. Amino acid sequence of the Bm947 protein, Figure S4. Schematic representation of the 300 bp region of homology among the *B. microti* RAP-1 like genes BMR1_03g00947 (947) and BMR1_03g00960 (960), Figure S5. Amino acid alignment between BmIPA48 (Bm) and PF3D7_1324300 (Pf), and Figure S6. Secondary structure prediction of BmIPA48using the software Phoebius.

Author Contributions: Conceptualization, R.G.B. and C.E.S.; Data curation, R.G.B. and C.E.S.; Formal analysis, R.G.B., J.T., C.B.M., L.F., R.E.M., M.F.-C., L.S., H.F.A. and C.E.S.; Funding acquisition, R.G.B., C.B.M., L.F., R.E.M., M.F.-C. and C.E.S.; Investigation, R.G.B., J.T., C.B.M., L.F., R.E.M., M.F.-C., L.S., H.F.A. and C.E.S.; Methodology, R.G.B., J.T., C.B.M., L.F., M.F.-C., L.S., H.F.A. and C.E.S.; Software, R.G.B., M.F.-C., L.S. and C.E.S.; Validation, R.G.B., J.T., C.B.M., L.F., R.E.M., M.F.-C., L.S., H.F.A. and C.E.S.; Writing—original draft, R.G.B., J.T., M.F.-C., L.S. and C.E.S.; Writing—review & editing, R.G.B., J.T., C.B.M., L.F., R.E.M., M.F.-C., L.S., H.F.A. and C.E.S. All authors have read and agreed to the published version of the manuscript.

Funding: RB is supported by the USDA National Institute of Food and Agriculture (NIFA) (Award Number: 2020-67015-31809; Proposal Number: 2019-05375, Accession Number: 1022541. Work supported by ARS-USDA CRIS 2090-32000-039-000-D. CBM research is supported by NIH grants AI123321, AI138139, AI152220 and AI136118, the Steven and Alexandra Cohen Foundation and Global Lyme Alliance. The financial support of MFC and LS by INTA (Instituto Nacional de Tecnologia Agropecuaria) projects 2019-PD-E5-I102-001 and 2019-PE-E5-I109-001 is acknowledged. REM is supported by ATCC's Internal Research and Development Program.

Institutional Review Board Statement: Not applicable.

Informed Consent Statement: As mentioned in the Material and Methods section, unidentified human patient serum samples used in this study were submitted to Fuller Laboratories from Labcorp, NC for anti-*B. microti* IgG determination. No clinical data were provided for any of the specimens.

Data Availability Statement: Not applicable.

Acknowledgments: The authors would like to acknowledge Sezayi Ozubek, Paul Lacy, Jacob Laughery, Manuel Rojas (DVM), and Jinna Navas for productive discussions and technical assistance.

Conflicts of Interest: The authors declare no conflict of interest.

References

1. Schnittger, L.; Rodriguez, A.E.; Florin-Christensen, M.; Morrison, D.A. Babesia: A world emerging. *Infect. Genet. Evol.* **2012**, *12*, 1788–1809. [CrossRef]
2. Jalovecka, M.; Hajdusek, O.; Sojka, D.; Kopacek, P.; Malandrin, L. The Complexity of Piroplasms Life Cycles. *Front. Cell. Infect. Microbiol.* **2018**, *8*, 248. [CrossRef] [PubMed]
3. Jalovecka, M.; Sojka, D.; Ascencio, M.; Schnittger, L. *Babesia* Life Cycle-When Phylogeny Meets Biology. *Trends Parasitol.* **2019**, *35*, 356–368. [CrossRef]
4. Yang, Y.; Christie, J.; Köster, L.; Du, A.; Yao, C. Emerging Human Babesiosis with "Ground Zero" in North America. *Microorganisms* **2021**, *9*, 440. [CrossRef]
5. Karshima, S.N.; Karshima, M.N.; Ahmed, M.I. Animal reservoirs of zoonotic *Babesia* species: A global systematic review and meta-analysis of their prevalence, distribution and species diversity. *Vet. Parasitol.* **2021**, *298*, 109539. [CrossRef] [PubMed]
6. Lobo, C.A.; Singh, M.; Rodriguez, M. Human babesiosis: Recent advances and future challenges. *Curr. Opin. Hematol.* **2020**, *27*, 399–405. [CrossRef] [PubMed]
7. Tang, T.T.M.; Tran, M.-H. Transfusion transmitted babesiosis: A systematic review of reported cases. *Transfus. Apher. Sci.* **2020**, *59*, 102843. [CrossRef] [PubMed]
8. Alkishe, A.; Raghavan, R.; Peterson, A. Likely geographic distributional shifts among medically important tick species and tick-associated diseases under climate change in North America: A review. *Insects* **2021**, *12*, 225. [CrossRef]
9. Tufts, D.M.; A Diuk-Wasser, M. Vertical Transmission: A vector-independent transmission pathway of *Babesia microti* in the natural reservoir host. *Peromyscus. Leucopus. J. Infect. Dis.* **2020**, *223*, 1787–1795. [CrossRef] [PubMed]
10. White, D.J.; Talarico, J.; Chang, H.-G.; Birkhead, G.S.; Heimberger, T.; Morse, D.L. Human babesiosis in New York State. *Arch. Intern. Med.* **1998**, *158*, 2149–2154. [CrossRef]
11. Gubbels, M.-J.; Duraisingh, M.T. Evolution of apicomplexan secretory organelles. *Int. J. Parasitol.* **2012**, *42*, 1071–1081. [CrossRef] [PubMed]
12. Robert-Paganin, J.; Xu, X.-P.; Swift, M.F.; Auguin, D.; Robblee, J.P.; Lu, H.; Fagnant, P.M.; Krementsova, E.B.; Trybus, K.M.; Houdusse, A.; et al. The actomyosin interface contains an evolutionary conserved core and an ancillary interface involved in specificity. *Nat. Commun.* **2021**, *12*, 1–11. [CrossRef]
13. Ben Chaabene, R.; Lentini, G.; Soldati-Favre, D. Biogenesis and discharge of the rhoptries: Key organelles for entry and hijack of host cells by the Apicomplexa. *Mol. Microbiol.* **2020**, *115*, 453–465. [CrossRef]
14. Thekkiniath, J.; Kilian, N.; Lawres, L.; A Gewirtz, M.; Graham, M.M.; Liu, X.; Ledizet, M.; Ben Mamoun, C. Evidence for vesicle-mediated antigen export by the human pathogen. *Babesia Microti. Life Sci. Alliance.* **2019**, *2*, e201900382. [CrossRef] [PubMed]

15. Suarez, C.E.; Palmer, G.H.; Hotzel, I.; McElwain, T.F. Structure, sequence, and transcriptional analysis of the *Babesia bovis rap-1* multigene locus. *Mol. Biochem. Parasitol.* **1998**, *93*, 215–224. [CrossRef] [PubMed]
16. Kappmeyer, L.; Perryman, L.E.; Hines, S.A.; Baszler, T.V.; Katz, J.B.; Hennager, S.G.; Knowles, D.P. Detection of equine antibodies to *Babesia caballi* by recombinant *B. caballi* rhoptry-associated protein 1 in a competitive-inhibition enzyme-linked immunosorbent assay. *J. Clin. Microbiol.* **1999**, *37*, 2285–2290. [CrossRef]
17. Suarez, C.E.; Palmer, G.H.; Florin-Christensen, M.; Hines, S.A.; Hötzel, I.; McElwain, T.F. Organization, transcription, and expression of rhoptry associated protein genes in the *Babesia bigemina rap-1* locus. *Mol. Biochem. Parasitol.* **2003**, *127*, 101–112. [CrossRef]
18. Zhou, J.; Jia, H.; Nishikawa, Y.; Fujisaki, K.; Xuan, X. *Babesia gibsoni* rhoptry-associated protein 1 and its potential use as a diagnostic antigen. *Vet. Parasitol.* **2007**, *145*, 16–20. [CrossRef] [PubMed]
19. Terkawi, M.A.; Amornthep, A.; Ooka, H.; Aboge, G.; Jia, H.; Goo, Y.-K.; Nelson, B.; Yamagishi, J.; Nishikawa, Y.; Igarashi, I.; et al. Molecular characterizations of three distinct *Babesia gibsoni* rhoptry-associated protein-1s (RAP-1s). *Parasitology* **2009**, *136*, 1147–1160. [CrossRef] [PubMed]
20. Rodriguez, M.; Alhassan, A.; Ord, R.L.; Cursino-Santos, J.R.; Singh, M.; Gray, J.; Lobo, C.A. Identification and characterization of the RouenBd1987 *Babesia divergens* rhopty-associated protein 1. *PLoS ONE* **2014**, *9*, e107727. [CrossRef]
21. Yu, Q.; He, L.; Zhang, W.-J.; Cheng, J.-X.; Hu, J.-F.; Miao, X.-Y.; Huang, Y.; Fan, L.-Z.; Khan, M.K.; Zhou, Y.-Q.; et al. Molecular cloning and characterization of *Babesia orientalis* rhoptry-associated protein 1. *Vet. Parasitol.* **2014**, *205*, 499–505. [CrossRef] [PubMed]
22. Niu, Q.; Bonsergent, C.; Guan, G.; Yin, H.; Malandrin, L. Sequence and organization of the rhoptry-associated-protein-1 (rap-1) locus for the sheep hemoprotozoan *Babesia* sp. BQ1 Lintan (*B. motasi* phylogenetic group). *Vet. Parasitol.* **2013**, *198*, 24–38. [CrossRef] [PubMed]
23. Niu, Q.; Marchand, J.; Yang, C.; Bonsergent, C.; Guan, G.; Yin, H.; Malandrin, L. Rhoptry-associated protein (rap-1) genes in the sheep pathogen *Babesia* sp. Xinjiang: Multiple transcribed copies differing by 3′ end repeated sequences. *Vet. Parasitol.* **2015**, *211*, 158–169. [CrossRef] [PubMed]
24. Shaw, M.K. Cell invasion by *Theileria* sporozoites. *Trends Parasitol.* **2003**, *19*, 2–6. [CrossRef]
25. Yokoyama, N.; Suthisak, B.; Hirata, H.; Matsuo, T.; Inoue, N.; Sugimoto, C.; Igarashi, I. Cellular localization of *Babesia bovis* merozoite rhoptry-associated protein 1 and its erythrocyte-binding activity. *Infect. Immun.* **2002**, *70*, 5822–5826. [CrossRef] [PubMed]
26. Suarez, C.E.; Laughery, J.M.; Bastos, R.G.; Johnson, W.C.; Norimine, J.; Asenzo, G.; Brown, W.C.; Florin-Christensen, M.; Goff, W.L. A novel neutralization sensitive and subdominant RAP-1-related antigen (RRA) is expressed by *Babesia bovis* merozoites. *Parasitology* **2011**, *138*, 809–818. [CrossRef] [PubMed]
27. Moreno, R.; Pöltl-Frank, F.; Stüber, D.; Matile, H.; Mutz, M.; Weiss, N.A.; Pluschke, G. Rhoptry-associated protein 1-binding monoclonal antibody raised against a heterologous peptide sequence inhibits *Plasmodium falciparum* growth in vitro. *Infect. Immun.* **2001**, *69*, 2558–2568. [CrossRef] [PubMed]
28. Ushe, T.C.; Palmer, G.H.; Sotomayor, L.; Figueroa, J.V.; Buening, G.M.; E Perryman, L.; McElwain, T.F. Antibody response to a *Babesia bigemina* rhoptry-associated protein 1 surface-exposed and neutralization-sensitive epitope in immune cattle. *Infect. Immun.* **1994**, *62*, 5698–5701. [CrossRef]
29. Mosqueda, J.; McElwain, T.F.; Stiller, D.; Palmer, G.H. *Babesia bovis* Merozoite surface antigen 1 and rhoptry-associated protein 1 are expressed in sporozoites, and specific antibodies inhibit sporozoite attachment to erythrocytes. *Infect. Immun.* **2002**, *70*, 1599–1603. [CrossRef]
30. Norimine, J.; Suarez, C.E.; McElwain, T.F.; Florin-Christensen, M.; Brown, W.C. Immunodominant epitopes in *Babesia bovis* rhoptry-associated protein 1 that elicit memory CD4(+)-T-lymphocyte responses in *B. bovis*-immune individuals are located in the amino-terminal domain. *Infect. Immun.* **2002**, *70*, 2039–2048. [CrossRef] [PubMed]
31. Boonchit, S.; Xuan, X.; Yokoyama, N.; Goff, W.L.; Waghela, S.D.; Wagner, G.; Igarashi, I. Improved enzyme-linked immunosorbent assay using c-terminal truncated recombinant antigens of *Babesia bovis* rhoptry-associated protein-1 for detection of specific antibodies. *J. Clin. Microbiol.* **2004**, *42*, 1601–1604. [CrossRef] [PubMed]
32. Boonchit, S.; Alhassan, A.; Chan, B.; Xuan, X.; Yokoyama, N.; Ooshiro, M.; Goff, W.L.; Waghela, S.D.; Wagner, G.; Igarashi, I. Expression of C-terminal truncated and full-length *Babesia bigemina* rhoptry-associated protein 1 and their potential use in enzyme-linked immunosorbent assay. *Vet. Parasitol.* **2006**, *137*, 28–35. [CrossRef] [PubMed]
33. Suarez, C.E.; Noh, S. Emerging perspectives in the research of bovine babesiosis and anaplasmosis. *Vet. Parasitol.* **2011**, *180*, 109–125. [CrossRef] [PubMed]
34. Niu, Q.; Liu, Z.; Yang, J.; Yu, P.; Pan, Y.; Zhai, B.; Luo, J.; Moreau, E.; Guan, G.; Yin, H. Expression analysis and biological characterization of *Babesia* sp. BQ1 (Lintan) (*Babesia motasi*-like) rhoptry-associated protein 1 and its potential use in serodiagnosis via ELISA. *Parasites Vectors.* **2016**, *9*, 1–14. [CrossRef] [PubMed]
35. Silva, J.C.; Cornillot, E.; McCracken, C.; Usmani-Brown, S.; Dwivedi, A.; Ifeonu, O.O.; Crabtree, J.; Gotia, H.T.; Virji, A.Z.; Reynes, C.; et al. Genome-wide diversity and gene expression profiling of *Babesia microti* isolates identify polymorphic genes that mediate host-pathogen interactions. *Sci. Rep.* **2016**, *6*, 35284. [CrossRef] [PubMed]
36. Magni, R.; Luchini, A.; Liotta, L.; Molestina, R.E. Analysis of the *Babesia microti* proteome in infected red blood cells by a combination of nanotechnology and mass spectrometry. *Int. J. Parasitol.* **2018**, *49*, 139–144. [CrossRef] [PubMed]

37. Magni, R.; Luchini, A.; Liotta, L.; Molestina, R.E. Proteomic analysis reveals pathogen-derived biomarkers of acute babesiosis in erythrocytes, plasma, and urine of infected hamsters. *Parasitol. Res.* **2020**, *119*, 2227–2235. [CrossRef]
38. Moreno-Hagelsieb, G.; Trevino, V.; Perez-Rueda, E.; Smith, T.F.; Collado-Vides, J. Transcription unit conservation in the three domains of life: A perspective from *Escherichia coli*. *Trends Genet.* **2001**, *17*, 175–177. [CrossRef]
39. Florin-Christensen, M.; Suarez, C.E.; Hines, S.A.; Palmer, G.H.; Brown, W.C.; McElwain, T.F. The *Babesia bovis* merozoite surface antigen 2 locus contains four tandemly arranged and expressed genes encoding immunologically distinct proteins. *Infect. Immun.* **2002**, *70*, 3566–3575. [CrossRef]
40. Suarez, C.E.; Norimine, J.; Lacy, P.; McElwain, T.F. Characterization and gene expression of *Babesia bovis* elongation factor-1α. *Int. J. Parasitol.* **2006**, *36*, 965–973. [CrossRef] [PubMed]
41. Silva, M.G.; Knowles, D.P.; Mazuz, M.L.; Cooke, B.M.; Suarez, C.E. Stable transformation of *Babesia bigemina* and *Babesia bovis* using a single transfection plasmid. *Sci. Rep.* **2018**, *8*, 1–9. [CrossRef]
42. Suarez, C.E.; Palmer, G.H.; Jasmer, D.P.; Hines, S.A.; Perryman, L.E.; McElwain, T.F. Characterization of the gene encoding a 60-kilodalton *Babesia bovis* merozoite protein with conserved and surface exposed epitopes. *Mol. Biochem. Parasitol.* **1991**, *46*, 45–52. [CrossRef]
43. Paing, M.M.; Tolia, N.H. multimeric assembly of host-pathogen adhesion complexes involved in apicomplexan invasion. *PLOS Pathog.* **2014**, *10*, e1004120. [CrossRef] [PubMed]
44. Kyte, J.; Doolittle, R.F. A simple method for displaying the hydropathic character of a protein. *J. Mol. Biol.* **1982**, *157*, 105–132. [CrossRef]
45. Bastos, R.G.; Franceschi, V.; Tebaldi, G.; Connelley, T.; Morrison, W.I.; Knowles, D.P.; Donofrio, G.; Fry, L.M. Molecular and antigenic properties of mammalian cell-expressed *Theileria parva* antigen Tp9. *Front. Immunol.* **2019**, *10*, 897. [CrossRef] [PubMed]
46. Jackson, A.P.; Otto, T.; Darby, A.; Ramaprasad, A.; Xia, D.; Echaide, I.E.; Farber, M.; Gahlot, S.; Gamble, J.; Gupta, D.; et al. The evolutionary dynamics of variant antigen genes in *Babesia* reveal a history of genomic innovation underlying host-parasite interaction. *Nucleic Acids Res.* **2014**, *42*, 7113–7131. [CrossRef] [PubMed]
47. A Brayton, K.; Lau, A.; Herndon, D.R.; Hannick, L.; Kappmeyer, L.; Berens, S.J.; Bidwell, S.L.; Brown, W.C.; Crabtree, J.; Fadrosh, D.; et al. Genome sequence of *Babesia bovis* and comparative analysis of apicomplexan hemoprotozoa. *PLoS Pathog.* **2007**, *3*, e148. [CrossRef] [PubMed]
48. Yamagishi, J.; Asada, M.; Hakimi, H.; Tanaka, T.Q.; Sugimoto, C.; Kawazu, S.-I. Whole-genome assembly of *Babesia ovata* and comparative genomics between closely related pathogens. *BMC Genom.* **2017**, *18*, 1–9. [CrossRef]
49. Tarigo, J.L.; Scholl, E.H.; Bird, D.; Brown, C.C.; Cohn, L.A.; Dean, G.A.; Levy, M.G.; Doolan, D.L.; Trieu, A.; Nordone, S.K.; et al. A novel candidate vaccine for *Cytauxzoonosis* inferred from comparative apicomplexan genomics. *PLoS ONE* **2013**, *8*, e71233. [CrossRef]
50. Pain, A.; Renauld, H.; Berriman, M.; Murphy, L.; Yeats, C.A.; Weir, W.; Kerhornou, A.; Aslett, M.; Bishop, R.; Bouchier, C.; et al. Genome of the host-cell transforming parasite *Theileria annulata* compared with *T. parva*. *Science* **2005**, *309*, 131–133. [CrossRef] [PubMed]
51. Kappmeyer, L.S.; Thiagarajan, M.; Herndon, D.R.; Ramsay, J.D.; Caler, E.; Djikeng, A.; Gillespie, J.J.; Lau, A.O.; Roalson, E.H.; Silva, J.C.; et al. Comparative genomic analysis and phylogenetic position of *Theileria equi*. *BMC Genom.* **2012**, *13*, 603. [CrossRef] [PubMed]
52. Hayashida, K.; Hara, Y.; Abe, T.; Yamasaki, C.; Toyoda, A.; Kosuge, T.; Suzuki, Y.; Sato, Y.; Kawashima, S.; Katayama, T.; et al. Comparative genome analysis of three eukaryotic parasites with differing abilities to transform leukocytes reveals key mediators of *Theileria*-induced leukocyte transformation. *mBio* **2012**, *3*, e00204-12. [CrossRef] [PubMed]
53. Gardner, M.J.; Bishop, R.; Shah, T.; de Villiers, E.P.; Carlton, J.M.; Hall, N.; Ren, Q.; Paulsen, I.T.; Pain, A.; Berriman, M.; et al. Genome sequence of *Theileria parva*, a bovine pathogen that transforms lymphocytes. *Science* **2005**, *309*, 134–137. [CrossRef]
54. Jones, D.T.; Taylor, W.R.; Thornton, J. The rapid generation of mutation data matrices from protein sequences. *Bioinformatics* **1992**, *8*, 275–282. [CrossRef]
55. Saitou, N.; Nei, M. The neighbor-joining method: A new method for reconstructing phylogenetic trees. *Mol. Biol. Evol.* **1987**, *4*, 406–425. [CrossRef]
56. Kumar, S.; Stecher, G.; Tamura, K. MEGA7: Molecular evolutionary genetics analysis version 7.0 for bigger datasets. *Mol. Biol. Evol.* **2016**, *33*, 1870–1874. [CrossRef] [PubMed]

pathogens

MDPI

Review

Treatment of Human Babesiosis: Then and Now

Isaline Renard and **Choukri Ben Mamoun** *

Department of Internal Medicine, Section of Infectious Diseases, Yale School of Medicine, New Haven, CT 06520, USA; isaline.renard@yale.edu
* Correspondence: choukri.benmamoun@yale.edu

Abstract: Babesiosis is an emerging tick-borne disease caused by apicomplexan parasites of the genus *Babesia*. With its increasing incidence worldwide and the risk of human-to-human transmission through blood transfusion, babesiosis is becoming a rising public health concern. The current arsenal for the treatment of human babesiosis is limited and consists of combinations of atovaquone and azithromycin or clindamycin and quinine. These combination therapies were not designed based on biological criteria unique to *Babesia* parasites, but were rather repurposed based on their well-established efficacy against other apicomplexan parasites. However, these compounds are associated with mild or severe adverse events and a rapid emergence of drug resistance, thus highlighting the need for new therapeutic strategies that are specifically tailored to *Babesia* parasites. Herein, we review ongoing babesiosis therapeutic and management strategies and their limitations, and further review current efforts to develop new, effective, and safer therapies for the treatment of this disease.

Keywords: babesiosis; *Babesia microti*; *Babesia duncani*; parasite; therapy; atovaquone; endochin-like quinolones (ELQs)

Citation: Renard, I.; Ben Mamoun, C. Treatment of Human Babesiosis: Then and Now. *Pathogens* **2021**, *10*, 1120. https://doi.org/10.3390/pathogens10091120

Academic Editors: Estrella Montero, Jeremy Gray, Cheryl Ann Lobo and Luis Miguel González

Received: 30 July 2021
Accepted: 27 August 2021
Published: 1 September 2021

1. Introduction

Human babesiosis is a rapidly emerging tick-born infectious disease caused by intraerythrocytic parasites of the genus *Babesia*. Of several hundred *Babesia* species identified so far, only a few are known to infect humans. These include *Babesia microti*, *Babesia duncani*, *Babesia divergens* and *divergens*-like species, *Babesia crassa*-like, and *Babesia venatorum* [1]. In the United States, most cases of human babesiosis have been attributed to infection with *B. microti*, but sporadic cases due to infection with *B. duncani* and *B. divergens*-like MO1 have also been reported. In Europe, *B. divergens* used to be the main species responsible for infection in humans. However, recent studies suggest that *B. microti* and *B. venatorum* are now more prevalent than *B. divergens* [2]. In China, human babesiosis is mainly caused by *B. microti* and *B. venatorum*, and in the rest of the world, only a few sporadic cases have been reported and were mostly linked to *B. microti* infection [2].

Babesia spp. are apicomplexan parasites that infect the host red blood cells and are transmitted to mammals by tick vectors (Figure 1). The species of ticks involved in the transmission of *Babesia* pathogens vary depending on the geographical area and parasite species [1,2]. During the life cycle of *Babesia*, humans are typically accidental hosts, and most infections are linked to a tick route of transmission [1,2]. However, an increasing number of transfusion-transmitted babesiosis cases have been reported in the US over the past 2–3 decades, making *Babesia* infections a major public health concern [1,3–6]. In 2011, human babesiosis became a nationally notifiable disease in the US [5] and as one of the most common transfusion-transmitted pathogens in the US, *B. microti* was added to the list of significant threats to the blood supply [3,4]. In addition to human-to-human transmission through blood transfusion, several reports have also established the possibility of transplacental transmission from mother to child [1].

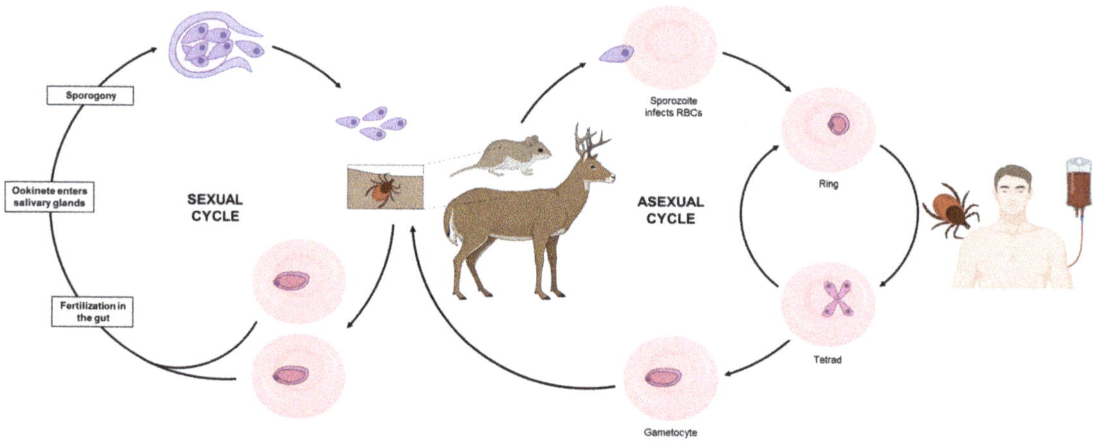

Figure 1. Cycle of transmission of the most common *Babesia* species, *B. microti*. During a blood meal, an infected tick introduces merozoites into the host (mouse or deer, for example). Free merozoites enter red blood cells and undergo asexual replication. While in the blood, some parasites differentiate into male and female gametocytes (not morphologically recognizable by light microscopy). These gametocytes are then taken up by a tick during a blood meal and differentiate into gametes. While in the gut, gametes fuse to form a zygote, that will subsequently undergo meiotic and several mitotic divisions to form sporozoites that are then transmitted to a mammalian host. Humans are typically accidental hosts and become infected through the bite of an infected tick. Human to human transmission is also possible via blood transfusion.

In most individuals, babesiosis remains asymptomatic or presents with mild flu-like symptoms [1,2]. However, in more susceptible populations, such as the elderly, asplenic, or immunocompromised individuals, the disease can become severe and even life-threatening, with symptoms such as severe anemia, acute respiratory distress, organ failure, and death [1,2].

In the following sections, we describe the current treatment and management of *Babesia*-infected patients and their limitations. Furthermore, we report on the development and evaluation of novel and highly promising antibabesial therapies.

2. Current Treatments against Human Babesiosis

The current arsenal for the treatment of human babesiosis relies principally on four drugs: atovaquone, azithromycin, clindamycin, and quinine. Atovaquone is used to treat several human diseases, including *Pneumocystis jirovecii* pneumonia [7], toxoplasmosis [8], and malaria (in combination with proguanil (Malarone) [9]. In apicomplexan parasites, atovaquone targets the cytochrome bc_1 complex of the mitochondrial electron transport chain (Figures 2 and 3) [10–13]. Azithromycin is a relatively broad-spectrum antibiotic indicated for the treatment of numerous bacterial infections, such as those caused by *Staphylococcus* spp. [14–16] and *Legionella* spp. [17]. The antibiotic is also used for the treatment of toxoplasmosis [12] and, in combination with other drugs, for the treatment of malaria [18]. Azithromycin is a well-characterized protein synthesis inhibitor, which in apicomplexan parasites targets the translation machinery in the apicoplast (Figure 2) [19–21]. It is worth noting that azithromycin was found to have a "delayed death" effect, in which parasite division produces viable daughter cells that are subsequently unable to divide in the following cycle [19,21,22]. Clindamycin is another antibiotic commonly used for the treatment of various bacterial infections [23] and repurposed for the treatment of parasitic infections. In combination with quinine, clindamycin is used for the treatment of both malaria and babesiosis [24–26]. Several reports have suggested that clindamycin acts in a similar way as azithromycin and targets protein synthesis in the apicoplast (Figure 2) [19,21,22]. Furthermore, selection of clindamycin-resistant *T. gondii* parasites showed cross-resistance to azithromycin, further suggesting a common target [27]. Quinine is a widely used antimalarial agent, typically administered in combination with an antibiotic such as clindamycin or doxycycline [28]. However, the drug is poorly tolerated and, as such, tends to be replaced by alternative drugs with fewer side-effects [28,29]. In malaria parasites, several modes of action for quinine have been proposed. The most commonly reported mechanism of action involves the disruption of hemozoin formation, resulting in accumulation of free ferriprotoporphyrin IX, a by-product of hemoglobin degradation, which is deleterious to parasite growth [30–32]. Confocal imaging using fluorescent derivatives of quinine and its structural analogues, quinidine and chloroquine, have shown accumulation of the probes in the digestive vacuole, consistent with the activity of this compound in this organelle [32,33]. Unlike *Plasmodium* parasites, *Babesia* species lack a digestive vacuole, do not degrade hemoglobin, and do not produce hemozoin. Therefore, the mode of action of quinine against *Babesia* parasites is likely to be different from that in *Plasmodium*. Interestingly, fluorescent probes were found to bind to phospholipids and to accumulate in membranous structures, including the parasite plasma membrane, the endoplasmic reticulum, and the mitochondrion, suggesting that quinine may inactivate specific biological functions in these organelles [32,33]. Another proposed hypothesis is that quinine acts as a DNA intercalator [34–36]. However, the lack of fluorescence in the nucleus reported by Woodland et al. seem to refute interactions with DNA as a potential mode of action [32,33]. More recently, a study in *P. falciparum* using thermal shift assays suggested that the purine nucleoside phosphorylase (PfPNP) might also be a target of quinine [37].

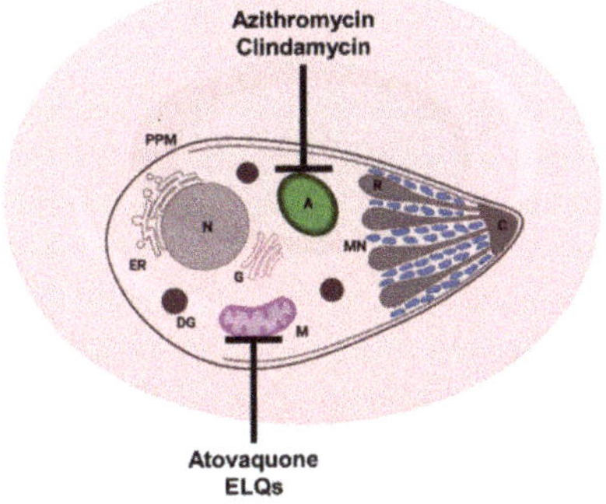

Figure 2. Schematic representation of a *Babesia*-infected red blood cell and sites of action of some approved and experimental drugs. Azithromycin and clindamycin target the apicoplast; atovaquone and ELQs target the mitochondrion. A: apicoplast, C: conoid + polar rings, DG: dense granule, ER: endoplasmic reticulum, G: Golgi apparatus, M: mitochondrion, MN: microneme, PPM: parasite plasma membrane and R: rhoptry.

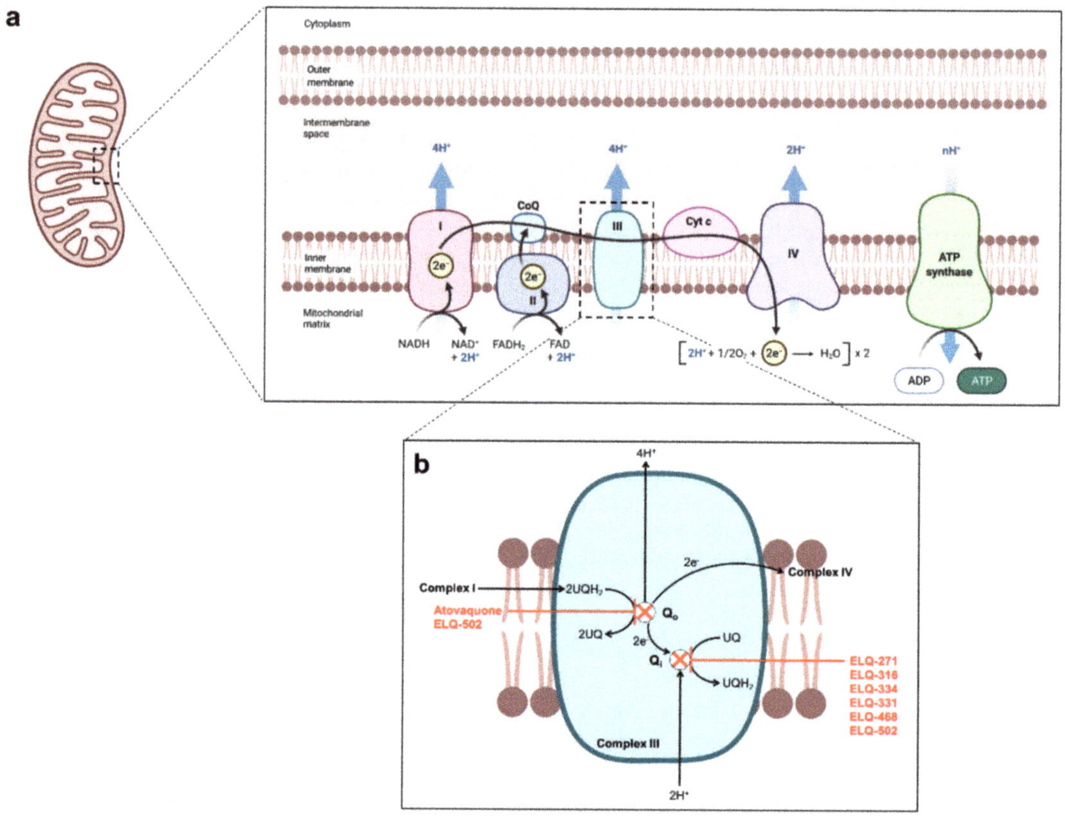

Figure 3. Proposed mechanism of action of atovaquone and endochin-like quinolones in *Babesia* mitochondrion. (**a**) Schematic representation the mitochondrial electron transfer chain. (**b**) Schematic representation of the parasite bc_1 complex with proposed mode of action of atovaquone and ELQs.

The severity of babesiosis depends mainly on the host's immune status, the presence of risk factors and the *Babesia* species responsible for the infection. In symptomatic patients, babesiosis usually manifests with flu-like symptoms such as fever, fatigue, chills, sweats, and headache [38]. For this moderate form of the disease, typically associated with a low parasitemia level (<4%) [26], no hospital admission is required and a 7–10-day treatment course of oral atovaquone + azithromycin (500 mg azithromycin on day 1, followed by 250 mg on subsequent days + 750 mg b.i.d. atovaquone) is recommended [26,38]. Babesiosis typically resolves within seven days from the start of the treatment, but asymptomatic, low level parasitemia may persist for up to one year [26]. Monitoring of persistent parasitemia in immunocompetent individuals following treatment is usually not necessary. However, given the risk of transmission of *Babesia* parasites through blood transfusion, these patients are excluded as blood donors [3]. Immunocompromised individuals are more at risk of developing a severe form of babesiosis, resulting in complications such as acute respiratory distress syndrome, disseminated intravascular coagulation, severe hemolytic anemia, organ failure, splenic rupture, relapse, and death [2,26]. A combination of oral clindamycin + quinine (600 mg + 650 mg, every 8 h) is the standard of care for the treatment of severe babesiosis [26,38]. However, this treatment regimen is frequently associated with serious side effects, such as hearing loss, vertigo, and tinnitus. In some cases, these side effects can be so severe that dose reduction or discontinuation of treatment is required [38]. Recently, it has been demonstrated that a combination of atovaquone + azithromycin is also suitable for the treatment of severe babesiosis, displaying comparable efficacy to clindamycin + quinine with fewer side effects [39]. Although atovaquone + azithromycin is now the preferred course of treatment for severe babesiosis, the standard 7–10-day treatment regimen of oral atovaquone + azithromycin is usually not enough to eliminate *Babesia* infection. Higher doses, longer treatment duration, and in some cases intravenous administration is required to clear the infection [26]. It is also worth noting that the use of immunosuppressive agents such as Rituximab to treat prior illnesses (B cell lymphoid malignancies, rheumatoid arthritis, etc.) may lead to babesiosis relapse and extended persistence of *Babesia* parasites [40–42].

One downside of a prolonged treatment regimen and dose escalation is the risk of developing drug resistance. Previous reports have established the emergence of mutations in the cytochrome b (Cytb) of *Babesia* parasites in humans and animal models following treatment with atovaquone [11,42,43]. In 2016, Lemieux et al. examined clinical isolates of relapsing babesiosis and identified a methionine to isoleucine mutation (M134I) in the Q_o site (atovaquone-binding site) of the BmCytb [43]. This same mutation was observed in a murine model of *B. microti* infection [11], as well as in other apicomplexan parasites, such as *P. falciparum* and *T. gondii* [43]. Later, Simon et al. reported a Y272C mutation in the BmCytb Q_o site in a patient presenting with relapsed *B. microti* infection following an atovaquone + azithromycin treatment course [42]. In both cases, these mutations have been shown to impact the atovaquone-binding domain [44] and appear to be associated with decreased sensitivity to the drug [42,43]. With regard to azithromycin resistance, sequencing of clinical isolates obtained from patients with relapsing babesiosis identified mutations in the ribosomal protein subunit L4 (RPL4) encoded by the apicoplast genome [42,43]. Lemieux et al. identified three substitutions in the RPL4: R86H, R86C and S73L [43]. Simon et al. observed the same R86C mutation in a patient presenting with relapsing babesiosis following atovaquone + azithromycin treatment [42]. Similar mutations associated with azithromycin resistance have been reported in *P. falciparum* [20] and *S. pneumoniae* [45] RPL4. Alternative management strategies for human babesiosis in the case of persistent relapse include the use of different drug combinations such as atovaquone + azithromycin + clindamycin, atovaquone + clindamycin, atovaquone + proguanil, or atovaquone + azithromycin + clindamycin + quinine [26,41,46,47]. The introduction of other drugs such as doxycycline, moxifloxacin, pentamidine, trimethoprim-sulfamethoxazole or artemisinin to treatment regimens with the standard therapies was also reported [40,48]. A recent study in a small cohort of patients suffering from Lyme disease and babesiosis co-infection suggested improvement, and in some cases remission, following one course of disulfiram monotherapy [49]. In patients with high parasitemia (>10%), exchange transfusion is recommended and often results in a rapid reduction of the parasite load [26,50].

Despite clinical evidence that atovaquone, azithromycin, clindamycin and quinine can be used to manage human babesiosis, preclinical evaluation of these drugs in different models of *Babesia* infection has not demonstrated unanimous results with regards to their efficacy. Clindamycin showed only limited activity at a dose of 300 mg/kg (p.o.) in *B. microti*-infected Mongolian jirds [51]. When evaluated in *B. microti*-infected hamster, a course of 150 mg/kg (i.m. or p.o.) of clindamycin resulted in a two-fold decrease in peak parasitemia. Similar results were obtained when clindamycin was administered in combination with quinine [52]. AbouLaila et al. reported a ~three-fold decrease in peak parasitemia following i.p. injection of 500 mg/kg of clindamycin in *B. microti*-infected Balb/c mice [53]. Another study using the same Balb/c model of *B. microti* infection showed that oral administration of clindamycin at 25, 50, and 100 mg/kg did not lead to reduction of parasite burden [54]. Similar results were obtained by Lawres et al. following oral administration of 10 or 50 mg/kg of clindamycin to immunocomprimized mice infected with *B. microti* [11]. The consensus seems to be more apparent in the case of quinine, where most studies report no effect on parasitemia following administration of quinine as a single drug [11,52,54]. Interestingly, a combination of clindamycin + quinine was reported to achieve up to 70% suppression of parasitemia [55] and result in a faster resolution of parasitemia compared to clindamycin alone [52], suggesting a potential synergy between the two drugs. Preclinical investigation of azithromycin efficiency against *Babesia* parasites also yielded inconsistent results. In *B. microti*-infected Balb/c mice, a four-day treatment course with azithromycin at 25, 50, and 100 mg/kg was found to be potent, resulting in 75–96% suppression of parasitemia [54]. In contrast, the evaluation of azithromycin in *B. microti*-infected SCID mice showed no effect on parasitemia at 10 and 50 mg/kg after a seven-day treatment course [11]. Similar results were obtained in *B. microti*-infected hamsters, where 150 mg/kg azithromycin treatment regimen, administered daily for almost two weeks, showed no apparent effect on parasitemia [56]. Out of the four clinically used drugs in the treatment of babesiosis, only atovaquone seems to consistently show high potency against *Babesia* parasites [11,56–59]. Studies carried out in *B. microti*-infected hamsters and SCID mice reported fast clearance of parasitemia following treatment with atovaquone [11,56]. However, recrudescence due to atovaquone-resistant parasites was observed [11,56]. In *B. microti*-infected hamsters, a combination therapy of atovaquone + azithromycin resulted in rapid clearance of parasitemia without recrudescence [56]. In a lethal model of *B. microti* infection in hamsters, atovaquone monotherapy was found to be superior to a combination of clindamycin + quinine, resulting in low to undetectable parasitemia and extended survival [58]. Potency of atovaquone was also demonstrated in *B. divergens* [59] and *B. duncani* [57] models, with IC_{50} values in the low nanomolar range. In gerbils, although prophylaxis experiments were not successful, a dose of atovaquone as low as 0.5 mg/kg was found to efficiently prevent *B. divergens* infection, so long as daily treatment was maintained several days post-infection [59]. In the case of *B. duncani*, a treatment course of 10 mg/kg atovaquone resulted in a clear reduction of parasitemia and 80% survival using a mouse model of lethal infection [57]. The results derived from the evaluation of atovaquone, azithromycin, clindamycin, and quinine in preclinical models of babesiosis are summarized in Table 1.

While combinations of atovaquone + azithromycin and clindamycin + quinine have been used for more than 20 years for the treatment of human babesiosis [60], the efficacy of these drugs and their primary modes of action in *Babesia* parasites have only recently started to be elucidated.

Table 1. Reported efficacy of atovaquone, azithromycin, clindamycin and quinine in animal models of babesiosis.

Drug	Treatment Regimen	Model	Effect	Ref.
Atovaquone	20 mg/kg (p.o.), 5 d	*B. microti* Balb/c mice	~5.7 × reduction in peak parasitemia.	[61]
	25 mg/kg (p.o.), 4 d	*B. microti* Balb/c mice	77% suppression of parasitemia at DPI 9.	[54]
	50 mg/kg (p.o.), 4 d	*B. microti* Balb/c mice	87% suppression of parasitemia at DPI 9.	[54]
	100 mg/kg (p.o.), 4 d	*B. microti* Balb/c mice	93% suppression of parasitemia at DPI 9.	[54]
	10 mg/kg (p.o.), 7 d	*B. microti* SCID mice	Parasitemia clearance followed by recrudescence by D5-9 post-treatment.	[11]
	10 mg/kg (p.o.), 10 d	*B. microti* SCID mice	Parasitemia clearance followed by recrudescence by D14 post-treatment.	[57]
	10 mg/kg (p.o.), 10 d	*B. duncani* C3H/HeJ mice	Parasitemia clearance followed by recrudescence by D10 post-treatment. 80% survival.	[57]

Table 1. *Cont.*

Drug	Treatment Regimen	Model	Effect	Ref.
Azithromycin	25 mg/kg (p.o.), 4 d	*B. microti* Balb/c mice	75% suppression of parasitemia at DPI 9.	[54]
	50 mg/kg (p.o.), 4 d	*B. microti* Balb/c mice	96% suppression of parasitemia at DPI 9.	[54]
	100 mg/kg (p.o.), 4 d	*B. microti* Balb/c mice	95% suppression of parasitemia at DPI 9.	[54]
	10 mg/kg (p.o.), 7 d	*B. microti* SCID mice	No effect.	[11]
	50 mg/kg (p.o.), 7 d	*B. microti* SCID mice	No effect.	[11]
Clindamycin	300 mg/kg (p.o.), 5d	*B. microti* Mongolian jirds	9.4% suppression of parasitemia at DPI 9.	[51]
	150 mg/kg (i.m.), 8d	*B. microti* Golden hamsters	~2× reduction in peak parasitemia.	[52]
	150 mg/kg (p.o.), 8d	*B. microti* Golden hamsters	~2× reduction in peak parasitemia.	[52]
	500 mg/kg (i.p.), 5d	*B. microti* Balb/c mice	~3.2× reduction in peak parasitemia.	[53]
	25 mg/kg (p.o.), 4 d	*B. microti* Balb/c mice	No effect.	[54]
	50 mg/kg (p.o.), 4 d	*B. microti* Balb/c mice	No effect.	[54]
	100 mg/kg (p.o.), 4 d	*B. microti* Balb/c mice	No effect.	[54]
	10 mg/kg (p.o.), 7 d	*B. microti* SCID mice	No effect.	[11]
	50 mg/kg (p.o.), 7 d	*B. microti* SCID mice	No effect.	[11]
Quinine	125 mg/kg (s.c.), 8d	*B. microti* Golden hamsters	No effect.	[52]
	250 mg/kg (p.o.), 8d	*B. microti* Golden hamsters	No effect.	[52]
	25 mg/kg (p.o.), 4 d	*B. microti* Balb/c mice	No effect.	[54]
	50 mg/kg (p.o.), 4 d	*B. microti* Balb/c mice	No effect.	[54]
	100 mg/kg (p.o.), 4 d	*B. microti* Balb/c mice	No effect.	[54]
	10 mg/kg (p.o.), 7 d	*B. microti* SCID mice	No effect.	[11]
	50 mg/kg (p.o.), 7 d	*B. microti* SCID mice	No effect.	[11]
	100 mg/kg (p.o.), 7 d	*B. microti* SCID mice	No effect.	[11]

3. In Vitro and In Vivo Models for the Evaluation of Novel Anti-*Babesia* Therapies

Evaluation of the potency of novel drugs for the treatment of human babesiosis has proven challenging due to the absence of a continuous in vitro culture system for *B. microti*, the main causative agent of human babesiosis. A *B. microti* short-term ex vivo system has been used previously for growth inhibition assays [11,62]. However, this culture system is not amenable for high-throughput screening of large libraries of compounds. Despite the current challenges faced in the development of a stable *B. microti* in vitro culture system, this parasite can easily be propagated in rodents, such as mice [63–65], hamsters [66], and gerbils [51]. Two very distinct profiles of *B. microti* infection in preclinical models have been observed, depending on the immune status of the host. In immunocompetent animals, such as Balb/c mice, golden hamsters, or gerbils, the parasitemia typically rises within a few days following infection, reaches a peak (40–60% parasitemia), and then resolves on its own [63–65]. In immunocompromised animals, such as SCID and rag2D mice, the parasitemia rises and then plateaus at ~50–80% parasitemia [11,57,63]. Immunocompromized mice infected with *B. microti* maintain high parasitemia levels over time but do not succumb to infection [11,57,63]. Although the most commonly used *B. microti* preclinical models (described above) are non-lethal, one research group reported the use of a lethal model of *B. microti* infection in hamsters using the ATCC30222 strain [58,67]. In this model, parasite inoculation results in fulminating disease reaching 90% parasitemia and almost 100% mortality by DPI 12 [58,67]. This model of infection was previously used to evaluate the potency of atovaquone [58].

In vitro culture of *B. divergens*, a species known to infect humans and cattle [1], has been established in mammalian erythrocytes and can be used for the evaluation of potential drug candidates [59,68–73]. An in vivo model of *B. divergens* is available in gerbils [74,75] and has been used for the evaluation of potential antibabesial drugs [59,76]. Multiple other rodent species such as rats, mice, hamsters or guinea pigs were tested for the establishment of infection, but none developed parasitemia [74].

The first in-vitro culture system of *B. duncani* in hamster red blood cells was established in 1994 [77]. More recently an adapted protocol of *B. duncani* culture in hamster RBCs was reported using another culture medium [78]. The authors also investigated alternate RBC sources such as mouse, rat, horse or cow. None of these RBCs were able to sustain *B. duncani* growth [78]. In 2018, Abraham et al. reported the first continuous in vitro culture system for *B. duncani* in human erythrocytes [79]. The development of this system allowed for the high-throughput screening of novel derivatives for the treatment of human babesiosis [57]. *B. duncani* can be propagated in hamsters and typically results in fatal infection following the development of pulmonary edema and respiratory distress [80,81]. However, to the best of our knowledge, the *B. duncani* hamster model was not used for the assessment of potential antibabesial drugs. *B. duncani* infection can also be established in mice and is associated with a fatal outcome in specific mouse genetic backgrounds [82,83]. Similar to the hamster model, *B. duncani*-infected mice present with pulmonary edema, leading to respiratory distress and death [83]. Interestingly, it was shown that susceptibility to acute babesiosis following *B. duncani* infection is significantly influenced by the gender and genetic background of the animal [82]. Recently, Chiu et al. presented the first use of a lethal model of *B. duncani* infection in mice for the evaluation of novel promising candidates for the treatment of human babesiosis [57]. The different models of in vitro and in vivo *B. microti*, *B. divergens*, and *B. duncani* available for the evaluation of novel therapeutics are summarized in Table 2.

Table 2. Current in vitro and in vivo systems available for *B. microti*, *B. divergens* and *B. duncani* propagation.

***Babesia* Species**	**In Vitro System**	**In Vivo Model**
B. microti	Short-term ex vivo system [11,62]	Mice [63–65], hamsters [58,66,67], gerbils [51]
B. divergens	Continuous in vitro culture system in human RBCs [69]	Gerbils [74,75]
B. duncani	Continuous in vitro culture system in hamster [77,78] and human [79] RBCs	Mice [57,82,83], hamsters [80,81]

Overall, there is a wide variety of *Babesia* models available. However, finding complementary systems can prove challenging. Even though *B. microti* accounts for the majority of human babesiosis cases, the absence of a continuous in vitro culture system makes it challenging to use this species for drug discovery purposes. On the other hand, *B. divergens* can be used for in vitro drug screening. However, it's in vivo model using gerbils may not be widely accessible. Considering this, *B. duncani* appears as the *Babesia* species of choice for drug development. The availability of a stable in vitro culture system in human red blood cells allows for high-throughput screening of large libraries of candidates, offering the possibility to conduct detailed structure–activity relationship studies. Furthermore, the availability of a reproducible model of *B. duncani* lethal infection in immunocompetent mice offers a reasonably affordable option to assess promising drug candidates.

4. Novel Therapies under Investigation for the Treatment of Human Babesiosis

The recent effort to develop new therapeutics for the treatment of human babesiosis has mostly focused on repurposing known anti-piroplasm agents. A large library of antimalarial drugs, such as artesunate, artemether, dihydroartemisinin, chloroquine, mefloquine, piperaquine, halofantrine, lumefantrine, pyrimethamine, and pyronaridine, has been assessed against *B. microti* but failed to demonstrate much, if any, efficacy against parasite load at the selected dose [51,54,55]. Other antimalarials such as primaquine, pentaquine and robenidine showed potent parasitemia suppression in *B. microti*-infected animals [51,54]. Screening of the Malaria Box, a 400-compound library with known antimalarial activity [84], led to the identification of nine compounds with low micromolar/nanomolar potency (2.1 μM to 160 nM) against *B. divergens* cultured in human erythrocytes [71]. To the best of our knowledge, no further evaluation of the most promising candidates has been reported so far. More recent screenings of the Malaria Box and the Pathogen Box (400 compounds active against neglected diseases) also reported 38 and nine compounds, respectively, with nanomolar potency against *Babesia* species responsible for bovine (*B. bovis* and *B. bigemina*) and equine (*B. caballi*) babesiosis [85,86]. The two most promising compounds identified from the Pathogen Box screening were further assessed in *B. microti*-infected Balb/c mice and showed significant reduction of peak parasitemia [85].

Over the recent years, a large number of drugs, including actinonin [87], atranorin [61], N-acetyl-L-cystein [88], chalcone-4-hydrate [89], trans-chalcone [89], cryptolepine [90], ellagic acid [91], eflornithine [92], fusidic acid [93], gossypol [94], gedunin [95], hydroxyurea [92], luteolin [87,95], nimbolide [95], pepstatin A [96], xanthohumol [94], fluoroquinolone derivatives (enrofloxacin, enoxacin, norfloxacin, ofloxacin, trovafloxacin) [97,98], ciprofloxacin and some of its novel derivatives [53,99], and natural extracts of *Syzygium aromaticum* [100], *Camellia sinensis* [100], *Cinnamomum verum* [101], *Olea europaea*, and *Acacia laeta* [102] have been assessed for antibabesial properties. The in vitro evaluation of these derivatives was mainly carried out against the species responsible for bovine and equine babesiosis and revealed, in most cases, growth inhibition in the micromolar range. In vivo evaluation of these compounds was typically performed in *B. microti*-infected hamsters or Balb/c mice. In most cases, diminution and/or delay in peak parasitemia was observed, but none of the monotherapies displayed high potency against *B. microti* [61,90–92,94,97,100,101]. Although some of these compounds could turn out to be promising for veterinary use, they are unlikely to be accepted for clinical use based on their poor selectivity indices. Despite this fact, some of these drugs could be investigated as starting points for structural optimization for the development of novel antibabesial agents.

Out of the multiple derivatives recently reported with potent anti-*Babesia* efficacy, tafenoquine, clofazimine, and endochin-like quinolones are probably the most promising drugs.

Tafenoquine, previously known as WR238605, is an 8-aminoquinoline. In 2018, tafenoquine was approved by FDA for the radical cure of *Plasmodium vivax* infection and for chemoprophylaxis of malaria [103]. Several research groups have investigated the potential of tafenoquine against *Babesia* parasites [55,104–106]. In 1997, Marley et al. reported that a twice daily injection of Tafenoquine (i.m.) at 52 mg/kg for four days resulted in 100% parasitemia suppression by day 3 post-drug removal in *B. microti*-infected golden hamsters [55]. Furthermore, a subpassage experiment was carried out to determine whether parasitologic cure was achieved. None of the animals that received blood from tafenoquine-treated hamsters became parasitemic after six weeks post-administration, indicating that treatment resulted in complete cure of *B. microti* infection [55]. More recently, Mordue et al. evaluated tafenoquine in *B. microti*-infected SCID mice [106]. When parasitemia reached ~10%, mice were administered with a single dose of 20 mg/kg of tafenoquine (p.o.). By day 4 post-treatment, parasitemia level was undetectable in tafenoquine-treated animals and remained so until the end of the experiment (day 18 post-treatment). To assess whether the lack of detection of parasites in blood smears was indicative of cure, blood collected from tafenoquine-treated animals at day 18 PT was injected in naive SCID mice. The newly inoculated animals developed detectable parasitemia within one week. Interestingly administration of a single dose of 20 mg/kg tafenoquine (p.o.) resulted in undetectable parasitemia within four days, indicating that the parasites remained sensitive to tafenoquine. In the case where mice were kept beyond day 18 PT, recrudescence was observed day 37 PT. In a separate experiment, *B. microti*-infected mice were treated with a first dose of 25 mg/kg of tafenoquine (p.o.) when parasitemia reached ~20%, followed by a second dose of 12.5 mg/kg of tafenoquine (p.o.) three days later to account for the decrease of plasma concentration. By day 5 after administration of the first dose, parasitemia was below detection level and remained so until day 28 PT. Subpassage of blood collected at day 28 PT in naïve SCID mice resulted in detectable parasitemia with nine days post-inoculation. Overall, although no radical cure was achieved in these experiments, a single oral dose of tafenoquine was found efficient to rapidly reduce parasitemia burden. It is also worth noting that despite the recrudescence observed following treatment, re-emerging parasites did not develop resistance to tafenoquine and remained susceptible to the drug [106]. In 2020, Carvalho et al. investigated tafenoquine in *B. microti*-infected Balb/c mice. Potent inhibition was observed following administration of 10 mg/kg of tafenoquine (three doses on alternate days, p.o.) or of a combination of 10 mg/kg of tafenoquine (three doses on alternate days, p.o.) + 25 mg/kg artesunate (five daily doses, i.p.), starting at day 4 post-infection [104]. In both cases, a ~5.6-fold reduction in peak parasitemia was observed and parasitemia was undetectable from DPI 9 by examination of Giemsa-stained thin-blood smears and remained so until the end of the study (DPI 30). However, except for one animal from the tafenoquine + artesunate treatment group, all mice remained positive for *B. microti* infection by PCR at DPI 27. Interestingly, subpassage of blood collected from tafenoquine-treated mice in a naïve Balb/c mouse resulted in the development of parasitemia, whereas the mouse receiving blood from combination-treated animals remained negative [104].

Based on the results described above (summarized in Table 3), tafenoquine could be an interesting drug candidate for further evaluation for the treatment of human babesiosis. With its extended half-life in humans (12–17 days) [106], only a few doses may be required, thus limiting the development of drug resistance. One downside, however, is that tafenoquine causes severe hemolytic anemia in patients with glucose-6-phosphate dehydrogenase (G6PD) deficiency [105,107,108], and as a result its use is contraindicated in such cases. While the exact mechanism of action of tafenoquine in *Babesia* parasites remains unknown, one hypothesis is that the 8-aminoquinoline mediates oxidative stress within the parasite without damaging the host red blood cells of individuals with active G6PD [105]. The latter enzyme plays a key role in the production of NADPH and protects red blood cells from damage by reactive oxygen species (ROS). In the case of G6PD deficiency, NADPH is at a level that is not enough to protect the RBCs from tafenoquine-induced oxidative stress [105].

Table 3. Preclinical evaluation of promising new therapeutics for the treatment of human babesiosis: tafenoquine, clofazimine and endochin-like quinolones (ELQs).

Drug	Treatment Regimen	Model	Effect	Ref.
ELQ-271	10 mg/kg (p.o.), 7 d	*B. microti* SCID mice	Parasitemia clearance followed by recrudescence by D12 post-treatment.	[11]
ELQ-316	10 mg/kg (p.o.), 7 d	*B. microti* SCID mice	Parasitemia clearance followed by recrudescence by D12 post-treatment.	[11]

Table 3. *Cont.*

Drug	Treatment Regimen	Model	Effect	Ref.
ELQ-334	10 mg/kg (p.o.), 7 d	*B. microti* SCID mice	Parasitemia clearance followed by recrudescence by D16 post-treatment.	[11]
ELQ-334 + Atovaquone	10 + 10 mg/kg (p.o.), 7 d	*B. microti* SCID mice	Parasitemia clearance throughout experiment.	[11]
ELQ-502	10 mg/kg (p.o.), 5 d	*B. microti* SCID mice	Parasitemia clearance followed by recrudescence by D17 post-treatment.	[109]
	10 mg/kg (p.o.), 10 d	*B. microti* SCID mice	Parasitemia clearance throughout study (DPI 91).	[57]
	10 mg/kg (p.o.), 10 d	*B. duncani* C3H/HeJ mice	Parasitemia clearance throughout study (DPI 91). 100% survival.	[57]
ELQ-502 + Atovaquone	10 + 10 mg/kg (p.o.), 10 d	*B. microti* SCID mice	Parasitemia clearance throughout study (DPI 91).	[109]
	10 + 10 mg/kg (p.o.), 10 d	*B. duncani* C3H/HeJ mice	Parasitemia clearance throughout study (DPI 91). 100% survival	[109]
Tafenoquine	52 mg/kg (i.m.), 4 d (b.i.d.)	*B. microti* Golden hamsters	100% suppression of parasitemia at D3 post-treatment. Reinfection of clean hamster negative.	[55]
	13 mg/kg (i.m.), 4 d (b.i.d.)	*B. microti* Golden hamsters	99% suppression of parasitemia at D3 post-treatment.	[55]
	3.25 mg/kg (i.m.), 4 d (b.i.d.)	*B. microti* Golden hamsters	91% suppression of parasitemia at D3 post-treatment.	[55]
	52 mg/kg (i.m.), 2 d (b.i.d.)	*B. microti* Golden hamsters	99% suppression of parasitemia at D3 post-treatment.	[55]
	20 mg/kg (p.o.), 1 d	*B. microti* SCID mice	Parasitemia clearance followed by recrudescence by D37 post-treatment.	[106]
	25 mg/kg (p.o.), 1 d, + 12.5 mg/kg (p.o.), 1 d (4 d after 1st dose)	*B. microti* SCID mice	Parasitemia clear through D28 post-treatment. Reinfection of "clean" mice positive.	[106]
	10 mg/kg (p.o.), 3 d	*B. microti* Balb/c mice	~5.6× reduction in peak parasitemia.	[104]
Clofazimine	20 mg/kg (p.o.), 52 d	*B. microti* Balb/c mice	Parasitemia clear through DPI 90 (smear + PCR negative).	[110]
	20 mg/kg (p.o.), 7 d	*B. microti* Balb/c mice	Parasitemia clearance followed by recrudescence on DPI 26, unresponsive to a 2nd course of clofazimine 20 mg/kg (p.o.) (14 d).	[110]

Clofazimine is an antibiotic used to treat leprosy [111] and drug-resistant tuberculosis [112]. In 2016, Tuvshintulga et al. reported that clofazimine has potent antibabesial effect, following its evaluation in *B. microti*-infected Balb/c mice. A five-day treatment course of 20 mg/kg clofazimine administered either i.p. or p.o. led to suppression of parasitemia by more than 80%, with a slightly superior efficacy when administered orally [113]. Interestingly, although no parasites could be detected by blood smears, blood, heart, spleen, kidney, and liver samples obtained from clofazimine-treated animals tested positive for the presence of *B. microti* ss-rRNA at DPI 40. Consistently, subpassage of blood collected from clofazimine-treated animals in naïve mice resulted in reinfection [113]. It is worth noting that no toxicity was observed in mice during treatment administration. Furthermore, daily administration of 200–300 mg for >30 months for the treatment drug-resistant tuberculosis in humans was well tolerated [114]. More recently, the same research group reported on the efficacy of clofazimine in *B. microti*-infected SCID mice [110]. The continuous administration of clofazimine from DPI 4 to 57 at a daily dose of 20 mg/kg resulted in undetectable parasitemia by examination of blood smears from DPI 14 onward. Parasite DNA could no longer be detected by PCR from DPI 54 until the end of the study (DPI 90), suggesting that this seven-week treatment course is efficient in curing *B. microti* infection [110]. *B. microti*-infected SCID mice treated with 20 mg/kg clofazimine for seven days (DPI4-10) showed no parasitemia by DPI 24. However, recrudescence was observed from DPI 26. Initiation of a second treatment course of clofazimine failed to clear parasitemia, suggesting that the rise of recrudescent parasites was associated with development of clofazimine resistance. Blood samples obtained from two mice that developed recrudescence were sub-passaged in naïve Balb/c mice, which subsequently underwent a five-day clofazimine treatment course. Interestingly, clofazimine successfully impacted the rise of parasitemia in one case, but not in the other [110]. Sequencing analysis established that, unlike atovaquone, clofazimine does not target the cytochrome b of the parasite. As a result, atovaquone-resistant parasites were generated in SCID mice and then propagated in Balb/c mice. A two-week course of 20 mg/kg clofazimine successfully cleared infection in all the mice. However, a relapse was observed in some of the animals, which responded to a second two-week course of a higher dose of clofazimine (40 mg/kg) [110]. Based on these results, clofazimine appears as a promising candidate for the treatment of human babesiosis. Due to the risk of development of drug resistance with a short-term monotherapy, it would be interesting to evaluate the efficacy of clofazimine when combined with a partner drug such as atovaquone. Results derived from the preclinical evaluation of clofazimine are summarized in Table 3.

A novel class of compounds, endochin-like quinolones (ELQs) has recently been reported with high potency against *B. microti* and *B. duncani* [11,57]. Previously reported for their high potency against other apicomplexan parasites such as *Plasmodium* [115–125], *Toxoplasma* [126,127] and *Leishmania* [128], ELQs have been shown to target the cytochrome bc_1 complex of the parasites (Figure 3) [117,120,122,128–130]. In 2016, Lawres et al. demonstrated potency of ELQ-271 and ELQ-316 in the short-term ex vivo culture system of *B. microti* as well as in the in vivo SCID model of *B. microti* infection. In *B. microti*-infected mice, a seven-day oral administration of 10 mg/kg of ELQ-271 or ELQ-316 resulted in clearance of parasitemia, followed by recrudescence by day 12 post-drug removal [11]. Due to the high crystallinity and low aqueous solubility of this class of compounds, which precludes administration of higher doses, a prodrug of ELQ-316, ELQ-334, was designed by esterification of the carbonyl group present in the quinolone core of the molecule [11,115,116,127]. This strategy led to improved aqueous solubility and increased plasma concentration of the drug following administration of molar equivalents [11,115,116,127]. Administration of ELQ-334 as a monotherapy at 10 mg/kg in *B. microti*-infected mice resulted to slightly extended clearance of parasitemia compared to treatment with ELQ-271 and ELQ-316. However, re-emerging parasitemia was observed by day 16 post-drug removal. In all cases, recrudescence was accompanied by a GCT $\rightarrow$ GTT mutation in the Q_i site of the parasite's cytochrome bc_1 complex, resulting in an Ala to Val substitution at codon 218 [11]. Since monotherapy is not the ideal treatment regimen, a combination of ELQ-334 + atovaquone was evaluated and resulted in complete clearance of parasitemia with no recrudescence following administration of doses as low as 5 + 5 mg/kg [11]. More recently, Chiu et al. reported the screening of a new library of ELQ derivatives against *B. duncani* and identified three potent ELQ prodrugs: ELQ-331 (IC_{50} = 141 ± 22 nM), ELQ- 468 (IC_{50} = 15 ± 1 nM), and ELQ-502 (IC_{50} = 6 ± 2 nM). The previously reported ELQ-316 and its prodrug, ELQ-

334 were also assessed against *B. duncani* and showed IC_{50} values of 136 ± 1 nM and 193 ± 66 nM, respectively [57].

Further evaluation of the lead candidate, ELQ-502, showed low toxicity in mammalian cells, and thus a highly desirable therapeutic index (>833). ELQ-502 was assessed in *B. duncani*- and *B. microti*-infected mice as a single drug (10 mg/kg) and in combination with atovaquone (10 + 10 mg/kg). Following a 10-day treatment course, both the mono- and the combination therapies resulted in radical cure with no recrudescence, and in the case of *B. duncani*-infected mice, 100% survival [57]. Interestingly, a shorter treatment duration with ELQ-502 alone at 10 mg/kg in *B. microti*-infected mice resulted in recrudescence [109]. Similarly to the results obtained following treatment with ELQ-271, ELQ-316, and ELQ-334, recrudescence following ELQ-502 shorter treatment duration was associated with GCT → GTT mutation in the Q_i site of the *BmCytb* [109]. Results obtained from the evaluation of ELQ derivatives are summarized in Table 3.

5. Conclusions and Considerations for Future Drug Development

Human babesiosis is an emerging tick-borne disease of rising incidence and a major public health concern. The current therapies for the treatment of human babesiosis are based on drugs already in use against other apicomplexan parasites and tend to be associated with significant adverse effects and/or the development of drug resistance. Moreover, the evaluation of these drugs, namely atovaquone, azithromycin, clindamycin, and quinine, in animal models of babesiosis has raised concerned about their efficacy in achieving parasite elimination. In light of these findings, the need for novel treatments specifically designed to tackle *Babesia* infection becomes apparent. Over the past decades, there has been a growing effort to develop such therapies. Based on their potency, selectivity, and ability to eliminate infection with no recrudescence when combined with atovaquone, endochin-like quinolones (ELQs) appear to be the most promising candidates to advance the treatment of human babesiosis. With regard to the identification of novel molecules with potency against human babesiosis, it could be interesting to establish a standardized protocol for the evaluation of new candidates, in order to facilitate a comparison of results between different research centers. A consensus protocol agreed upon by members of the community and one that follows standard methods for efficacy and safety using established in vitro cell culture assays and in vivo mouse models is warranted.

Author Contributions: Conceptualization, C.B.M. and I.R.; writing-original draft preparation, I.R; writing-review and editing, I.R. and C.B.M.; supervision, C.B.M.; funding acquisition, C.B.M. All authors have read and agreed to the published version of the manuscript.

Funding: CBM research is supported by NIH grants (AI-123321, AI-138139, AI-152220, AI-153100, AI136138 and the Steven & Alexandra Cohen Foundation and the Global Lyme Alliance).

Institutional Review Board Statement: Not applicable.

Informed Consent Statement: Not applicable.

Data Availability Statement: No new data were created. The information presented in this review article are from published reports available in public databases.

Conflicts of Interest: The authors declare no conflict of interest.

References

1. Krause, P.J. Human babesiosis. *Int. J. Parasit.* **2019**, *49*, 165–174. [CrossRef] [PubMed]
2. Madison-Antenucci, S.; Kramer, L.D.; Gebhardt, L.L.; Kauffman, E. Emerging Tick-Borne Diseases. *Clin. Microbiol. Rev.* **2020**, *33*, 34. [CrossRef]
3. Levin, A.E.; Krause, P.J. Transfusion-transmitted babesiosis: Is it time to screen the blood supply? *Curr. Opin. Hematol.* **2016**, *23*, 573–580. [CrossRef] [PubMed]
4. Lobo, C.A.; Singh, M.; Rodriguez, M. Human babesiosis: Recent advances and future challenges. *Curr. Opin. Hematol.* **2020**, *27*, 399–405. [CrossRef] [PubMed]

5. Moritz, E.D.; Winton, C.S.; Tonnetti, L.; Townsend, R.L.; Berardi, V.P.; Hewins, M.E.; Weeks, K.E.; Dodd, R.Y.; Stramer, S.L. Screening for *Babesia microti* in the U. S. Blood Supply. *N. Engl. J. Med.* **2016**, *375*, 2236–2245. [CrossRef] [PubMed]
6. Tonnetti, L.; Townsend, R.L.; Dodd, R.Y.; Stramer, S.L. Characteristics of transfusion-transmitted *Babesia microti*, American Red Cross 2010–2017. *Transfusion* **2019**, *59*, 2908–2912. [CrossRef]
7. Mantadakis, E. *Pneumocystis jirovecii* Pneumonia in Children with Hematological Malignancies: Diagnosis and Approaches to Management. *J. Fungi* **2020**, *6*, 331. [CrossRef] [PubMed]
8. Dunay, I.R.; Gajurel, K.; Dhakal, R.; Liesenfeld, O.; Montoya, J.G. Treatment of Toxoplasmosis: Historical Perspective, Animal Models, and Current Clinical Practice. *Clin. Microbiol. Rev.* **2018**, *31*, e00057-17. [CrossRef]
9. Nixon, G.L.; Moss, D.M.; Shone, A.E.; Lalloo, D.G.; Fisher, N.; O'Neill, P.M.; Ward, S.A.; Biagini, G.A. Antimalarial pharmacology and therapeutics of atovaquone. *J. Antimicrob. Chemother.* **2013**, *68*, 977–985. [CrossRef]
10. Jacobsen, L.; Husen, P.; Solov'yov, I.A. Inhibition Mechanism of Antimalarial Drugs Targeting the Cytochrome bc1 Complex. *J. Chem. Inf. Modeling* **2021**, *61*, 1334–1345. [CrossRef]
11. Lawres, L.A.; Garg, A.; Kumar, V.; Bruzual, I.; Forquer, I.P.; Renard, I.; Virji, A.Z.; Boulard, P.; Rodriguez, E.X.; Allen, A.J.; et al. Radical cure of experimental babesiosis in immunodeficient mice using a combination of an endochin-like quinolone and atovaquone. *J. Exp. Med.* **2016**, *213*, 1307–1318. [CrossRef]
12. Montazeri, M.; Mehrzadi, S.; Sharif, M.; Sarvi, S.; Shahdin, S.; Daryani, A. Activities of anti-*Toxoplasma* drugs and compounds against tissue cysts in the last three decades (1987 to 2017), a systematic review. *Parasitol. Res.* **2018**, *117*, 3045–3057. [CrossRef]
13. Vaidya, A.B.; Mather, M.W. Atovaquone resistance in malaria parasites. *Drug Resist. Updates* **2000**, *3*, 283–287. [CrossRef]
14. Daniel, R. Azithromycin, erythromycin and cloxacillin in the treatment of infections of skin and associated soft tissues. European Azithromycin Study Group. *J. Int. Med. Res.* **1991**, *19*, 433–445. [CrossRef]
15. Dinwiddie, R. Anti-inflammatory therapy in cystic fibrosis. *J. Cyst. Fibros.* **2005**, *4* (Suppl. S2), 45–48. [CrossRef] [PubMed]
16. Ladhani, S.; Garbash, M. Staphylococcal skin infections in children: Rational drug therapy recommendations. *Paediatr. Drugs* **2005**, *7*, 77–102. [CrossRef] [PubMed]
17. Carratala, J.; Garcia-Vidal, C. An update on *Legionella*. *Curr. Opin. Infect. Dis.* **2010**, *23*, 152–157. [CrossRef]
18. Van Eijk, A.M.; Terlouw, D.J. Azithromycin for treating uncomplicated malaria. *Cochrane Database Syst. Rev.* **2011**, *2011*, Cd006688. [CrossRef] [PubMed]
19. Chakraborty, A. Understanding the biology of the *Plasmodium falciparum* apicoplast; an excellent target for antimalarial drug development. *Life Sci.* **2016**, *158*, 104–110. [CrossRef] [PubMed]
20. Sidhu, A.B.S.; Sun, Q.G.; Nkrumah, L.J.; Dunne, M.W.; Sacchettini, J.C.; Fidock, D.A. In vitro efficacy, resistance selection, and structural modeling studies implicate the malarial parasite apicoplast as the target of azithromycin. *J. Biol. Chem.* **2007**, *282*, 2494–2504. [CrossRef] [PubMed]
21. Beckers, C.J.M.; Roos, D.S.; Donald, R.G.K.; Luft, B.J.; Schwab, J.C.; Cao, Y.; Joiner, K.A. Inhibition of cytoplasmic and organellar protein synthesis in *Toxoplasma gondii*. Implications for the target of macrolide antibiotics. *J. Clin. Investig.* **1995**, *95*, 367–376. [CrossRef]
22. Dahl, E.L.; Rosenthal, P.J. Multiple antibiotics exert delayed effects against the *Plasmodium falciparum* anicoplast. *Antimicrob. Agents Chemother.* **2007**, *51*, 3485–3490. [CrossRef]
23. Murphy, P.B.; Bistas, K.G.; Le, J.K. Clindamycin. In *StatPearls*; StatPearls Publishing: Treasure Island, FL, USA, 2021.
24. Griffith, K.S.; Lewis, L.S.; Mali, S.; Parise, M.E. Treatment of malaria in the United States: A systematic review. *Jama* **2007**, *297*, 2264–2277. [CrossRef]
25. Lell, B.; Kremsner, P.G. Clindamycin as an antimalarial drug: Review of clinical trials. *Antimicrob. Agents Chemother.* **2002**, *46*, 2315–2320. [CrossRef] [PubMed]
26. Smith, R.P.; Hunfeld, K.P.; Krause, P.J. Management strategies for human babesiosis. *Expert Rev. Anti-Infect. Ther.* **2020**, *18*, 625–636. [CrossRef] [PubMed]
27. Pfefferkorn, E.R.; Borotz, S.E. Comparison of mutants of *Toxoplasma gondii* selected for resistance to azithromycin, spiramycin, or clindamycin. *Antimicrob. Agents Chemother.* **1994**, *38*, 31–37. [CrossRef]
28. Talapko, J.; Škrlec, I.; Alebić, T.; Jukić, M.; Včev, A. Malaria: The Past and the Present. *Microorganisms* **2019**, *7*, 179. [CrossRef] [PubMed]
29. Tse, E.G.; Korsik, M.; Todd, M.H. The past, present and future of anti-malarial medicines. *Malar. J.* **2019**, *18*, 93. [CrossRef] [PubMed]
30. Sullivan, D.J., Jr.; Gluzman, I.Y.; Russell, D.G.; Goldberg, D.E. On the molecular mechanism of chloroquine's antimalarial action. *Proc. Natl. Acad. Sci. USA* **1996**, *93*, 11865–11870. [CrossRef]
31. Tang, Y.Q.; Ye, Q.; Huang, H.; Zheng, W.Y. An Overview of Available Antimalarials: Discovery, Mode of Action and Drug Resistance. *Curr. Mol. Med.* **2020**, *20*, 583–592. [CrossRef] [PubMed]
32. Woodland, J.G.; Hunter, R.; Smith, P.J.; Egan, T.J. Shining new light on ancient drugs: Preparation and subcellular localisation of novel fluorescent analogues of *Cinchona* alkaloids in intraerythrocytic *Plasmodium falciparum*. *Org. Biomol. Chem.* **2017**, *15*, 589–597. [CrossRef]
33. Woodland, J.G.; Hunter, R.; Smith, P.J.; Egan, T.J. Chemical Proteomics and Super-resolution Imaging Reveal That Chloroquine Interacts with *Plasmodium falciparum* Multidrug Resistance-Associated Protein and Lipids. *ACS Chem. Biol.* **2018**, *13*, 2939–2948. [CrossRef] [PubMed]

34. Punihaole, D.; Workman, R.J.; Upadhyay, S.; Van Bruggen, C.; Schmitz, A.J.; Reineke, T.M.; Frontiera, R.R. New Insights into Quinine-DNA Binding Using Raman Spectroscopy and Molecular Dynamics Simulations. *J. Phys. Chem. B* **2018**, *122*, 9840–9851. [CrossRef] [PubMed]
35. Golan, D.E.; Armstrong, E.J.; Armstrong, A.W.; Tashjian, A.H. *Principles of Pharmacology: The Pathophysiologic Basis of Drug Therapy*, 3rd ed.; Lippincott Williams & Wilkins: Philadelphia, PA, USA, 2012; pp. 1–1956.
36. Percário, S.; Moreira, D.R.; Gomes, B.A.; Ferreira, M.E.; Gonçalves, A.C.; Laurindo, P.S.; Vilhena, T.C.; Dolabela, M.F.; Green, M.D. Oxidative stress in malaria. *Int. J. Mol. Sci.* **2012**, *13*, 16346–16372. [CrossRef]
37. Dziekan, J.M.; Yu, H.; Chen, D.; Dai, L.; Wirjanata, G.; Larsson, A.; Prabhu, N.; Sobota, R.M.; Bozdech, Z.; Nordlund, P. Identifying purine nucleoside phosphorylase as the target of quinine using cellular thermal shift assay. *Sci. Transl. Med.* **2019**, *11*. [CrossRef]
38. Krause, P.J.; Auwaerter, P.G.; Bannuru, R.R.; Branda, J.A.; Falck-Ytter, Y.T.; Lantos, P.M.; Lavergne, V.; Meissner, H.C.; Osani, M.C.; Rips, J.G.; et al. Clinical Practice Guidelines by the Infectious Diseases Society of America (IDSA): 2020 Guideline on Diagnosis and Management of Babesiosis. *Clin. Infect. Dis.* **2021**, *72*, 185–189. [CrossRef] [PubMed]
39. Kletsova, E.A.; Spitzer, E.D.; Fries, B.C.; Marcos, L.A. Babesiosis in Long Island: Review of 62 cases focusing on treatment with azithromycin and atovaquone. *Ann. Clin. Microbiol. Antimicrob.* **2017**, *16*, 7. [CrossRef] [PubMed]
40. Krause, P.J.; Gewurz, B.E.; Hill, D.; Marty, F.M.; Vannier, E.; Foppa, I.M.; Furman, R.R.; Neuhaus, E.; Skowron, G.; Gupta, S.; et al. Persistent and relapsing babesiosis in Immunocompromised patients. *Clin. Infect. Dis.* **2008**, *46*, 370–376. [CrossRef] [PubMed]
41. Raffalli, J.; Wormser, G.P. Persistence of babesiosis for >2 years in a patient on rituximab for rheumatoid arthritis. *Diagn. Microbiol. Infect. Dis.* **2016**, *85*, 231–232. [CrossRef]
42. Simon, M.S.; Westblade, L.F.; Dziedziech, A.; Visone, J.E.; Furman, R.R.; Jenkins, S.G.; Schuetz, A.N.; Kirkman, L.A. Clinical and Molecular Evidence of Atovaquone and Azithromycin Resistance in Relapsed *Babesia microti* Infection Associated with Rituximab and Chronic Lymphocytic Leukemia. *Clin. Infect. Dis.* **2017**, *65*, 1222–1225. [CrossRef]
43. Lemieux, J.E.; Tran, A.D.; Freimark, L.; Schaffner, S.F.; Goethert, H.; Andersen, K.G.; Bazner, S.; Li, A.; McGrath, G.; Sloan, L.; et al. A global map of genetic diversity in *Babesia microti* reveals strong population structure and identifies variants associated with clinical relapse. *Nat. Microbiol.* **2016**, *1*, 7. [CrossRef]
44. Birth, D.; Kao, W.C.; Hunte, C. Structural analysis of atovaquone-inhibited cytochrome *bc(1)* complex reveals the molecular basis of antimalarial drug action. *Nat. Commun.* **2014**, *5*, 11. [CrossRef]
45. Doktor, S.Z.; Shortridge, V.D.; Beyer, J.M.; Flamm, R.K. Epidemiology of macrolide and/or lincosamide resistant *Streptococcus pneumoniae* clinical isolates with ribosomal mutations. *Diagn. Microbiol. Infect. Dis.* **2004**, *49*, 47–52. [CrossRef]
46. Li, Y.J.; Stanley, S.; Villalba, J.A.; Nelson, S.; Gelfand, J. Case Report: Overwhelming *Babesia* Parasitemia Successfully Treated Promptly with RBC Apheresis and Triple Therapy with Clindamycin, Azithromycin, and Atovaquone. *Open Forum Infect. Dis.* **2020**, *7*, 3. [CrossRef]
47. Vyas, J.M.; Telford, S.R.; Robbins, G.K. Treatment of refractory *Babesia microti* infection with atovaquone-proguanil in an HIV-infected patient: Case report. *Clin. Infect. Dis.* **2007**, *45*, 1588–1590. [CrossRef]
48. Man, S.Q.; Qiao, K.; Cui, J.; Feng, M.; Fu, Y.F.; Cheng, X.J. A case of human infection with a novel *Babesia* species in China. *Infect. Dis. Poverty* **2016**, *5*, 6. [CrossRef]
49. Gao, J.C.; Gong, Z.D.; Montesano, D.; Glazer, E.; Liegner, K. "Repurposing" Disulfiram in the Treatment of Lyme Disease and Babesiosis: Retrospective Review of First 3 Years' Experience in One Medical Practice. *Antibiotics* **2020**, *9*, 868. [CrossRef]
50. Radcliffe, C.; Krause, P.J.; Grant, M. Repeat exchange transfusion for treatment of severe babesiosis. *Transfus. Apher. Sci.* **2019**, *58*, 638–640. [CrossRef] [PubMed]
51. Ruebush, T.K.; Contacos, P.G.; Steck, E.A. Chemotherapy of *Babesia microti* infections in Mongolian Jirds. *Antimicrob. Agents Chemother.* **1980**, *18*, 289–291. [CrossRef] [PubMed]
52. Rowin, K.S.; Tanowitz, H.B.; Wittner, M. Therapy of Experimental Babesiosis. *Ann. Intern. Med.* **1982**, *97*, 556–558. [CrossRef]
53. AbouLaila, M.; Munkhjargal, T.; Sivakumar, T.; Ueno, A.; Nakano, Y.; Yokoyama, M.; Yoshinari, T.; Nagano, D.; Katayama, K.; El-Bahy, N.; et al. Apicoplast-Targeting Antibacterials Inhibit the Growth of *Babesia* Parasites. *Antimicrob. Agents Chemother.* **2012**, *56*, 3196–3206. [CrossRef]
54. Yao, J.M.; Zhang, H.B.; Liu, C.S.; Tao, Y.; Yin, M. Inhibitory effects of 19 antiprotozoal drugs and antibiotics on *Babesia microti* infection in BALB/c mice. *J. Infect. Dev. Ctries.* **2015**, *9*, 1004–1010. [CrossRef] [PubMed]
55. Marley, S.E.; Eberhard, M.L.; Steurer, F.J.; Ellis, W.L.; McGreevy, P.B.; Ruebush, T.K. Evaluation of selected antiprotozoal drugs in the *Babesia microti*-hamster model. *Antimicrob. Agents Chemother.* **1997**, *41*, 91–94. [CrossRef] [PubMed]
56. Wittner, M.; Lederman, J.; Tanowitz, H.B.; Rosenbaum, G.S.; Weiss, L.M. Atovaquone in the treatment of *Babesia microti* infections in hamsters. *Am. J. Trop. Med. Hyg.* **1996**, *55*, 219–222. [CrossRef]
57. Chiu, J.E.; Renard, I.; Pal, A.C.; Singh, P.; Vydyam, P.; Thekkiniath, J.; Kumar, M.; Gihaz, S.; Pou, S.; Winter, R.W.; et al. Effective Therapy Targeting Cytochrome *bc(1)* Prevents *Babesia* Erythrocytic Development and Protects from Lethal Infection. *Antimicrob. Agents Chemother.* **2021**, *65*, AAC-00662. [CrossRef] [PubMed]
58. Hughes, W.T.; Oz, H.S. Successful Prevention and Treatment of Babesiosis with Atovaquone. *J. Infect. Dis.* **1995**, *172*, 1042–1046. [CrossRef] [PubMed]
59. Pudney, M.; Gray, J.S. Therapeutic efficacy of atovaquone against the bovine intraerythrocytic parasite, *Babesia divergens*. *J. Parasitol.* **1997**, *83*, 307–310. [CrossRef] [PubMed]
60. Krause, P.J. Babesiosis. *Med. Clin. North. Am.* **2002**, *86*, 361–373. [CrossRef]

61. Beshbishy, A.M.; Batiha, G.E.S.; Alkazmi, L.; Nadwa, E.; Rashwan, E.; Abdeen, A.; Yokoyama, N.; Igarashi, I. Therapeutic Effects of Atranorin towards the Proliferation of *Babesia* and *Theileria* Parasites. *Pathogens* **2020**, *9*, 127. [CrossRef]
62. Chen, D.; Copeman, D.B.; Hutchinson, G.W.; Burnell, J. Inhibition of growth of cultured *Babesia microti* by serum and macrophages in the presence or absence of T cells. *Parasitol. Int.* **2000**, *48*, 223–231. [CrossRef]
63. Matsubara, J.; Koura, M.; Kamiyama, T. Infection of Immunodeficient Mice with a Mouse-Adapted Substrain of the Gray Strain of *Babesia microti. J. Parasitol.* **1993**, *79*, 783–786. [CrossRef]
64. Ruebush, M.J.; Hanson, W.L. Susceptibility of 5 Strains of Mice to *Babesia microti* of Human Origin. *J. Parasitol.* **1979**, *65*, 430–433. [CrossRef]
65. Skariah, S.; Arnaboldi, P.; Dattwyler, R.J.; Sultan, A.A.; Gaylets, C.; Walwyn, O.; Mulhall, H.; Wu, X.; Dargham, S.R.; Mordue, D.G. Elimination of *Babesia microti* Is Dependent on Intraerythrocytic Killing and CD4(+) T Cells. *J. Immunol.* **2017**, *199*, 633–642. [CrossRef]
66. Hu, R.J.; Yeh, M.T.; Hyland, K.E.; Mather, T.N. Experimental *Babesia microti* infection in golden hamsters: Immunoglobulin G response and recovery from severe hemolytic anemia. *J. Parasitol.* **1996**, *82*, 728–732. [CrossRef]
67. Oz, H.S.; Hughes, W.T. Acute fulminating babesiosis in hamsters infected with *Babesia microti. Int. J. Parasit.* **1996**, *26*, 667–670. [CrossRef]
68. Chauvin, A.; Valentin, A.; Malandrin, L.; L'Hostis, M. Sheep as a new experimental host for *Babesia divergens. Vet. Res.* **2002**, *33*, 429–433. [CrossRef] [PubMed]
69. Gorenflot, A.; Brasseur, P.; Precigout, E.; Lhostis, M.; Marchand, A.; Schrevel, J. Cytological and immunological responses to *Babesia-divergens* in different hosts- Ox, gerbil, man. *Parasitol. Res.* **1991**, *77*, 3–12. [CrossRef] [PubMed]
70. Musa, N.B.; Phillips, R.S. The adaptation of 3 isolates of *Babesia-divergens* to continuous culture in rat erythrocytes. *Parasitology* **1991**, *103*, 165–170. [CrossRef] [PubMed]
71. Paul, A.S.; Moreira, C.K.; Elsworth, B.; Allred, D.R.; Duraisingh, M.T. Extensive Shared Chemosensitivity between Malaria and Babesiosis Blood-Stage Parasites. *Antimicrob. Agents Chemother.* **2016**, *60*, 5059–5063. [CrossRef] [PubMed]
72. Vayrynen, R.; Tuomi, J. Continuous in vitro cultivation of *Babesia divergens. Acta Vet. Scand.* **1982**, *23*, 471–472. [CrossRef]
73. Zintl, A.; Westbrook, C.; Mulcahy, G.; Skerrett, H.E.; Gray, J.S. Invasion, and short- and long-term survival of *Babesia divergens* (Phylum Apicomplexa) cultures in non-bovine sera and erythrocytes. *Parasitology* **2002**, *124*, 583–588. [CrossRef] [PubMed]
74. Entrican, J.H.; Williams, H.; Cook, I.A.; Lancaster, W.M.; Clark, J.C.; Joyner, L.P.; Lewis, D. Babesiosis in man- Report of a case from scotland with observations on the infecting strain. *J. Infect.* **1979**, *1*, 227–234. [CrossRef]
75. Gray, J.S. Chemotherapy of *Babesia divergens* in the gerbil, Meriones unguiculatus. *Res. Vet. Sci.* **1983**, *35*, 318–324. [CrossRef]
76. Brasseur, P.; Lecoublet, S.; Kapel, N.; Favennec, L.; Ballet, J.J. In vitro evaluation of drug susceptibilities of *Babesia divergens* isolates. *Antimicrob. Agents Chemother.* **1998**, *42*, 818–820. [CrossRef]
77. Thomford, J.W.; Conrad, P.A.; Telford, S.R.; Mathiesen, D.; Bowman, B.H.; Spielman, A.; Eberhard, M.L.; Herwaldt, B.L.; Quick, R.E.; Persing, D.H. Cultivation and Phylogenetic Characterization of a Newly Recognized Human Pathogenic Protozoan. *J. Infect. Dis.* **1994**, *169*, 1050–1056. [CrossRef]
78. McCormack, K.A.; Alhaboubi, A.; Pollard, D.A.; Fuller, L.; Holman, P.J. In vitro cultivation of *Babesia duncani* (Apicomplexa: Babesiidae), a zoonotic hemoprotozoan, using infected blood from Syrian hamsters (*Mesocricetus auratus*). *Parasitol. Res.* **2019**, *118*, 2409–2417. [CrossRef] [PubMed]
79. Abraham, A.; Brasov, I.; Thekkiniath, J.; Kilian, N.; Lawres, L.; Gao, R.Y.; DeBus, K.; He, L.; Yu, X.; Zhu, G.; et al. Establishment of a continuous in vitro culture of *Babesia duncani* in human erythrocytes reveals unusually high tolerance to recommended therapies. *J. Biol. Chem.* **2018**, *293*, 19974–19981. [CrossRef] [PubMed]
80. Dao, A.H.; Eberhard, M.L. Pathology of acute fatal babesiosis in hamsters experimentally infected with the WA-1 strain of *Babesia. Lab. Investig.* **1996**, *74*, 853–859.
81. Wozniak, E.J.; Lowenstine, L.J.; Hemmer, R.; Robinson, T.; Conrad, P.A. Comparative pathogenesis of human WA1 and *Babesia microti* isolates in a Syrian hamster model. *Lab. Anim. Sci.* **1996**, *46*, 507–515. [PubMed]
82. Aguilar-Delfin, I.; Homer, M.J.; Wettstein, P.J.; Persing, D.H. Innate resistance to *Babesia* infection is influenced by genetic background and gender. *Infect. Immun.* **2001**, *69*, 7955–7958. [CrossRef] [PubMed]
83. Hemmer, R.M.; Wozniak, E.J.; Lowenstine, L.J.; Plopper, C.G.; Wong, V.; Conrad, P.A. Endothelial cell changes are associated with pulmonary edema and respiratory distress in mice infected with the WA1 human *Babesia* parasite. *J. Parasitol.* **1999**, *85*, 479–489. [CrossRef] [PubMed]
84. Spangenberg, T.; Burrows, J.N.; Kowalczyk, P.; McDonald, S.; Wells, T.N.C.; Willis, P. The Open Access Malaria Box: A Drug Discovery Catalyst for Neglected Diseases. *PLoS ONE* **2013**, *8*, 8. [CrossRef]
85. Nugraha, A.B.; Tuvshintulga, B.; Guswanto, A.; Tayebwa, D.S.; Rizk, M.A.; Gantuya, S.; Batiha, G.E.; Beshbishy, A.M.; Sivakumar, T.; Yokoyama, N.; et al. Screening the Medicines for Malaria Venture Pathogen Box against piroplasm parasites. *Int. J. Parasitol.-Drugs Drug Resist.* **2019**, *10*, 84–90. [CrossRef] [PubMed]
86. Rizk, M.A.; El-Sayed, S.A.; El-Khodery, S.; Yokoyama, N.; Igarashi, I. Discovering the in vitro potent inhibitors against *Babesia* and *Theileria* parasites by repurposing the Malaria Box: A review. *Vet. Parasitol.* **2019**, *274*, 10. [CrossRef] [PubMed]
87. Rizk, M.A.; El-Sayed, S.A.; AbouLaila, M.; Tuvshintulga, B.; Yokoyama, N.; Igarashi, I. Large-scale drug screening against *Babesia divergens* parasite using a fluorescence-based high-throughput screening assay. *Vet. Parasitol.* **2016**, *227*, 93–97. [CrossRef] [PubMed]

88. Rizk, M.A.; El-Sayed, S.A.; AbouLaila, M.; Yokoyama, N.; Igarashi, I. Evaluation of the inhibitory effect of N-acetyl-L-cysteine on *Babesia* and *Theileria* parasites. *Exp. Parasitol.* **2017**, *179*, 43–48. [CrossRef] [PubMed]
89. Batiha, G.E.; Beshbishy, A.M.; Tayebwa, D.S.; Adeyemi, O.S.; Shaheen, H.; Yokoyama, N.; Igarashi, I. The effects of trans-chalcone and chalcone 4 hydrate on the growth of *Babesia* and *Theileria*. *PLoS Negl. Trop. Dis.* **2019**, *13*, e0007030. [CrossRef]
90. Batiha, G.E.; Beshbishy, A.M.; Alkazmi, L.M.; Nadwa, E.H.; Rashwan, E.K.; Yokoyama, N.; Igarashi, I. In vitro and in vivo growth inhibitory activities of cryptolepine hydrate against several *Babesia* species and Theileria equi. *PLoS Negl. Trop. Dis.* **2020**, *14*, 15. [CrossRef]
91. Beshbishy, A.M.; Batiha, G.E.; Yokoyama, N.; Igarashi, I. Ellagic acid microspheres restrict the growth of *Babesia* and *Theileria* in vitro and *Babesia microti* in vivo. *Parasit Vectors* **2019**, *12*, 269. [CrossRef]
92. Batiha, G.E.; Beshbishy, A.M.; Adeyemi, O.S.; Nadwa, E.; Rashwan, E.; Yokoyama, N.; Igarashi, I. Safety and efficacy of hydroxyurea and eflornithine against most blood parasites *Babesia* and *Theileria*. *PLoS ONE* **2020**, *15*, 15. [CrossRef]
93. Salama, A.A.; AbouLaila, M.; Moussa, A.A.; Nayel, M.A.; Ei-Sify, A.; Terkawi, M.A.; Hassan, H.Y.; Yokoyama, N.; Igarashi, I. Evaluation of in vitro and in vivo inhibitory effects of fusidic acid on *Babesia* and *Theileria* parasites. *Vet. Parasitol.* **2013**, *191*, 1–10. [CrossRef] [PubMed]
94. Guo, J.Y.; Luo, X.Y.; Wang, S.; He, L.; Zhao, J.L. Xanthohumol and Gossypol Are Promising Inhibitors against *Babesia microti* by In Vitro Culture via High-Throughput Screening of 133 Natural Products. *Vaccines* **2020**, *8*, 613. [CrossRef] [PubMed]
95. Rizk, M.A.; El-Sayed, S.A.; Terkawi, M.A.; Youssef, M.A.; El Said, E.E.; Elsayed, G.; El-Khodery, S.; El-Ashker, M.; Elsify, A.; Omar, M.; et al. Optimization of a Fluorescence-Based Assay for Large-Scale Drug Screening against *Babesia* and *Theileria* Parasites. *PLoS ONE* **2015**, *10*, 15. [CrossRef]
96. Munkhjargal, T.; AbouLaila, M.; Terkawi, M.A.; Sivakumar, T.; Ichikawa, M.; Davaasuren, B.; Nyamjargal, T.; Yokoyama, N.; Igarashi, I. Inhibitory Effects of Pepstatin A and Mefloquine on the Growth of *Babesia* Parasites. *Am. J. Trop. Med. Hyg.* **2012**, *87*, 681–688. [CrossRef] [PubMed]
97. Rizk, M.A.; AbouLaila, M.; El-Sayed, S.A.S.; Guswanto, A.; Yokoyama, N.; Igarashi, I. Inhibitory effects of fluoroquinolone antibiotics on *Babesia divergens* and *Babesia microti*, blood parasites of veterinary and zoonotic importance. *Infect. Drug Resist.* **2018**, *11*, 1605–1615. [CrossRef]
98. Omar, M.A.; Salama, A.; Elsify, A.; Rizk, M.A.; Al-Aboody, M.S.; AbouLaila, M.; El-Sayed, S.A.; Igarashi, I. Evaluation of in vitro inhibitory effect of enoxacin on *Babesia* and *Theileria* parasites. *Exp. Parasitol.* **2016**, *161*, 62–67. [CrossRef]
99. Batiha, G.E.S.; Tayebwa, D.S.; Beshbishy, A.M.; N'Da, D.D.; Yokoyama, N.; Igarashi, I. Inhibitory effects of novel ciprofloxacin derivatives on the growth of four *Babesia* species and *Theileria equi*. *Parasitol. Res.* **2020**, *119*, 3061–3073. [CrossRef]
100. Batiha, G.E.-S.; Beshbishy, A.M.; Tayebwa, D.S.; Shaheen, H.M.; Yokoyama, N.; Igarashi, I. Inhibitory effects of Syzygium aromaticum and Camellia sinensis methanolic extracts on the growth of *Babesia* and *Theileria* parasites. *Ticks Tick-Borne Dis.* **2019**, *10*, 949–958. [CrossRef]
101. Batiha, G.E.; Beshbishy, A.M.; Guswanto, A.; Nugraha, A.; Munkhjargal, T.; M Abdel-Daim, M.; Mosqueda, J.; Igarashi, I. Phytochemical Characterization and Chemotherapeutic Potential of *Cinnamomum verum* Extracts on the Multiplication of Protozoan Parasites In Vitro and In Vivo. *Molecules* **2020**, *25*, 996. [CrossRef]
102. Beshbishy, A.M.; Batiha, G.E.S.; Adeyemi, O.S.; Yokoyama, N.; Igarashi, I. Inhibitory effects of methanolic Olea europaea and acetonic Acacia laeta on growth of *Babesia* and *Theileria*. *Asian Pac. J. Trop. Med.* **2019**, *12*, 425–434. [CrossRef]
103. Frampton, J.E. Tafenoquine: First Global Approval. *Drugs* **2018**, *78*, 1517–1523. [CrossRef]
104. Carvalho, L.J.M.; Tuvshintulga, B.; Nugraha, A.B.; Sivakumar, T.; Yokoyama, N. Activities of artesunate-based combinations and tafenoquine against *Babesia bovis* in vitro and *Babesia microti* in vivo. *Parasites Vectors* **2020**, *13*, 9. [CrossRef] [PubMed]
105. Liu, M.; Ji, S.; Kondoh, D.; Galon, E.M.; Li, J.; Tomihari, M.; Yanagawa, M.; Tagawa, M.; Adachi, M.; Asada, M.; et al. Tafenoquine Is a Promising Drug Candidate for the Treatment of Babesiosis. *Antimicrob. Agents Chemother.* **2021**, *65*, e0020421. [CrossRef]
106. Mordue, D.G.; Wormser, G.P. Could the Drug Tafenoquine Revolutionize Treatment of *Babesia microti* Infection? *J. Infect. Dis.* **2019**, *220*, 442–447. [CrossRef] [PubMed]
107. Chu, C.S.; Hwang, J. Tafenoquine: A toxicity overview. *Expert Opin. Drug Saf.* **2021**, *20*, 349–362. [CrossRef]
108. Rueangweerayut, R.; Bancone, G.; Harrell, E.J.; Beelen, A.P.; Kongpatanakul, S.; Möhrle, J.J.; Rousell, V.; Mohamed, K.; Qureshi, A.; Narayan, S.; et al. Hemolytic Potential of Tafenoquine in Female Volunteers Heterozygous for Glucose-6-Phosphate Dehydrogenase (G6PD) Deficiency (*G6PD Mahidol Variant*) versus G6PD-Normal Volunteers. *Am. J. Trop. Med. Hyg* **2017**, *97*, 702–711. [CrossRef]
109. Chiu, J.E.; Renard, I.; George, S.; Pal, A.; Alday, H.; Narasimhan, S.; Riscoe, M.K.; Doggett, J.S.; Ben Mamoun, C. Cytochrome b Drug Resistance Mutation Decreases *Babesia* Fitness in the Tick Stages but not the Mammalian Erythrocytic Cycle. *J. Infect. Dis.* **2021**. [CrossRef] [PubMed]
110. Tuvshintulga, B.; Vannier, E.; Tayebwa, D.S.; Gantuya, S.; Sivakumar, T.; Guswanto, A.; Krause, P.J.; Yokoyama, N.; Igarashi, I. Clofazimine, a Promising Drug for the Treatment of *Babesia microti* Infection in Severely Immunocompromised Hosts. *J. Infect. Dis.* **2020**, *222*, 1027–1036. [CrossRef]
111. Riccardi, N.; Giacomelli, A.; Canetti, D.; Comelli, A.; Intini, E.; Gaiera, G.; Diaw, M.M.; Udwadia, Z.; Besozzi, G.; Codecasa, L.; et al. Clofazimine: An old drug for never-ending diseases. *Future Microbiol.* **2020**, *15*, 557–566. [CrossRef]
112. Jang, J.G.; Chung, J.H. Diagnosis and treatment of multidrug-resistant tuberculosis. *Yeungnam Univ. J. Med.* **2020**, *37*, 277–285. [CrossRef]

113. Tuvshintulga, B.; AbouLaila, M.; Davaasuren, B.; Ishiyama, A.; Sivakumar, T.; Yokoyama, N.; Iwatsuki, M.; Otoguro, K.; Omura, S.; Igarashi, I. Clofazimine Inhibits the Growth of *Babesia* and *Theileria* Parasites In Vitro and In Vivo. *Antimicrob. Agents Chemother.* **2016**, *60*, 2739–2746. [CrossRef]
114. Mitnick, C.D.; Shin, S.S.; Seung, K.J.; Rich, M.L.; Atwood, S.S.; Furin, J.J.; Fitzmaurice, G.M.; Viru, F.A.A.; Appleton, S.C.; Bayona, J.N.; et al. Comprehensive treatment of extensively drug-resistant tuberculosis. *N. Engl. J. Med.* **2008**, *359*, 563–574. [CrossRef]
115. Frueh, L.; Li, Y.X.; Mather, M.W.; Li, Q.G.; Pou, S.; Nilsen, A.; Winter, R.W.; Forquer, I.P.; Pershing, A.M.; Xie, L.H.; et al. Alkoxycarbonate Ester Prodrugs of Preclinical Drug Candidate ELQ-300 for Prophylaxis and Treatment of Malaria. *ACS Infect. Dis.* **2017**, *3*, 728–735. [CrossRef] [PubMed]
116. Miley, G.P.; Pou, S.; Winter, R.; Nilsen, A.; Li, Y.X.; Kelly, J.X.; Stickles, A.M.; Mather, M.W.; Forquer, I.P.; Pershing, A.M.; et al. ELQ-300 Prodrugs for Enhanced Delivery and Single-Dose Cure of Malaria. *Antimicrob. Agents Chemother.* **2015**, *59*, 5555–5560. [CrossRef]
117. Nilsen, A.; LaCrue, A.N.; White, K.L.; Forquer, I.P.; Cross, R.M.; Marfurt, J.; Mather, M.W.; Delves, M.J.; Shackleford, D.M.; Saenz, F.E.; et al. Quinolone-3-Diarylethers: A New Class of Antimalarial Drug. *Sci. Transl. Med.* **2013**, *5*, 13. [CrossRef] [PubMed]
118. Nilsen, A.; Miley, G.P.; Forquer, I.P.; Mather, M.W.; Katneni, K.; Li, Y.X.; Pou, S.; Pershing, A.M.; Stickles, A.M.; Ryan, E.; et al. Discovery, Synthesis, and Optimization of Antimalarial 4(1H)-Quinolone-3-Diarylethers. *J. Med. Chem.* **2014**, *57*, 3818–3834. [CrossRef]
119. Smilkstein, M.J.; Pou, S.; Krollenbrock, A.; Bleyle, L.A.; Dodean, R.A.; Frueh, L.; Hinrichs, D.J.; Li, Y.X.; Martinson, T.; Munar, M.Y.; et al. ELQ-331 as a prototype for extremely durable chemoprotection against malaria. *Malar. J.* **2019**, *18*, 17. [CrossRef] [PubMed]
120. Stickles, A.M.; de Almeida, M.J.; Morrisey, J.M.; Sheridan, K.A.; Forquer, I.P.; Nilsen, A.; Winter, R.W.; Burrows, J.N.; Fidock, D.A.; Vaidya, A.B.; et al. Subtle Changes in Endochin-Like Quinolone Structure Alter the Site of Inhibition within the Cytochrome *bc(1)* Complex of *Plasmodium falciparum*. *Antimicrob. Agents Chemother.* **2015**, *59*, 1977–1982. [CrossRef]
121. Stickles, A.M.; Smilkstein, M.J.; Morrisey, J.M.; Li, Y.X.; Forquer, I.P.; Kelly, J.X.; Pou, S.; Winter, R.W.; Nilsen, A.; Vaidya, A.B.; et al. Atovaquone and ELQ-300 Combination Therapy as a Novel Dual-Site Cytochrome *bc(1)* Inhibition Strategy for Malaria. *Antimicrob. Agents Chemother.* **2016**, *60*, 4853–4859. [CrossRef] [PubMed]
122. Stickles, A.M.; Ting, L.M.; Morrisey, J.M.; Li, Y.X.; Mather, M.W.; Meermeier, E.; Pershing, A.M.; Forquer, I.P.; Miley, G.P.; Pou, S.; et al. Inhibition of Cytochrome *bc(1)* as a Strategy for Single-Dose, Multi-Stage Antimalarial Therapy. *Am. J. Trop. Med. Hyg.* **2015**, *92*, 1195–1201. [CrossRef] [PubMed]
123. Van Schalkwyk, D.A.; Riscoe, M.K.; Pou, S.; Winter, R.W.; Nilsen, A.; Duffey, M.; Moon, R.W.; Sutherland, C.J. Novel Endochin-Like Quinolones Exhibit Potent In Vitro Activity against *Plasmodium knowlesi* but Do Not Synergize with Proguanil. *Antimicrob. Agents Chemother.* **2020**, *64*, 8. [CrossRef]
124. Winter, R.; Kelly, J.X.; Smilkstein, M.J.; Hinrichs, D.; Koop, D.R.; Riscoe, M.K. Optimization of endochin-like quinolones for antimalarial activity. *Exp. Parasitol.* **2011**, *127*, 545–551. [CrossRef]
125. Winter, R.W.; Kelly, J.X.; Smilkstein, M.J.; Dodean, R.; Hinrichs, D.; Riscoe, M.K. Antimalarial quinolones: Synthesis, potency, and mechanistic studies. *Exp. Parasitol.* **2008**, *118*, 487–497. [CrossRef]
126. Doggett, J.S.; Nilsen, A.; Forquer, I.; Wegmann, K.W.; Jones-Brando, L.; Yolken, R.H.; Bordon, C.; Charman, S.A.; Katneni, K.; Schultz, T.; et al. Endochin-like quinolones are highly efficacious against acute and latent experimental toxoplasmosis. *Proc. Natl. Acad. Sci. USA* **2012**, *109*, 15936–15941. [CrossRef] [PubMed]
127. Doggett, J.S.; Schultz, T.; Miller, A.J.; Bruzual, I.; Pou, S.; Winter, R.; Dodean, R.; Zakharov, L.N.; Nilsen, A.; Riscoe, M.K.; et al. Orally Bioavailable Endochin-Like Quinolone Carbonate Ester Prodrug Reduces *Toxoplasma gondii* Brain Cysts. *Antimicrob. Agents Chemother.* **2020**, *64*, 13. [CrossRef]
128. Ortiz, D.; Forquer, I.; Boitz, J.; Soysa, R.; Elya, C.; Fulwiler, A.; Nilsen, A.; Polley, T.; Riscoe, M.K.; Ullman, B.; et al. Targeting the Cytochrome *bc(1)* Complex of *Leishmania* Parasites for Discovery of Novel Drugs. *Antimicrob. Agents Chemother.* **2016**, *60*, 4972–4982. [CrossRef] [PubMed]
129. Alday, P.H.; Bruzual, I.; Nilsen, A.; Pou, S.; Winter, R.; Ben Mamoun, C.; Riscoe, M.K.; Doggett, J.S. Genetic Evidence for Cytochrome *b Q(i)* Site Inhibition by 4(1*H*)-Quinolone-3-Diarylethers and Antimycin in *Toxoplasma gondii*. *Antimicrob. Agents Chemother.* **2017**, *61*, 8. [CrossRef] [PubMed]
130. Song, Z.; Iorga, B.I.; Mounkoro, P.; Fisher, N.; Meunier, B. The antimalarial compound ELQ-400 is an unusual inhibitor of the *bc(1)* complex, targeting both *Q(o)* and *Q(i)* sites. *FEBS Lett.* **2018**, *592*, 1346–1356. [CrossRef] [PubMed]

pathogens

MDPI

Article

An Alternative Culture Medium for Continuous In Vitro Propagation of the Human Pathogen *Babesia duncani* in Human Erythrocytes

Pallavi Singh, Anasuya C. Pal and Choukri Ben Mamoun *

Department of Internal Medicine, Section of Infectious Diseases, Yale School of Medicine, New Haven, CT 06519, USA; pallavi.singh@yale.edu (P.S.); anasuya.chattopadhyay@yale.edu (A.C.P.)
* Correspondence: choukri.benmamoun@yale.edu; Tel.: +1-203-737-1972

Abstract: Continuous propagation of *Babesia duncani* in vitro in human erythrocytes and the availability of a mouse model of *B. duncani* lethal infection make this parasite an ideal model to study *Babesia* biology and pathogenesis. Two culture media, HL-1 and Claycomb, with proprietary formulations are the only culture media known to support the parasite growth in human erythrocytes; however, the HL-1 medium has been discontinued and the Claycomb medium is often unavailable leading to major interruptions in the study of this pathogen. To identify alternative media conditions, we evaluated the growth of *B. duncani* in various culture media with well-defined compositions. We report that the DMEM-F12 culture medium supports the continuous growth of the parasite in human erythrocytes to levels equal to those achieved in the HL-1 and Claycomb media. We generated new clones of *B. duncani* from the parental WA-1 clinical isolate after three consecutive subcloning events in this medium. All clones showed a multiplication rate in vitro similar to that of the WA-1 parental isolate and cause fatal infection in C3H/HeJ mice. The culture medium, which can be readily reconstituted from its individual components, and the tools and resources developed here will facilitate the study of *B. duncani*.

Keywords: parasite; babesiosis; *Babesia duncani*; in vitro culture; erythrocytes; DMEM-F12; virulence

Citation: Singh, P.; Pal, A.C.; Mamoun, C.B. An Alternative Culture Medium for Continuous In Vitro Propagation of the Human Pathogen *Babesia duncani* in Human Erythrocytes. *Pathogens* **2022**, *11*, 599. https://doi.org/10.3390/pathogens11050599

Academic Editors: Estrella Montero, Jeremy Gray, Cheryl Ann Lobo and Luis Miguel González

Received: 4 May 2022
Accepted: 19 May 2022
Published: 20 May 2022

1. Introduction

The rapid emergence of tick-borne disease cases in the United States as well as other parts of the world poses a great threat to human health, thereby highlighting the need to develop novel disease diagnosis tools and novel effective therapies to treat the disease as well as strategic plans to control pathogen transmission [1]. One such disease is human babesiosis, which is caused by intraerythrocytic apicomplexan parasites of the genus *Babesia*. Human babesiosis infections are often asymptomatic or display mild flu-like symptoms in healthy individuals [2–4]. However, the disease can become severe and fatal in immunocompromised, asplenic and elderly individuals, with symptoms ranging from acute respiratory distress, hemolytic anemia, multiple organ failure and possibly death [2–4].

Several *Babesia* species have been associated with infection in humans. They include *Babesia microti* [5], *Babesia duncani* [4,6,7], *Babesia divergens* [8], *Babesia divergens* MO1 [9], *Babesia crassa*-like [10], *Babesia venatorum* [11] and *Babesia odocoilei* [12]. *B. microti* is responsible for the majority of reported clinical babesiosis cases whereas WA-1 and WA-1-type *B. duncani* cases have so far been documented primarily in Washington state and California [3,4,6].

Babesia parasites are transmitted to humans primarily through a bite from an infected tick or through blood transfusion [3], but transplacental transmission from mother to child can also occur [3,13].

Babesia spp. are phylogenetically related to *Plasmodium* spp., the causal agents of human malaria [14,15]. Both *Babesia* and *Plasmodium* spp. are obligate intracellular parasites with a complex life cycle which involves an invertebrate vector (ticks or mosquitoes) and a vertebrate host (humans). The intraerythrocytic life of *Babesia* parasites starts following invasion of red blood cells (RBCs) by free circulating merozoites. Following cell invasion, each merozoite develops and multiplies to form four daughter parasites, which subsequently exit the infected RBC (iRBC) through the process of egress. The egressed merozoites continue to infect new RBCs and increase their numbers exponentially. The repeated rounds of invasion and egress into and from the human RBCs (hRBCs) are responsible for the clinical manifestations of human babesiosis.

Efforts to control the disease through the development of novel therapeutics heavily rely on understanding the biological processes that control the development of the parasites within the host RBCs. A recent study has demonstrated the successful establishment of an in vitro culture system for the propagation of *B. duncani* in hRBCs [16]. This continuous in vitro culture system made it possible for the first time to conduct large-scale screening of chemical libraries to assess the efficacy of novel drugs, as well as to study drug–drug interactions [17]. In addition to its ability to propagate in human erythrocytes in vitro, *B. duncani* can also infect mice and causes lethal infection in both immunocompetent and immunocompromised animals. The severity of the disease and survival outcome in mice depends heavily on the genetic background and the infectious dose [18]. A combined *B. duncani* continuous in vitro culture in hRBCs and in vivo lethal infection in mice is referred to as the in culture-in mouse (ICIM) model of duncani infection and represents an ideal system to study and address several critical questions related to intraerythrocytic parasitism, host-parasite interactions, parasite virulence and disease pathogenesis [18]. The ICIM model provides a strong foundation to develop novel therapeutic strategies against babesiosis as well as diseases caused by other apicomplexan parasites.

The success of establishment of an in vitro culture system of apicomplexan parasites depends on the nutritional requirements of the parasite. While some parasites can be propagated in basic cell culture medium such as RPMI (*Plasmodium falciparum*) or DMEM (*Toxoplasma gondii*), others require special medium such as LIT (*Trypanosoma cruzi*) [19] and NNN (*Leishmania*) [20]. Since its inception, the *B. duncani* continuous in vitro culture system in hRBCs relied on two commercially manufactured media, HL-1 (Lonza) and Claycomb (Sigma) [21]. The high cost of these complex media and the frequent shortages, which were further exacerbated by the COVID-19 pandemic, have significantly impacted the advancement of *Babesia* research. Furthermore, the composition of the HL-1 medium is unknown, and the culture medium has been unavailable since March 2021 and has now been discontinued by the manufacturer as of March 2022. Whereas the composition of the Claycomb medium was previously reported [21], the specific source of the base medium is not known and several protein components, such as growth factors, used as supplements in the medium are expensive. To overcome all these challenges, this study was conducted to identify an alternate growth medium that can support the in vitro growth of *B. duncani* in human red blood cells. Here we report that DMEM-F12 medium supports continuous in vitro culture of *B. duncani* in human red blood cells to levels identical to those achieved with HL-1 and Claycomb media. The lower cost of this culture medium and the availability of its constituent formulation, which makes it possible to make it entirely from individual components in any research lab, now eliminates completely the challenges caused by media shortages or discontinuations.

2. Results

2.1. DMEM-F12 Medium Supports the In Vitro growth of B. duncani WA-1 in Human RBCs

To identify defined nutritional conditions that could support continuous in vitro propagation of *B. duncani* WA-1 clinical isolate in human RBCs, several growth media with known formulations were tested as base media, including RPMI, DMEM and DMEM-F12 from various sources, and parasite growth was compared to that under Claycomb medium. All base media were supplemented as indicated in Table 1 to build the complete culture media. The rate of parasite multiplication was determined by initiating parasite cultures in different growth media at 0.5% parasitemia in A^+ human RBCs (5% hematocrit (HC) (day 0)) using a preculture of *B. duncani* propagated in Claycomb-based medium and washed extensively in each of the four complete media. The parasitemia was monitored by light microscopy every third day (day 3, day 6, day 9, day 12 and day 15) and the cultures were diluted to 0.5% parasitemia on days 3, 6 and 9. Monitoring of parasite counts by light microscopy showed that *B. duncani* parasitemia increased to similar levels in Claycomb- and DMEM-F12-based media on days 3, 6, 9, 12 and 15 (Figure 1A). However, in both RPMI- or DMEM-based complete media, *B. duncani* parasitemia showed modest increase during the first cycle of continuous growth ending on day 3 post-inoculation but no significant increase was detected during the following cycles ending on day 6, day 9, day 12 and day 15 (Figure 1A). Parasite morphology was identical in both DMEM-F12- and Claycomb-based media with all developmental stages represented under both growth conditions (Figure 1B). The proportion of infected red blood cells with rings, double rings, filamentous forms and tetrads throughout the intraerythrocytic cycle was comparable in both media with no significant differences ($p \geq 0.99$, two-way ANOVA) observed between the different developmental stages in the two media (Figure 1C).

Table 1. Constituents of the culture media that support continuous growth of *B. duncani* in human RBCs in vitro.

	Complete Claycomb Medium	Complete DMEM-F12 Medium	Complete HL-1 Medium
Base Medium	Claycomb Medium (Sigma: Cat. No.: 51800C)	DMEM-F12 Medium (Lonza: Cal. No.: BE04-687F/U1)	HL-1 Medium (LonzaTM: Discontinued)
Supplements	20% Fetal Bovine Serum (Heat Inactivated) (Gibco, Cat. No.: 10438-026) 1× of HT media supplement (50×) (Sigma, Cat. No.: H0137-10VL) 1× of L-Glutamine (200 mM; 100×) (Gibco, Cat. No.: 25030-081) 1× of Antimycotic-Antibiotic (100×) (Gibco, Cat. No.: 15240-062) 1× of Gentamicin (10 mg/mL; 100×) (Gibco, Cat. No.: 15710-072)		

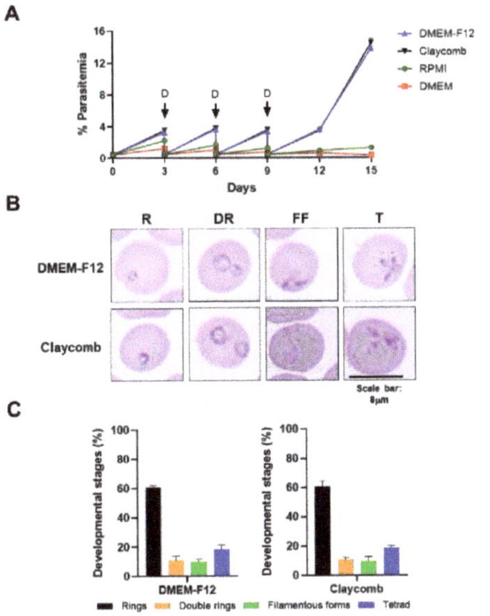

Figure 1. In vitro culture of *B. duncani* WA-1 in different growth media. (**A**) Growth of *B. duncani* WA-1

over a 15-day period in human RBCs with culture dilution at day 3, day 6 and day 9. Arrows (**D**) indicate when cultures were diluted to 0.5% parasitemia as determined by counting of Giemsa-stained blood smears. A total of 2500–3500 RBCs were counted. (**B**) Representative images of Giemsa-stained smears of *B. duncani* WA-1 infected human erythrocytes on day 15 in DMEM-F12 or Claycomb media showing different infection forms. R, rings; DR, double rings; FF, filamentous forms, T, tetrads. (**C**) Graph represents percentages of different parasite development stages as identified in DMEM-F12 or Claycomb media. Data presented as mean ± SD of two independent experiments performed in biological duplicates. No significant differences ($p \geq 0.99$, two-way ANOVA) were observed between the different developmental stages in the two media.

2.2. Derivation of New Lines of *B. duncani* WA-1 Clinical Isolate

The *B. duncani* WA-1 clinical isolate was cryopreserved from blood collected in 1991 from a patient from Washington state [22]. The sample was found to be highly virulent following inoculation into hamsters and caused acute infection and death in animals [23]. WA-1 was subsequently used to inoculate both hamsters and mice to study the immune response to *B. duncani* as well as to grow the parasite in vitro in human or hamster red blood cells. To ensure the clonality of the parasite, we conducted three consecutive limiting dilution cloning of the WA-1 isolate in the DMEM-F12-based complete culture medium as shown in Figure 2. Each dilution cloning was conducted in a 96-well plate format with 0.3 infected red blood cell per well at 5% HC. Culture medium was changed every third day and the parasitemia was monitored after 14 days by light microscopy of Giemsa-stained blood smears. Six individual clones were isolated in the first round of cloning, three of which were subjected to the second round of limiting dilution cloning. Three individual clones were isolated in the second round of cloning and were subjected to a third round of limiting dilution cloning. The last three clones isolated are referred to as BdWA1-301, BdWA1-302 and BdWA1-303. Comparison of growth kinetics in DMEM-F12-based medium showed that all clones have similar growth patterns in vitro in hRBCs compared to the BdWA-1 parental isolate as determined by parasitemia count determined by light microscopy (Figure 2B) or by increased incorporation of SYBR Green in parasite DNA (Figure 2C). No significant differences were found in the parasitemia counts by microscopy ($p \geq 0.1$, two-way ANOVA) or by SYBR Green I incorporation ($p \geq 0.6$, two-way ANOVA) between *B. duncani* parental isolate and three GenIII clones. Additionally, an immunofluorescence assay performed to localize a predicted heat shock protein, BdHSP70 (ID#: BdWA1_001707), using affinity-purified antisera showed that the localization of this protein in all three clones follows the same pattern as the parental clone, indicating that there are no major differences in the protein expression between these clonal lines (Figure 3A).

2.3. New *B. duncani* Clones Are Virulent in Mice

Our recent work on the *B. duncani* ICIM model demonstrated the infectivity of in vitro cultured parental BdWA-1 clinical isolate when inoculated into mice [18]. To assess whether the newly cloned BdWA1-301, BdWA1-302 and BdWA1-303 parasites are still virulent in mice, the parasites were propagated in vitro in human red blood cells and injected by the intravenous (IV) route into female C3H/HeJ mice ($n = 3$/clone). Parasitemia was monitored by determining parasite counts in Giemsa-stained thin blood smears made from blood collected from infected mice. As shown in Figure 3B, all three clones led to establishment of parasitemia in mice starting at DPI3 demonstrating the infectivity of all third generation *B. duncani* clones. Peak parasitemia in all mice ranged between 3.6% and 5.2% at DPI 7 at which point all mice became moribund and were euthanized. No significant differences between the parasitemia levels were observed ($p > 0.2$, two-way ANOVA) between the different infected groups.

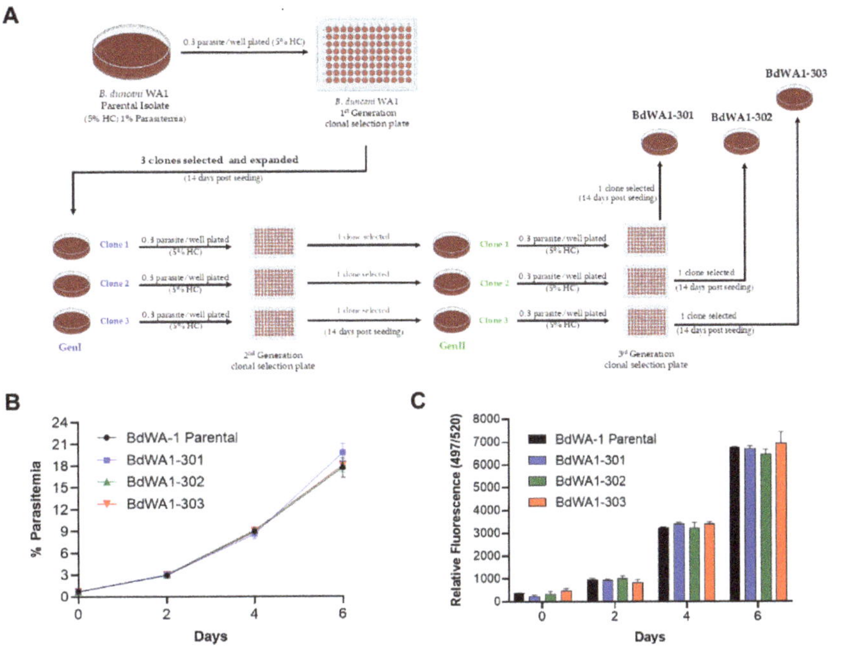

Figure 2. Limiting dilution cloning of *B. duncani* parental isolate and growth comparison of triple cloned and in vitro cultured *B. duncani* WA-1 clones to parental isolate. (**A**) Schematic representation of limiting dilution cloning of *B. duncani* WA-1 parasites. The parental clinical *B. duncani* WA-1 parasite was subcloned by three consecutive limiting dilution steps to produce first, second and third generation clones. (**B**,**C**) Multiplication rate of BdWA1-301, BdWA-2 and BdWA-3 clones in human RBCs in DMEM-F12-based complete culture medium. The multiplication rate of the third generation clones was compared to that of the parental BdWA-1 strain and determined by microscopic examination of Giemsa-stained smears from samples collected at the indicated time points (**B**) and using the SYBR Green I incorporation assay (**C**). The data represent mean ± SD of biological duplicates. No significant differences were found in the parasitemia counts by microscopy ($p \geq 0.1$, two-way ANOVA) or by SYBR Green I incorporation ($p \geq 0.6$, two-way ANOVA) between *B. duncani* parental isolate and three GenIII clones.

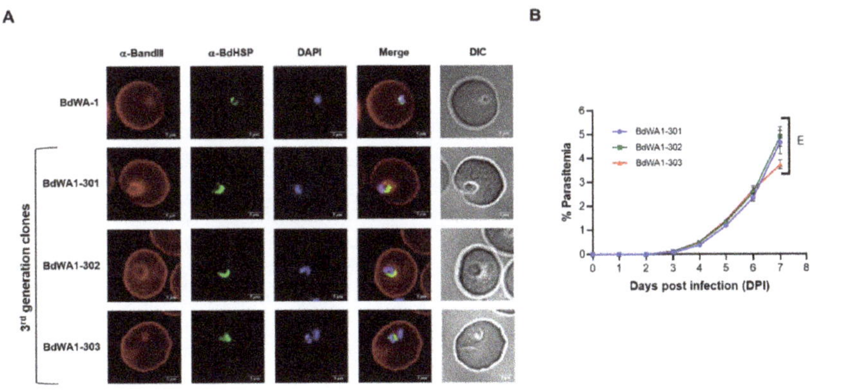

Figure 3. Cloned *B. duncani* WA-1 parasites show similar expression profile of *B. duncani* protein and

maintain virulence in in vivo mouse model. (**A**) Subcellular localization of a putative BdHSP70 (ID#: BdWA1_001707) protein of *B. duncani* in the parental isolate and third generation clones. Images show immunofluorescence staining of BdHSP70 protein with polyclonal antibodies raised against the protein in rabbits followed by Alexa Fluor 488 conjugated anti-rabbit immunoglobulin secondary antibodies on fixed human RBCs infected with either BdWA-1 or third generation clones BdWA1-301, BdWA1-302 and BdWA1-303. DAPI was used to label parasite DNA. Human RBCs were stained with an anti-BandIII antibody followed by Rhodamine conjugated anti-human secondary antibody. Bars, 5 µm. (**B**) Evaluation of the virulence of third generation BdWA1-301, BdWA-2 and BdWA-3 clones in C3H/HeJ mice (three mice per clone) following intravenous administration of 10^7 infected human RBCs. The multiplication rate of the third generation clones was determined by microscopic examination of Giemsa-stained smears of mouse blood collected at the indicated time points and no significant differences between the parasitemia levels were observed ($p > 0.2$, two-way ANOVA) between the different infected groups. E, euthanized.

3. Discussion

In this short communication, we report the identification of DMEM-F12-based culture medium as an alternative growth medium for continuous propagation of *B. duncani* in human red blood cells. No parasite adaptation was required when shifting the parasite from Claycomb or HL1-based media to DMEM-F12. Furthermore, we have now successfully propagated *B. duncani* in continuous in vitro culture in human red blood cells in this medium for several months. The discovery of the DMEM-F12 medium will help the *Babesia* research community overcome the major challenges faced over the past several years as a result of frequent shortages by the manufacturers of the HL-1 and Claycomb media. These two media were first reported to be suitable for propagation of the parasite in human and hamster red blood cells in vitro [16,24]. However, their specific constituents were not disclosed by the manufacturers. While media shortages were common before the COVID-19 pandemic, the situation worsened during the pandemic with backorders for both media announced for several months. To add "insult to injury", one of the manufacturers announced discontinuation of the HL-1 medium. Faced with these challenges, we scrambled to reconstitute the Claycomb medium from the constituents reported in the original report by Claycomb and colleagues for propagation of human HL-1 cardiomyocytes [21,25]. This growth condition uses DMEM as a base medium supplemented with proteins and lipids; however, the specific DMEM used was not indicated [21]. When reconstituted based on reported formulation and using different commercially available DMEM media, no growth of *B. duncani* could be achieved in culture. Interestingly, we found that DMEM-F12-based culture medium, without the supplements used in the Claycomb media, was sufficient to support the continuous growth of *B. duncani* in hRBCs. This finding suggests that *B. duncani* relies on specific nutrients from its environment for survival within human red blood cells and some of these nutrients are present in the DMEM-F12 but not the standard DMEM medium. Analysis of the components of these two media identified several nutrients that are present in DMEM-F12 but absent in DMEM. These include six amino acids (alanine, asparagine, aspartic acid, cysteine, glutamic acid and proline), two vitamins (biotin and cobalamin) and four inorganic salts (cupric sulfate, ferric sulfate, magnesium chloride and zinc sulfate) as well as hypoxanthine, thymidine, linoleic acid, lipoic acid and putrescine. A new study is now underway to determine which of these nutrients is critical for *B. duncani* survival in human red blood cells. The reliance of *B. duncani* on host nutrients for survival is shared with other intraerythrocytic parasites such as the human malaria parasite *P. falciparum* [26,27]. The malaria parasite relies heavily on a large number of nutrients such as carbohydrates, lipid precursors and vitamins for survival within human erythrocytes. The transporters and metabolic enzymes involved in the uptake and utilization of these nutrients are considered attractive targets for the development of new antimalarial drugs [26,28–31]. Future efforts to identify the nutrients required for *Babesia* survival in human erythrocytes and to understand their mechanism of uptake and utilization are warranted.

The discovery that DMEM-F12 supports the continuous growth of *B. duncani* in vitro is also important for two other reasons. First, DMEM-F12 is more affordable than the HL-1 and Claycomb media. Second, the availability of a detailed composition of the DMEM-F12 medium makes it possible to reconstitute it entirely from individual constituents in any research lab thus preventing any possible disruptions that could occur in the future due to manufacturers' shortages or discontinuations.

Finally, we report the isolation of three third generation clones of *B. duncani* from the WA-1 clinical isolate. These clones represent an important resource for the scientific community as more scientists become interested in the biology, pathogenesis and virulence of *Babesia* parasites. The ability of *B. duncani* to grow continuously in vitro in human red blood cells and to cause severe disease and fatal infection in mice (ICIM model [18]) is unique among apicomplexan parasites that infect human red blood cells and creates an unprecedented opportunity to evaluate the efficacy of experimental drugs in vitro and in mice to accelerate research towards the development of effective antiparasitic therapies [3,17,18].

The tools and resources reported in this communication are available to the research community through direct requests and will be shared with BEI Resources for wider distribution.

4. Materials and Methods

4.1. In Vitro Parasite Culture of *B. duncani* WA-1 in Different Growth Media

B. duncani parasites were cultured in vitro as reported previously [16]. Parasite growth was monitored and evaluated in the following media: DMEM (Thermo Fisher, 11995-065, Waltham, MA, USA), DMEM-F12 (Lonza, BE04-687/U1, Basel, Switzerland), RPMI (Thermo Fisher, 11875-093) and Claycomb (Sigma, 51800C, Grand Island, NY, USA). All media were supplemented with 20% heat-inactivated FBS (Gibco, 10438-026, Waltham, MA, USA), 1× of 50× HT Media Supplement Hybrid-Max ™ (Sigma, H0137), 1× of 100× (200 mM) L-Glutamine (Gibco, 25030-081), 1× of 100× Antibiotic-Antimycotic (Gibco, 15240-062) and 1× of 100× (10 mg/mL) Gentamicin (Gibco, 15710-072).

4.2. In Vitro Culture of *B. duncani* in Human RBCs

In vitro propagation of *B. duncani* in hRBCs was carried out as previously reported by Abraham et al. [16] and Chiu et al. [17]. Parasitemia was monitored either by light microscopy examination of Giemsa-stained blood smears or by fluorescence detection of SYBR Green I [16].

4.3. Cloning of *B. duncani* WA-1 Clinical Isolate

In vitro culture of *B. duncani* WA-1 clinical isolate was initiated in A^+ human RBCs in DMEM-F12 medium at 0.5% parasitemia and 5% hematocrit (HC). The parasites were allowed to grow for 2 days and the parasitemia was measured by Giemsa-stained blood smears on day 2. The culture was serially diluted to obtain 30 parasites in 20 mL volume at 5% HC. Then, 200 μL of this parasite suspension was plated per well of a 96-well plate. This GenI cloning plate was subjected to medium change on every third day. To determine which wells of the 96-well plate contain parasites, the parasitemia estimation was performed using SYBR Green-I based fluorescence assay on day 14. Then, 25 μL of culture per well of the 96-well plate was mixed with 25 μL of SYBR Green-I lysis buffer consisting of 20 mM Tris, pH 7.4, 5 mM EDTA, 0.008% saponin, 0.08% Triton X-100 and 1X SYBR Green-I (Molecular Probes, 10,000X solution in DMSO, Eugene, OR, USA). Additionally, the uninfected human RBCs (5% HC, 25 μL volume) were used as a negative control. The SYBR Green-I measurement plates were incubated in dark at 37 °C for 1 h. Following this, the plates were read on a BioTek Synergy MX fluorescence plate reader with an excitation of 497 nm and emission of 520 nm. Using readings from uninfected human RBC as a background, the readings for different wells of GenI cloning plate were calculated to determine which wells of the 96-well plate contained parasites (higher SYBR Green-I readings in comparison to the negative control). After identification of the wells containing parasite clones, Giemsa smears were prepared from the same wells and observed under light microscopy to confirm the presence of the parasites. Following this, six GenI *B. duncani* clones were picked and expanded to 1 mL cultures. The clones were allowed to grow to a parasitemia of 2%. Three out of six clones were chosen to perform a second round of limiting dilution cloning using the same steps as described above for GenI cloning. On the 14th day, the GenII clonal plates were screened for parasites using SYBR Green-I based assay. Three Gen II clones were picked, expanded to 1 mL cultures and allowed to grow to 2% parasitemia. Finally, these three GenII clones were subjected to a final third round of limiting dilution cloning and three GenIII clones were obtained after day 14. These three GenIII clones were named as BdWA1-301, BdWA1-302 and BdWA1-303.

4.4. Comparison of In Vitro growth of B. duncani WA-1 and Clonal Lines BdWA1-301, BdWA1-302 and BdWA1-303

In vitro cultures of BdWA-1, BdWA1-301, BdWA1-302 and BdWA1-303 parasites were initiated in A^+ human RBCs in DMEM-F12 medium at 0.75% parasitemia and 5% HC. The parasites were allowed to grow for 6 days, and the media was changed after every 24 h. The parasitemia was measured by SYBR Green I based assay as well as counting of Giemsa-stained blood smears on day 2, day 4 and day 6. Data were analyzed using Graphpad Prism version 9.3.1 software. Error bar represents mean ± SD of two independent experiments performed in biological duplicates.

4.5. Immunofluorescence Assay

Thin blood smears from in vitro cultures of BdWA1-301, BdWA1-302, BdWA1-303 and Bd WA-1 parental isolate were prepared on glass slides (640-001T, DOT Scientific, Tokyo, Japan) and fixed with chilled methanol (9070-05, JT Baker) for 15 min at −20 °C. The smears were air-dried and blocked in 3% BSA in PBS buffer (A9418, Sigma) for 1 h at room temperature. Following this, the smears were incubated with rabbit polyclonal anti-HSP70 (BdWA1_001707) antibodies (1:200 dilution) and mouse monoclonal anti-Band3 antibody (1:500) (Sigma, B9277) for 1 h at room temperature. This was followed by three washes in 1X PBS containing 0.05% Tween (PBST) and three washes in 1X PBS, 5 min each. Subsequently, the smears were incubated with goat anti-rabbit IgG antibodies conjugated to Alexa Fluor 488 (1:500 dilution) (A-11008, Life Technologies) and goat anti-mouse IgG (H+L) antibodies conjugated to Rhodamine (1:500 dilution) (31660, Invitrogen, Waltham, MA, USA) for 1 h at room temperature. This was followed by three washes in 1X PBST and three washes in 1X PBS. Coverslips were then mounted on the slides using Vectashield mounting medium containing DAPI (H-1200-10, Vector Laboratories, Burlingame, CA, USA) and observed under Nikon ECLIPSE TE2000-E microscope. A 100X oil immersion objective was used for image acquisition. Excitation at 465–495 nm was used to detect Alexa Fluor 488 positive cells; excitation at 510–560 nm was used to detect Rhodamine positive cells and excitation at 340–380 nm was used to detect DAPI positive cells. The images were acquired using MetaVue with 1392 × 1040 pixel as the chosen image size and subsequently analyzed using ImageJ.

4.6. Ethics Statement

All animal experiments were approved by the Institutional Animal Care and Use Committees (IACUC) at Yale University (Protocol #2020-07689). Animals were acclimatized for 1 week after arrival before the start of an experiment. Animals that showed signs of distress or appeared moribund were humanly euthanized using approved protocols.

4.7. Virulence Assays in Mice

To assess the virulence of third generation *B. duncani* clones, 6-to-8-week-old female C3H/HeJ mice (The Jackson Laboratories, Bar Harbor, ME, USA) were inoculated with 1×10^7 iRBC of BdWA1-301, BdWA1-302 or BdWA1-303 (n = 3/clone) by the IV route.

Parasitemia was monitored over time by light microscopic examination of Giemsa-stained blood smears. Moribund mice were humanely euthanized.

Author Contributions: Investigation, methodology, formal analysis, visualization, writing—original draft, review and editing, P.S. and A.C.P.; conceptualization, supervision, funding acquisition, project administration, writing—original draft, review and editing, C.B.M. All authors have read and agreed to the published version of the manuscript.

Funding: This work was supported by the National Institutes of Health AI138139, AI152220 and AI136118 to Ben Mamoun. Research on babesiosis in the Ben Mamoun Lab is also supported by grants from the Steven and Alexandra Cohen Foundation, and the Global Lyme Alliance.

Institutional Review Board Statement: All animal studies conducted were approved by the Institutional Animal Care and Use Committees (IACUC) at Yale University (Protocol #2020-07689).

Informed Consent Statement: Not Applicable.

Data Availability Statement: Not applicable.

Acknowledgments: We thank Jae-Yeon Choi and Meenal Chand for providing the affinity-purified anti-BdWA1_001707 polyclonal antibodies used in this study.

Conflicts of Interest: None of the named authors have any conflict of interest, financial or otherwise.

References

1. Paules, C.I.; Marston, H.D.; Bloom, M.E.; Fauci, A.S. Tickborne diseases-confronting a growing threat. *N. Engl. J. Med.* **2018**, *379*, 701–703. [CrossRef] [PubMed]
2. Allred, D.R.; Ben Mamoun, C. Babesiosis. In *eLS*; John Wiley & Sons, Ltd.: Chichester, UK, 2018.
3. Renard, I.; Ben Mamoun, C. Treatment of human babesiosis: Then and now. *Pathogens* **2021**, *10*, 1120. [CrossRef] [PubMed]
4. Kjemtrup, A.M.; Conrad, P.A. Human babesiosis: An emerging tick-borne disease. *Int. J. Parasitol.* **2000**, *30*, 1323–1337. [CrossRef]
5. Vannier, E.; Krause, P.J. Human babesiosis. *N. Engl. J. Med.* **2012**, *366*, 2397–2407. [CrossRef] [PubMed]
6. Herwaldt, B.L.; Kjemtrup, A.M.; Conrad, P.A.; Barnes, R.C.; Wilson, M.; McCarthy, M.G.; Sayers, M.H.; Eberhard, M.L. Transfusion-transmitted babesiosis in Washington state: First reported case caused by a WA1-type parasite. *J. Infect. Dis.* **1997**, *175*, 1259–1262. [CrossRef]
7. Kjemtrup, A.M.; Lee, B.; Fritz, C.L.; Evans, C.; Chervenak, M.; Conrad, P.A. Investigation of transfusion transmission of a WA1-type babesial parasite to a premature infant in California. *Transfusion* **2002**, *42*, 1482–1487. [CrossRef]
8. Hildebrandt, A.; Zintl, A.; Montero, E.; Hunfeld, K.P.; Gray, J. Human babesiosis in Europe. *Pathogens* **2021**, *10*, 1165. [CrossRef]
9. Herwaldt, B.; Persing, D.H.; Precigout, E.A.; Goff, W.L.; Mathiesen, D.A.; Taylor, P.W.; Eberhard, M.L.; Gorenflot, A.F. A fatal case of babesiosis in Missouri: Identification of another piroplasm that infects humans. *Ann. Intern. Med.* **1996**, *124*, 643–650. [CrossRef]
10. Jia, N.; Zheng, Y.C.; Jiang, J.F.; Jiang, R.R.; Jiang, B.G.; Wei, R.; Liu, H.B.; Huo, Q.B.; Sun, Y.; Chu, Y.L.; et al. Human babesiosis caused by a *Babesia crassa*-like pathogen: A case series. *Clin. Infect. Dis.* **2018**, *67*, 1110–1119. [CrossRef]
11. Jiang, J.F.; Zheng, Y.C.; Jiang, R.R.; Li, H.; Huo, Q.B.; Jiang, B.G.; Sun, Y.; Jia, N.; Wang, Y.W.; Ma, L.; et al. Epidemiological, clinical, and laboratory characteristics of 48 cases of *Babesia venatorum* infection in China: A descriptive study. *Lancet Infect. Dis.* **2015**, *15*, 196–203. [CrossRef]
12. Scott, J.D.; Sajid, M.S.; Pascoe, E.L.; Foley, J.E. Detection of *Babesia odocoilei* in humans with babesiosis symptoms. *Diagnostics* **2021**, *11*, 947. [CrossRef] [PubMed]
13. Walker, S.; Coray, E.; Ginsberg-Peltz, J.; Smith, L. A five-week-old twin with profound anemia: A case report of asymmetric congenital babesiosis. *Cureus* **2022**, *14*, e22774. [CrossRef] [PubMed]
14. Cornillot, E.; Hadj-Kaddour, K.; Dassouli, A.; Noel, B.; Ranwez, V.; Vacherie, B.; Augagneur, Y.; Bres, V.; Duclos, A.; Randazzo, S.; et al. Sequencing of the smallest Apicomplexan genome from the human pathogen *Babesia microti*. *Nucleic Acids Res.* **2012**, *40*, 9102–9114. [CrossRef] [PubMed]
15. Silva, J.C.; Cornillot, E.; McCracken, C.; Usmani-Brown, S.; Dwivedi, A.; Ifeonu, O.O.; Crabtree, J.; Gotia, H.T.; Virji, A.Z.; Reynes, C.; et al. Genome-wide diversity and gene expression profiling of *Babesia microti* isolates identify polymorphic genes that mediate host-pathogen interactions. *Sci. Rep.* **2016**, *6*, 35284. [CrossRef] [PubMed]
16. Abraham, A.; Brasov, I.; Thekkiniath, J.; Kilian, N.; Lawres, L.; Gao, R.; DeBus, K.; He, L.; Yu, X.; Zhu, G.; et al. Establishment of a continuous in vitro culture of *Babesia duncani* in human erythrocytes reveals unusually high tolerance to recommended therapies. *J. Biol. Chem.* **2018**, *293*, 19974–19981. [CrossRef]
17. Chiu, J.E.; Renard, I.; Pal, A.C.; Singh, P.; Vydyam, P.; Thekkiniath, J.; Kumar, M.; Gihaz, S.; Pou, S.; Winter, R.W.; et al. Effective therapy targeting cytochrome *bc1* prevents *Babesia* erythrocytic development and protects from lethal infection. *Antimicrob. Agents Chemother.* **2021**, *65*, e0066221. [CrossRef]

18. Pal, A.C.; Renard, I.; Singh, P.; Vydyam, P.; Chiu, J.E.; Pou, S.; Winter, R.W.; Dodean, R.; Frueh, L.; Nilsen, A.C.; et al. *Babesia duncani* as a model organism to study the development, virulence and drug susceptibility of intraerythrocytic parasites in vitro and in vivo. *J. Infect. Dis.* **2022**. [CrossRef]
19. Camargo, E.P. Growth and differentiation in *Trypanosoma cruzi*. I. Origin of metacyclic trypanosomes in liquid media. *Rev. Inst. Med. Trop. Sao Paulo* **1964**, *6*, 93–100.
20. Limoncu, M.E.; Balcioglu, I.C.; Yereli, K.; Ozbel, Y.; Ozbilgin, A. A new experimental in vitro culture medium for cultivation of *Leishmania* species. *J. Clin. Microbiol.* **1997**, *35*, 2430–2431. [CrossRef]
21. White, S.M.; Constantin, P.E.; Claycomb, W.C. Cardiac physiology at the cellular level: Use of cultured hl-1 cardiomyocytes for studies of cardiac muscle cell structure and function. *Am. J. Physiol. Heart Circ. Physiol.* **2004**, *286*, H823–H829. [CrossRef]
22. Quick, R.E.; Herwaldt, B.L.; Thomford, J.W.; Garnett, M.E.; Eberhard, M.L.; Wilson, M.; Spach, D.H.; Dickerson, J.W.; Telford, S.R., 3rd; Steingart, K.R.; et al. Babesiosis in Washington state: A new species of *babesia*? *Ann. Intern. Med.* **1993**, *119*, 284–290. [CrossRef] [PubMed]
23. Dao, A.H.; Eberhard, M.L. Pathology of acute fatal babesiosis in hamsters experimentally infected with the WA-1 strain of *Babesia*. *Lab. Investig.* **1996**, *74*, 853–859. [PubMed]
24. McCormack, K.A.; Alhaboubi, A.; Pollard, D.A.; Fuller, L.; Holman, P.J. In vitro cultivation of *Babesia duncani* (Apicomplexa: Babesiidae), a zoonotic hemoprotozoan, using infected blood from Syrian hamsters (*Mesocricetus auratus*). *Parasitol. Res.* **2019**, *118*, 2409–2417. [CrossRef] [PubMed]
25. Claycomb, W.C.; Lanson, N.A., Jr.; Stallworth, B.S.; Egeland, D.B.; Delcarpio, J.B.; Bahinski, A.; Izzo, N.J., Jr. Hl-1 cells: A cardiac muscle cell line that contracts and retains phenotypic characteristics of the adult cardiomyocyte. *Proc. Natl. Acad. Sci. USA* **1998**, *95*, 2979–2984. [CrossRef]
26. Downie, M.J.; Kirk, K.; Mamoun, C.B. Purine salvage pathways in the intraerythrocytic malaria parasite *Plasmodium falciparum*. *Eukaryot. Cell* **2008**, *7*, 1231–1237. [CrossRef]
27. Zuzarte-Luis, V.; Mota, M.M. Parasite sensing of host nutrients and environmental cues. *Cell Host Microbe* **2018**, *23*, 749–758. [CrossRef]
28. Augagneur, Y.; Jaubert, L.; Schiavoni, M.; Pachikara, N.; Garg, A.; Usmani-Brown, S.; Wesolowski, D.; Zeller, S.; Ghosal, A.; Cornillot, E.; et al. Identification and functional analysis of the primary pantothenate transporter, PfPAT, of the human malaria parasite *Plasmodium falciparum*. *J. Biol. Chem.* **2013**, *288*, 20558–20567. [CrossRef]
29. Downie, M.J.; El Bissati, K.; Bobenchik, A.M.; Nic Lochlainn, L.; Amerik, A.; Zufferey, R.; Kirk, K.; Ben Mamoun, C. Pfnt2, a permease of the equilibrative nucleoside transporter family in the endoplasmic reticulum of *Plasmodium falciparum*. *J. Biol. Chem.* **2010**, *285*, 20827–20833. [CrossRef]
30. El Bissati, K.; Downie, M.J.; Kim, S.K.; Horowitz, M.; Carter, N.; Ullman, B.; Ben Mamoun, C. Genetic evidence for the essential role of PfNT1 in the transport and utilization of xanthine, guanine, guanosine and adenine by *Plasmodium falciparum*. *Mol. Biochem. Parasitol.* **2008**, *161*, 130–139. [CrossRef]
31. El Bissati, K.; Zufferey, R.; Witola, W.H.; Carter, N.S.; Ullman, B.; Ben Mamoun, C. The plasma membrane permease PfNT1 is essential for purine salvage in the human malaria parasite *Plasmodium falciparum*. *Proc. Natl. Acad. Sci. USA* **2006**, *103*, 9286–9291. [CrossRef]

pathogens

Article

In Silico Survey and Characterization of *Babesia microti* Functional and Non-Functional Proteases

Monica Florin-Christensen [1,2,*], Sarah N. Wieser [1,2], Carlos E. Suarez [3,4] and Leonhard Schnittger [1,2]

1 Instituto de Patobiologia Veterinaria (IPVET), Centro de Investigaciones en Ciencias Veterinarias y Agronomicas, Instituto Nacional de Tecnología Agropecuaria (INTA), Hurlingham C1033AAE, Argentina; wieser.sarah@inta.gob.ar (S.N.W.); schnittger.leonhard@inta.gob.ar (L.S.)
2 Consejo Nacional de Investigaciones Científicas y Técnicas (CONICET), Buenos Aires C1033AAJ, Argentina
3 Animal Disease Research Unit, USDA-ARS, Pullman, WA 99163, USA; suarez@wsu.edu
4 Department of Veterinary Microbiology and Pathology, Washington State University, Pullman, WA 99163, USA
* Correspondence: jacobsen.monica@inta.gob.ar

Abstract: Human babesiosis caused by the intraerythrocytic apicomplexan *Babesia microti* is an expanding tick-borne zoonotic disease that may cause severe symptoms and death in elderly or immunocompromised individuals. In light of an increasing resistance of *B. microti* to drugs, there is a lack of therapeutic alternatives. Species-specific proteases are essential for parasite survival and possible chemotherapeutic targets. However, the repertoire of proteases in *B. microti* remains poorly investigated. Herein, we employed several combined bioinformatics tools and strategies to organize and identify genes encoding for the full repertoire of proteases in the *B. microti* genome. We identified 64 active proteases and 25 nonactive protease homologs. These proteases can be classified into cysteine (n = 28), serine (n = 21), threonine (n = 14), asparagine (n = 7), and metallopeptidases (n = 19), which, in turn, are assigned to a total of 38 peptidase families. Comparative studies between the repertoire of *B. bovis* and *B. microti* proteases revealed differences among sensu stricto and sensu lato *Babesia* parasites that reflect their distinct evolutionary history. Overall, this data may help direct future research towards our understanding of the biology and pathogenicity of *Babesia* parasites and to explore proteases as targets for developing novel therapeutic interventions.

Keywords: human babesiosis; *Babesia microti*; therapeutic drugs; peptidases

Citation: Florin-Christensen, M.; Wieser, S.N.; Suarez, C.E.; Schnittger, L. In Silico Survey and Characterization of *Babesia microti* Functional and Non-Functional Proteases. *Pathogens* **2021**, *10*, 1457. https://doi.org/10.3390/pathogens10111457

Academic Editors: Estrella Montero, Jeremy Gray, Cheryl Ann Lobo and Luis Miguel González

Received: 18 September 2021
Accepted: 6 November 2021
Published: 10 November 2021

1. Introduction

Human babesiosis caused by *Babesia microti* is a malaria-like tick-borne zoonotic disease, first described in the 1950s in the USA, with an increasing number of cases reported ever since in this and other countries around the world [1]. Infections proceed asymptomatic or are accompanied by mild or moderate signs in immunocompetent patients but often lead to severe disease and even death in neonates and the elderly or immunocompromised adults [2].

Some wild rodents act as natural reservoirs of *B. microti*, where the parasite is transmitted both by bites of *Ixodes* sp. ticks, as well as transplacentally [3,4]. Humans are dead-end hosts and suffer accidental infections mainly through tick bites. Transplacental and blood transfusion-related transmissions have also been documented [1,5,6].

Currently, there is no specific therapy for *B. microti* human babesiosis [7]. The recommended therapeutic drugs to treat *B. microti* infections are azithromycin plus atovaquone as the first choice or a combination of clindamycin and quinine as an alternative [7,8]. However, the reported appearance of *B. microti* parasites resistant to the first two drugs in chronically infected patients and the negative side effects of the latter two call for the development of alternative therapeutic strategies and increased investments in this field [2,7–10].

B. microti belongs to the Apicomplexa phylum and, as such, has a mandatory parasitic lifestyle that alternates between its definitive tick host and its intermediate mammalian hosts. Complex physiological processes and molecular interactions between the pathogen and host are needed for invasion, egress, parasite development in the tick stages, and migration processes that lead to the completion of the parasite life cycle and its efficient perpetuation and dissemination. Among the molecules involved in these events, parasite proteases, i.e., enzymes that catalyze proteolytic cleavages, are bound to be of paramount importance [2,11,12].

Indeed, proteases of the model Apicomplexan protozoans *Toxoplasma gondii* and *Plasmodium falciparum* have been shown to participate in several essential physiological processes, including nutrient acquisition and processing, invasion and egress from host cells, protein recycling, posttranslational processing, and signal transduction, among others [13–15]. Due to their vital roles and the fact that they show low or no identity with host-encoded peptidases, parasite proteases have been proposed as potential drug targets and/or vaccine candidates [16–20]. In the case of *Babesia* spp., the importance of peptidases for parasite survival and their potential as therapeutic targets are highlighted by several studies showing that different protease inhibitors significantly impede parasite growth in vitro and/or in vivo [21–25].

The present study aims to shortlist the proteases encoded in the *B. microti* genome by organizing the information available in the MEROPS protease database, as well as identifying additional peptidases by homology searches for paralogs within the *B. microti* genome and orthologs of previously described active proteases of *B. bovis* [26]. We also tested the hypothesis that the repertoires of functional proteases encoded in the genomes of *B. bovis* and *B. microti* differ, possibly due to the peculiarities displayed in their life cycles and their different phylogenetic placements [27,28]. The information recorded in this study can be applied to future research aimed at understanding the biology of this emergent pathogen and designing new therapeutic interventions.

2. Results and Discussion

2.1. Survey of *B. microti* Proteases

The present study shows that the *B. microti* genome encodes for at least 64 active proteases and 25 non active protease homologs. These proteases belong to the cysteine ($n = 28$), serine ($n = 21$), threonine ($n = 14$), aspartic ($n = 7$), and metallopeptidase ($n = 19$) types, which, in turn, are assigned to a total of 38 peptidase families (Table 1).

The classification into peptidase types refers to the nature of the nucleophile in the hydrolytic reaction, which can be the thiol of a cysteine in cysteine peptidases, the hydroxyl of a serine, or a threonine residue in serine and threonine peptidases, respectively, or water bound to aspartic acid or to a metal ion in aspartic and metallopeptidases, respectively. An additional protease group has been described, the glutamic peptidases, in which the nucleophile is water bound to a glutamic acid residue, but these enzymes are absent in Apicomplexan protozoa. Peptidases of each type are assigned into families according to sequence similarities. Non active protease homologs are characterized by bearing a conserved protease domain but lacking in the active site one or more of the critical amino acids needed for catalysis [29].

Table 1. Proteases belonging to the aspartic, cysteine, threonine, serine, and metallopeptidase types encoded by *B. microti*.

Type	Family	Protein Id	GenBank Annotation	Gene Locus	MEROPS Annotation	Type and Position of Peptidase Domain	Active Side Residues (Active Proteases)	Transcriptomic/ Proteomic Data
Aspartic proteases	A1	XP_021337483	Cathepsin E-B	BMR1_01G02485 BBM_I02485	MER1133958—subfamily A1A unassigned peptidases	PTZ00165 aspartyl protease 82-403	D110, Y158, D307	T
		XP_021337801	Pepsin A	BmR1_04g07350 BBM_III07350	MER0383113 MER1136315 subfamily A1A unassigned peptidases	cd05471 pepsin_like 109-417	D128, F173, D324	T
		XP_021338468	Eukaryotic aspartyl protease	BMR1_03g00915 BBM_III00915	MER1142805 MER0383316 subfamily A1A unassigned peptidases	cd05471 pepsin_like 133-473	D160, F205, D373	T
		XP_021338748	Eukaryotic aspartyl protease	BMR1_03g03850 BBM_III03850	MER0384385 subfamily A1A unassigned peptidases	PTZ00165 aspartyl protease 88-401	D106, Y160, D310	T
		XP_021337625	Plasmepsin V	BmR1_04g05270 BBM_III05270	MER0495838 subfamily A1B unassigned peptidases	cl11403 pepsin_retropepsin _like aspartate proteases 167-502	D198, Y253, D388	T
	A22B	XP_021338622	Signal peptide peptidase	BMR1_03g02475 BBM_III02475	MER0323102 subfamily A22B unassigned peptidases	cl01342 Peptidase_A22B Superfamily 27-225	D115, D156	T
	A28	XP_021337501	DNA damage-inducible protein 1	BMR1_01G02675 BBM_I02675	MER0321004 subfamily A28A unassigned peptidases	cd05479 RP_DDI; retropepsin-like domain of DNA damage inducible protein 221-342	D231	T

Table 1. *Cont.*

Type	Family	Protein Id	GenBank Annotation	Gene Locus	MEROPS Annotation	Type and Position of Peptidase Domain	Active Side Residues (Active Proteases)	Transcriptomic/ Proteomic Data
Cysteine proteases	C1A	XP_021338611	Cathepsin C	BMR1_03g02385 BBM_III02385	MER0345528 Subfamily C1A unassigned peptidases	PTZ00049 cathepsin C-like protein 273-483	Q274, C280, H44, D466	T
		XP_012647584	Cysteine proteinase	BMR1_01G02595 BBM_I02595	MER0701894 Non-peptidase homolog	PTZ00200 cysteine proteinase 296-475	Inactive	T
		XP_012650559	Papain family cysteine protease	BmR1_04g09925 BBM_III09925	MER0344826 subfamily C1A unassigned peptidases	cd02248 Peptidase_C1A 236-444	Q252, C258, H38, N410	T/H
		XP_012650562	Papain family cysteine protease	BmR1_04g09940 BBM_III09940	-	cd02248 Peptidase_C1A 236-444	Q252, C258, H38, N410	T
		XP_012647628	Papain family cysteine protease	BMR1_01G02825 BBM_I02825	MER0345177 Unassigned peptidase	PTZ00200 cysteine proteinase 324-538	Q342, C348, H48, N503	T
	C2	XP_021337703	Calpain family cysteine protease	BmR1_04g06080 BBM_III06080	MER0348343 subfamily C2A unassigned peptidases	cl00051 CysPc Superfamily 72-354	Q96, C102, H293, N313	T
	C12	XP_021337460	ubiquitin carboxyl-terminal hydrolase L3	BMR1_01G02185 BBM_I02185	MER0342930 MER1171398 family C12 non-peptidase homologs	cl08306 Peptidase_C12 Superfamily 8-224	Inactive	T

Table 1. *Cont.*

Type	Family	Protein Id	GenBank Annotation	Gene Locus	MEROPS Annotation	Type and Position of Peptidase Domain	Active Side Residues (Active Proteases)	Transcriptomic/ Proteomic Data
	C13	XP_012650207	GPI-anchored transamidase	BmR1_04g08080 BBM_III08080	MER0674277 glycosylphosphatidylinositol:protein transamidase	cl00042 CASc Superfamily 391-639	H532, C574	T
	C14	XP_012648342	Caspase domain	BMR1_02g02900 BBM_II02900	MER0393785 subfamily C14B unassigned peptidases	cl00042 CASc Superfamily 48-168	Inactive	T
	C19	XP_012647713	U4/U6.U5 tri-snRNP-associated protein 2	BMR1_01G03245 BBM_I03245	MER0711213 family C19 non-peptidase homologs	cd02669 Peptidase_C19M 158-365	Inactive	T
		XP_012649658	Ubiquitin carboxyl-terminal hydrolase 25	BmR1_04g05260 BBM_III05260	MER0706972 family C19 unassigned peptidases	cl37989 UCH Superfamily 839-1135	N842, C847, H1084, D1105	T
		XP_021337689	Ubiquitin carboxyl-terminal hydrolase	BmR1_04g05926 BBM_III05930	MER0710229 family C19 non-peptidase homologs	cl37989 Ubiquitin carboxyl-terminal hydrolase	Inactive	T
		XP_021338067	Ubiquitin carboxyl-terminal hydrolase 5/13	BMR1_02g00955 BBM_II00955	MER0708474 family C19 unassigned peptidases	cl34941 UBP14 Superfamily 184-673	N315, C321, H751, N746	T
	C26	XP_012647696	CTP synthase	BMR1_01G03155 BBM_I03155	-	cl33465 CTP synthase 4-570	C398, H540	T
		XP_021337469	carbamoyl-phosphate synthase// aspartate carbamoyltransferase	BMR1_01G02285 BBM_I02285	-	cl36884 CPSaseII_lrg Superfamily 459-1571	C334, H407	T

Table 1. *Cont.*

Type	Family	Protein Id	GenBank Annotation	Gene Locus	MEROPS Annotation	Type and Position of Peptidase Domain	Active Side Residues (Active Proteases)	Transcriptomic/ Proteomic Data
	C44	XP_012650079	glucosamine–fructose-6-phosphate aminotransferase	BmR1_04g07400 BBM_III07400	-	cl36542 PTZ00295 super family	C40	T
	C48	XP_012648199	sentrin-specific protease 1	BMR1_02g02160 BBM_II02160	MER0378492 family C48 unassigned peptidases	cl23802 Peptidase_C48 Superfamily 191-358	H279, D298, Q347, C353	T
		XP_021337449	sentrin-specific protease 2	BMR1_01G02005 BBM_I02005	MER0378539 family C48 unassigned peptidases	cl23802 Peptidase_C48 Superfamily 377-660	H453, D583, Q642, C648	T
	C54	XP_021337321	autophagy-related protein 4	BMR1_01G00840 BBM_I00840	-	cl04056 Peptidase family C54 34-256	Y32, C69, D218, H220	T
	C56	XP_012649637	4-methyl-5(b-hydroxyethyl)-thiazole monophosphate biosynthesis	BmR1_04g05155 BBM_III05155	MER0385822 family C56 non-peptidase homologs	cl00020 GAT_1 superfamily 45′207	Inactive	T/H
	C78	XP_021337753	Peptidase family C78	BmR1_04g06690 BBM_III06690	MER0393880 family C78 unassigned peptidases	cl06790 Peptidase family C78 486-677	Y498, C510, D634, H636	T
	C85A	XP_021337245	Ubiquitin thioesterase otu2	BMR1_01G00165 BBM_I00165	MER0743969 subfamily C85A unassigned peptidases	cl9932 OTU Superfamily OTU-like cysteine protease 65-186	D65, C68, H185	T

Table 1. *Cont.*

Type	Family	Protein Id	GenBank Annotation	Gene Locus	MEROPS Annotation	Type and Position of Peptidase Domain	Active Side Residues (Active Proteases)	Transcriptomic/ Proteomic Data
	C86	XP_021338227	Josephin	BMR1_02g02671 BBM_II02675	MER0399903 family C86 unassigned peptidases	cl20229 Josephin Superfamily 1-121	Inactive	T
	C97	XP_021338702	PPPDE putative peptidase domain	BMR1_03g03275 BBM_III03275	MER0746696 family C97 unassigned peptidases	cl05462 Peptidase_C97 154-283	H193, C274	T
	C115	XP_021337547	Protein FAM63A	BMR1_01G03140 BBM_I03140	MER0933699 family C115 homologs, unassigned	cl04510 MINDY_DUB 4-256	Q21, C27, H 211	T
Threonine proteases	T1A	XP_012647140	20S proteasome subunit alpha 1	BMR1_01G00290 BBM_I00290	MER1091683—subfamily T1A unassigned peptidases	cd03754 protea-some_alpha_type_6 29-150	T38	T/M
		XP_012650489	20S proteasome subunit alpha 2	BmR1_04g09560 BBM_III09560	MER1089221—subfamily T1A unassigned peptidases	cd03750 protea-some_alpha_type_2 61-224	T62	T
		XP_021337746	20S proteasome subunit alpha 3	BmR1_04g06615 BBM_III06615	MER1088544—subfamily T1A unassigned peptidases	PTZ00246 proteasome subunits alpha 32-188	T33	T
		XP_021337745	20S proteasome subunit alpha 4	BmR1_04g06610 BBM_III06610	-	cl00467 proteasome_alpha_type_7 3-209	T32	T

Table 1. *Cont.*

Type	Family	Protein Id	GenBank Annotation	Gene Locus	MEROPS Annotation	Type and Position of Peptidase Domain	Active Side Residues (Active Proteases)	Transcriptomic/ Proteomic Data
		XP_012649604	20S proteasome subunit alpha 5	BmR1_04g04985 BBM_III04985	MER1363164—subfamily T1A Non-peptidase homologs	Cd03753 proteasome_alpha_type_5 35-204	Inactive	T
		XP_012650085	20S proteasome subunit alpha 6	BmR1_04g07427 BBM_III07427	MER1089259—subfamily T1A unassigned peptidases	cd03749 protea-some_alpha_type_1 36-205	T33	T
		XP_021338656	20S proteasome subunit alpha 7	BMR1_03g02775 BBM_III02775	-	cl00467 Ntn_hydrolase Superfamily 6-214	Inactive?	T
		XP_012648315	20S proteasome subunit beta 1	BMR1_02g02760 BBM_II02760	-	cl00467 Ntn_hydrolase Superfamily 29-268	T31	T
		XP_012649453	20S proteasome subunit beta 2	BMR1_03g04210 BBM_III04210	MER0378485—proteasome subunit beta2	Cd03763 Proteasome_beta_type_7 73-254	T73	T
		XP_012649873	20S proteasome subunit beta 3	BmR1_04g06340 BBM_III06340	MER0376976—proteasome subunit beta 3	cd03759 protea-some_beta_type_3 5-191	Inactive?	T
		XP_012647857	20S proteasome subunit beta 4	BMR1_02g00410 BBM_II00410	-	Cd03758 proteasome_beta_type_2 1-152	Inactive?	T/M

Table 1. *Cont.*

Type	Family	Protein Id	GenBank Annotation	Gene Locus	MEROPS Annotation	Type and Position of Peptidase Domain	Active Side Residues (Active Proteases)	Transcriptomic/ Proteomic Data
		XP_021338777	20S proteasome subunit beta 5	BMR1_03g04170 BBM_III04170	MER0376387—subfamily T1A unassigned peptidases	cd03761 protea-some_beta_type_5 24-226	T28	T
		XP_012650322	20S proteasome subunit beta 6	BmR1_04g08685 BBM_III08685	MER1090686—subfamily T1A unassigned peptidases	cl00467 Ntn_hydrolase Superfamily 13-197	T13	T
		XP_021337419	20S proteasome subunit beta 7	BMR1_01G01780 BBM_I01780	MER1088514—subfamily T1A non-peptidase homologs	cl00467 Ntn_hydrolase Superfamily 11-150	Inactive	T
Metallo proteases	M01	XP_012648031	aminopeptidase N	BMR1_02g01305 BBM_II01305	MER0335312—M1 aminopeptidase	PRK14015 pepN aminopeptidase N 366-533	E423, Y506 metal ligand(s): H422, H426, E445	T/M
	M3A	XP_021338435	Mitochondrial intermediate peptidase	BMR1_03g00560 BBM_III00560	MER0817287—family M3 unassigned peptidases	cl14813 GluZincin Superfamily Gluzin Peptidase family 49-519	E482 metal ligand(s): H481, H485, E510	T/M
	M16B	XP_021338255	Probable zinc protease PqqL	BMR1_02g02935 BBM_II02935	MER0925233—subfamily M16A unassigned peptidases	COG0612 PqqL Predicted Zn-dependent peptidase 14-164	E40, E116 metal ligand(s): H37, H41, E123	T
		XP_021337876	Mitochondrial processing peptidase	BmR1_04g08505 BBM_III08505	MER0392117—subfamily M16B non-peptidase homologs	COG0612 PqqL Predicted Zn-dependent peptidase 51-251	Inactive	T/H

Table 1. *Cont.*

Type	Family	Protein Id	GenBank Annotation	Gene Locus	MEROPS Annotation	Type and Position of Peptidase Domain	Active Side Residues (Active Proteases)	Transcriptomic/ Proteomic Data
	M16C	XP_021338005	Mitochondrial processing peptidase	BMR1_02g00260 BBM_II00260	MER0391438–MER0764852 mitochondrial processing peptidase beta-subunit	COG0612 PqqL Predicted Zn-dependent peptidase 49-253	E90, E160 metal ligand(s): H87, H91, E167	T/H
		XP_012650528	peptidase M16 inactive domain containing	BmR1_04g09765 BBM_III09765	MER0393094—subfamily M16C unassigned peptidases	PTZ00432 falcilysin 78-550	E89, E164 metal ligand(s): H86, H90, E203	T
		XP_021338727	Uncharacterized protein C05D11.1	BMR1_03g03610 BBM_III03610	MER0393111—subfamily M16C non-peptidase homologs	COG1026 Cym1 Zn-dependent peptidase, M16 family 54-450	Inactive	T
	M17	XP_021338349	leucyl aminopeptidase	BMR1_02g03960 BBM_II03960	MER0340008—family M17 unassigned peptidases	PRK00913 multifunctional aminopeptidase a154-499	K300,R376 metal ligand(s): A288, D293, D312, H372, Q374	T/H
	M18	XP_021338536	aminopeptidase	BMR1_03g01710 BBM_III01710	MER0340957–MER1122391 aspartyl aminopeptidase	cl14876 Zinc_peptidase_like_Supe 12-481	D95, E296 metal ligand(s): H93, D255, E297, D355, H449	T/H
	M24A	XP_021337644	methionyl aminopeptidase	BmR1_04g05525 BBM_III05525	-	PTZ00053 methionine aminopetidase 2 9-447	H199 metal ligand(s): D230, H299, E332,E427	T

Table 1. *Cont.*

Type	Family	Protein Id	GenBank Annotation	Gene Locus	MEROPS Annotation	Type and Position of Peptidase Domain	Active Side Residues (Active Proteases)	Transcriptomic/ Proteomic Data
		XP_021337770	methionyl aminopeptidase	BmR1_04g06870 BBM_III06870	MER0394794—methionyl aminopeptidase 1	cd1086 MetAP1 Methionine Aminopeptidase 70-312	H143 metal ligand(s): D160, D171, H234, E267,H298	T
		XP_021337427	methionyl aminopeptidase	BMR1_01G01855 BBM_I01855	MER0395783—subfamily M24A unassigned peptidases	cd1086 MetAP1 Methionine Aminopeptidase 146-514	H219 metal ligand(s): D243, D254, H423, E455, E486	T
		XP_012649271	methionyl aminopeptidase	BMR1_03g03300 BBM_III03300	MER0394867—methionyl aminopeptidase 1	PLN03158 methionine aminopeptidase 105-356	H179 metal ligand(s): D196, D207, H270, E303, E334	T
	M24B	XP_012650004	Xaa-Pro aminopeptidase	BmR1_04g07005 BBM_III07005	-	cd01066 X-Prolyl Aminopeptidase	H382,H468,H491 metal ligand(s): D401, D412, H472, E509, E523	T
	M41 *	XP_021338270	Peptidase family M41	BMR1_02g03060 BBM_II03060	MER0363780—PF14_0616 g.p.	TIGR01241 FtsH_fam ATP-dependent metalloprotease FtsH 431-647	E482 metal ligand(s): H481, H485, D558	T/H
		XP_021338301	AFG3 family protein	BMR1_02g03370 BBM_II03370	MER0363828—family M41 unassigned peptidases	TIGR01241 FtsH_fam ATP-dependent metalloprotease FtsH 461-682	E515 metal ligand(s): H514, H518, D581	T/H

Table 1. *Cont.*

Type	Family	Protein Id	GenBank Annotation	Gene Locus	MEROPS Annotation	Type and Position of Peptidase Domain	Active Side Residues (Active Proteases)	Transcriptomic/ Proteomic Data
		XP_012648901	ATPase family associated with various cellular activities	BMR1_03g01455 BBM_III01455	MER0362824—family M41 unassigned peptidases	TIGR01241 FtsH_fam ATP-dependent metalloprotease FtsH 355-575	E406 metal ligand(s): H405, H409, D484	T
	M48A	XP_012650086	STE24 endopeptidase	BmR1_04g07429 BBM_III07429	MER0347520—subfamily M48A unassigned peptidases	cd07343 M48A_Zmpste24p_lilke Peptidase M48 subfamily A 170-441	E304 metal ligand(s): H303, H307, E382	T/H
	M67	XP_021338577	26S proteasome regulatory subunit N11	BMR1_03g02055 BBM_III02055	MER0393303—subfamily M67A unassigned peptidases	cd08069 MPN_RPN11_CSN5 Mov34/MPN/PAD-1 family proteasomal regulatory protein Rpn11 and signalosome complex subunits CSN5 25-314	E52 metal ligand(s): S113, P115, D126	T
Serine proteases	S1B	XP_021338066	Protease Do-like 9	BMR1_02g00945 BBM_II00945	MER0960997—subfamily S1B unassigned peptidases	Pfam13365Trypsin_2 78-230	H93, D124, S202	T
		XP_021337263	hypothetical protein	BMR1_01G00280 BBM_I00280	-	cl34357 Protease II 105-542	S536, D592, H628	T

Table 1. *Cont.*

Type	Family	Protein Id	GenBank Annotation	Gene Locus	MEROPS Annotation	Type and Position of Peptidase Domain	Active Side Residues (Active Proteases)	Transcriptomic/ Proteomic Data
	S09	XP_012649807	Alpha/beta hydrolase domain-containing protein 17C	BmR1_04g06005 BBM_III06005	-	cl27027 Fermentation-respiration switch protein FrsA, has esterase activity, DUF1100 family 102-312	S179, D260, H292	T
		XP_021338600	alpha/beta hydrolase, putative	BMR1_03g02286 BBM_III2290	-	Fermentation-respiration switch protein FrsA, has esterase activity, DUF1100 family 120-256	S142, D194, H246	T
		XP_012650025	alpha/beta hydrolase domain-containing protein 17B	BmR1_04g07110 BBM_III07110	-	cl27027 Fermentation-respiration switch protein FrsA, has esterase activity, DUF1100 family 35-220	S125, D189, H217	T
	S12	XP_012649063	aarF domain-containing kinase	BMR1_03g02265 BBM_III02265	MER1005027—family S12 non-peptidase homologs	cl21491 Transpeptidase superfamily 554-737	Inactive	T

Table 1. *Cont.*

Type	Family	Protein Id	GenBank Annotation	Gene Locus	MEROPS Annotation	Type and Position of Peptidase Domain	Active Side Residues (Active Proteases)	Transcriptomic/ Proteomic Data
	S14	XP_012648206	ATP-dependent Clp protease, protease subunit	BMR1_02g02195 BBM_II02195	MER0359175—family S14 unassigned peptidases	Cd07017 S14_ClpP_2 Caseinolytic protease (ClpP) 41-228	S135, H160, D209	T
		XP_021337686	Clp protease	BmR1_04g05887 BBM_III05890	MER0359717 family S14 non-peptidase homologs	cd07017 caseinolytic protease (ClpP) 50-227	Inactive	T
	S16	XP_012649081	Lon protease homolog 1 mitochondrial	BMR1_03g02350 BBM_III02350	MER0361396—family S16 unassigned peptidases	cl36736 Ion endopeptidase La 835-1038	S946, K989	T/H
	S26	XP_021338290	mitochondrial inner membrane protease subunit 1	BMR1_02g03240 BBM_II03240	MER1047726—subfamily S26A non-peptidase homologs	Cd06530 S26_SPase_I 64-102	Inactive	T
		XP_012650493	signal peptidase, endoplasmic reticulum-type	BmR1_04g09580 BBM_III09580	MER0334095—signalase (animal) 21 kDa component	cl10465 Peptidase_S24_S26 Superfamily 52-169	S63, H101	T/M
	S33	XP_012648716	cardiolipin-specific phospholipase	BMR1_03g00525 BBM_III00525	-	cl21494 Abhydrolase_1 98-327	S172, D292, H350	T
	S54	XP_021338360	Rhomboid-like protease 6	BMR1_02g04085 BBM_II04085	MER1084044—family S54 unassigned peptidases	cl21536 Rhomboid Superfamily 363-474	S391, H452	T
		XP_021338239	ROM4	BMR1_02g02777 BBM_II02780	MER0374041—family S54 unassigned peptidases	cl21536 Rhomboid Superfamily 177-339	S270, H322	T

Table 1. *Cont.*

Type	Family	Protein Id	GenBank Annotation	Gene Locus	MEROPS Annotation	Type and Position of Peptidase Domain	Active Side Residues (Active Proteases)	Transcriptomic/ Proteomic Data
		XP_021338238	ROM3 (a)	BMR1_02g02776 BBM_II02775	-	c21536 Rhomboid Superfamily 205-337	S273, H325	T
		XP_012650510	hypothetical protein BmR1_04g09675 (b)	BmR1_04g09675 BBM_III09675	MER1083102—family S54 non-peptidase homologs	cl21536 Rhomboid Superfamily 139-357	S287, H342	T
		XP_021338098	hypothetical protein BMR1_02g01230 (c)	BMR1_02g01230 BBM_II01230	-	cl21536 Rhomboid Superfamily 267-458	Inactive	T
		XP_012647608	Der1-like family	BMR1_01G02725 BBM_I02725	-	cl21536 Rhomboid Superfamily 11-202	Inactive	T
		XP_012650093	Der1-like family	BmR1_04g07462 BBM_III07462	-	cl21536 Rhomboid Superfamily 87-295	Inactive	T/H
		XP_012649979	Derlin 2/3	BmR1_04g06880 BBM_III06880	-	cl21536 Rhomboid Superfamily 12-205	Inactive	T
	S59 *	XP_012650001	Nucleoporin autopeptidase	BmR1_04g06990 BBM_III06990	MER1071845—family S59 non-peptidase homologs	pfam04096 Nucleoporin2 444-579	Inactive	T

Protease types are color-coded: blue: aspartic, light yellow: cysteine, orange: threonine, gray: metallo, and yellow: serine proteases, with darker colors for peptidases predicted as active. The relevant amino acid positions in the active site needed for catalytic activity are included for each active protease. Inactive proteases have a predicted protease domain but lack one or more of the functional amino acids. Paralog groups within each family are underlined. When more than a paralog group is present in a family, different underlining styles are used for each group. (a) ROM4, (b) ROM7 (active protease, wrongly predicted as inactive in MEROPS), and (c) ROM8 [29]. (*) Paralogs of the M41 and the S59 families lacking peptidase domains are shown separately (Supplementary Tables S1 and S2). T: Transcribed genes in the intraerythrocytic stage [30]. H or M: High or medium levels of protein expression detected in Reference [31].

Twenty of the proteases presented in this study are not included in the MEROPS database and were identified by homology searches. In addition, five of the proteases listed in Table 1 presented duplicated MEROPS entries, likely because of the use of different sources of peptide sequences in this database (Table 1). On the other hand, a number of *B. microti* proteases have been annotated in GenBank as hypothetical proteins, uncharacterized proteins, or following the designation of another conserved domain also present in the sequences, and they are, thus, not identifiable by searches using keywords such as protease or peptidase. Importantly, despite the exhaustive search carried out to produce the list presented in Table 1, the presence of additional protease-coding genes in the *B. microti* genome that passed inadvertently in this study cannot be ruled out. In addition, it should be noted that the predicted catalytic activity for some threonine proteases (Table 1) could not be determined beyond doubt and needs to be confirmed experimentally.

All of the listed active and non active proteases are transcribed in *B. microti* merozoites suggesting they likely fulfill a relevant functional role in this parasite stage [30]. In addition, 17 active and non active proteases were identified in the proteomic profile of *B. microti* during the acute infection of a hamster model (Table 1) [31]. Proteases that remained undetected might be expressed in low amounts at the intraerythrocytic stage or bear physicochemical characteristics that preclude detection by the experimental approach employed in this study [31].

Localization predictor algorithms located most of the identified proteases in the cytoplasm. Four proteases were predicted as extracellular and six as lysosomal. The latter might reach the extracellular milieu by the fusion of vacuoles with the plasma membrane as has been shown for *Tetrahymena thermophila*, a free-living protozoon belonging together with Apicomplexa to Alveolata. However, this mechanism has not been demonstrated for *Babesia* spp. [32]. Other predicted locations include the nucleus, the mitochondria, a plastid (which would correspond to the apicoplast, in this case), the plasma membrane, the endoplasmic reticulum, the Golgi apparatus, and the peroxisomes (Supplementary Table S3). Importantly, these predictions are only tentative until they have been experimentally confirmed. Additionally, the used algorithm is not able to predict the location of proteases in Apicomplexa-specific secretory organelles, such as rhoptries and micronemes, where the trafficking of proteases has been shown to occur in *Plasmodium* and *Toxoplasma* [33].

2.2. *Aspartic Proteases*

Seven aspartic proteases were found in the *B. microti*-predicted proteome, all of which bear the aspartate and, in the case of the A1 family, also the phenylalanine or tyrosine residues in their active sites, needed to display catalytic activity (Table 1).

Interestingly, a recent transcriptomics study involving four of the five A1 aspartic protease genes of *B. microti* showed stage-associated expression for two of them. Thus, while BmR1_01G02485 (encoding cathepsin E-B or ASP2) displayed higher expression in mouse blood intraerythrocytic stages than in the stages present in *I. ricinus* gut or salivary glands, the opposite was true for BmR1_03g03850 (encoding ASP6). These results suggest a role for ASP2 in processes connected to the asexual reproduction of the parasite and/or gametocyte formation and, for ASP6, in zygote and/or kinete development, kinete dissemination in tick tissues, including salivary glands, and sporogony. For the other two studied A1 aspartic protease-encoding genes, BmR1_04g07350 and BmR1_04g05270, corresponding to ASP3 and ASP5, respectively, expression was similar in the three stages, suggesting a role in invasion both of erythrocytes and tick cells or in other cellular processes such as secretion or the trafficking of proteins [34].

Aspartic proteases have been proposed as chemotherapeutic targets against *B. microti*. Indeed, the aspartic protease inhibitors Lopinavir and Atazanavir, which are well-tolerated drugs used in HIV patients, were shown to be potent suppressors of *B. microti* infection in vitro, as well as in vivo, in a mouse model [24]. It is unknown which parasite aspartic protease is affected by these inhibitors, but one candidate is the signal peptide peptidase (SPP, XP_021338622), which has a critical role in the maintenance of the homeostasis of the endoplasmic reticulum. Consistent with this view, in the case of *P. falciparum*, these inhibitors were effective in blocking SPP activity and in vitro parasite growth [24,35]. Notably, *B. microti* and *Plasmodium* sp. SPP proteins are orthologous (results not shown) but do not have a counterpart in *B. bovis* (Supplementary Table S4) or any other *Babesia* sp. (not shown).

Hemoglobin is certainly the main protein source available for the nutrition of intraerythrocytic parasites. The sequential steps for hemoglobin degradation by *Plasmodium* sp., as described by Guzman et al. 1994 [36], start with the unwinding of the molecule and partial digestion by aspartic proteases, followed by cysteine protease cleavage, which yields protein fragments that are finally degraded by exopeptidases, generating free amino acids useful for parasite nutrition. In *Plasmodium* sp., the first part of this process takes place in the food vacuole and involves the aspartic proteases Plasmepsins I-IV and is then followed by the action of papain-like cysteine proteases in the erythrocyte cytoplasm [37]. There is no evidence that a food vacuole is present in *B. microti*, and consistent with its absence, Plasmepsins I-IV homologs cannot be found in this parasite. The lack of these enzymes has been used as an argument to postulate that *B. microti* is not able to degrade hemoglobin [38]. However, it may be hypothesized that other *B. microti* aspartyl proteases of the A1 family (Table 1), likely secreted to the erythrocyte cytoplasm, are able to initiate hemoglobin degradation, such as pepsin A (XP_021337801), predicted to have a signal peptide and, thus, be exported to the erythrocyte cytoplasm (Supplementary Table S3). To find out whether this is the case or there is an alternative protein source available for the nutrition of the intraerythrocytic trophozoite and merozoite stages would need experimental exploration.

2.3. Cysteine Proteases

Cysteine proteinases are involved in the essential biological roles of Apicomplexan parasites [13,39,40]. They are present in *B. microti* with at least 27 members, of which 18 are predicted to be catalytically active (Table 1).

In *P. falciparum*, the papain-like falcipain-2 and falcipain-3 peptidases of the C1A family have attracted the most attention among cysteine proteases as potential therapeutic targets against malaria [41]. As mentioned above, these enzymes participate in hemoglobin degradation in the intraerythrocytic stage of the parasite, and, in addition, falcipain-2 has been shown to cleave erythrocyte cytoskeletal proteins during egress from the host cell [42,43]. Falcipain-2 orthologs have been characterized in *B. bovis*, *B. bigemina*, and *B. ovis* and have been named bovipain-2, babesipain, and ovipain-2, respectively. Similar to their *P. falciparum* counterpart, they are expressed inside merozoites and also released to the erythrocyte cytoplasm, consistent with the dual role described for falcipain-2 [44–47]. The significant impairment of the in vitro growth of *B. ovis* and *B. bovis* merozoites by antibodies against ovipain-2 and a papain-like C1A cysteine protease, respectively, indicate a relevant role of this type of enzymes in the propagation of the asexual stages of *Babesia* spp. [47,48].

The *B. microti* ortholog of falcipain-2 (XP_012650559) has four paralogs (three active proteases and one non-protease homolog), one of which is 100% identical (XP_012650562; Table 1). The corresponding genes for these two identical proteins are located on the same strand of chromosome 3, separated by a ~5 kb intergenic region, where two unrelated genes are found in the opposite strand. Predictor algorithms localized XP_012650559 and XP_012650562, either within lysosomes or other vacuoles or secreted through a non classical pathway (Supplementary Table S3). This predicted localization agrees well with that described for their counterparts in *B. bovis*, *B. bigemina*, and *B. ovis* [44–48]. In a recent study, an enzymatically active recombinant form of *B. microti* XP_012650559 (rBmCYP) was expressed in *E. coli*. The activity of rBmCYP against a fluorescent peptide was significantly inhibited by recombinant forms of the cysteine protease inhibitors cystatins 1 and 2 of *Riphicephalus haemaphysaloides* ticks [49]. Although *R. haemaphysaloides* is not a typical *B. microti*-transmitting tick, it has been suggested as a potential vector for this parasite in China [50]. These results coincide with the inhibition exerted by *R. microplus* cystatins on a *B. bovis* C1A cysteine protease and suggest the involvement of these enzymes in tick host–pathogen interactions [51]

Interestingly, the phylogenetic analysis of C1A cysteine protease paralog profiles of piroplasmids of the *Babesia*, *Theileria* and *Cytauxzoon* genera corroborates the assignment of analyzed species into Clades I–VI according to their 18S rRNA gene sequences [27,52].

2.4. Serine Proteases

At least thirteen functional serine proteases and eight non functional protease homologs belonging to nine families are encoded in the *B. microti* genome (Table 1).

A prominent group of serine proteases is constituted by the S54 family, which consists of rhomboid proteases (ROMs). ROMs were first described in *Drosophila melanogaster* and later shown to be present in all kingdoms of life, fulfilling various relevant roles, including cell signaling in animals, quorum sensing in bacteria, homeostasis regulation in mitochondria, and the dismantling of adhesion complexes in apicomplexan protozoa. They are characterized by having six to seven transmembrane domains and their active site embedded in the lipid bilayer [53,54].

ROMs have been thoroughly studied in the apicomplexans *Toxoplasma gondii* and *Plasmodium* spp. The former encodes ROM1–6, according to the nomenclature defined by Dowse and Soldati, 2005 [55], all of which have, with exception of ROM2, homologs in *P. falciparum*. The latter parasite has four additional ROMs that are not present in *T. gondii*, designated ROM7–10 [56,57]. *T. gondii* and *Plasmodium* sp. ROM4 proteases were shown to cleave parasite adhesins, thus dismantling the adhesive junctions formed between the membranes of the host and parasite, a process needed for parasite internalization into the host cell [53,57]. Due to their critical role in invasion, ROMs are regarded as potential targets for therapeutic interventions against apicomplexans [58]. Indeed, two ROM4 inhibitors were shown to specifically block the *P. falciparum* invasion of human erythrocytes [59]. Additionally, experimental vaccine formulations based on *T. gondii* and *Emeria tenella* ROM4 were able to partially protect mice and chickens, respectively, against challenges [20,60].

In a recent study, ROM-coding genes were identified in the genomes of several piroplasmids and shown to belong exclusively to the ROM4, ROM6, ROM7, and ROM8 types. While the latter three were always present in a single copy, two to five ROM4 paralogs could be found depending on the piroplasmid lineage analyzed [61]. *B. microti* has two ROM4 paralogs, one of which (XP_021338238) has been misannotated as "ROM3" in GenBank (Table 1). ROM4 proteinases are found exclusively throughout the phylum Apicomplexa, which is consistent with their predicted role in invasion of the host cell, a critical mechanism for these obligate parasites [56]. ROM6, on the other hand, is the only piroplasmid rhomboid not exclusive to apicomplexans and has been shown to participate in various processes, including mitochondrial homeostasis, apoptosis, and the electron transport chain [62]. Accordingly, a mitochondrial localization was predicted for *B. microti* ROM6 (XP_021338360; Supplementary Table S3). *B. microti* ROM7 (XP_012650510) and ROM8

(XP_021338098) were predicted to localize in the membranes of the endoplasmic reticulum and the Golgi apparatus, respectively (Supplementary Table S3). These two types of ROMs are present in *Plasmodium* sp. and piroplasmids but not in other apicomplexans. Their functions are unknown but could be related to processes shared by all Aconoidasida, such as those that take place during the intraerythrocytic stage [61]. Finally, three members of the "derlin" subfamily were found in *B. microti* (Table 1). Derlins are catalytically inactive members of the Rhomboid Superfamily and were first described in yeast and later found in mammals and other organisms. Their function is still unclear, but it has been suggested that they could be part of a channel through which misfolded proteins are retro-translocated from the endoplasmic reticulum to the cytoplasm prior to their ubiquitination and degradation [63].

Notably, for *B. bovis*, one of the ROM-encoding genes (XP_001610128) was found to be significantly higher expressed in the parasite stages present in the hemolymph of *Rhipicephalus microplus* ticks as compared to the stages present in bovine blood, suggesting that the role of this protease is mostly associated with the development of the parasite in the tick [64]. It remains to be analyzed whether a similar scenario takes place for the corresponding orthologs in *B. microti* and other piroplasmids.

In an early study, the serine protease activity of *B. bovis* merozoite homogenates was found to be higher in two virulent than in two avirulent strains from Australia, and thus, these proteases were postulated as virulence determinants [65]. However, in a later study, all the genes encoding for active proteases ($n = 66$) were shown to be present and transcribed to similar levels in the asexual blood stages of a *B. bovis* virulent parental strain and an attenuated strain, obtained by successive blood passages in splenectomized bovines [26]. These data suggest that the virulent/attenuated phenotype in this parasite is not related to a different peptidase gene content or to changes in the transcriptional levels of any peptidase-coding gene. To establish whether or not parasite serine or other types of proteases are virulence determinants in *Babesia* spp. will need further experimental evidence, but in any case, their relevance for pathogenicity is based on the vital role they probably fulfill in the parasitic lifestyle.

2.5. Metalloproteases

Metalloproteases contain a metal ion at their active site, which acts as a catalyst in the hydrolysis of peptide bonds, and are represented by at least 17 active and two non active protease homologs in *B. microti* (Table 1) [29].

Among them, methionine aminopeptidases (MAPs), which are present with four members in *B. microti* (M24A family, Table 1), take care of the N-terminal methionine excision from polypeptides, general metabolism of amino acids and proteins, and regulation processes that imply the activation and inactivation of biologically active peptides [66]. Inhibitors of MAPs significantly reduced the in vitro growth of *P. falciparum*, *B. bovis*, *B. bigemina*, *B. caballi*, and *T. equi*, highlighting a relevant role of MAPs in the survival of these parasites [23,67]. Moreover, *B. microti*-infected mice treated with MAP inhibitors reached significantly lower parasitemia levels than untreated mice [23]. Additionally, one of the *B. microti* MAPs (XP_012649271) was tested in mice as a potential vaccine candidate for human babesiosis. Immunization with an *E. coli*-expressed recombinant form of this MAP induced a Th1 immune response characterized by IgG2a antibody titers and IFN-γ production, and provided partial protection against the challenge with *B. microti* [68]. Although the number of boosters and protein amounts needed to achieve this effect would not be practical to apply in humans, these results suggest a potential usefulness of MAPs in future vaccine formulations against *B. microti*.

2.6. Threonine Proteases and the Proteasome

The proteasome is a cylindrically shaped large complex of proteins in charge of degrading intracellular proteins destined for destruction that have been tagged with polyubiquitin chains, thereby controlling many cellular processes, such as cell cycle progression and cell signaling [69,70]. All *B. microti* threonine proteases are proteasome constituents (seven alpha and seven beta 20S proteasome subunits, Table 1). Additionally, a metalloprotease with a proteasome regulatory function is also listed among the *B. microti* proteases (XP_021338577 of the M67 family), while assignment of other proteases to this structure needs experimental confirmation. Due to their vital role in cell physiology, drugs targeting proteasome functions have been proposed as therapeutics against several parasitic diseases [71–73]. In the case of *Babesia* sp., the proteasome inhibitors epoxyketones and boronic acid were shown to reduce the chymotrypsin activity of the proteasome in lysates of *B. divergens* in vitro cultures, leading to the accumulation of poli-ubiquinated proteins and, also, impeding parasite growth in vitro [24]. One of the epoxyketones, carfilzomib, was also assayed in *B. microti*-infected mice. Carfilzomib is a covalent and irreversible peptide inhibitor of the β5 subunit of the human proteasome approved for the clinical treatment of multiple myeloma [74]. Blood lysates of *B. microti*-infected mice treated with carfilzomib also showed the accumulation of poli-ubiquinated proteins as compared to untreated mice. Moreover, carfilzomib treatment reduced the peak parasitemia levels without apparent toxic effects in the treated mice. Although the dose required to eliminate the parasite would be toxic when applied in humans, these studies indicate that specifically targeting the *B. microti* proteasome would be a possible chemotherapeutic approach against this parasite [24].

2.7. Comparison between B. microti and B. bovis Functional Proteases

The genome of *B. microti* is the smallest among Apicomplexans and encodes 7% less genes compared to that of *B. bovis*. This difference is mainly due to the large *vesa* and *SmORF* multigene families present in *B. bovis*, which are absent in *B. microti* [38]. These two gene families encode for highly variable proteins that are involved in escaping the immune system of the vertebrate host and cytoadhesion [75,76]. It remains unknown whether strategies to escape effectors of the immune system exist in *B. microti*. However, cytoadhesion, especially affecting brain capillaries, has not been described as a major pathogenic mechanism for this parasite [2]. Other unraveled differences include the lack of spherical body proteins in *B. microti*, consistent with a reduced apical complex [38]. Additionally, contrary to *B. bovis*, *B. microti* does not have an oligosaccharyl transferase in charge of transferring a $(NAcGlc)_2$ moiety from a lipid-linked oligosaccharide to a nascent protein destined for the secretory pathway in the endoplasmic reticulum. Thus, a significant difference among *B. bovis* and *B. microti* is the lack of ability of the latter to produce N-glycosylated proteins [77].

In the present study, we hypothesized that the differences between *B. bovis* and *B. microti* include the repertoire of active proteases encoded in their genomes. By orthology searches, we observed that most *B. bovis* active proteases have an ortholog in *B. microti* (Supplementary Table S4). The lack of orthology was connected in all but two cases to the expansion of a protease-coding ancestor gene into different numbers of paralogs, which most likely took place after the separation of the most recent common ancestor (MRCA) of *B. bovis* and *B. microti*, and thus, they differentiate both species. However, the S8 family of serine proteases is present with a single member, a subtilisin-like protein (XP_001610126), only in *B. bovis* but is absent in *B. microti*. The *B. bovis* subtilisin-like protein gene is syntenic with orthologous genes in *B. divergens*, *B. ovata*, and *Babesia* sp. Xinjang (data not shown). Importantly, characterization of the subtilisin-like protein of *B. divergens* showed that it localizes to dense granules and contains neutralization-sensitive B-cell epitopes, consistent with a relevant role in the invasion or establishment of the parasite in the infected erythrocyte, as observed for subtilisin-1 and subtilisin-2 in *P. falciparum* [78–80]. The other case is *B. microti* SPP aspartic protease (XP_021338622), which is absent in *B.*

bovis and other *Babesia* spp., as mentioned above. The identification of genes absent in *B. microti* and present in other *Babesia* spp. or vice versa can allow comprehending the minimum protein dotation needed to fulfill a basic *Babesia* sp. life cycle, as well as to identify which proteins are associated with species-specific peculiarities and can also be exploited for differential diagnosis, therapeutic, and vaccine developments. *B. bovis* and *B. microti* share important similarities in their life cycles, namely being tick-transmitted and having an asexual reproduction stage exclusively within the erythrocytes of their vertebrate hosts. However, they differ in tick and vertebrate host species, as well as by the presence or absence of transovarial transmission in the tick. Transovarial transmission is, indeed, a trademark of the "true" babesias or *Babesia* sensu stricto, such as *B. bovis*, while those members of the *Babesia* genus that do not have this trait, such as *B. microti*, are considered *Babesia* sensu lato [27,28,81]. These differences are undoubtedly connected with the evolutionary history of *B. bovis* and *B. microti*, which can be clearly visualized by their phylogenetic placement into two distant clades (Clades VI and I, respectively, according to Schnittger et al., 2012 and 2021 [27,28].

2.8. Non-Peptidase Homologs

At least 25 non-peptidase homologs are encoded in the *B. microti* genome (Table 1). A conserved protease domain can be predicted in their sequences, but they lack one or more of the catalytically relevant amino acids. Non-peptidase homologs are commonly found among living organisms and believed to have evolved from catalytically active enzymes. They have lost their catalytic capacity but developed new functions, such as competitive inhibition regulating their active counterparts or even completely new non-protease-related activities [82,83]. An extreme case of loss of function is observed with a group of paralogs of *B. microti* that include three metalloproteases of the M41 family and 14 other non-protease members. Different from other non-peptidase homologs, the latter do not have a recognizable protease active site region. According to their conserved domains, their functions include the hydrolysis of nucleoside triphosphates, fusion of vesicles, intracellular transport, and proteasome regulation (Supplementary Table S1).

2.9. Conclusions and Perspectives

Proteases are attractive targets against a large number of infectious agents, since many of them are druggable and participate in essential biological processes of pathogenic virus, bacteria, protozoa, and fungi [84]. Indeed, several protease inhibitors are commercially available, and some are successfully employed in the treatment of HIV and Hepatitis C [85,86]. The use of protease inhibitors against other relevant viruses, such as dengue and SARS-CoV-2, has also been postulated [87,88].

The present study was aimed at organizing the available information of *B. microti* proteases and extending the array of identified peptidases encoded in its genome. This information is expected to set the stage for future research directed to understand the biology and pathogenicity of this parasite and to explore proteases as targets for developing novel therapeutic interventions. Recent advances in *B. microti* gene editing will permit exploring the functional relevance of selected proteases [89,90]. In addition, the application of computer-based inhibitor screening and the use of optimized pipelines to test drug efficacies using in vitro cultures and animal models allows obtaining new therapeutics against human babesiosis in a relatively short period of time [34,91,92].

3. Materials and Methods

The proteases of *B. microti*, R1 strain, presented in this study were identified by three different search approaches: (i) extracting and organizing the data available for this parasite in the MEROPS database (www.ebi.ac.uk/merops/, accessed on 1 September 2021) [29], (ii) the identification of homologs of *B. bovis* proteases predicted as active, as reported by Mesplet et al. (2011) [26], and (iii) the search for paralogs of *B. microti* proteases identified in (i) and (ii). Orthology between *B. bovis* and *B. microti* proteases was defined using a BLASTp bidirectional best hit (BBH) approach [93]. Paralogs within the *B. microti* genome were determined by BLASTp (blast.ncbi.nlm.nih.gov/Blast.cgi, accessed on 1 September 2021), considering a threshold E value of 0.05. Peptidase domain names and locations were obtained from the Conserved Domains database of the NCBI.

For those proteases included in the MEROPS database and predicted as active, the relevant amino acids of the catalytic site were identified using the data available at this website. For the proteases not included in the MEROPS database, alignments of *B. bovis* and *B. microti* orthologs were carried out by Clustal omega [94] (https://www.ebi.ac.uk/Tools/msa/clustalo/, accessed on 1 September 2021), and the relevant amino acids described for *B. bovis* in MEROPS were manually identified for the corresponding *B. microti* protease. The non-peptidase homologs included those described as such in the MEROPS database. In addition, the peptidases not present in MEROPS were listed as non-peptidase homologs whenever one or more of the catalytically relevant amino acid residues at the homologous positions were missing upon alignment with the sequence of an active proteinase homolog.

The presence of transcripts and translated proteins in the blood parasite stages was evaluated in PiroplasmaDB [95] (piroplasmadb.org/piro/app, accessed on 10.09.2021) and in the proteomic database provided in Reference [31], respectively. The subcellular location of each protease was evaluated by the presence of a signal peptide (SignalP 5.0 server, www.cbs.dtu.dk/services/SignalP/, accessed on 10 September 2021) [96] and transmembrane domains [97] (TMHMM server, www.cbs.dtu.dk/services/TMHMM/, accessed on 10 September 2021) and using the localization predictor DeepLoc-1.0 [98] (www.cbs.dtu.dk/services/DeepLoc/, accessed on 10 September 2021) with the settings for eukaryotic sequences.

Supplementary Materials: The following are available online at https://www.mdpi.com/article/10.3390/pathogens10111457/s1, Table S1: M41 metalloprotease paralogue family of *B. microti*, Table S2: S59 paralogue family of *B. microti*, Table S3: Predicted subcellular localization of *B. microti* proteases, Table S4: Comparison between the repertoire of *B. microti* and *B. bovis* proteases predicted as active at least in one of either species.

Author Contributions: Conceptualization, M.F.-C. and L.S.; investigation: M.F.-C. and S.N.W.; original draft preparation: M.F.-C.; and writing—reviewing and editing: C.E.S., S.N.W., L.S., and M.F.-C. All authors have read and agreed to the published version of the manuscript.

Funding: We acknowledge the support of projects 2019-PD-E5-I102, 2019-PE-E5-I109, and 2019-PE-E5-I105 from the National Institute of Agricultural Technology (INTA, Argentina) and CRIS 2090-32000-039-000-D from ARS-USDA (USA). SNW received a doctoral fellowship from Consejo Nacional de Investigaciones Científicas y Técnicas (CONICET, Argentina).

Institutional Review Board Statement: Not applicable.

Informed Consent Statement: Not applicable.

Data Availability Statement: Not applicable.

Conflicts of Interest: The authors declare no competing interests.

References

1. Yang, Y.; Christie, J.; Köster, L.; Du, A.; Yao, C. Emerging Human Babesiosis with "Ground Zero" in North America. *Microorganisms* **2021**, *9*, 440. [CrossRef]
2. Vannier, E.; Krause, P.J. Human Babesiosis. *N. Engl. J. Med.* **2012**, *366*, 2397–2407. [CrossRef] [PubMed]
3. Tołkacz, K.; Bednarska, M.; Alsarraf, M.; Dwużnik, D.; Grzybek, M.; Welc-Falęciak, R.; Behnke, J.M.; Bajer, A. Prevalence, Genetic Identity and Vertical Transmission of *Babesia microti* in Three Naturally Infected Species of Vole, Microtus Spp. (Cricetidae). *Parasites Vectors* **2017**, *10*, 1–12. [CrossRef]
4. Tufts, D.M.; Diuk-Wasser, M.A. Transplacental Transmission of Tick-Borne *Babesia microti* in Its Natural Host Peromyscus Leucopus. *Parasites Vectors* **2018**, *11*, 1–9. [CrossRef]
5. Iyer, S.; Goodman, K. Congenital Babesiosis From Maternal Exposure: A Case Report. *J. Emerg. Med.* **2019**, *56*, e39–e41. [CrossRef]
6. Stanley, J.; Stramer, S.L.; Erickson, Y.; Cruz, J.; Gorlin, J.; Janzen, M.; Rossmann, S.N.; Straus, T.; Albrecht, P.; Pate, L.L.; et al. Detection of *Babesia* RNA and DNA in Whole Blood Samples from US Blood Donations. *Transfusion* **2021**. [CrossRef]
7. Renard, I.; Ben Mamoun, C. Treatment of Human Babesiosis: Then and Now. *Pathogens* **2021**, *10*, 1120. [CrossRef] [PubMed]
8. Krause, P.J.; Auwaerter, P.G.; Bannuru, R.R.; Branda, J.A.; Falck-Ytter, Y.T.; Lantos, P.M.; Lavergne, V.; Meissner, H.C.; Osani, M.C.; Rips, J.G.; et al. Clinical Practice Guidelines by the Infectious Diseases Society of America (IDSA): 2020 Guideline on Diagnosis and Management of Babesiosis. *Clin. Infect. Dis.* **2021**, *72*, e49–e64. [CrossRef] [PubMed]
9. Wormser, G.P.; Prasad, A.; Neuhaus, E.; Joshi, S.; Nowakowski, J.; Nelson, J.; Mittleman, A.; Aguero-Rosenfeld, M.; Topal, J.; Krause, P.J. Emergence of Resistance to Azithromycin-Atovaquone in Immunocompromised Patients with *Babesia microti* Infection. *Clin. Infect. Dis.* **2010**, *50*, 381–386. [CrossRef] [PubMed]
10. Simon, M.S.; Westblade, L.F.; Dziedziech, A.; Visone, J.E.; Furman, R.R.; Jenkins, S.G.; Schuetz, A.N.; Kirkman, L.A. Clinical and Molecular Evidence of Atovaquone and Azithromycin Resistance in Relapsed *Babesia microti* Infection Associated With Rituximab and Chronic Lymphocytic Leukemia. *Clin. Infect. Dis.* **2017**, *65*, 1222–1225. [CrossRef] [PubMed]
11. Florin-Christensen, M.; Schnittger, L. Piroplasmids and Ticks: A Long-Lasting Intimate Relationship. *Front. Biosci.* **2009**, *14*, 3064–3073. [CrossRef] [PubMed]
12. Antunes, S.; Rosa, C.; Couto, J.; Ferrolho, J.; Domingos, A. Deciphering Babesia-Vector Interactions. *Front. Cell. Infect. Microbiol.* **2017**, *7*, 429. [CrossRef] [PubMed]
13. Klemba, M.; Goldberg, D.E. Biological Roles of Proteases in Parasitic Protozoa. *Annu. Rev. Biochem.* **2003**, *71*, 275–305. [CrossRef] [PubMed]
14. Cai, H.; Kuang, R.; Gu, J.; Wang, Y. Proteases in Malaria Parasites—A Phylogenomic Perspective. *Curr. Genom.* **2011**, *12*, 417–427. [CrossRef] [PubMed]
15. Lilburn, T.G.; Cai, H.; Zhou, Z.; Wang, Y. Protease-Associated Cellular Networks in Malaria Parasite *Plasmodium falciparum*. *BMC Genom.* **2011**, *12*, 1–16. [CrossRef]
16. Rosenthal, P.; Sijwali, P.; Singh, A.; Shenai, B. Cysteine Proteases of Malaria Parasites: Targets for Chemotherapy. *Curr. Pharma. Des.* **2002**, *8*, 1659–1672. [CrossRef]
17. Li, H.; Child, M.A.; Bogyo, M. Proteases as Regulators of Pathogenesis: Examples from the Apicomplexa. *Biochim. Biophys. Acta (BBA)-Proteins Proteom.* **2012**, *1824*, 177–185. [CrossRef]
18. Pandey, K.C. Centenary Celebrations Article: Cysteine proteases of human malaria parasites. *J. Parasit. Dis.* **2011**, *35*, 94–103. [CrossRef]
19. Sedwick, C. Plasmepsin V, a Secret Weapon Against Malaria. *PLoS Biol.* **2014**, *12*, e1001898. [CrossRef]
20. Zhang, N.-Z.; Xu, Y.; Wang, M.; Petersen, E.; Chen, J.; Huang, S.-Y.; Zhu, X.-Q. Protective Efficacy of Two Novel DNA Vaccines Expressing Toxoplasma Gondii Rhomboid 4 and Rhomboid 5 Proteins against Acute and Chronic Toxoplasmosis in Mice. *Expert Rev. Vaccines* **2015**, *14*, 1289–1297. [CrossRef]
21. Okubo, K.; Yokoyama, N.; Govind, Y.; Alhassan, A.; Igarashi, I. *Babesia bovis*: Effects of Cysteine Protease Inhibitors on in vitro Growth. *Exp. Parasitol.* **2007**, *117*, 214–217. [CrossRef] [PubMed]
22. AbouLaila, M.; Nakamura, K.; Govind, Y.; Yokoyama, N.; Igarashi, I. Evaluation of the in Vitro Growth-Inhibitory Effect of Epoxomicin on *Babesia* Parasites. *Vet. Parasitol.* **2010**, *167*, 19–27. [CrossRef] [PubMed]
23. Munkhjargal, T.; Ishizaki, T.; Guswanto, A.; Takemae, H.; Yokoyama, N.; Igarashi, I. Molecular and Biochemical Characterization of Methionine Aminopeptidase of *Babesia bovis* as a Potent Drug Target. *Vet. Parasitol.* **2016**, *221*, 14–23. [CrossRef]
24. Jalovecka, M.; Hartmann, D.; Miyamoto, Y.; Eckmann, L.; Hajdusek, O.; O'Donoghue, A.J.; Sojka, D. Validation of *Babesia* Proteasome as a Drug Target. *Int. J. Parasitol. Drugs Drug Res.* **2018**, *8*, 394–402. [CrossRef] [PubMed]
25. Schwake, C.; Baldwin, M.R.; Bachovchin, W.; Hegde, S.; Schiemer, J.; Okure, C.; Levin, A.E.; Vannier, E.; Hanada, T.; Chishti, A.H. HIV Protease Inhibitors Block Parasite Signal Peptide Peptidases and Prevent Growth of *Babesia microti* Parasites in Erythrocytes. *Biochem. Biophys. Res. Commun.* **2019**, *517*, 125–131. [CrossRef]
26. Mesplet, M.; Palmer, G.H.; Pedroni, M.J.; Echaide, I.; Florin-Christensen, M.; Schnittger, L.; Lau, A.O.T. Genome-Wide Analysis of Peptidase Content and Expression in a Virulent and Attenuated *Babesia bovis* Strain Pair. *Mol. Biochem. Parasitol.* **2011**, *179*, 111–113. [CrossRef] [PubMed]
27. Schnittger, L.; Rodriguez, A.E.; Florin-Christensen, M.; Morrison, D.A. *Babesia*: A World Emerging. *Infect. Genet. Evol.* **2012**, *12*, 1788–1809. [CrossRef]

28. Schnittger, L.; Ganzinelli, S.; Bhoora, R.; Omondi, D.; Nijhof, A.M.; Florin-Christensen, M. The Piroplasmida *Babesia, Cytauxzoon,* and *Theileria* in Farm and Companion Animals: Species Compilation, Molecular Phylogeny, and Evolutionary Insights. *Parasitol. Res.* **2021**. under revision.
29. Rawlings, N.D.; Bateman, A. How to Use the MEROPS Database and Website to Help Understand Peptidase Specificity. *Protein Sci.* **2021**, *30*, 83–92. [CrossRef]
30. Silva, J.C.; Cornillot, E.; McCracken, C.; Usmani-Brown, S.; Dwivedi, A.; Ifeonu, O.O.; Crabtree, J.; Gotia, H.T.; Virji, A.Z.; Reynes, C.; et al. Genome-Wide Diversity and Gene Expression Profiling of *Babesia microti* Isolates Identify Polymorphic Genes That Mediate Host-Pathogen Interactions. *Sci. Rep.* **2016**, *6*, 1–15. [CrossRef]
31. Magni, R.; Luchini, A.; Liotta, L.; Molestina, R.E. Analysis of the *Babesia microti* proteome in infected red blood cells by a combination of nanotechnology and mass spectrometry. *Int. J. Parasitol.* **2019**, *49*, 139–144. [CrossRef]
32. Florin-Christensen, M.; Florin-Christensen, J.; Tiedtke, A.; Rasmussen, L. New aspects of extracellular hydrolytic enzymes in lower eukaryotes. *Eur. J. Cell Biol.* **1989**, *48*, 1–4.
33. Binder, E.M.; Kim, K. Location, location, location: Trafficking and function of secreted proteases of *Toxoplasma* and *Plasmodium*. *Traffic* **2004**, *5*, 914–924. [CrossRef]
34. Šnebergerová, P.; Bartošová-Sojková, P.; Jalovecká, M.; Sojka, D. Plasmepsin-like Aspartyl Proteases in *Babesia*. *Pathogens* **2021**, *10*, 1241. [CrossRef] [PubMed]
35. Li, X.; Chen, H.; Bahamontes-Rosa, N.; Kun, J.F.J.; Traore, B.; Crompton, P.D.; Chishti, A.H. *Plasmodium falciparum* Signal Peptide Peptidase Is a Promising Drug Target against Blood Stage Malaria. *Biochem. Biophys. Res. Commun.* **2009**, *380*, 454–459. [CrossRef] [PubMed]
36. Gluzman, I.Y.; Francis, S.E.; Oksman, A.; Smith, C.E.; Duffin, K.L.; Goldberg, D.E. Order and Specificity of the *Plasmodium falciparum* Hemoglobin Degradation Pathway. *J. Clin. Investig.* **1994**, *93*, 1602–1608. [CrossRef]
37. Nasamu, A.S.; Polino, A.J.; Istvan, E.S.; Goldberg, D.E. Malaria Parasite Plasmepsins: More than Just Plain Old Degradative Pepsins. *J. Biolog. Chem.* **2020**, *295*, 8425–8441. [CrossRef] [PubMed]
38. Cornillot, E.; Hadj-Kaddour, K.; Dassouli, A.; Noel, B.; Ranwez, V.; Vacherie, B.; Augagneur, Y.; Brès, V.; Duclos, A.; Randazzo, S.; et al. Sequencing of the Smallest Apicomplexan Genome from the Human Pathogen *Babesia Microti*. *Nucleic Acids Res.* **2012**, *40*, 9102–9114. [CrossRef]
39. Kim, K. Role of Proteases in Host Cell Invasion by *Toxoplasma gondii* and Other Apicomplexa. *Acta Tropica* **2004**, *91*, 69–81. [CrossRef]
40. Cowman, A.F.; Crabb, B.S. Invasion of Red Blood Cells by Malaria Parasites. *Cell* **2006**, *124*, 755–766. [CrossRef]
41. Ettari, R.; Previti, S.; di Chio, C.; Zappalà, M. Falcipain-2 and Falcipain-3 Inhibitors as Promising Antimalarial Agents. *Curr. Med. Chem.* **2021**, *28*, 3010–3031. [CrossRef]
42. Hanspal, M.; Dua, M.; Takakuwa, Y.; Chishti, A.H.; Mizuno, A. *Plasmodium falciparum* Cysteine Protease Falcipain-2 Cleaves Erythrocyte Membrane Skeletal Proteins at Late Stages of Parasite DevelopmentPresented in Part in Abstract Form at the 43rd Annual Meeting of the American Society of Hematology, Orlando, FL, 2001. *Blood* **2002**, *100*, 1048–1054. [CrossRef]
43. Sijwali, P.S.; Rosenthal, P.J. Gene Disruption Confirms a Critical Role for the Cysteine Protease Falcipain-2 in Hemoglobin Hydrolysis by *Plasmodium falciparum*. *Proc. Natl. Acad. Sci. USA* **2004**, *101*, 4384–4389. [CrossRef]
44. Mesplet, M.; Echaide, I.; Dominguez, M.; Mosqueda, J.J.; Suarez, C.E.; Schnittger, L.; Florin-Christensen, M. Bovipain-2, the falcipain-2 ortholog, is expressed in intraerythrocytic stages of the tick-transmitted hemoparasite *Babesia bovis*. *Parasites Vectors* **2010**, *3*, 113. [CrossRef] [PubMed]
45. Martins, T.M.; Gonçalves, L.M.D.; Capela, R.; Moreira, R.; do Rosário, V.E.; Domingos, A. Effect of Synthesized Inhibitors on Babesipain-1, a New Cysteine Protease from the Bovine Piroplasm *Babesia bigemina*. *Transbound. Emerg. Dis.* **2010**, *57*, 68–69. [CrossRef] [PubMed]
46. Martins, T.M.; do Rosário, V.E.; Domingos, A. Expression and Characterization of the *Babesia bigemina* Cysteine Protease BbiCPL1. *Acta Tropica* **2012**, *121*, 1–5. [CrossRef]
47. Carletti, T.; Barreto, C.; Mesplet, M.; Mira, A.; Weir, W.; Shiels, B.; Oliva, A.G.; Schnittger, L.; Florin-Christensen, M. Characterization of a Papain-like Cysteine Protease Essential for the Survival of *Babesia ovis* Merozoites. *Ticks Tick-Borne Dis.* **2016**, *7*, 85–93. [CrossRef] [PubMed]
48. Lu, S.; Ascencio, M.E.; Torquato, R.J.S.; Florin-Christensen, M.; Tanaka, A.S. Kinetic Characterization of a Novel Cysteine Peptidase from the Protozoan *Babesia bovis*, a Potential Target for Drug Design. *Biochimie* **2020**, *179*, 127–134. [CrossRef]
49. Wei, N.; Du, Y.; Lu, J.; Zhou, Y.; Cao, J.; Zhang, H.; Gong, H.; Zhou, J. A Cysteine Protease of *Babesia microti* and Its Interaction with Tick Cystatins. *Parasitol. Res.* **2020**, *119*, 3013–3022. [CrossRef]
50. Wu, J.; Cao, J.; Zhou, Y.; Zhang, H.; Gong, H.; Zhou, J. Evaluation on Infectivity of *Babesia microti* to Domestic Animals and Ticks Outside the Ixodes Genus. *Front. Microbiol.* **2017**, *8*, 1915. [CrossRef]
51. Lu, S.; da Rocha, L.A.; Torquato, R.J.S.; da Silva Vaz Junior, I.; Florin-Christensen, M.; Tanaka, A.S. A Novel Type 1 Cystatin Involved in the Regulation of *Rhipicephalus microplus* Midgut Cysteine Proteases. *Ticks Tick-Borne Dis.* **2020**, *11*, 101374. [CrossRef]
52. Ascencio, M.E.; Florin-Christensen, M.; Mamoun, C.B.; Weir, W.; Shiels, B.; Schnittger, L. Cysteine Proteinase C1A Paralog Profiles Correspond with Phylogenetic Lineages of Pathogenic Piroplasmids. *Vet. Sci.* **2018**, *5*, 41. [CrossRef] [PubMed]
53. Dogga, S.K.; Soldati-Favre, D. Biology of Rhomboid Proteases in Infectious Diseases. *Semin. Cell Dev. Biol.* **2016**, *60*, 38–45. [CrossRef] [PubMed]

54. Düsterhöft, S.; Künzel, U.; Freeman, M. Rhomboid Proteases in Human Disease: Mechanisms and Future Prospects. *Biochim. Et Biophys. Acta (BBA)-Mol. Cell Res.* **2017**, *1864*, 2200–2209. [CrossRef] [PubMed]
55. Dowse, T.J.; Soldati, D. Rhomboid-like Proteins in Apicomplexa: Phylogeny and Nomenclature. *Trends Parasitol.* **2005**, *21*, 254–258. [CrossRef] [PubMed]
56. Santos, J.M.; Graindorge, A.; Soldati-Favre, D. New Insights into Parasite Rhomboid Proteases. *Mol. Biochem. Parasitol.* **2012**, *182*, 27–36. [CrossRef] [PubMed]
57. Lin, J.; Meireles, P.; Prudêncio, M.; Engelmann, S.; Annoura, T.; Sajid, M.; Chevalley-Maurel, S.; Ramesar, J.; Nahar, C.; Avramut, C.M.C.; et al. Loss-of-Function Analyses Defines Vital and Redundant Functions of the *Plasmodium* Rhomboid Protease Family. *Mol. Microbiol.* **2013**, *88*, 318–338. [CrossRef]
58. Urban, S. Making the Cut: Central Roles of Intramembrane Proteolysis in Pathogenic Microorganisms. *Nat. Rev. Microbiol.* **2009**, *7*, 411–423. [CrossRef]
59. Gandhi, S.; Baker, R.P.; Cho, S.; Stanchev, S.; Strisovsky, K.; Urban, S. Designed Parasite-Selective Rhomboid Inhibitors Block Invasion and Clear Blood-Stage Malaria. *Cell Chem. Biol.* **2020**, *27*, 1410–1424. [CrossRef]
60. Han, Y.; Zhou, A.; Lu, G.; Zhao, G.; Wang, L.; Guo, J.; Song, P.; Zhou, J.; Zhou, H.; Cong, H.; et al. Protection via a ROM4 DNA Vaccine and Peptide against *Toxoplasma gondii* in BALB/c Mice. *BMC Infect. Dis.* **2017**, *17*, 1–9. [CrossRef]
61. Gallenti, R.; Poklepovich, T.; Florin-Christensen, M.; Schnittger, L. The Repertoire of Serine Rhomboid Proteases of Piroplasmids of Importance to Animal and Human Health. *Int. J. Parasitol.* **2021**, *51*, 455–462. [CrossRef]
62. Lysyk, L.; Brassard, R.; Touret, N.; Lemieux, M.J. PARL Protease: A Glimpse at Intramembrane Proteolysis in the Inner Mitochondrial Membrane. *J. Mol. Biol.* **2020**, *432*, 5052–5062. [CrossRef] [PubMed]
63. Freeman, M. Proteolysis within the Membrane: Rhomboids Revealed. *Nat. Rev. Mol. Cell Biol.* **2004**, *5*, 188–197. [CrossRef] [PubMed]
64. Ueti, M.W.; Johnson, W.C.; Kappmeyer, L.S.; Herndon, D.R.; Mousel, M.R.; Reif, K.E.; Taus, N.S.; Ifeonu, O.O.; Silva, J.C.; Suarez, C.E.; et al. Transcriptome Dataset of *Babesia bovis* Life Stages within Vertebrate and Invertebrate Hosts. *Data Brief* **2020**, *33*, 106533. [CrossRef] [PubMed]
65. Wright, I.G.; Goodger, B.V.; Mahoney, D.F. Virulent and Avirulent Strains of *Babesia bovis*: The Relationship Between Parasite Protease Content and Pathophysiological Effect of the Strain. *J. Protozool.* **1981**, *28*, 118–120. [CrossRef]
66. Lowther, W.T.; Matthews, B.W. Structure and Function of the Methionine Aminopeptidases. *Biochim. Et Biophys. Acta (BBA)-Protein Struct. Mol. Enzymol.* **2000**, *1477*, 157–167. [CrossRef]
67. Naughton, J.A.; Nasizadeh, S.; Bell, A. Downstream Effects of Haemoglobinase Inhibition in *Plasmodium falciparum*-Infected Erythrocytes. *Mol. Biochem. Parasitol.* **2010**, *173*, 81–87. [CrossRef]
68. Munkhjargal, T.; Yokoyama, N.; Igarashi, I. Recombinant Methionine Aminopeptidase Protein of *Babesia microti*: Immunobiochemical Characterization as a Vaccine Candidate against Human Babesiosis. *Parasitol. Res.* **2016**, *115*, 3669–3676. [CrossRef] [PubMed]
69. Ciechanover, A. The Ubiquitin-Proteasome Proteolytic Pathway. *Cell* **1994**, *79*, 13–21. [CrossRef]
70. Bedford, L.; Paine, S.; Sheppard, P.W.; Mayer, R.J.; Roelofs, J. Assembly, Structure, and Function of the 26S Proteasome. *Trends Cell Biol.* **2010**, *20*, 391–401. [CrossRef]
71. Li, H.; Bogyo, M.; Fonseca, P.C.A. da The Cryo-EM Structure of the *Plasmodium falciparum* 20S Proteasome and Its Use in the Fight against Malaria. *FEBS J.* **2016**, *283*, 4238–4243. [CrossRef] [PubMed]
72. Bijlmakers, M.J. Ubiquitination and the Proteasome as Drug Targets in Trypanosomatid Diseases. *Front. Chem.* **2021**, *8*. [CrossRef] [PubMed]
73. Thomas, M.; Brand, S.; de Rycker, M.; Zuccotto, F.; Lukac, I.; Dodd, P.G.; Ko, E.-J.; Manthri, S.; McGonagle, K.; Osuna-Cabello, M.; et al. Scaffold-Hopping Strategy on a Series of Proteasome Inhibitors Led to a Preclinical Candidate for the Treatment of Visceral Leishmaniasis. *J. Med. Chem.* **2021**, *64*, 5905–5930. [CrossRef] [PubMed]
74. Kuhn, D.J.; Chen, Q.; Voorhees, P.M.; Strader, J.S.; Shenk, K.D.; Sun, C.M.; Demo, S.D.; Bennett, M.K.; van Leeuwen, F.W.B.; Chanan-Khan, A.A.; et al. Potent Activity of Carfilzomib, a Novel, Irreversible Inhibitor of the Ubiquitin-Proteasome Pathway, against Preclinical Models of Multiple Myeloma. *Blood* **2007**, *110*, 3281–3290. [CrossRef]
75. Allred, D.R.; Carlton, J.M.R.; Satcher, R.L.; Long, J.A.; Brown, W.C.; Patterson, P.E.; O'Connor, R.M.; Stroup, S.E. The Ves Multigene Family of *B. bovis* Encodes Components of Rapid Antigenic Variation at the Infected Erythrocyte Surface. *Mol. Cell* **2000**, *5*, 153–162. [CrossRef]
76. Ferreri, L.M.; Brayton, K.A.; Sondgeroth, K.S.; Lau, A.O.T.; Suarez, C.E.; McElwain, T.F. Expression and Strain Variation of the Novel "Small Open Reading Frame" (Smorf) Multigene Family in *Babesia bovis*. *Int. J. Parasitol.* **2012**, *42*, 131–138. [CrossRef]
77. Florin-Christensen, M.; Rodriguez, A.E.; Suárez, C.E.; Ueti, M.W.; Delgado, F.O.; Echaide, I.; Schnittger, L. N-Glycosylation in Piroplasmids: Diversity within Simplicity. *Pathogens* **2021**, *10*, 50. [CrossRef]
78. Montero, E.; Gonzalez, L.M.; Rodriguez, M.; Oksov, Y.; Blackman, M.J.; Lobo, C.A. A Conserved Subtilisin Protease Identified in *Babesia divergens* Merozoites. *J. Biol. Chem.* **2006**, *281*, 35717–35726. [CrossRef]
79. Harris, P.K.; Yeoh, S.; Dluzewski, A.R.; O'Donnell, R.A.; Withers-Martinez, C.; Hackett, F.; Bannister, L.H.; Mitchell, G.H.; Blackman, M.J. Molecular Identification of a Malaria Merozoite Surface Sheddase. *PLoS Pathogens* **2005**, *1*, e29. [CrossRef]

80. Koussis, K.; Withers-Martinez, C.; Yeoh, S.; Child, M.; Hackett, F.; Knuepfer, E.; Juliano, L.; Woehlbier, U.; Bujard, H.; Blackman, M.J. A Multifunctional Serine Protease Primes the Malaria Parasite for Red Blood Cell Invasion. *EMBO J.* **2009**, *28*, 725–735. [CrossRef]
81. Jalovecka, M.; Sojka, D.; Ascencio, M.; Schnittger, L. *Babesia* Life Cycle—When Phylogeny Meets Biology. *Trends Parasitol.* **2019**, *35*, 356–368. [CrossRef] [PubMed]
82. Todd, A.E.; Orengo, C.A.; Thornton, J.M. Sequence and Structural Differences between Enzyme and Nonenzyme Homologs. *Structure* **2002**, *10*, 1435–1451. [CrossRef]
83. Reynolds, S.L.; Fischer, K. Pseudoproteases: Mechanisms and Function. *Biochem. J.* **2015**, *468*, 17–24. [CrossRef]
84. Agbowuro, A.A.; Huston, W.M.; Gamble, A.B.; Tyndall, J.D.A. Proteases and protease inhibitors in infectious diseases. *Med. Care Res. Rev.* **2018**, *38*, 1295–1331. [CrossRef]
85. Fernández-Montero, J.V.; Barreiro, P.; Soriano, V. HIV protease inhibitors: Recent clinical trials and recommendations on use. *Expert Opin. Pharm.* **2009**, *10*, 1615–1629. [CrossRef]
86. Rowe, I.A.; Mutimer, D.J. Protease inhibitors for treatment of genotype 1 hepatitis C virus infection. *The BMJ* **2011**, *343*, d6972. [CrossRef]
87. Mushtaq, M.; Naz, S.; Parang, K.; Ul-Haq, Z. Exploiting Dengue Virus Protease as a Therapeutic Target; Current Status, Challenges and Future Avenues. *Curr. Med. Chem.* **2021**, in press. [CrossRef] [PubMed]
88. Srivastava, K.; Singh, M.K. Drug repurposing in COVID-19: A review with past, present and future. *Metab. Open* **2021**, *12*, 100121. [CrossRef]
89. Jaijyan, D.K.; Govindasamy, K.; Singh, J.; Bhattacharya, S.; Singh, A.P. Establishment of a stable transfection method in Babesia microti and identification of a novel bidirectional promoter of Babesia microti. *Sci. Rep.* **2020**, *10*, 15614. [CrossRef]
90. Liu, M.; Ji, S.; Rizk, M.A.; Adjou Moumouni, P.F.; Galon, E.M.; Li, J.; Li, Y.; Zheng, W.; Benedicto, B.; Tumwebaze, M.A.; et al. Transient Transfection of the Zoonotic Parasite *Babesia microti*. *Pathogens* **2020**, *9*, 108. [CrossRef]
91. Pérez, B.; Antunes, S.; Gonçalves, L.M.; Domingos, A.; Gomes, J.R.; Gomes, P.; Teixeira, C. Toward the discovery of inhibitors of babesipain-1, a *Babesia bigemina* cysteine protease: In vitro evaluation, homology modeling and molecular docking studies. *J. Comput. -Aided Mol. Des.* **2013**, *27*, 823–835. [CrossRef]
92. Yin, M.; Zhang, H.B.; Tao, Y.; Yao, J.M.; Liu, H.; Win, H.H.; Huo, L.L.; Jiang, B.; Chen, J.X. Optimization of an Evaluation Method for Anti-*Babesia microti* Drug Efficacy. *Acta Tropica* **2021**, *225*, 106179. [CrossRef]
93. Tatusov, R.L.; Koonin, E.V.; Lipman, D.J. A Genomic Perspective on Protein Families. *Science* **1997**, *278*, 631–637. [CrossRef] [PubMed]
94. Sievers, F.; Higgins, D.G. Clustal Omega for Making Accurate Alignments of Many Protein Sequences. *Protein Sci.* **2018**, *27*, 135–145. [CrossRef] [PubMed]
95. Aurrecoechea, C.; Barreto, A.; Brestelli, J.; Brunk, B.P.; Cade, S.; Doherty, R.; Fischer, S.; Gajria, B.; Gao, X.; Gingle, A.; et al. EuPathDB: The Eukaryotic Pathogen Database. *Nucleic Acids Res.* **2013**, *41*, D684–D691. [CrossRef]
96. Almagro Armenteros, J.J.; Tsirigos, K.D.; Sønderby, C.K.; Petersen, T.N.; Winther, O.; Brunak, S.; von Heijne, G.; Nielsen, H. SignalP 5.0 Improves Signal Peptide Predictions Using Deep Neural Networks. *Nat. Biotechnol.* **2019**, *37*, 420–423. [CrossRef]
97. Krogh, A.; Larsson, B.; von Heijne, G.; Sonnhammer, E.L.L. Predicting Transmembrane Protein Topology with a Hidden Markov Model: Application to Complete Genomes. *J. Mol. Biol.* **2001**. [CrossRef]
98. Almagro Armenteros, J.J.; Sønderby, C.K.; Sønderby, S.K.; Nielsen, H.; Winther, O. DeepLoc: Prediction of Protein Subcellular Localization Using Deep Learning. *Bioinformatics* **2017**, *33*, 3387–3395. [CrossRef]

pathogens
MDPI

Article

Plasmepsin-like Aspartyl Proteases in *Babesia*

Pavla Šnebergerová [1,2], Pavla Bartošová-Sojková [1], Marie Jalovecká [2] and Daniel Sojka [1,*]

[1] Institute of Parasitology, Biology Centre, Academy of Sciences of the Czech Republic, Branišovská 1160/31, CZ-37005 České Budějovice, Czech Republic; pavla.snebergerova@paru.cas.cz (P.Š.); bartosova@paru.cas.cz (P.B.-S.)
[2] Faculty of Science, University of South Bohemia in České Budějovice, Branišovská 1760c, CZ-37005 České Budějovice, Czech Republic; jalovecka@prf.jcu.cz
* Correspondence: sojka@paru.cas.cz

Abstract: Apicomplexan genomes encode multiple pepsin-family aspartyl proteases (APs) that phylogenetically cluster to six independent clades (A to F). Such diversification has been powered by the function-driven evolution of the ancestral apicomplexan AP gene and is associated with the adaptation of various apicomplexan species to different strategies of host infection and transmission through various invertebrate vectors. To estimate the potential roles of *Babesia* APs, we performed qRT-PCR-based expressional profiling of *Babesia microti* APs (BmASP2, 3, 5, 6), which revealed the dynamically changing mRNA levels and indicated the specific roles of individual BmASP isoenzymes throughout the life cycle of this parasite. To expand on the current knowledge on piroplasmid APs, we searched the EuPathDB and NCBI GenBank databases to identify and phylogenetically analyse the complete sets of APs encoded by the genomes of selected *Babesia* and *Theileria* species. Our results clearly determine the potential roles of identified APs by their phylogenetic relation to their homologues of known function—*Plasmodium falciparum* plasmepsins (PfPM I–X) and *Toxoplasma gondii* aspartyl proteases (TgASP1–7). Due to the analogies with plasmodial plasmepsins, piroplasmid APs represent valuable enzymatic targets that are druggable by small molecule inhibitors—candidate molecules for the yet-missing specific therapy for babesiosis.

Keywords: aspartyl protease; plasmepsin; apicomplexa; piroplasmida; *Babesia*

Citation: Šnebergerová, P.; Bartošová-Sojková, P.; Jalovecká, M.; Sojka, D. Plasmepsin-like Aspartyl Proteases in *Babesia*. *Pathogens* **2021**, *10*, 1241. https://doi.org/10.3390/pathogens10101241

Academic Editors: Estrella Montero, Jeremy Gray, Cheryl Ann Lobo and Luis Miguel González

Received: 3 August 2021
Accepted: 22 September 2021
Published: 26 September 2021

1. Introduction

Babesiosis (also known as piroplasmosis) is a malaria-like disease caused by the parasites from the genus *Babesia* of the apicomplexan order Piroplasmida. This order was initially represented by three separated lineages—*Babesia*, *Theileria*, and *Cytauxzoon*—but more recent phylogenetic analyses have indicated approximately six lineages of Piroplasmida, out of which the approximately 100 *Babesia* species are represented in at least three distinct clades [1]. Analogously to their malaria-causing relatives (genus *Plasmodium*, order Haemosporidia), *Babesia* parasites are transmitted to their vertebrate hosts via a blood-feeding arthropod (tick), where they follow an asexual erythrocytic growth cycle. With the global distribution of ticks and their dynamically changing distribution in recent decades, babesiosis represents an important worldwide veterinary threat, and an emerging risk to humans [2].

Despite routine epidemiological surveillance, babesiosis has long been recognised as an economically important disease affecting livestock, with growing incidence in both domesticated and wildlife animals [3]. Bovine babesiosis, commonly called red water fever, is the economically most important arthropod-transmitted disease affecting cattle, causing mortalities, miscarriages, and decreased meat production [4]. Recently, increased attention has been devoted to the alarming increase in severe "dog babesiosis", caused mainly by *Babesia canis* transmitted by the ornate dog tick *Dermacentor reticulatus*, which has mosaic distribution throughout Europe [5]. Humans are accidental hosts of *Babesia*, but numerous factors indicate human babesiosis as an emerging zoonosis. The clinical features of human babesiosis are similar to malaria, and can be fatal, particularly in the elderly and in immunocompromised individuals [2]. The majority of human infections are reported from the USA, where the principal agent *Babesia microti* is the most commonly transmitted pathogen during blood transfusions [6,7]. Babesiosis is also an emerging problem in Europe, where *Ixodes ricinus*-transmitted *Babesia divergens* is considered the major causative agent of human babesiosis [8]. Incidence rates of human babesiosis are probably underestimated due to misdiagnosis of malaria in the overlapping distribution areas of these parasitic diseases [9].

Protection against bovine babesiosis is mostly based on the debatable vaccination of young cattle with attenuated parasites [10]. Treatment of human babesiosis is non-specific and relies on the combination of antimalarial drugs and antibiotics, such as atovaquone and azithromycin [6]. However, a remarkable increase in parasite resistance, together with significant numbers of relapsed immunocompromised and asplenic individuals [11], has made this widely used treatment regime less effective [12]. Alternative therapy with clindamycin and quinine is toxic and has never been tested in clinical trials. Reports of babesiosis within new geographical regions, as well as identifications of new *Babesia* species as agents of severe human disease, suggest rapid changes in *Babesia* spp. epidemiology, and make human babesiosis a serious public health concern [2]. Hence, novel approved drugs and veterinary control strategies based on *Babesia*-specific molecular targets are highly desirable [10,12].

Parasite-derived proteolytic enzymes (proteases) have been adapted for various functions connected with the parasitic lifestyle [13]. Aspartyl (aspartic, aspartate) proteases use an activated water molecule bound to one or more aspartate residues for catalysis of their peptide substrate. The peptidase database MEROPS [14] identifies five clans of aspartic proteases (AA, AC, AD, AE, and AF), each representing an independent evolution of the same active site and mechanisms. Proteases in the clan AA are either bilobed (family A1, the pepsin family) or homodimeric (all other families in the clan, including the A2 family of retropepsins) [15]. Each lobe consists of a single domain with a closed beta-barrel, and each lobe contributes one aspartate to form the active site. The monomers (retroviruses, retrotransposons, and badnaviruses) are structurally related to one lobe of the pepsin molecule. Due to their ability of specific cleavage within protein bonds, pepsin family (A1) aspartyl proteases (APs) have been evolutionary selected and adapted for unique cellular and physiological roles [16]. Apicomplexa, in contrast to metazoan parasites, have used rapid evolution of the single ancestral A1 protease, resulting in multiple AP-encoding genes being found in their genomes, as best represented by the 7 different APs of *Toxoplasma gondii* (TgASP1–7) [17] and 10 plasmepsin isoenzymes encoded by the genome of *P. falciparum* (PfPM I–X) [18]. The multiple Apicomplexan APs are phylogenetically clustered into six clearly distinguishable clades, tagged A–F. These clades reflect the function-driven evolution and various biological roles of these enzymes within the life cycle of these parasitic organisms [16,17]. Due to their essential roles and affordable selective targetability by small molecule inhibitors, APs have been considered and validated as valuable therapeutic targets [16,19].

In this work, we use the available EuPathDB and NCBI GenBank database records to identify and phylogenetically analyse the yet unrevealed plasmepsin and other apicomplexan AP homologues from selected *Babesia* and *Theileria* species. We estimate the roles of newly identified entries by their phylogenetic clustering to the six clades of apicomplexan APs, as well as their evolutionary relation to *P. falciparum* plasmepsins and *T. gondii* ASP homologues of known functions. Our estimation is supported by the dynamic expression profiling throughout selected life stages of *Babesia microti* using our previously developed *B. microti–Ixodes ricinus*–mouse acquisition model [20].

2. Results and Discussion

2.1. Expression Profiling of BmASPs Indicate Their Various Roles throughout the Life Cycle of Babesia microti

Based on the previously published phylogenetic analysis of parasite cathepsin D-like proteases [16], we initially assessed the expression dynamics of four identified *B. microti* APs (BmASPs) to estimate their potential roles within the life cycle of *B. microti*. This was enabled by the use of our established *B. microti* acquisition model, involving BALB/c mice and *I. ricinus* tick nymphs [20]. Our results clearly show *B. microti* ASP3 (BmASP3, BmR1_04g07350) to be the most abundantly expressed AP isoenzyme of the parasite intraerythrocytic stage (Figure 1A). This finding is in line with the phylogenetic clustering of BmASP3 to clade C of apicomplexan APs, together with the *P. falciparum* plasmepsins PfPM IX and PfPM X [21], and *T. gondii* ASP3 [22], which are the apical complex-associated proteases playing essential roles in parasite invasion and egress from the host cell (further discussed in Section 2.2.). Analogously to the clade C plasmepsins, BmASP3 is also expressed in *B. microti* stages developing in the midgut and salivary glands of *I. ricinus* nymphs (Figure 1B,C), indicating the potential involvement of BmASP3 in tick tissue invasion.

B. microti ASP6 (BmASP6; BMR1_03g03850) mRNA represents the relatively most abundant AP encoding mRNA (54%) in the gut of fully fed tick nymphs, and its abundance in this tissue remains strong even 6 days post the detachment of tick nymphs from their host (24%) (Figure 1B,C). This indicates the involvement of BmASP6 in *Babesia* zygote development and resembles the mRNA expression profile of the *P. falciparum* orthologue PM VII. This enzyme is present in all sexual stages of *P. falciparum* [23], although the protein first appears in diploid stages upon fertilization, presumably due to regulated protein translation [23]. Since BmASP6 is also expressed in *B. microti* stages developing in the tick midgut 6 days post tick detachment, we hypothesise its potential role during the *B. microti* zygote–kinete stage transition, and the subsequent development of kinetes occurring in the tick midgut wall. Supported by the predominant expression of BmASP6 in the salivary glands of fully fed and detached *I. ricinus* nymphs (Figure 1B,C), BmASP6 presumably plays a role in the dissemination of kinetes to other tick tissues, including salivary glands, and subsequently in the early phase of *B. microti* sporogony. The BmASP6 *T. gondii* orthologue TgASP6 is expressed in sporulated oocyst-containing haploid sporozoites [17]. Since piroplasms do not create oocysts in tick midguts, and sporogony occurs in tick salivary glands, we speculate that BmASP6 might be synthesised as a precursor during early sporogony, and that the enzyme could be catalytically activated upon tick feeding. Mature BmASP6 might thus be involved in the release of sporozoites to tick saliva and/or sporozoite invasion of host red blood cells.

Interestingly, the clade B member *B. microti* ASP2 (BmASP2, BMR1_01G02485) is relatively more expressed in *B. microti* blood stages. This contrasts with its orthologue PfPM VI, which is specifically expressed in the vector stages, and is involved in the correct transition of sporozoites from the oocyst [24]. BmASP2 is relatively lowly expressed in monitored tick stages (Figure 1B,C), while it appears abundant (up to 27%) in host blood (Figure 1A). Thus, BmASP2 might be already produced in gametocytes in host blood, and the protein is first produced upon fertilization in tick midguts due to regulated translation in the same manner as the clade E PfPM VII [23]. Alternatively, it might play a different role during the *B. microti* life cycle than its orthologue PfPM VI [25].

The clade D member *B. microti* ASP5 (BmASP5, BmR1_04g05270), the PEXEL (TEXEL)-cleaving *P. falciparum* PM V [26,27], and *T. gondii* ASP5 [27,28] orthologue, are expressed throughout all three selected timepoints of the *B. microti* life cycle (Figure 1). Since the exported proteins of *B. microti* were proposed to lack the PEXEL-like motifs [29] and their trafficking is most likely mediated via vesicles [30], BmASP5 supposedly plays other roles throughout the parasite life cycle, e.g., in the intracellular trafficking of proteins to specific organelles [31], in the development of gametocytes analogous to PfPM V [32], or in the secretion of proteins interacting with tick tissues during transmission. However, the role of

B. microti PEXEL processing should not be fully excluded, as only more complex studies on the *B. microti* secretome can fully address this point in the future.

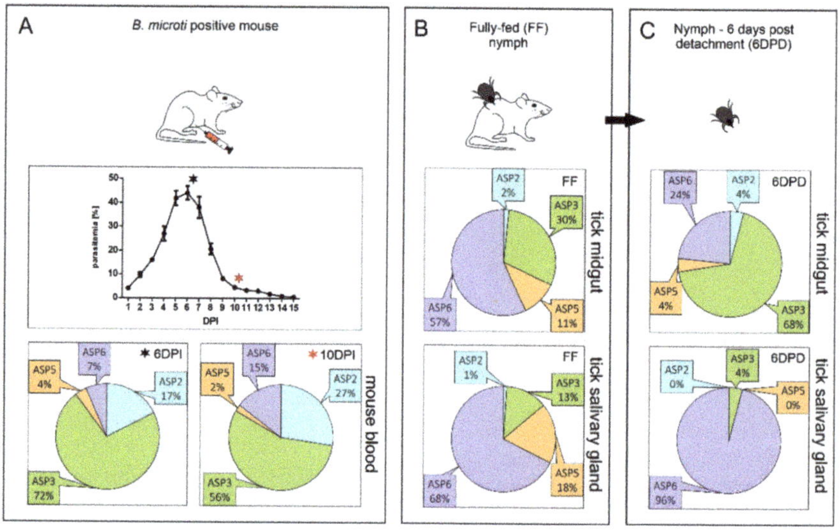

Figure 1. Dynamic expression profile of aspartyl proteases (BmAPs) during the life cycle of *B. microti*. The qPCR results were obtained with cDNA templates prepared from the total RNA isolated: *A*—from mouse blood on the 6th (red asterisk) and 10th (black asterisk) days post parasite injection; *B*—from infected midgut and salivary glands of *I. ricinus* nymphs at fully fed tick stage; *C*—6 days post detachment of *I. ricinus* nymphs from the host. DPI: days post-injection; FF: fully fed stage; 6DPD: 6 days post detachment; ASP2: BmASP2 (BMR1_01G02485, clade B); ASP3: BmASP3a (BmR1_04g07350, clade C); ASP5: BmASP5 (BmR1_04g05270, clade D); ASP6: BmASP6 (BMR1_03g03850, clade E). Relative expression of individual BmASP-encoding mRNAs was counted as percentage ratios of the BmASP mRNA with the highest Ct value (100%) for each cDNA template. The obtained ratios were used to create the pie charts (100% total).

2.2. Data-Mining and Phylogenetic Analysis of Piroplasmid APs Reveals the Presence of Multiple AP Isoenzymes Clustering to Several Apicomplexan AP Clades

2.2.1. Clade A

Our data search throughout available Piroplasmida sequence databases did not reveal a single AP isoenzyme that would cluster into clade A (Figure 2) represented by the digestive vacuole-residing hemoglobinolytic *Plasmodium falciparum* plasmepsins I, II, and IV (PfPM I, PfPM II, and PfPM IV), or the histo-aspartyl protease (HAP/PfPM III) [33]. This clade has apparently formed under the evolutionary demand to digest host haemoglobin. Although both apicomplexan sister orders Haemosporida and Piroplasmida are obligate intracellular parasites whose propagation strictly depends on nutrients provided by the host cell [34], their feeding mechanisms likely differ, which is also reflected in their classification: *Plasmodium* spp. intraerythrocytic stages digest a substantial amount (up to 80%) of host cell haemoglobin (Hb) [35]. Hb proteolysis releases heme, and globin serves as a source of free amino acids. During Hb digestion within the acidic environment of the food vacuole (FV), clade F plasmepsins tightly cooperate with cysteine proteases—falcipains, metalloprotease falcilysin, and other aminopeptidases that complete the degradation process [36]. The digestive plasmepsins are the most closely related isoenzymes among the 10 *P. falciparum* plasmepsins; they share 50–70% amino acid identity, and their encoding genes are located together on one chromosome [37]. Interestingly, the plasmodial species outside the primate-infecting group of *P. falciparum* encode for a single digestive plasmepsin, analogous to PfPM IV [37]. The heme moiety originating from host Hb does not appear to be metabolised or recycled; instead, it is aggregated and polymerised to the dark pigmented hemozoin (Hz) (the name of the order Haemosporida) [38–40].

In contrast to *Plasmodium* spp., piroplasms degrade little if any Hb during host erythrocyte infection, and no pigmented Hz is formed [41–43]. Knowledge of the exact routes of nutrient uptake and processing remains rather unclear and is mainly based on electron microscopy observations of trophozoites. The FV formation via cytostome has been observed in *Theileria* spp., where the optical density of this vacuole indicated potential Hb presence [44]. In addition, *T. equi* possibly uses another tubular feeding structure that is formed via the invagination of an erythrocyte plasma membrane enclosing only a minor amount of ingested cytoplasmic material [45]. *Babesia* does not possess a cytostome; thus, the true FV that emerges from its constriction cannot be formed. The ovoid bodies in *Babesia* trophozoites, initially considered to be true FVs, have since been recognized as invaginations of host cell cytoplasm [46]. In *B. microti*—the basal piroplasmid species (*Babesia microti*-like group)—the obscure coiled structure that protrudes from the parasite into the host cytoplasm has been observed and speculated to contain digestive enzymes. Similarly, possible haemoglobin-containing vesicles were also observed from *B. divergens* trophozoites, indicating—yet not confirming—the endocytic uptake of hemoglobin from the cytoplasm of host erythrocytes [47]. The role of hemoglobin invaginations in trophozoites of different species of *Babesia* remains unclear, but could be relevant to the biology of piroplasms, e.g., by limited digestion of hemoglobin providing the essential source of heme to these heme auxotrophic organisms. Moreover, the special organelle of *B. microti* allegedly contains ferritin, which may be used as a nutrient source for *Babesia* [46]. Although piroplasms do not encode direct homologues of Hb-digesting plasmepsins, they do encode several papain-like cysteine proteases [36]. However, these orthologues of hemoglobinolytic *Plasmodium* spp. falcipains have not yet been subjected to biochemical and functional characterization that would reliably validate their contribution to Hb digestion in erythrocyte-residing piroplasms. Thus far, the only evidence of their essential role in the survival of *Babesia* spp. parasites has come from the observation of a hampering effect on *B. bovis* erythrocyte invasion and in vitro replication by cysteine protease inhibitors [48], and from the lowered parasitemia observed in *B. ovis* erythrocyte cultures exposed to antibodies against ovipain-2, the *B. ovis* orthologue of falcipain-2 from *P. falciparum* [49]. The same applies to the falcilysin protein family represented by one or two isoenzymes in *Babesia* and *Theileria*, respectively [36]. A homologue of the *P. falciparum* heme detoxification protein (HDP) has already been identified in *Babesia* and *Theileria*. However, this homologue supposedly plays a different role than in *Plasmodium* spp., since piroplasms do not form the hemozoin pigment [36]. Overall, the molecular basis of feeding and catabolic metabolism in piroplasms, and the involvement of individual aspartyl and cysteine proteases in protein digestion, remain unclear, and should be addressed by future experimental studies.

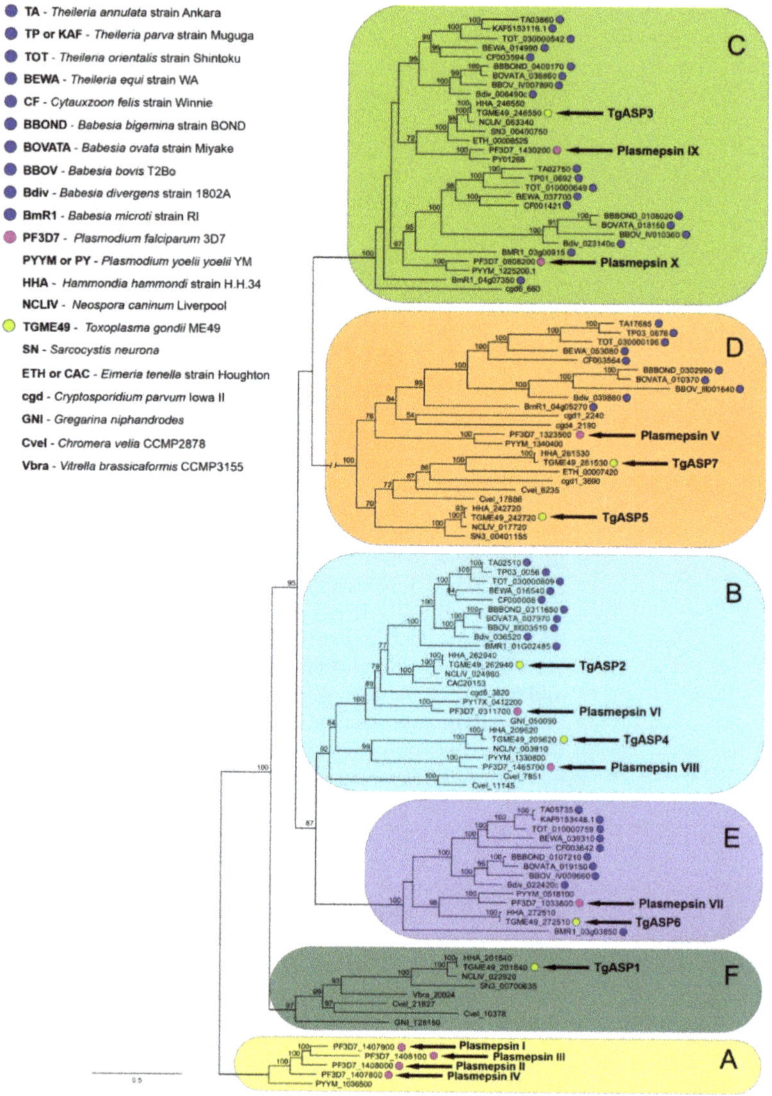

Figure 2. Phylogenetic tree of apicomplexan pepsin family aspartyl proteases (AP). Data-mined APs from selected piroplasmid species cluster into previously determined clades A–F together with their apicomplexan homologues. The image displays the unrooted maximum likelihood phylogenetic tree of 106 selected apicomplexan AP sequences, including those from the basal free-living species *Vitrella brassicaformis* and *Chromera velia;* clades A–F are tagged and highlighted with colours. Sequences were retrieved from EuPathDB and GenBank, and the source organisms are indicated (upper left). Nodal supports were calculated from 1000 bootstrap replicates; those lower than 50 are not depicted. For better orientation within the tree, the 7 *Toxoplasma gondii* ASPs and the 10 *Plasmodium falciparum* plasmepsins are highlighted (arrows: yellow-green and magenta dots, respectively). Data-mined piroplasmid APs are tagged with dark blue dots. Note: The branch leading to clade D was shortened to 25% of its original length for optimal image display. Multiple alignment data are accessible as an online supplementary file at Mendeley Data, link: http://dx.doi.org/10.17632/ds3f2j32ny.1, accessed on 23 September 2021.

2.2.2. Clade B

Clade B is an independent cluster originally recognized as the ancestral group of apicomplexan APs by Jean et al. [50]. Some members of this group—for example, the proteases of *T. gondii* (TgASP2 and TgASP4), *Eimeria tenella* (eimepsin), *Cryptosporidium parvum* (EAK89992), and *Theileria annulata* (TA02510)—are predicted to be GPI-anchored, while plasmepsins VI and VIII lack a sufficiently long hydrophobic region at the C-terminus for the GPI anchor prediction [17]. Our analyses confirm the phylogenetic relation of clades B and E (discussed below) and highlight the existence of three subclusters within the clade B. In addition to the basal subgroup represented by the two *Chromera velia* isoenzymes, the two other independent subgroups are represented by plasmepsin VI (PM VI)/TgASP2 and plasmepsin VIII (PM VIII)/TgASP4, respectively (Figure 2). Interestingly, all analysed piroplasmid species encode for a single clade B AP orthologue clustering with the first listed group of PM VI/TgASP2. Analogously to PM VI, no GPI anchor is predicted in this enzyme (data not shown). Clade B member plasmepsins, studied mostly in the rodent malaria parasite *Plasmodium berghei*, are primarily expressed in oocysts and sporozoites—the parasite transmission stages [24,51]. They play a role in midgut sporozoite development. Functional genomic analyses involving gene disruptions did not confirm the essential roles of these enzymes for the blood stages of malaria [24,52], but the *pm vi* gene knockout did affect sporozoite development from oocysts, resulting in an unsuccessful transmission of the parasite through the mosquito vector [24]. The role of the plasmepsin VI piroplasmid orthologues might thus be connected to the penetration and migration of piroplasmid stages through tick tissues, offering a suitable target to develop transmission-blocking therapy. However, our dynamic expression profiling (Figure 1) analysis controversially revealed a higher abundance of BmASP2-encoding mRNA in the blood stages of *B. microti* in comparison to the tick tissue isolates. This might be explained by the expression of clade B piroplasmid APs already encoding mRNA in gametocytes in host blood, and by regulated protein translation of the clade B AP enzyme later in tick tissues (upon fertilization).

The *P. berghei pm viii* gene knockout lineage developed in the mosquito midgut, but it showed a limited ability of the parasites to egress from oocysts. This was accompanied by a drastic decrease in the number of salivary gland and haemolymph sporozoites with a defect in gliding motility, leading to the block of transmission to hosts [51]. Interestingly, the egress phenotype mirrors that seen with PfPM X knockout lineages in intraerythrocytic parasites (see below). We propose that the reason piroplasms do not possess a direct homologue of the PfPM VIII/TgASP4 subclade is because they do not create—and do not need to egress from—oocysts in the tick gut tissue.

2.2.3. Clade C

In recent years, Clade C of apicomplexan APs has gained a lot of attention, as this group of enzymes have been demonstrated as regulators of invasion and egress of host cells. This clade comprises *P. falciparum* plasmepsins IX and X (PfPM IX and PfPM X), and their *T. gondii* homologue TgASP3 [21,22]. Our analysis clearly identified two different isoenzymes clustering to two groups of clade C piroplasmid APs. While the first piroplasmid group (here termed *Babesia* ASP3b) firmly clusters together with PfPM X (bootstrap value of 97), and its members might thus be considered as the PfPM X direct orthologues, the sister relationship of the second piroplasmid cluster (here termed *Babesia* ASP3a) and the PM IX + TgASP3 group is not well supported (bootstrap value <50). Clade C APs are believed to undergo self-catalytic activation, upon which they proteolytically process/activate a vast number of protein precursors associated with secretory organelles of the apical complex (AC) [19,22,53]. Thus, PfPM IX and PfPM X are the major self-activating maturases standing at the top of the proteolytic machinery regulating *P. falciparum* cell invasion and egress [54]. Although the mechanism of invasion and egress employing the secretory and non-secretory parts of the AC is relatively conserved among apicomplexan parasites, species-specific alterations of the generic mechanisms have evolved [55,56]. *Babesia* and *Plasmodium* replicate solely inside host erythrocytes, and the invasion process involves initial attachment of the parasite to the host cell via a receptor-ligand-mediated interaction [57]. Both parasites interact with glycophorin receptors on the RBC surface, although their surface adhesins differ [58,59]. *Plasmodium* merozoites attach via merozoite surface proteins (MSPs), erythrocyte-binding ligands (EBLs), and reticulocyte binding-like homologues (RHs)—protein families [60] that undergo proteolytic shedding by PfPM X [53]. Proteins of the merozoite surface antigen (MSA) family that are found on the *Babesia* merozoite surface also undergo processing by a yet unidentified sheddase [61]. This role supposedly might be played by the newly identified *Babesia* ASP3b isoenzyme. Similarly, *Theileria*'s surface coat is shed by an undescribed protease, suggesting an identical role of the *Theileria* ASP3b orthologues [62]. Initial attachment of the parasite to the host erythrocyte is followed by the reorientation of the apical tip towards the host cell, and the establishment of the moving (tight) junction (MJ) [63]. The components of MJ—such as the parasite membrane-associated apical membrane antigen 1 (AMA1) and the host cell membrane-anchored rhoptry neck protein complex serving as a ligand structure—are also conserved among piroplasms [63,64]. In *P. falciparum*, AMA1 is directly cleaved by PfPM X, and subsequently shed via PfPM X-activated integral membrane serine protease subtilisin 2 (SUB2) [21]. Since AMA1 of *Babesia* parasites is also proteolytically processed at several positions [65–67], we propose that ASP3b might be analogously involved in AMA1 maturation. However, this concept needs to be experimentally validated because other proteases, such as the intramembrane-cleaving rhomboids that have been identified from *Babesia* [68], cannot be excluded as *Babesia* AMA-1 sheddases working in the same manner as shown in *T. gondii* tachyzoites [69]. Moving junction protein orthologues are most likely dispensable for the non-motile merozoites of *Theileria* that enter the host cell in any orientation via a passive process known as zippering [64,70]. Thus, processing of *Theileria* AMA1 via the *Theileria* ASP3b homologues might be crucial in different motile invasive stages [71]. Upon its internalization within the host cell, *P. falciparum* remains surrounded by parasitophorous vacuole membrane (PVM) and undergoes schizogony. Later, exoneme-specific serine protease subtilisin 1 (PfSUB1), which is cleaved both autocatalytically and by PfPM X, is in charge of PVM lysis, erythrocyte plasma membrane poration, and red blood cell rupture [72]. Only minutes prior to the merozoite's egress from the erythrocyte, PfSUB1 is secreted into the parasitophorous vacuole (PV) space, where it cleaves the pseudoprotease serine repeat antigen 5 (SERA5)—the negative regulator of *P. falciparum* egress [72,73]—as well as other PV-resident proteins important for egress [74]. Additionally, PfSUB1 initiates the primary processing of merozoite surface protein complex (MSP1/6/7) [75,76]. Piroplasmid genomes encode for a single subtilisin-like protease that is believed to represent the direct orthologue of PfSUB1. This protease presumably undergoes analogous post-translation processing during secretory transport [77]. However, the analogy in identical protein substrate cleavage by *Plasmodium* and piroplasmid SUB1 proteases [78], as well as the involvement of the activated SUB1 enzyme in *Babesia* and *Theileria* parasite egress from erythrocytes, remains to be experimentally confirmed. Notably, PfPM X mRNA is also transcribed in gametocytes, while the protein can be found in gametes, zygotes, and ookinetes. In the late stage of ookinete development, PfPM X cleaves the cell-traversal protein of ookinetes and sporozoites (CelTOS) [21]. This processing is necessary for ookinetes to pass through arthropod cells to the site of oocyst formation. Moreover, the disruption of CelTOS abolishes liver infection by *P. berghei* sporozoites [79]. As CelTOS is conserved among apicomplexan parasites [80], we propose that its processing by clade C APs plays an important role during the transmission of piroplasmid species through their tick vectors.

PfPM IX, the second *P. falciparum* protease member of the apicomplexan clade C APs, has been previously confirmed to be a key maturase involved in erythrocyte invasion by *P. falciparum* merozoites [21]. However, more recent contributions have speculated as to its multifaceted role throughout the malaria parasite life cycle [53]. PfPM IX processes rhoptry-associated protein 1 (RAP1) and rhoptry neck protein 3 (RON3), which are released into the PV during invasion and later aid the parasite's development within the PV [81,82]. The translation initiation of PM IX has been suggested during *P. berghei* gamete development in mosquitos, where PM IX cleaves merozoite thrombospondin-related anonymous protein (MTRAP), enabling the release of gametes from host erythrocytes [83]. When mosquitoes were infected with PbMTRAP knockout gametocytes, the oocyst formation was aborted. In addition, these gametocytes were unable to form ookinetes (the motile form of zygote) in vitro. Particularly, TRAP is a conserved family of proteins that are involved in the gliding motility of apicomplexan parasites, and are also found in *Babesia* [68,83]. This suggests that piroplasmid APs branching together with PM IX might be involved in the development of zygotes and kinetes within tick tissues, as indicated by the expression of BmASP3 mRNA following the detachment of tick nymphs from the host (Figure 1C).

2.2.4. Clade D

Clade D is the most derived group of apicomplexan APs within our phylogenetic analysis (Figure 2); it consists of distant relatives of the human β-site amyloid precursor protein-cleaving enzyme (BACE) [27]—the major beta secretase generating amyloid-β peptides in the neurons. BACE is also responsible for the generation of the amyloid-β peptides that aggregate in the brains of Alzheimer's patients and, thus, represents a valuable target for drug development [84]. These proteases have a long C-terminal extension with a trans-membrane domain that serves for their anchoring to membranes. The most studied member of this clade is PfPM V—a *P. falciparum* endoplasmic reticulum (ER)-resident protease that has been demonstrated to cleave proteins containing the *Plasmodium* export element RxLxE/Q/D (PEXEL) motif [26]. These effector proteins are then secreted through the PV surrounding the parasite during the intracellular infection and multiplication to host erythrocytes [26,27]. PfPM V has also been shown to be essential for gametocyte development [32]. Thus, specific inhibition of PfPM V activity appears to be a highly convenient therapy targeting both the asexual and sexual stages of malaria [32,85]. Interesting findings have been made with PM V's corresponding *T. gondii* orthologue TgASP5—a Golgi-resident AP that processes TEXEL (*T. gondii* PEXEL-like) motif containing dense-granule proteins (GRAs) [86]. Analogously to its orthologue PfPM V, TgASP5 plays an important role during intracellular parasite survival and multiplication [87], as well as modulation of host cell responses [28]. Another *T. gondii* isoenzyme, TgASP7, which also clusters within clade D, is not expressed in the tachyzoite stage, and its functional role remains unknown [17].

Our phylogenetic analysis revealed piroplasmid clade D APs to be a single subgroup that clusters alongside *Cryptosporidium* and *Plasmodium* PM V. Thus, we propose that they play a similar role in the secretory pathway of piroplasms—the cleavage of PEXEL-like containing proteins in the ER of the cell—although we expect significant differences due to the different strategy of piroplasms in persisting inside infected cells. Shortly upon host cell invasion, *Babesia* and *Theileria* parasites are surrounded by a PVM that is derived from the host cell cytoplasmic membrane, but unlike the *Plasmodium* and *Toxoplasma* PVM, it starts its disintegration after parasite internalization [31,88,89]. It has been discussed previously that the PVM breaks down either because piroplasms are not able to incorporate lipids into the PVM during parasite intracellular growth, or because they have developed this strategy as a more convenient way to transport effector proteins into infected host cells in order to alter their morphology and physiology [90]. The persistence of piroplasms directly in host cell cytoplasm is thus different to *P. falciparum* residing in the PV surrounded by the PVM. In the malaria parasite, the PEXEL-containing protein precursors are cleaved by the ER-resident PM V immediately upon their translation. This facilitates them for export to the PV, PVM, and all the way to the host cell [26]. The PEXEL-motif-containing exportome of *P. falciparum* is estimated to include ~463 proteins [26]. On the other hand, TgASP5 recognizes only several identified TEXEL-motif-harbouring proteins, but also appears to be important for the trafficking of other (non-TEXEL)-secreted proteins during intracellular infection with *T. gondii* tachyzoites [91]. Both *Plasmodium* and *Toxoplasma* use sophisticated protein transporting complexes PTEX (plasmodium translocon of exported proteins) and the MYR translocon, respectively, which are incorporated into the PVM [92,93]. Unsurprisingly, piroplasms do not encode for components of the *Plasmodium* translocon machinery [29], with the single exception of the PTEX complex protein component HSP101, which is expressed across all piroplasms [62].

The PEXEL-like motif (PLM) has also been recognized in various piroplasmid proteins. This supports the above-given hypothesis of functional analogy between the piroplasmid clade D APs and plasmodial PM V enzymes [94]. PLM has been recognized in *B. bovis* variant erythrocyte surface antigens (VESAs) [95] involved in erythrocyte adhesion and antigenic variation of the red blood cell surface—sophisticated parasite-driven mechanisms enabling the infected erythrocytes to evade host immune responses [96]. VESA1-like proteins have also been described from the genomes of other piroplasmid species—the *Babesia* sensu stricto group [97], and the *B. microti*-like group [98]—indicating that VESA processing by clade D APs might be an immunoevasive strategy shared across *Babesia* species. Small open reading frame protein families (SmORFs) and spherical body protein-2 protein family members (SBP2) also contain PLM [94]. While SmORFs are also involved in erythrocyte adhesion [95,96], SBP2 proteins concentrate under the red blood cell cytoplasmic membrane and are believed to alternate the red blood cell surface [99]. Although PLM has not yet been detected in *Theileria* [62,97], the apparent conservation of clade D APs within the phylum suggests the preserved mode of protein processing across Piroplasmida. Further studies on clade D APs should further elucidate the exact role of these enzymes in the trafficking mechanisms of *Babesia* spp. effector proteins affecting infected host cells.

2.2.5. Clade E

This group of apicomplexan APs is clearly determined by our phylogenetic analysis as the sister clade to clade B, which includes PM VII and TgASP6 (Figure 2). PM VII is thus sometimes classified together with clade B PM VI and PM VIII as the transmission-stage plasmepsins [37]. PM VII is produced in the ookinetes of *P. falciparum*, supposedly upon fertilization, as PM VII is not detected in *P. falciparum* gametocytes [23]. Its role remains unknown—it has been proven to be disposable for the parasite, as the PM VII knockout had no effect on any stage of the *P. berghei* life cycle [23]. However, the authors of this study also note that redundancy exists among transmission-stage-expressed plasmepsins—and especially clade B member PM VIII, which shares a similar expression profile with PM VII, may thus compensate for its loss of function [100]. This would probably not be the case for piroplasms, which do not possess direct homologues of PM VIII, but produce a single clade E AP orthologue. If the clade B PM VI orthologues play a role in regulating sporogony in tick salivary glands, the remaining function for clade E piroplasmid APs might thus insist in parasite invasion of tick tissues upon zygote formation. This is in accordance with the obtained expression profile of BmASP6 in stages developing within the vector midgut (Figure 1). However, some role of BmASP6 and other clade E piroplasmid APs in sporogony should not be fully excluded, as BmASP6 mRNA is also present in the salivary glands of infected tick nymphs (Figure 1).

2.2.6. Clade F

This is a diverse group of apicomplexan APs first identified in our 2016 contribution [16], and now once more confirmed by our current phylogenetic analysis (Figure 2). This group is represented by TgASP1 and its coccidian homologues, as well as some APs of gregarines and free-living basal Apicomplexa. TgASP1 is an enzyme associated with the secretory pathway in non-dividing cells, which re-localizes in close proximity to the nascent inner membrane complex (IMC) of daughter cells during replication [17]. However, it's role is non-vital for *T. gondii* [101], and Haemosporida and Piroplasmida genomes apparently do not encode any of the clade F homologues as they might have lost these disposable proteases as a part of their adaptation to the parasitic lifestyle and the evolution of specific intracellular multiplication mechanisms differing from *T. gondii* endodyogeny [102].

3. Conclusions

Babesia and other Piroplasmida encode for several pepsin (cathepsin-D-like) family AP isoenzymes. Their phylogenetic relation to malarial plasmepsins and analogous enzymes from other apicomplexan parasites enable the prediction of their various roles within the lifecycle of these erythrocyte-infecting parasites (Figure 3). These roles are associated with their different protein structures, time-expression profiles, and intracellular localization. As these enzymes have been long considered and recently validated as great therapeutic targets for malaria, they are worthy of scientific attention when proposing novel therapeutic strategies for babesiosis (piroplasmosis).

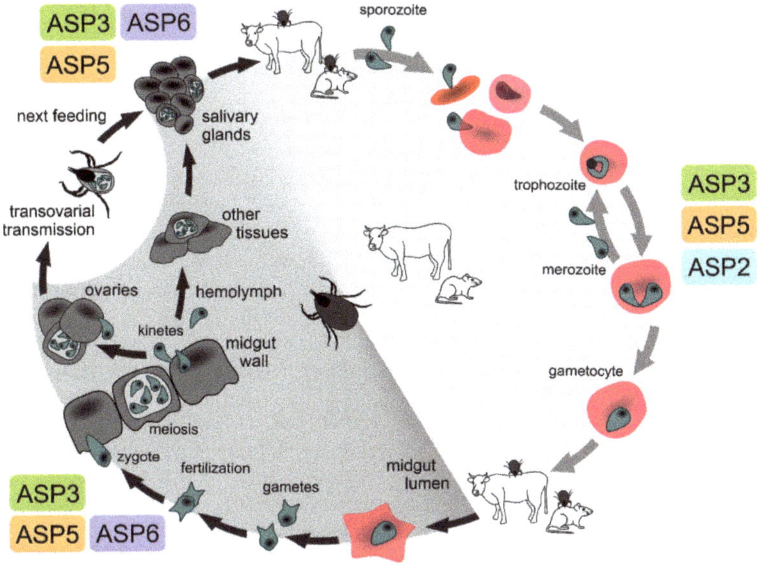

Figure 3. The role of *Babesia* plasmepsin-like APs marked within the generic life cycle of *Babesia* parasites. Sporozoites are transmitted from the salivary glands of an infected tick to the vertebrate host bloodstream during tick feeding. They invade red blood cells, where they start asexual multiplication (merogony). The cyclic egress and invasion of host red blood cells by haploid merozoites represents the intraerythrocytic cycle, causing the symptoms of babesiosis in vertebrates by time the first sexual stages (gametocytes) occur in the bloodstream. When another naïve tick feeds on the infected host, gametocytes are ingested with the blood meal, mature, and produce gametes in the tick gut lumen (gamogony). Newly developed gametes fuse in a zygote, which passes through the peritrophic matrix into tick gut epithelial cells. Meiotic division and subsequent mitosis give rise to primary kinetes, which invade and multiply in different tick tissues. Newly emerged secondary kinetes undergo multiplication in salivary glands (sporogony). Upon the tick metamorphosis, motile sporozoites are transmitted to the host with the blood meal (transstadial transmission). Secondary kinetes of *Babesia* sensu stricto species are capable of invading and multiplying within adult female ovaries and can be transmitted to the larval progeny (transovarial transmission), while the *Babesia microti*-like group parasites are transmitted solely transstadially [25]. The colour-marked text notes indicate the positions in the *Babesia* life cycle positions where the five aspartyl proteases ASP2, ASP3a, ASP3b, ASP5, and ASP6 supposedly play their herein-deduced roles. White background: part of *Babesia* life cycle occurring in the vertebrate host; grey background: part of *Babesia* life cycle occurring within the tick vector.

4. Materials and Methods

4.1. *B. microti* Propagation in Mice

B. microti (Franca) Reichenow (strain Peabody mjr) was obtained from ATCC (ATTC® PRA-99™, USA). Two BABL/c mice, supplied by Charles River Laboratories (VELAZ), were intraperitoneally injected with 150 μL of *B. microti*-infected murine blood (50% parasitemia, 800 × 10^6 of infected red blood cells). One mouse was kept under general anaesthesia, and the blood was collected from the carotid artery into sodium citrate-phosphate-dextrose solution (ratio 1:25, Sigma-Aldrich) on the 6th day post injection (6DPI) according to 50% parasitemia. Similarly, the blood was obtained from the second mouse when parasitemia dropped to 5% on the 10th day post injection (10DPI). The murine experiment was performed repeatedly to confirm the results of expression profiling. All laboratory animals were treated in accordance with the Animal Protection Law of the Czech Republic No. 246/1992 Sb., ethics approval No. 25/2018.

4.2. RNA Isolation from Tick Tissues and Murine Blood Cells

Pathogen-free *Ixodes ricinus* nymphs were obtained from the in-house breeding facility of the Institute of Parasitology, BC CAS, Ceske Budejovice, Czech Republic. Twenty individuals were placed on one *B. microti*-positive BABL/c mouse in the acute phase of infection (1–4DPI, Figure 1A) and allowed to feed until repletion (around 72 h). The fully fed (FF) nymphs were collected and surface-sterilized by washing in 3% H_2O_2, 70% ethanol, and distilled water (each wash 30 s). Ticks were separated into two groups: first group of 10 nymphs was dissected immediately (FF stage), while the other 10 individuals were kept at room temperature in a humid chamber until they were dissected on the 6th day post detachment (6DPD). Dissection of tick tissues (salivary glands and midguts) was performed under a stereomicroscope (Olympus) on wax dishes with diethyl pyrocarbonate (DEPC)-treated cold phosphate-buffered saline (PBS), and then transferred into RA1 buffer (NucleoSpin RNA II Kit, Macherey-Nagel, Düren, Germany) supplemented with β-mercaptoethanol (Sigma-Aldrich). Prior to the extraction, the collected tissues were homogenised using an insulin syringe. Total RNA was extracted from the pool of midguts and salivary glands originating from 10 individual ticks via the NucleoSpin RNA II Kit, following the protocol provided by the manufacturer (Macherey-Nagel, Düren, Germany). Murine blood total RNA was isolated using the previously described protocol [103]. Samples were collected from two timepoints at 6 and 10 DPI. The quality and concentration of total RNA were checked by gel electrophoresis and determined using a NanoDrop UV spectrophotometer (Thermo Fisher Scientific; Waltham, MA, USA), and RNA samples were stored at −80 °C.

4.3. Quantitative RT-PCR

Reverse transcription was performed from 1 μg of total RNA isolate using the Transcriptor High-Fidelity cDNA Synthesis Kit (Roche Diagnostics GmbH; Mannheim, Germany). The resulting cDNA was used as a template for the quantitative real-time PCR (qRT-PCR) using a LightCycler 480 (Roche Diagnostics GmbH), the Fast Star Universal SYBR Green Master Mix (Roche Diagnostics GmbH), and according primer pairs BmASP2 forward: 5′-TCCGGCGTCTATTGAAGAGT-3′/BmASP2 reverse: 5′-TGAACCGGTGTCAAAA ACAA-3′; BmASP3 forward: 5′-GGAAGCTTGGGGAGTCTGTA-3′/BmASP3 reverse: 5′-TGTGCTCCCTGTGTCGAATA-3′; BmASP5 forward: 5′-GCCCAAACACCACCAACTAT-3′/BmASP5 reverse: 5′-CACCAAATGCGAGATACACG-3′; BmASP6 forward: 5′-GATTGG GCTTCCCAAACAC-3′/BmASP6 reverse: 5′-ATCCGCCAGTTGAATCTTTG-3′. All qRT-PCR amplifications were performed in technical triplicates. Relative expressions were calculated using the mathematical model of the ΔCt method [104] and normalized to *B. microti* actin (GenBank XM_012791652; primers—BmActin forward: 5′-GGCCTACTCACAGCCCT TTA-3′/BmActin reverse: 5′-ACAGGGTTGTAGAGTGTTGGTT-3′). To express the representation of all isoenzymes as a percentage per time point, the ASP with the highest Ct value was set as 100%, and the values for other ASP isoenzymes were accordingly recalculated. The algorithm applied later adjusted the values to fit the total of 100% in a pie chart.

4.4. Phylogenetic Analysis

The dataset used for the phylogenetic analysis comprised 106 AP protein sequences of representatives from the phylum Apicomplexa, and related *Vitrella* and *Chromera* spp. Clade F involving digestive plasmepsins served as an outgroup. All sequences were retrieved from either GenBank or EuPathDB using the blastp and tblastn BLAST algorithms and an E-value cutoff of 10^{-5}. Alignment was constructed in Geneious Prime 2020.1.2. using MAFFT v7.017 [105] with the default parameters for the gap opening penalty (1.53) and the offset value (0.123). The protein sequences were crosschecked for the presence of DTG/DTG or DTG/DSG aspartic protease motifs. Poorly aligned N- (signal peptide included) and C-termini were manually trimmed, which resulted in the final alignment comprising 324 amino acid positions. The phylogenetic tree was reconstructed via maximum likelihood (ML) method in IQ-TREE v1.6.12 [106], using the WAG + F + I + G4 model selected by ModelFinder [107]. Bootstraps were based on 1000 replicates. The tree was visualized in Geneious Prime v2019.0.4 and graphically modified in CorelDRAW graphic suite 2020.

Supplementary Materials: The multiple alignment data used to construct the maximum likelihood tree in Figure 2 are accessible online at Mendeley Data, link: http://dx.doi.org/10.17632/ds3f2j32ny.1, accessed on 23 September 2021.

Author Contributions: P.Š. and D.S. designed and performed the experiments, performed the analyses, and wrote the original draft; P.B.-S. supervised phylogenetic analysis, its visualization and interpretation, and reviewed and edited the manuscript; M.J. designed the expression profiling experiments, performed qPCR, and reviewed and edited the manuscript. All authors have read and agreed to the published version of the manuscript.

Funding: This work was primarily supported by the grant Czech Science Foundation (GA CR) project No. 20-05736S, and the ERDF/ESF Centre for research of pathogenicity and virulence of parasites (No.CZ.02.1.01/0.0/0.0/16_019/0000759). P.Š. was additionally supported by an internal grant from the University of South Bohemia GAJU No. 120/2021/P. D.S. and P.B-S. were additionally supported by the grant number LTAUSA17201 from the Ministry of Education, Youth, and Sports of the Czech Republic.

Institutional Review Board Statement: All animal experiments were carried out in accordance with the Animal Protection Law of the Czech Republic No. 246/1992 Sb., ethics approval No. 34/2018, and protocols approved by the responsible committee of the Institute of Parasitology, Biology Centre of the Czech Academy of Sciences.

Informed Consent Statement: Not applicable.

Data Availability Statement: All data are either contained within the manuscript and supporting information or available from the corresponding author on reasonable request.

Acknowledgments: We would like to thank Luïse Robbertse, David Hartmann, and Dominika Reichensdörferová for their initial help with *Babesia* parasites, and their previous involvement in apicomplexan-AP-related topics. We would also like to thank to the head of the laboratory of Vector Immunology, IoP BC CAS, Ceske Budejovice, Petr Kopáček, for his continuous support.

Conflicts of Interest: The authors declare no conflict of interest.

References

1. Jalovecka, M.; Sojka, D.; Ascencio, M.; Schnittger, L. Babesia life cycle–when phylogeny meets biology. *Trends Parasitol.* **2019**, *35*, 356–368. [CrossRef]
2. Vannier, E.; Krause, P.J. Babesiosis. In *Hunter's Tropical Medicine and Emerging Infectious Diseases*; Elsevier: Amsterdam, The Netherlands, 2020; pp. 799–802.
3. Schnittger, L.; Rodriguez, A.E.; Florin-Christensen, M.; Morrison, D.A. Babesia: A world emerging. *Infect. Genet. Evol.* **2012**, *12*, 1788–1809. [CrossRef]

4. Florin-Christensen, M.; Suarez, C.E.; Rodriguez, A.E.; Flores, D.A.; Schnittger, L. Vaccines against bovine babesiosis: Where we are now and possible roads ahead. *Parasitology* **2014**, *141*, 1563–1592. [CrossRef]
5. Rubel, F.; Brugger, K.; Pfeffer, M.; Chitimia-Dobler, L.; Didyk, Y.M.; Leverenz, S.; Dautel, H.; Kahl, O. Geographical distribution of *Dermacentor marginatus and Dermacentor reticulatus* in Europe. *Ticks Tick-Borne Dis.* **2016**, *7*, 224–233. [CrossRef]
6. Vannier, E.; Krause, P.J. Human babesiosis. *N. Engl. J. Med.* **2012**, *366*, 2397–2407. [CrossRef]
7. Lobo, C.A.; Cursino-Santos, J.R.; Alhassan, A.; Rodrigues, M. Babesia: An emerging infectious threat in transfusion medicine. *PLoS Pathog.* **2013**, *9*, e1003387. [CrossRef]
8. Lempereur, L.; Shiels, B.; Heyman, P.; Moreau, E.; Saegerman, C.; Losson, B.; Malandrin, L. A retrospective serological survey on human babesiosis in Belgium. *Clin. Microbiol. Infect.* **2015**, *21*, 96.e91–96.e97. [CrossRef] [PubMed]
9. Arsuaga, M.; González, L.M.; Padial, E.S.; Dinkessa, A.W.; Sevilla, E.; Trigo, E.; Puente, S.; Gray, J.; Montero, E. Misdiagnosis of babesiosis as malaria, Equatorial Guinea, 2014. *Emerg. Infect. Dis.* **2018**, *24*, 1588–1589. [CrossRef]
10. Rathinasamy, V.; Poole, W.A.; Bastos, R.G.; Suarez, C.E.; Cooke, B.M. Babesiosis vaccines: Lessons learned, challenges ahead, and future glimpses. *Trends Parasitol.* **2019**, *35*, 622–635. [CrossRef] [PubMed]
11. Lemieux, J.E.; Tran, A.D.; Freimark, L.; Schaffner, S.F.; Goethert, H.; Andersen, K.G.; Bazner, S.; Li, A.; McGrath, G.; Sloan, L. A global map of genetic diversity in *Babesia microti* reveals strong population structure and identifies variants associated with clinical relapse. *Nat. Microbiol.* **2016**, *1*, 1–7. [CrossRef] [PubMed]
12. Simon, M.S.; Westblade, L.F.; Dziedziech, A.; Visone, J.E.; Furman, R.R.; Jenkins, S.G.; Schuetz, A.N.; Kirkman, L.A. Clinical and molecular evidence of atovaquone and azithromycin resistance in relapsed *Babesia microti* infection associated with rituximab and chronic lymphocytic leukemia. *Clin. Infect. Dis.* **2017**, *65*, 1222–1225. [CrossRef]
13. McKerrow, J.H.; Caffrey, C.; Kelly, B.; Loke, P.n.; Sajid, M. Proteases in parasitic diseases. *Annu. Rev. Pathol. Mech. Dis.* **2006**, *1*, 497–536. [CrossRef]
14. Rawlings, N.D.; Bateman, A. How to use the MEROPS database and website to help understand peptidase specificity. *Protein Sci.* **2021**, *30*, 83–92. [CrossRef]
15. Barrett, A.J.; Rawlings, N.D.; Salvesen, G.; Woessner, J.F. Handbook of proteolytic enzymes introduction. In *Handbook of Proteolytic Enzymes*, 3rd ed.; Elsevier: Abingdon, UK, 2012; ISBN 9780123822208.
16. Sojka, D.; Hartmann, D.; Bartošová-Sojková, P.; Dvořák, J. Parasite cathepsin D-like peptidases and their relevance as therapeutic targets. *Trends Parasitol.* **2016**, *32*, 708–723. [CrossRef]
17. Shea, M.; Jäkle, U.; Liu, Q.; Berry, C.; Joiner, K.A.; Soldati-Favre, D. A family of aspartic proteases and a novel, dynamic and cell-cycle-dependent protease localization in the secretory pathway of *Toxoplasma Gondii. Traffic* **2007**, *8*, 1018–1034. [CrossRef]
18. Coombs, G.H.; Goldberg, D.E.; Klemba, M.; Berry, C.; Kay, J.; Mottram, J.C. Aspartic proteases of *Plasmodium falciparum* and other parasitic protozoa as drug targets. *Trends Parasitol.* **2001**, *17*, 532–537. [CrossRef]
19. Burrows, J.N.; Soldati-Favre, D. Targeting plasmepsins—an achilles' heel of the malaria parasite. *Cell Host Microbe* **2020**, *27*, 496–498. [CrossRef] [PubMed]
20. Jalovecka, M.; Urbanova, V.; Sojka, D.; Malandrin, L.; Sima, R.; Kopacek, P.; Hajdusek, O. Establishment of *Babesia microti* laboratory model and its experimental application. In Proceedings of the 9. Tick and Tick-borne Pathogen Conference and 1st Asia Pacific Rickettsia Conference, Cairns, Australia, 20 August 2017; p. 140.
21. Pino, P.; Caldelari, R.; Mukherjee, B.; Vahokoski, J.; Klages, N.; Maco, B.; Collins, C.R.; Blackman, M.J.; Kursula, I.; Heussler, V. A multistage antimalarial targets the plasmepsins IX and X essential for invasion and egress. *Science* **2017**, *358*, 522–528. [CrossRef]
22. Dogga, S.K.; Mukherjee, B.; Jacot, D.; Kockmann, T.; Molino, L.; Hammoudi, P.-M.; Hartkoorn, R.C.; Hehl, A.B.; Soldati-Favre, D. A druggable secretory protein maturase of Toxoplasma essential for invasion and egress. *Elife* **2017**, *6*, e27480. [CrossRef] [PubMed]
23. Li, F.; Bounkeua, V.; Pettersen, K.; Vinetz, J.M. *Plasmodium falciparum* ookinete expression of plasmepsin VII and plasmepsin X. *Malar. J.* **2016**, *15*, 1–10. [CrossRef] [PubMed]
24. Ecker, A.; Bushell, E.S.; Tewari, R.; Sinden, R.E. Reverse genetics screen identifies six proteins important for malaria development in the mosquito. *Mol. Microbiol.* **2008**, *70*, 209–220. [CrossRef] [PubMed]
25. Jalovecka, M.; Hajdusek, O.; Sojka, D.; Kopacek, P.; Malandrin, L. The complexity of piroplasms life cycles. *Front. Cell. Infect. Microbiol.* **2018**, *8*, 248. [CrossRef]
26. Boddey, J.A.; Carvalho, T.G.; Hodder, A.N.; Sargeant, T.J.; Sleebs, B.E.; Marapana, D.; Lopaticki, S.; Nebl, T.; Cowman, A.F. Role of plasmepsin V in export of diverse protein families from the *Plasmodium falciparum* exportome. *Traffic* **2013**, *14*, 532–550. [CrossRef] [PubMed]
27. Russo, I.; Babbitt, S.; Muralidharan, V.; Butler, T.; Oksman, A.; Goldberg, D.E. Plasmepsin V licenses Plasmodium proteins for export into the host erythrocyte. *Nature* **2010**, *463*, 632–636. [CrossRef]
28. Coffey, M.J.; Dagley, L.F.; Seizova, S.; Kapp, E.A.; Infusini, G.; Roos, D.S.; Boddey, J.A.; Webb, A.I.; Tonkin, C.J. Aspartyl protease 5 matures dense granule proteins that reside at the host-parasite interface. *Toxoplasma Gondii. MBio* **2018**, *9*, e01718–e01796. [CrossRef] [PubMed]
29. Silva, J.C.; Cornillot, E.; McCracken, C.; Usmani-Brown, S.; Dwivedi, A.; Ifeonu, O.O.; Crabtree, J.; Gotia, H.T.; Virji, A.Z.; Reynes, C.; et al. Genome-wide diversity and gene expression profiling of *Babesia microti* isolates identify polymorphic genes that mediate host-pathogen interactions. *Sci. Rep.* **2016**, *6*, 35284. [CrossRef]

30. Thekkiniath, J.; Kilian, N.; Lawres, L.; Gewirtz, M.A.; Graham, M.M.; Liu, X.; Ledizet, M.; Mamoun, C.B. Evidence for vesicle-mediated antigen export by the human pathogen *Babesia Microti*. *Life Sci. Alliance* **2019**, *2*, e201900382. [CrossRef]
31. Rudzinska, M.A.; Trager, W.; Lewengrub, S.J.; Gubert, E. An electron microscopic study of *Babesia microti* invading erythrocytes. *Cell Tissue Res.* **1976**, *169*, 323–334. [CrossRef]
32. Jennison, C.; Lucantoni, L.; O'Neill, M.T.; McConville, R.; Erickson, S.M.; Cowman, A.F.; Sleebs, B.E.; Avery, V.M.; Boddey, J.A. Inhibition of plasmepsin V activity blocks *Plasmodium falciparum* gametocytogenesis and transmission to mosquitoes. *Cell Rep.* **2019**, *29*, 3796–3806.e3794. [CrossRef]
33. Liu, J.; Gluzman, I.Y.; Drew, M.E.; Goldberg, D.E. The role of *Plasmodium falciparum* food vacuole plasmepsins. *J. Biol. Chem.* **2005**, *280*, 1432–1437. [CrossRef]
34. Votýpka, J.; Modrý, D.; Oborník, M.; Šlapeta, J.; Lukeš, J. Apicomplexa. *Handb. Protists* **2017**, *2*, 567–624.
35. Rinehart, M.T.; Park, H.S.; Walzer, K.A.; Chi, J.-T.A.; Wax, A. Hemoglobin consumption by *P. falciparum* in individual erythrocytes imaged via quantitative phase spectroscopy. *Sci. Rep.* **2016**, *6*, 1–9. [CrossRef]
36. Ponsuwanna, P.; Kochakarn, T.; Bunditvorapoom, D.; Kümpornsin, K.; Otto, T.D.; Ridenour, C.; Chotivanich, K.; Wilairat, P.; White, N.J.; Miotto, O. Comparative genome-wide analysis and evolutionary history of haemoglobin-processing and haem detoxification enzymes in malarial parasites. *Malar. J.* **2016**, *15*, 1–14. [CrossRef]
37. Nasamu, A.S.; Polino, A.J.; Istvan, E.S.; Goldberg, D.E. Malaria parasite plasmepsins: More than just plain old degradative pepsins. *J. Biol. Chem.* **2020**, *295*, 8425–8441. [CrossRef]
38. Rosenthal, P.J.; Meshnick, S.R. Hemoglobin catabolism and iron utilization by malaria parasites. *Mol. Biochem. Parasitol.* **1996**, *83*, 131–139. [CrossRef]
39. Lew, V.L.; Tiffert, T.; Ginsburg, H. Excess hemoglobin digestion and the osmotic stability of *Plasmodium falciparum*–infected red blood cells. *Blood* **2003**, *101*, 4189–4194. [CrossRef] [PubMed]
40. Chugh, M.; Sundararaman, V.; Kumar, S.; Reddy, V.S.; Siddiqui, W.A.; Stuart, K.D.; Malhotra, P. Protein complex directs hemoglobin-to-hemozoin formation in *Plasmodium falciparum*. *Proc. Natl. Acad. Sci. USA* **2013**, *110*, 5392–5397. [CrossRef] [PubMed]
41. Park, H.; Hong, S.-H.; Kim, K.; Cho, S.-H.; Lee, W.-J.; Kim, Y.; Lee, S.-E.; Park, Y. Characterizations of individual mouse red blood cells parasitized by *Babesia microti* using 3-D holographic microscopy. *Sci. Rep.* **2015**, *5*, 1–11. [CrossRef]
42. Lempereur, L.; Beck, R.; Fonseca, I.; Marques, C.; Duarte, A.; Santos, M.; Zúquete, S.; Gomes, J.; Walder, G.; Domingos, A. Guidelines for the detection of Babesia and Theileria parasites. *Vector-Borne Zoonotic Dis.* **2017**, *17*, 51–65. [CrossRef]
43. Cursino-Santos, J.R.; Singh, M.; Senaldi, E.; Manwani, D.; Yazdanbakhsh, K.; Lobo, C.A. Altered parasite life-cycle processes characterize *Babesia divergens* infection in human sickle cell anemia. *Haematologica* **2019**, *104*, 2189. [CrossRef]
44. Fawcett, D.W.; Conrad, P.A.; Grootenhuis, J.G.; Morzaria, S.P. Ultrastructure of the intra-erythrocytic stage of Theileria species from cattle and waterbuck. *Tissue Cell* **1987**, *19*, 643–655. [CrossRef]
45. Guimarães, A.M.; Lima, J.D.; Ribeiro, M.F. Ultrastructure of *Babesia equi* trophozoites isolated in Minas Gerais, Brazil. *Pesqui. Vet. Bras.* **2003**, *23*, 101–104. [CrossRef]
46. Rudzinska, M.A. Ultrastructure of intraerythrocytic *Babesia microti* with emphasis on the feeding mechanism. *J. Protozool.* **1976**, *23*, 224–233. [CrossRef] [PubMed]
47. Conesa, J.J.; Sevilla, E.; Terrón, M.C.; González, L.M.; Gray, J.; Pérez-Berná, A.J.; Carrascosa, J.L.; Pereiro, E.; Chichón, F.J.; Luque, D.; et al. Four-dimensional characterizationof the *Babesia divergens* asexual life cycle, from the trophozoite to the multiparasite stage. *MSphere* **2020**, *5*, e00928-20. [CrossRef]
48. Okubo, K.; Yokoyama, N.; Govind, Y.; Alhassan, A.; Igarashi, I. *Babesia bovis*: Effects of cysteine protease inhibitors on in vitro growth. *Exp. Parasitol.* **2007**, *117*, 214–217. [CrossRef]
49. Carletti, T.; Barreto, C.; Mesplet, M.; Mira, A.; Weir, W.; Shiels, B.; Oliva, A.G.; Schnittger, L.; Florin-Christensen, M. Characterization of a papain-like cysteine protease essential for the survival of *Babesia ovis* merozoites. *Ticks Tick-Borne Dis.* **2016**, *7*, 85–93. [CrossRef] [PubMed]
50. Jean, L.; Long, M.; Young, J.; Péry, P.; Tomley, F. Aspartyl proteinase genes from apicomplexan parasites: Evidence for evolution of the gene structure. *Trends Parasitol.* **2001**, *17*, 491–498. [CrossRef]
51. Mastan, B.S.; Narwal, S.K.; Dey, S.; Kumar, K.A.; Mishra, S. *Plasmodium berghei* plasmepsin VIII is essential for sporozoite gliding motility. *Int. J. Parasitol.* **2017**, *47*, 239–245. [CrossRef]
52. Banerjee, R.; Liu, J.; Beatty, W.; Pelosof, L.; Klemba, M.; Goldberg, D.E. Four plasmepsins are active in the *Plasmodium falciparum* food vacuole, including a protease with an active-site histidine. *Proc. Natl. Acad. Sci. USA* **2002**, *99*, 990–995. [CrossRef]
53. Favuzza, P.; de Lera Ruiz, M.; Thompson, J.K.; Triglia, T.; Ngo, A.; Steel, R.W.; Vavrek, M.; Christensen, J.; Healer, J.; Boyce, C. Dual plasmepsin-targeting antimalarial agents disrupt multiple stages of the malaria parasite life cycle. *Cell Host Microbe* **2020**, *27*, 642–658.e612. [CrossRef] [PubMed]
54. Sojka, D.; Šnebergerová, P.; Robbertse, L. Protease inhibition—an established strategy to combat infectious diseases. *Int. J. Mol. Sci.* **2021**, *22*, 5762. [CrossRef]
55. Meissner, M.; Ferguson, D.J.; Frischknecht, F. Invasion factors of apicomplexan parasites: Essential or redundant? *Curr. Opin. Microbiol.* **2013**, *16*, 438–444. [CrossRef] [PubMed]
56. Frénal, K.; Dubremetz, J.-F.; Lebrun, M.; Soldati-Favre, D. Gliding motility powers invasion and egress in Apicomplexa. *Nat. Rev. Microbiol.* **2017**, *15*, 645–660. [CrossRef]

57. Chauvin, A.; Moreau, E.; Bonnet, S.; Plantard, O.; Malandrin, L. Babesia and its hosts: Adaptation to long-lasting interactions as a way to achieve efficient transmission. *Vet. Res.* **2009**, *40*, 1–18. [CrossRef]
58. Lobo, C.-A. *Babesia divergens* and *Plasmodium falciparum* use common receptors, glycophorins A and B, to invade the human red blood cell. *Infect. Immun.* **2005**, *73*, 649–651. [CrossRef] [PubMed]
59. Malpede, B.M.; Tolia, N.H. Malaria adhesins: Structure and function. *Cell. Microbiol.* **2014**, *16*, 621–631. [CrossRef] [PubMed]
60. Beeson, J.G.; Drew, D.R.; Boyle, M.J.; Feng, G.; Fowkes, F.J.; Richards, J.S. Merozoite surface proteins in red blood cell invasion, immunity and vaccines against malaria. *FEMS Microbiol. Rev.* **2016**, *40*, 343–372. [CrossRef]
61. Mosqueda, J.; McElwain, T.F.; Palmer, G.H. *Babesia bovis* merozoite surface antigen 2 proteins are expressed on the merozoite and sporozoite surface, and specific antibodies inhibit attachment and invasion of erythrocytes. *Infect. Immun.* **2002**, *70*, 6448–6455. [CrossRef] [PubMed]
62. Woods, K.; Perry, C.; Brühlmann, F.; Olias, P. Theileria's strategies and effector mechanisms for host cell transformation: From invasion to immortalization. *Front. Cell Dev. Biol.* **2021**, *9*, 972. [CrossRef]
63. Lobo, C.A.; Rodriguez, M.; Cursino-Santos, J.R. Babesia and red cell invasion. *Curr. Opin. Hematol.* **2012**, *19*, 170–175. [CrossRef]
64. Besteiro, S.; Dubremetz, J.F.; Lebrun, M. The moving junction of apicomplexan parasites: A key structure for invasion. *Cell. Microbiol.* **2011**, *13*, 797–805. [CrossRef] [PubMed]
65. Montero, E.; Rodriguez, M.; Oksov, Y.; Lobo, C.A. *Babesia divergens* apical membrane antigen 1 and its interaction with the human red blood cell. *Infect. Immun.* **2009**, *77*, 4783–4793. [CrossRef]
66. Moitra, P.; Zheng, H.; Anantharaman, V.; Banerjee, R.; Takeda, K.; Kozakai, Y.; Lepore, T.; Krause, P.J.; Aravind, L.; Kumar, S. Expression, purification, and biological characterization of *Babesia microti* apical membrane antigen 1. *Infect. Immun.* **2015**, *83*, 3890–3901. [CrossRef]
67. Gaffar, F.R.; Yatsuda, A.P.; Franssen, F.F.; de Vries, E. Erythrocyte invasion by *Babesia bovis* merozoites is inhibited by polyclonal antisera directed against peptides derived from a homologue of *Plasmodium falciparum* apical membrane antigen 1. *Infect. Immun.* **2004**, *72*, 2947–2955. [CrossRef] [PubMed]
68. González, L.M.; Estrada, K.; Grande, R.; Jiménez-Jacinto, V.; Vega-Alvarado, L.; Sevilla, E.; Barrera, J.; Cuesta, I.; Zaballos, Á.; Bautista, J.M.; et al. Comparative and functional genomics of the protozoan parasite *Babesia divergens* highlighting the invasion and egress processes. *PLoS Negl. Trop. Dis.* **2019**, *13*, e0007680. [CrossRef]
69. Buguliskis, J.S.; Brossier, F.; Shuman, J.; Sibley, L.D. Rhomboid 4 (ROM4) affects the processing of surface adhesins and facilitates host cell invasion by *Toxoplasma gondii*. *PLoS Pathog.* **2010**, *6*, e1000858. [CrossRef]
70. Shaw, M.K. Cell invasion by Theileria sporozoites. *Trends Parasitol.* **2003**, *19*, 2–6. [CrossRef]
71. Shaw, M.K. Theileria development and host cell invasion. In *Theileria*; Springer: Boston, MA, USA, 2002; pp. 1–22.
72. Thomas, J.A.; Tan, M.S.; Bisson, C.; Borg, A.; Umrekar, T.R.; Hackett, F.; Hale, V.L.; Vizcay-Barrena, G.; Fleck, R.A.; Snijders, A.P. A protease cascade regulates release of the human malaria parasite *Plasmodium falciparum* from host red blood cells. *Nat. Microbiol.* **2018**, *3*, 447–455. [CrossRef]
73. Collins, C.R.; Hackett, F.; Atid, J.; Tan, M.S.Y.; Blackman, M.J. The *Plasmodium falciparum* pseudoprotease SERA5 regulates the kinetics and efficiency of malaria parasite egress from host erythrocytes. *PLoS Pathog.* **2017**, *13*, e1006453. [CrossRef]
74. Withers-Martinez, C.; Strath, M.; Hackett, F.; Haire, L.F.; Howell, S.A.; Walker, P.A.; Christodoulou, E.; Dodson, G.G.; Blackman, M.J. The malaria parasite egress protease SUB1 is a calcium-dependent redox switch subtilisin. *Nat. Commun.* **2014**, *5*, 1–11. [CrossRef]
75. Das, S.; Hertrich, N.; Perrin, A.J.; Withers-Martinez, C.; Collins, C.R.; Jones, M.L.; Watermeyer, J.M.; Fobes, E.T.; Martin, S.R.; Saibil, H.R. Processing of *Plasmodium falciparum* merozoite surface protein MSP1 activates a spectrin-binding function enabling parasite egress from RBCs. *Cell Host Microbe* **2015**, *18*, 433–444. [CrossRef] [PubMed]
76. Koussis, K.; Withers-Martinez, C.; Yeoh, S.; Child, M.; Hackett, F.; Knuepfer, E.; Juliano, L.; Woehlbier, U.; Bujard, H.; Blackman, M.J. A multifunctional serine protease primes the malaria parasite for red blood cell invasion. *EMBO J.* **2009**, *28*, 725–735. [CrossRef]
77. Montero, E.; Gonzalez, L.M.; Rodriguez, M.; Oksov, Y.; Blackman, M.J.; Lobo, C.A. A conserved subtilisin protease identified in *Babesia divergens* merozoites. *J. Biol. Chem.* **2006**, *281*, 35717–35726. [CrossRef]
78. Lempereur, L.; Larcombe, S.D.; Durrani, Z.; Karagenc, T.; Bilgic, H.B.; Bakirci, S.; Hacilarlioglu, S.; Kinnaird, J.; Thompson, J.; Weir, W.; et al. Identification of candidate transmission-blocking antigen genes in *Theileria annulata* and related vector-borne apicomplexan parasites. *BMC Genom.* **2017**, *18*, 438. [CrossRef] [PubMed]
79. Kariu, T.; Ishino, T.; Yano, K.; Chinzei, Y.; Yuda, M. CelTOS, a novel malarial protein that mediates transmission to mosquito and vertebrate hosts. *Mol. Microbiol.* **2006**, *59*, 1369–1379. [CrossRef] [PubMed]
80. Jimah, J.R.; Salinas, N.D.; Sala-Rabanal, M.; Jones, N.G.; Sibley, L.D.; Nichols, C.G.; Schlesinger, P.H.; Tolia, N.H. Malaria parasite CelTOS targets the inner leaflet of cell membranes for pore-dependent disruption. *Elife* **2016**, *5*, e20621. [CrossRef]
81. Baldi, D.L.; Andrews, K.T.; Waller, R.F.; Roos, D.S.; Howard, R.F.; Crabb, B.S.; Cowman, A.F. RAP1 controls rhoptry targeting of RAP2 in the malaria parasite *Plasmodium Falciparum*. *EMBO J.* **2000**, *19*, 2435–2443. [CrossRef]
82. Low, L.M.; Azasi, Y.; Sherling, E.S.; Garten, M.; Zimmerberg, J.; Tsuboi, T.; Brzostowski, J.; Mu, J.; Blackman, M.J.; Miller, L.H. Deletion of *Plasmodium falciparum* protein RON3 affects the functional translocation of exported proteins and glucose uptake. *MBio* **2019**, *10*, e01419–e01460. [CrossRef]

83. Bargieri, D.Y.; Thiberge, S.; Tay, C.L.; Carey, A.F.; Rantz, A.; Hischen, F.; Lorthiois, A.; Straschil, U.; Singh, P.; Singh, S. Plasmodium merozoite TRAP family protein is essential for vacuole membrane disruption and gamete egress from erythrocytes. *Cell Host Microbe* **2016**, *20*, 618–630. [CrossRef] [PubMed]
84. Cai, H.; Wang, Y.; McCarthy, D.; Wen, H.; Borchelt, D.R.; Price, D.L.; Wong, P.C. BACE1 is the major β-secretase for generation of Aβ peptides by neurons. *Nat. Neurosci.* **2001**, *4*, 233–234. [CrossRef]
85. Sleebs, B.E.; Lopaticki, S.; Marapana, D.S.; O'Neill, M.T.; Rajasekaran, P.; Gazdik, M.; Günther, S.; Whitehead, L.W.; Lowes, K.N.; Barfod, L. Inhibition of Plasmepsin V activity demonstrates its essential role in protein export, PfEMP1 display, and survival of malaria parasites. *PLoS Biol.* **2014**, *12*, e1001897. [CrossRef] [PubMed]
86. Curt-Varesano, A.; Braun, L.; Ranquet, C.; Hakimi, M.A.; Bougdour, A. The aspartyl protease TgASP5 mediates the export of the Toxoplasma GRA16 and GRA24 effectors into host cells. *Cell. Microbiol.* **2016**, *18*, 151–167. [CrossRef] [PubMed]
87. Hammoudi, P.-M.; Jacot, D.; Mueller, C.; Di Cristina, M.; Dogga, S.K.; Marq, J.-B.; Romano, J.; Tosetti, N.; Dubrot, J.; Emre, Y.; et al. Fundamental roles of the Golgi-associated Toxoplasma aspartyl protease, ASP5, at the host-parasite interface. *PLoS Pathog.* **2015**, *11*, e1005211. [CrossRef]
88. Asada, M.; Goto, Y.; Yahata, K.; Yokoyama, N.; Kawai, S.; Inoue, N.; Kaneko, O.; Kawazu, S.-I. Gliding motility of *Babesia bovis* merozoites visualized by time-lapse video microscopy. *PLoS ONE* **2012**, *7*, e35227. [CrossRef] [PubMed]
89. Repnik, U.; Gangopadhyay, P.; Bietz, S.; Przyborski, J.M.; Griffiths, G.; Lingelbach, K. The apicomplexan parasite *Babesia divergens* internalizes band 3, glycophorin A and spectrin during invasion of human red blood cells. *Cell. Microbiol.* **2015**, *17*, 1052–1068. [CrossRef] [PubMed]
90. Matz, J.M.; Beck, J.R.; Blackman, M.J. The parasitophorous vacuole of the blood-stage malaria parasite. *Nat. Rev. Microbiol.* **2020**, *18*, 379–391. [CrossRef] [PubMed]
91. Egea, P.F. Crossing the vacuolar rubicon: Structural insights into effector protein trafficking in apicomplexan parasites. *Microorganisms* **2020**, *8*, 865. [CrossRef]
92. Ho, C.-M.; Beck, J.R.; Lai, M.; Cui, Y.; Goldberg, D.E.; Egea, P.F.; Zhou, Z.H. Malaria parasite translocon structure and mechanism of effector export. *Nature* **2018**, *561*, 70–75. [CrossRef]
93. Cygan, A.M.; Theisen, T.C.; Mendoza, A.G.; Marino, N.D.; Panas, M.W.; Boothroyd, J.C. Coimmunoprecipitation with MYR1 identifies three additional proteins within the *Toxoplasma gondii* parasitophorous vacuole required for translocation of dense granule effectors into host cells. *Msphere* **2020**, *5*, e00819–e00858. [CrossRef]
94. Hakimi, H.; Templeton, T.J.; Sakaguchi, M.; Yamagishi, J.; Miyazaki, S.; Yahata, K.; Uchihashi, T.; Kawazu, S.-I.; Kaneko, O.; Asada, M. Novel *Babesia bovis* exported proteins that modify properties of infected red blood cells. *PLoS Pathog.* **2020**, *16*, e1008917. [CrossRef]
95. Pellé, K.G.; Jiang, R.H.; Mantel, P.Y.; Xiao, Y.P.; Hjelmqvist, D.; Gallego-Lopez, G.M.; OTLau, A.; Kang, B.H.; Allred, D.R.; Marti, M. Shared elements of host-targeting pathways among apicomplexan parasites of differing lifestyles. *Cell. Microbiol.* **2015**, *17*, 1618–1639. [CrossRef] [PubMed]
96. Suarez, C.E.; Alzan, H.F.; Silva, M.G.; Rathinasamy, V.; Poole, W.A.; Cooke, B.M. Unravelling the cellular and molecular pathogenesis of bovine babesiosis: Is the sky the limit? *Int. J. Parasitol.* **2019**, *49*, 183–197. [CrossRef] [PubMed]
97. Jackson, A.P.; Otto, T.D.; Darby, A.; Ramaprasad, A.; Xia, D.; Echaide, I.E.; Farber, M.; Gahlot, S.; Gamble, J.; Gupta, D. The evolutionary dynamics of variant antigen genes in Babesia reveal a history of genomic innovation underlying host–parasite interaction. *Nucleic Acids Res.* **2014**, *42*, 7113–7131. [CrossRef]
98. Cornillot, E.; Hadj-Kaddour, K.; Dassouli, A.; Noel, B.; Ranwez, V.; Vacherie, B.; Augagneur, Y.; Brès, V.; Duclos, A.; Randazzo, S. Sequencing of the smallest Apicomplexan genome from the human pathogen *Babesia microti*. *Nucleic Acids Res.* **2012**, *40*, 9102–9114. [CrossRef]
99. Guo, J.; Hu, J.; Sun, Y.; Yu, L.; He, J.; He, P.; Nie, Z.; Li, M.; Zhan, X.; Zhao, Y. A novel *Babesia orientalis* 135-kilodalton spherical body protein like: Identification of its secretion into cytoplasm of infected erythrocytes. *Parasites Vectors* **2018**, *11*, 1–10. [CrossRef] [PubMed]
100. Mastan, B.S.; Kumari, A.; Gupta, D.; Mishra, S.; Kumar, K.A. Gene disruption reveals a dispensable role for plasmepsin VII in the *Plasmodium berghei* life cycle. *Mol. Biochem. Parasitol.* **2014**, *195*, 10–13. [CrossRef] [PubMed]
101. Polonais, V.; Shea, M.; Soldati-Favre, D. *Toxoplasma gondii* aspartic protease 1 is not essential in tachyzoites. *Exp. Parasitol.* **2011**, *128*, 454–459. [CrossRef]
102. Francia, M.E.; Striepen, B. Cell division in apicomplexan parasites. *Nat. Rev. Microbiol.* **2014**, *12*, 125–136. [CrossRef] [PubMed]
103. Jalovecka, M.; Bonsergent, C.; Hajdusek, O.; Kopacek, P.; Malandrin, L. Stimulation and quantification of *Babesia divergens* gametocytogenesis. *Parasites Vectors* **2016**, *9*, 439. [CrossRef]
104. Pfaffl, M.W. A new mathematical model for relative quantification in real-time RT–PCR. *Nucleic Acids Res.* **2001**, *29*, e45. [CrossRef]
105. Kearse, M.; Moir, R.; Wilson, A.; Stones-Havas, S.; Cheung, M.; Sturrock, S.; Buxton, S.; Cooper, A.; Markowitz, S.; Duran, C. Geneious Basic: An integrated and extendable desktop software platform for the organization and analysis of sequence data. *Bioinformatics* **2012**, *28*, 1647–1649. [CrossRef] [PubMed]
106. Trifinopoulos, J.; Nguyen, L.-T.; von Haeseler, A.; Minh, B.Q. W-IQ-TREE: A fast online phylogenetic tool for maximum likelihood analysis. *Nucleic Acids Res.* **2016**, *44*, W232–W235. [CrossRef] [PubMed]
107. Kalyaanamoorthy, S.; Minh, B.Q.; Wong, T.K.; Von Haeseler, A.; Jermiin, L.S. ModelFinder: Fast model selection for accurate phylogenetic estimates. *Nat. Methods* **2017**, *14*, 587–589. [CrossRef] [PubMed]

MDPI
St. Alban-Anlage 66
4052 Basel
Switzerland
Tel. +41 61 683 77 34
Fax +41 61 302 89 18
www.mdpi.com

Pathogens Editorial Office
E-mail: pathogens@mdpi.com
www.mdpi.com/journal/pathogens

www.ingramcontent.com/pod-product-compliance
Lightning Source LLC
LaVergne TN
LVHW070148100526
838202LV00015B/1911
9783036544724